Springer-Verlag Italia Srl.

A. Gullo (Ed.)

Anaesthesia, Pain, Intensive Care and Emergency Medicine - A.P.I.C.E.

Proceedings of the

16th Postgraduate Course in Critical Care Medicine
Trieste, Italy - November 16-20, 2001

Springer

Prof. ANTONINO GULLO, M.D.
Head, Department of Clinical Sciences
Section of Anaesthesia, Intensive Care and Pain Clinic
Trieste University School of Medicine
Trieste, Italy

Originally published by Springer-Verlag Italia, Milano in 2002

http://www.springer.de

ISBN 978-88-470-0176-3   ISBN 978-88-470-2099-3 (eBook)
DOI 10.1007/978-88-470-2099-3

SPIN 10858730

Table of Contents

OBSTETRICS

Authors Index

Ajmone Cat C.
Department of Anaesthesia and Intensive Care, S. Camillo-Forlanini Hospital, Rome (Italy)

Alexander R.
Department of Anaesthesia and Intensive Care, Worcester Acute Hospitals NHS Trust, The Worcester Royal Infirmary, Worcester (U.K.)

Allaria B.
Intensive Care Unit, National Institute for the Study and Treatment of Tumours, Milan (Italy)

Almeida de Oliveira S.
Heart Thoracic Division, Heart Institute, FMUSP Clinical Hospital, São Paulo (Brazil)

Auler J.O.C.
Department of Anaesthesiology, Heart Institute, FMUSP Clinical Hospital, São Paulo (Brazil)

Banti S.
Department of Anaesthesia and Intensive Care, IRCCS Burlo Garofolo Hospital, Trieste (Italy)

Baumgartner C.
Department of Anaesthesia and General Intensive Care Medicine, University of Vienna, Vienna (Austria)

Berlot G.
Department of Clinical Sciences, Section of Anaesthesia, Intensive Care and Pain Clinic, Trieste University School of Medicine, Trieste (Italy)

Bigatello L.M.
Department of Anaesthesia and Critical Care, Massachusetts General Hospital, Harvard Medical School, Boston, Massachusetts (U.S.A.)

Biolo G.
Department of Clinical, Morphological and Technological Sciences, Division of Internal Medicine, University of Trieste, Trieste (Italy)

Bird F.M.
Bird Institute of Biomedical Technology, Sandpoint, Idaho (U.S.A.)

Blanch L.
Critical Care Centre, Sabadell Hospital, Parc Taulí University Institute, Sabadell (Spain)

Boezeman H.
Department of Clinical Neurophysiology, St. Antonius Hospital, Nieuwegein (The Netherlands)

Boyd O.F.
Department of Intensive Care, The Royal Sussex County Hospital, Brighton (U.K.)

Brandolese R.
Intensive Care Unit, Multidisciplinary Rehabilitation Centre, Padua City Hospital, Padua (Italy)

Brett S.J.
Department of Anaesthesia and Intensive Care, Hammersmith and Queen Charlotte's Hospital, London (U.K.)

Brisinda G.
Department of Surgery, Division of Organ Transplantation, Catholic University, University Hospital "A. Gemelli" and CNR, Rome (Italy)

Busoni P.
Department of Anaesthesia and Intensive Care, A. Meyer Hospital, Florence (Italy)

Caironi P.
Department of Anaesthesia and Intensive Care, Milan University, Maggiore Hospital, Milan (Italy)

Camorcia M.
Department of Anaesthesia, AfaR – CRCCS Fatebenefratelli General Hospital, Rome (Italy)

Candiani A.
Institute of Anaestehsiology and Intensive Care, University of Brescia, Spedali Civili, Brescia (Italy)

Capogna G.
Department of Anaesthesia, AfaR – CRCCS Fatebenefratelli General Hospital, Rome (Italy)

Carli F.
Department of Anaesthesia, McGill University Health Centre, Montreal, Quebec (Canada)

Castagneto M.
Department of Surgery, Division of Organ Transplantation, Catholic University, University Hospital "A. Gemelli" and CNR, Rome (Italy)

Cavaglià M.
Department of Anaesthesiology and Intensive Care, University "A. Avogadro" of Eastern Piedmont, Novara (Italy)

Cerchiari E.
Department of Anaesthesia and Intensive Care, S. Camillo-Forlanini Hospital, Rome (Italy)

Chierego M.L.
Department of Clinical Sciences, Section of Anaesthesia, Intensive Care and Pain Clinic, Trieste University School of Medicine, Trieste (Italy)

Colombo G.
Department of Clinical and Biologic Sciences, Insubria University, Varese (Italy)

Crowhurst J.A.
Department of Anaesthesia and Intensive Care, Hammersmith and Queen Charlotte's Hospital, London (U.K.)

D'Amato L.
Department of Surgical, Anaesthesiological and Emergency Sciences, Naples University "Federico II", Naples (Italy)

Dallan L.A.
Heart Thoracic Division, Heart Institute, FMUSP Clinical Hospital, São Paulo (Brazil)

De Blasio E.
Intensive Care Unit "Marchiafava", Emergency Department, S. Camillo-Forlanini Hospital, Rome (Italy)

de Haan P.
Department of Anaesthesiology, Onze Lieve Vrouwe Gasthuis, Amsterdam (The Netherlands)

De Robertis E.
Department of Anaesthesia and Intensive Care, Naples University "Federico II", Naples (Italy)

Della Corte F.
Department of Anaesthesiology and Intensive Care, University "A. Avogadro" of Eastern Piedmont, Novara (Italy)

Douglas J.
Department of Anaesthesia, British Columbia's Women's Hospital and University of British Columbia, Vancouver, British Columbia (Canada)

Drakulovic M.
Respiratory Intensive Care Unit, Department of Pneumology, Clinical Institute of Pneumology and Thoracic Surgery, Clinical Hospital, Institute of Biomedical Investigation Augusti Pi i Sunyer, University of Barcelona, Barcelona (Spain)

Fernandes C.R.
Department of Anaesthesiology, Heart Institute, FMUSP Clinical Hospital, São Paulo (Brazil)

Finsterer U.
Department of Anaesthesiology, Ludwig-Maximilians University, Munich (Germany)

Flabouris A.
Intensive Care Unit, Liverpool Hospital, University of New South Wales, Sydney (Australia)

Fontanesi L.
Department of Clinical Sciences, Section of Anaesthesia, Intensive Care and Pain Clinic, Trieste University School of Medicine, Trieste (Italy)

Frova G.
Department of Anaesthesia and Intensive Care, "Spedali Civili" Hospital, Brescia (Italy)

Galimberti G.
Department of Clinical Sciences, Section of Anaesthesia, Intensive Care and Pain Clinic, Trieste University School of Medicine, Trieste (Italy)

Gamberoni C.
Department of Anaesthesiology and Intensive Care, Insubria University, Varese (Italy)

Gattinoni L.
Department of Anaesthesia and Intensive Care, Milan University, Maggiore Hospital, Milan (Italy)

Giarratano A.
Department of Anaesthesiology and Intensive Care, Palermo University, Palermo (Italy)

Girardis M.
Department of Anaesthesia and Intensive Care, Modena General Hospital, Modena (Italy)

Giunta F.
Department of Anaesthesiology and Intensive Care, Pisa University, Pisa (Italy)

Gordini G.
Department of Intensive Care, 118 – Maggiore Hospital, Bologna (Italy)

Grocott M.
Surgical Outcomes Research Centre, University College, London (U.K.)

Gullo A.
Department of Clinical Sciences, Section of Anaesthesia, Intensive Care and Pain Clinic, Trieste University School of Medicine, Trieste (Italy)

Gurman G.M.
Division of Anaesthesiology, Soroka Medical Centre and Faculty of Health Sciences, Ben Gurion University of the Negev, Beer Sheva (Israel)

Hamilton M.
Centre for Anaesthesia, University College, London (U.K.)

Hammerle A.F.
Department of Anaesthesia and General Intensive Care Medicine, University of Vienna, Vienna (Austria)

Hedenstierna G.
Department of Clinical Physiology, University Hospital, Uppsala (Sweden)

Illievich U.M.
Department of Anaesthesiology and General Intensive Care, University of Vienna, Vienna (Austria)

Jakob S.M.
Department of Intensive Care Medicine, University Hospital, Bern (Switzerland)

Jonson B.
Department of Clinical Physiology, University Hospital, Lund (Sweden)

Josten C.
Department of Traumatology, University of Leipzig, Leipzig (Germany)

Kalkman C.J.
Department of Anaesthesiology, University Hospital, Utrecht (The Netherlands)

Kaplan L.J.
Departments of Surgery and Emergency Medicine, Medical College of Pennsylvania-Hahnemann University, Philadelphia, Pennsylvania (U.S.A.)

Kellum J.A.
Department of Critical Care Medicine, University of Pittsburgh Medical Center, Pittsburgh, Pennsylvania (U.S.A.)

Kesecioglu J.
Department of Intensive Care, University of Amsterdam, Academic Medical Centre, Amsterdam (The Netherlands)

Kovachev I.
Department of Anaesthesia and Intensive Care, University Hospital of Obstetrics and Gynaecology, Medical University, Sofia (Bulgaria)

Lachmann B.
Department of Anaesthesiology, Erasmus University Rotterdam, Rotterdam (The Netherlands)

Lapinsky S.E.
Intensive Care and Division of Respirology, Mount Sinai Hospital, Toronto, Ontario (Canada)

Latronico N.
Institute of Anaesthesiology and Intensive Care, University of Brescia, Spedali Civili, Brescia (Italy)

Lavoie J.-P.
School of Veterinary Medicine, University of Montreal, Ste Hyacinthe, Quebec (Canada)

Lingnau W.
Department of Anaesthesia and Critical Care Medicine, Leopold-Franzens-University, Innsbruck (Austria)

Lips J.
Department of Anaesthesiology, Academic Medical Centre, University of Amsterdam, Amsterdam (The Netherlands)

Lombardini C.
Department of Anaesthesia and Intensive Care, Modena General Hospital, Modena (Italy)

Lucangelo U.
Department of Clinical Sciences, Section of Anaesthesia, Intensive Care and Pain Clinic, Trieste University School of Medicine, Trieste (Italy)

Lumb P.D.
Department of Anaesthesiology, Keck School of Medicine at USC, Los Angeles, California (U.S.A.)

Lyons G.
Obstetric Anaesthesia, St. James' University Hospital, Leeds (U.K.)

Machata A.-M.
Department of Anaesthesiology and General Intensive Care, University of Vienna, Vienna (Austria)

Magder S.
Department of Medicine and Physiology, McGill University Hospital Centre, Montreal, Quebec (Canada)

Mangione S.
Department of Anaesthesiology and Intensive Care, Palermo University, Palermo (Italy)

Maria G.
Department of Surgery, Division of Organ Transplantation, Catholic University, University Hospital "A. Gemelli" and CNR, Rome (Italy)

Martin J.G.
Meakins-Christie Laboratories, Department of Medicine, McGill University, Montreal, Quebec (Canada)

McKeating E.G.
Department of Neuroanaesthesia and Critical Care, The Royal Preston Hospital, Preston (U.K.)

Melloni C.
Department of Anaesthesia and Intensive Care, Faenza Hospital, Faenza (Italy)

Menarini M.
Department of Intensive Care, 118 – Maggiore Hospital, Bologna (Italy)

Messeri A.
Department of Anaesthesia and Intensive Care, A. Meyer Hospital, Florence (Italy)

Minucci S.
Interventional Radiology, Department of Radiology, S. Camillo Forlanini Hospital, Rome (Italy)

Morgan T.J.
Intensive Care Facility, Royal Brisbane Hospital, Brisbane, Queensland (Australia)

Muchada R.
Department of Anaesthesia and Intensive Care, Eugène André Hospital, Lyon (France)

Muggia-Sullam M.
Department of Surgery, Hadassah Hebrew University Medical Centre, Jerusalem (Israel)

Murias G.
Critical Care Centre, Sabadell Hospital, Parc Taulí University Institute, Sabadell (Spain)

Mythen M.G.
Centre for Anaesthesia, University College, London (U.K.)

Nardi G.
Intensive Care Unit "Marchiafava", Emergency Department, S. Camillo-Forlanini Hospital, Rome (Italy)

Novak-Jankovic V.
Clinical Department of Anaesthesiology and Intensive Care, University Medical Centre, Ljubljana (Slovenia)

Paolicchi A.
Department of Anaesthesia and Intensive Care, Pisa Hospital, Pisa (Italy)

Parr M.J.A.
Intensive Care Unit, Liverpool Hospital, University of New South Wales, Sydney (Australia)

Pasetto A.
Department of Anaesthesia and Intensive Care, Modena General Hospital, Modena (Italy)

Paver Eržen V.
Clinical Department of Anaesthesiology and Intensive Care, University Medical Centre, Ljubljana (Slovenia)

Pellis T.
Department of Clinical Sciences, Section of Anaesthesia, Intensive Care and Pain Clinic, and The Institute of Critical Care Medicine, Palm Springs, California (U.S.A.)

Pelosi P.
Department of Anaesthesiology and Intensive Care, Insubria University, Varese (Italy)

Penney D.J.
Intensive Care Unit, Liverpool Hospital, University of New South Wales, Sydney (Australia)

Pino G.P.
Diagnostic Cardiology, Department of Cardiology, S. Camillo Forlanini Hospital, Rome (Italy)

Pittarello D.
Department of Pharmacology and Anaesthesiology, Padua General Hospital, Padua (Italy)

Poelma D.L.H.
Department of Anaesthesiology, Erasmus University Rotterdam, Rotterdam (The Netherlands)

Pozzi Mucelli F.
Radiology Department, University of Trieste, Trieste (Italy)

Primadei M.
Department of Pharmacology and Anaesthesiology, Padua General Hospital, Padua (Italy)

Rasmussen L.S.
Department of Anaesthesia, Copenhagen University Hospital, Rigshospitalet, Copenhagen (Denmark)

Rawal N.
Department of Anaesthesiology and Intensive Care, Örebro Medical Centre Hospital, Örebro (Sweden)

Rehm M.
Department of Anaesthesiology, Ludwig-Maximilians University, Munich (Germany)

Resta M.
Intensive Care Unit, National Institute for the Study and Treatment of Tumours, Milan (Italy)

Ricci Z.
Department of Nephrology, St. Bortolo Hospital, Vicenza (Italy)

Riccioni L.
Intensive Care Unit “Marchiafava”, Emergency Department, S. Camillo-Forlanini Hospital, Rome (Italy)

Robson V.
Department of Anaesthesia and Intensive Care, Hammersmith and Queen Charlotte’s Hospital, London (U.K.)

Rocco P.R.M.
Laboratory of Respiration Physiology, Carlos Chagas Filho Biophysics Institute, Federal University of Rio de Janeiro, Centre for Health Sciences, Rio de Janeiro (Brazil)

Ronco C.
Department of Nephrology, St. Bortolo Hospital, Vicenza (Italy)

Rupreht J.
Department of Anaesthesiology, University Hospital Rotterdam, Rotterdam (The Netherlands)

Russell I.F.
Department of Anaesthesia, Hull Royal Infirmary, Hull (U.K.)

Sarti A.
Department of Anaesthesia and Intensive Care, IRCCS Burlo Garofolo Hospital, Trieste (Italy)

Scarpa R.
Department of Anaesthesia and Intensive Care, IRCCS Burlo Garofolo Hospital, Trieste (Italy)

Scheibner L.
Intensive Care Unit, University of Leipzig, Leipzig (Germany)

Schepens M.A.
Department of Cardiothoracic Surgery, St. Antonius Hospital, Nieuwegein (The Netherlands)

Schmidt G.A.
Department of Clinical Medicine and Anaesthesia/Critical Care, University of Chicago, Chicago, Illinois (U.S.A.)

Schreiter D.
Intensive Care Unit, University of Leipzig, Leipzig (Germany)

Servillo G.
Department of Anaesthesia and Intensive Care, Naples University "Federico II", Naples (Italy)

Sganga G.
Department of Surgery, Division of Organ Transplantation, Catholic University, University Hospital "A. Gemelli" and CNR, Rome (Italy)

Silverstein J.H.
Department of Anaesthesiology, Mount Sinai School of Medicine, New York (U.S.A.)

Smilov I.
Department of Anaesthesia and Intensive Care, University Hospital of Obstetrics and Gynaecology, Medical University, Sofia (Bulgaria)

Sorbara C.
Department of Pharmacology and Anaesthesiology, Padua General Hospital, Padua (Italy)

Spiss C.K.
Department of Anaesthesiology and General Intensive Care, University of Vienna, Vienna (Austria)

Stefini R.
Institute of Neurosurgery, University of Brescia, Spedali Civili, Brescia (Italy)

Story D.A.
Department of Anaesthesia, Austin and Repatriation Medical Centre, Heidelberg, Victoria (Australia)

Sutcliffe A.J.
Department of Anaesthesia and Intensive Care, Queen Elizabeth Hospital, Birmingham (U.K.)

Tabor T.
Advisor to Florida Community College, Respiratory Physiology Programme, Jacksonville, Florida (U.S.A.)

Tang W.
The University of Southern California, Keck School of Medicine, Los Angeles, California (U.S.A.)

Tatschl C.
Department of Anaesthesia and General Intensive Care Medicine, University of Vienna, Vienna (Austria)

Tomasini A.
Department of Clinical Sciences, Section of Anaesthesia, Intensive Care and Pain Clinic, Trieste University School of Medicine, Trieste (Italy)

Torres A.
Respiratory Intensive Care Unit, Department of Pneumology, Clinical Institute of Pneumology and Thoracic Surgery, Clinical Hospital, Institute of Biomedical Investigation Augusti Pi i Sunyer, University of Barcelona, Barcelona (Spain)

Torri G.
Department of Anaesthesia and Intensive Care, University of San Raffaele, Milan (Italy)

Trayanov I.
Department of Anaesthesia and Intensive Care, University Hospital of Obstetrics and Gynaecology, Medical University, Sofia (Bulgaria)

Trevisanuto D.
Department of Paediatrics, Padua University Medical School, Padua (Italy)

Tufano R.
Department of Anaesthesia and Intensive Care, Naples University "Federico II", Naples (Italy)

van Dongen E.P.
Department of Anaesthesiology and Intensive Care, St. Antonius Hospital, Nieuwegein (The Netherlands)

Ventafridda V.
Floriani Foundation, Milan (Italy)

Vignazia G.L.
Department of Anaesthesiology and Intensive Care, University "A. Avogadro" of Eastern Piedmont, Novara (Italy)

Villagra A.
Critical Care Centre, Sabadell Hospital, Parc Taulí University Institute, Sabadell (Spain)

Volpe N.G.
Department of Anaesthesia and Intensive Care, Worcester Acute Hospitals NHS Trust, The Worcester Royal Infirmary, Worcester (U.K.)

Weksler N.
Division of Anaesthesiology, Soroka Medical Centre and Faculty of Health Sciences, Ben Gurion University of the Negev, Beer Sheva (Israel)

Zacchello F.
Department of Paediatrics, Padua University Medical School, Padua (Italy)

Zin W.A.
Laboratory of Respiration Physiology, Carlos Chagas Filho Biophysics Institute, Federal University of Rio de Janeiro, Centre for Health Sciences, Rio de Janeiro (Brazil)

Abbreviations

γ, surface tension

γGT, gamma-gluamyltranspeptidase

AAST, American Association for the Surgery of Trauma

ABF, aortic blood flow

ABS, apparent bicarbonate space

ACEIs, angiotensin-converting enzyme inhibitors

ACOG, American College of Obstetricians Gynecologists

ACTH, adrenocortitrophic hormone

ADH, antidiuretic hormone

ADL, activities of daily living

AED, automatic external defibrillator

AFE, amniotic fluid embolism

AG, anion gap

AIDS, acquired immunodeficiency syndrome

AIS, abbreviated injury scale

ALI, acute lung injury

ALS, advances life support

AMPA, alpha-amino-3-hydroxy-5-methyl-4-isoxazoleproprionate

ANH, acute normovolemic haemodilution

ANS, autonomic nervous system

AP, alkaline phosphatase

AP, arterial pressure

APACHE-II, Acute Physiology And Chronic Health Evaluation II

APOE, apolipoprotein E

APRV, airway pressure release ventilation

APS, Acute Pain Service

ARDS, acute respiratory distress syndrome

ARF, acute respiratory failure

ASA, American Society of Anesthesiologists

ASPIDS, aspirate dead space gas from the trachea

AT, abdominal trauma

A_{TOT}, total weak acid concentration

ATS, American Thoracic Society

BAI, blunt aortic injury

BCI, blunt cardiac injury

BCT, blunt cardiac trauma

BD, base deficit

BE, base excess

BEua, base excess caused by unmeasured strong anions

BP, blood pressure

BPI, bactericidial/permeability increasing protein

BUN, blood urea nitrogen

C/S, caesarean section

CAGB, coronary artery bypass grafting

CBF, cerebral blood flow

CCS, Canadian Cardiovascular Society

CDC, Centres for Disease Control

CEGA, combined epidural-general anaesthesia

CEMD, Confidential Enquiries into Maternal Deaths

CEMDEW or **CEMDUK**, Confidential Enquiry into maternal deaths of England and Wales (later United Kingdom)

CFAM, cerebral function analysing monitor

Cl_{CR}, creatinine clearance

CMV, continuous mechanical ventilation

CO, cardiac output

COP, colloid osmotic pressure

COPA, cuffed oropharyngeal airway

COPD, chronic obstructive pulmonary disease

COX, cyclooxygenase

CPAP, continuous positive airway pressure

CPB, cardiopulmonary bypass

CPP, cerebral perfusion pressure

CPR, cardiopulmonary resuscitation

CPRI, cardiopulmonary risk index

CRF, corticothropin releasing factor

CSA, continuous spinal anaesthesia

CSE, combined spinal epidural

CSF, cerebrospinal fluid

Cst, static compliance

CT, computed tomography

CTC, computed tomography of the chest

CTD, Common Technical Document

c-TnI, cardiac troponin I

CVI, ventilator/computer interface
CVP, central venous pressure
D/FRC, dynamic functional residual capacities
D, dialysance
DAP, diastolic arterial pressure
DCA, dichloroacetate
DCS, damage control surgery
DIC, disseminated intravascular coagulation
DKA, diabetic ketoacidosis
DO_2, oxygen delivery
DPL, diagnostic peritoneal lavage
DVDR, dynamic volumetric diffusive respiration
DVT, deep vein thrombosis
E, expiratory time
EAA, epidural anaesthesia and analgesia
EBM, evidence-based medicine
ECG, electrocardiogram
ECMO, extracorporeal membrane oxygenation
ECV, extracellular volume
ED, emergency department
EE, energy expenditure
EF, external fixation
EFPIA, European Federation of Pharmaceutical Industries and Associations
EFTA, European Free Trade Area
EKG, electrocardiogram
ELSO, Extracorporeal Life Support Organization
EMS, emergency medical services
ER, extraction ratio
ESBL, extended-spectrum beta-lactamase
ESG, endovascular stent-grafting
Est:cw, elastance of the chest wall
FAST, focussed abdominal sonogram for trauma
FDA, Food and Drug Administration
FF, filtration fraction
FiO_2, fraction inspired oxygen
FMH, foetomaternal haemorrhage
FRC, functional residual capacity
GA, general anaesthesia
GCS, Glasgow Coma Scale
GDM, gestational diabetes mellitus
GER, gastroesophageal reflux
GFR, glomerular filtration rate
GIT, gastrointestinal tract
GOS, Glasgow Outcome Scale
GOSE, Glasgow Outcome Scale Extended
H^+, hydrogen ions
HA-1A, human IgM monoclonal antibody
HARM, Harborview assessment for risk of mortality
HCMA, hyperchloraemic metabolic acidosis
HCO_3^-, bicarbonate ions
HDF, haemodiafiltration
HDU, High Dependency Units
HES, hydroxyethyl starch
HF, haemofiltration
HFPV, high frequency percussive ventilation
HFV, high frequency ventilation
HGH, human growth hormone
HICPAC, Hospital Infection Control Advisory Committee
HPT, haemopneumothorax
HPV, hypoxic pulmonary vasoconstriction
HR, heart rate
HT, haemothorax
HU, Hounsfield units
I:E, inspiration expiration ratio
IACS, intra-abdominal compartment syndrome
IADL, independent activities of daily living
IAP, intra-abdominal pressure
IASP, International Association for the Study of Pain
IBD, inflammatory bowel disease
ICD-9-CM, international classification of disease – 9th Rev.
ICH, International Conference on Harmonisation
ICISS, international classification disease-9 based injury severity score
ICP, intracranial pressure
ICU, intensive care unit
IFPMA, International Federation of Pharmaceutical Manufacturers Association
IL, interleukin
ILCOR, International Liaison Committee on Resuscitation
IMN, intramedullary nail fixation
IMV, intermittent mandatory ventilation

INCB, International Narcotics Control Board
ipH, intracellular pH
IPPB, intermittent positive pressure breathing
IPV®, intrapulmonary percussive ventilation
ISPOCD, International Study of Postoperative Cognitive Dysfunction
ISS, Injury Severity Score
IV, intravenous
JCAHO, Joint Commission on Accreditation of Healthcare Organizations
JHRCS, Johns Hopkins Risk Classification System
JPMA, Japan Pharmaceutical Manufacturers Association
LA, local anaesthetic
LAR, late allergic response
LIP, lower inflection point
LMA, laryngeal mask airway
LPS, lipopolysaccharide
LV, left ventricule
LVETi, left ventricular ejection time indexed to the HR
LVSWI, left ventricular stroke work index
MAC, minimum alveolar concentration
MAP, mean arterial pressure
MH, malignant hyperthermia
MHLW, Ministry of Health, Labor and Welfare, Japan
MHP, mentally handicapped patients
MI, myocardial infarction
MODS, multiple organ dysfunction syndrome
MOF, multiple organ failure
MRS, magnetic resonance spectroscopy
MRUPL, minimal required upper pressure limit
MT, major trauma
MTR, mass transfer rate
MV, mechanical ventilation
MVA, motor vehicle accidents
MVO_2, myocardial oxygen consumption
NACA-scale, National Advisory Committee of Aeronautics scale
NAIS, non adrenergic inhibitory system
NGT, nasogastric tube
NIBP, non-invasive blood pressure
NICO, non-invasive cardiac output
NICU, neuro-intensive care unit
NIH, National Institute of Health
NISS, new injury severity score
NMDA, N-methyl-D-aspartate
NNIS, National Nosocomial Infections Surveillance
NO, nitric oxide
NP, nosocomial pneumonia
NPE, neurogenic pulmonary oedema
NSAIDs, non-steroidal anti-inflammatory drugs
NTB, necrotising tracheo-bronchitis
OPS, Orthogonal Polarization Spectral
OR, operating room
P, pressure
PA, pulmonary artery
PACU, Postanaesthesia Care Unit
PAD, public access defibrillation
PAF, platelet-aggregating factor
PAFS, preoperative assessment of fitness score
PAI-1, plasminogen activator inhibitor-1
Paw, airway pressure
PAWP, peak airway pressure
PCA, patient-controlled analgesia
PCBF, pulmonary capillary blood flow
PCEA, patient-controlled epidural analgesia
PCV, packed cell volume
PCWP, pulmonary capillary wedge pressure
PDH, pyruvate dehydrogenase
PDPH, post dural puncture headache
PDSA, plan-do-study-act
PE, pulmonary embolism
PEA, pulseless electrical activity
PEEP, positive end expiratory pressure
PEEPi, intrinsic positive end-expiratory pressure
PEPi, pre-ejection period indexed to the HR
Pes, esophageal pressure
PET, positron emission tomography
PGE2, prostaglandin
pHi, intramucosal pH
PhRMA, Pharmaceutical Research and Manufacturers of America
PIE, pulmonary interstitial emphysema
PMN, polymorphonuclear granulocytes
POCD, postoperative cognitive dysfunction
POD, postoperative day

PONV, postoperative nausea and vomiting
POPC, paediatric overall performance category
PPF, plasma protein fraction
PPMs, potentially pathogenic micro-organisms
PPV, positive pressure ventilation
PRC, packet red cells
PRCO, partial rebreathing for cardiac output measurement
PRMD, post-resuscitation myocardial dysfunction
PT, percutaneous tracheostomy
PT, pneumothorax
PT, prothrombin time
PTA, post-traumatic amnesia
PTCA, percutaneous transluminal coronary angiography
PTS, Paediatric Trauma Score
PTT, partial thromboplastin time
P-V, pressure-volume
PVC, premature ventricular contraction
$PvCO_2$, venous carbon dioxide tension
PVE, plasma volume expansion
r, radius
RBC, red blood cell
RBF, renal blood flow
rBPI, recombinant bactercidal/permeability increasing protein
REACT, rapid early action for coronary treatment
rhGH, recombinant human growth hormone
Rmax,cw, contribution of total resistance of the chest wall
Rmax,L, increase in total resistance of the lung
Rmax,rs, increase in total resistance of the respiratory system
ROC, receiver operating characteristic curve
ROSC, return to spontaneous circulation
RPF, renal plasma flow
RR, respiration rate
rSO_2, regional oxygen saturation
r-tPA, recombinant tissue plasminogen activator
RTS, Revised Trauma Score
RVEDV, right ventricular end diastolic volume
RVSWI, right ventricular stroke work index
SA, status asthmaticus
SAP, systolic arterial pressure
$SBCO_2$, single breath CO_2
SCBF, spinal cord blood flow
SCPP, spinal cord perfusion pressure
SCUF, slow continuous ultra filtration
SDD, selective digestive decontamination
SEP, somatosensory evoked potentials
SGOT-SGTP, serum-glutamic-oxalacetic transaminase and serum glutamic-pyruvic transaminase
SID, strong ion difference
SIDa, "apparent" SID
SIDe, effective SID
SIG, strong ion gap
SIMV, synchronous inspiratory intermittent mandatory ventilation
SIRS, systemic inflammatory response syndrome
SjO_2, oxygen saturation in the jugular vein
SLTA, severe life-threatening asthma
SPECT, single photon emission tomography
SSA, single shot spinal anaesthesia
SSEP, somatosensory evoked potentials
STI, systolic time interval
STS, Society of Thoracic Surgery
SV, stroke volume
SVRI, systemic vascular resistance index
SW, stroke work
TAAA, thoracoabdominal aortic aneurysm
TAE, transcatheter arterial embolization
T-AT, thrombin-antithrombin III
TBI, traumatic brain injury
TBW, total body water
TCD, trans-cranial Doppler
TCI, target controlled infusion
tcMEP, transcranial electrical stimulation
TDCO, thermodilution cardiac output measurement
TED, transoesophageal echodoppler
TEE, transesophageal echocardiography
TFPI, tissue factor and pathway inhibitor
TGI, tracheal gas insufflation
THAM , Tris-hydroxymethyl aminomethane

TIVA, total intravenous anaesthesia

TLT, translaryngeal tracheostomy

TMRL, transmyocardial revascularization laser

TNF, tumour necrosis factor

TNFα, tumour necrosis factor-α

TPN, total parenteral nutrition

TPT, hypertensive pneumothorax

TRISS, trauma revised injury score

TS, Trauma Score

TSVR, total systemic vascular resistance

TTS, trauma thoracic severity score

TV, tidal volume

TX, thromboxane

UHDDS, Uniform Health Discharge Data Set

UI-D, uterine incision-delivery interval

UIP, upper inflection point

UNESCO, United Nations Educational, Scientific, and Cultural Organization

UOP, urine output

US, ultrasound

V/Q, ventilation/perfusion matching

VAP, ventilator associated pneumonia

VAS, visual analogue scale

Vc, central compartment

VCO_2, CO_2 production

$V_{D\,ALV}$, alveolar dead space

VD/VT, total dead space

VF, ventricular fibrillation

VILI, ventilatory-induced lung injury

VISA, vancomycin-intermediate *S. aureus*

VO_2, oxygen consumption

VPS, verbal pain scale

VRE, enterococci with resistance to vancomycin

VRSA, vancomycin-resistant *S. aureus*

V_T, tidal volume

VT, ventricular tachycardia

WBC, white blood cell count

WHO, World Health Organization

$W_{I,aw}$, work done to overcome the airway resistance

$W_{I,dyn,rs}$, dynamic components of lung and chest wall

$W_{I,PEEPi}$, work due to PEEPi

$W_{I,rs}$, inspiratory work done on the respiratory system

$W_{I,st,rs}$, static components of lung and chest wall

Δpes, difference in esophageal pressure

ΔPt, difference in tracheal pressure

$\Delta W_{I,rs}$, work due to the viscoelastic properties of the thoracic tissues and/or time constant inequality within the lungs

PREFACE

APICE 2001

APICE 2001 provides continuous updates of topics pertaining to critical care medicine. The foundations of this fascinating branch of medicine include basic and technological research, the progress of computer technology and the success of clinical pharmacology. Critical care medicine is no longer considered a pioneer activity for few experts, but a branch in which there is an interdisciplinary cooperation among researchers, health-care operators, nurses and technical staff who put their competence at the disposal of patients whose vital functions are potentially and often severely compromised. This edition has the objective of providing researchers and health-care operators with the most recent achievements in some important sectors. The volume is divided into six sections.

The first part is dedicated to topics which are key elements of critical care. It includes personal contributions on the learning process in the treatment of critically ill patients and updates on the monitoring of vital functions, ethical and legal aspects in the field of perioperative medicine, as well as some guidelines in the treatment of patients in line with the declaration of Helsinki.

The second section is dedicated to the lung. In particular, it includes some experimental and clinical experiences on important topics such as asthma and the experimental Acute Lung Injury model. Other important aspects which can improve the clinical approach to patients undergoing artificial ventilation are the need to optimise the ratio of ventilation to perfusion, the importance of alveolar recruitment and the role of ventilation in semirecumbency. This section also includes some interesting experiences regarding the monitoring of the respiratory function and the application of some ventilation support techniques with permissive hypercapnia and high-frequency percussive ventilation.

The third part is dedicated to trauma, an ever topical and important subject which, together with cardiovascular diseases, represents the very core of the emergency department. The role of the latter as training structure becomes increasingly important, both for the different competences it includes and the advanced technology which can guarantee high care standards.

The fourth section is dedicated to the acid-base balance, which is analysed in all its aspects, starting from the modern concept of homoeostasis and the physiopathological consequences of the different disorders of the acid-base system. Particularly important are the chapters regarding fluid therapy in the perioperative period, lactic acidosis and acid-base disorders during renal replacement therapy. In addition, the monitoring of intragastric pH provides important evidence of splanchnic dysfunction. The last chapter regards the never solved controversy crystalloids vs. colloids.

The fifth part is dedicated to perioperative medicine, which is an integral part of Critical Care. The most recent progresses of the organisational and clinical sectors are reported. In particular some chapters are dedicated to the treatment of postoperative pain.

The sixth section is dedicated to obstetrics and deals with the need to customize the different anaesthetic techniques. Various authoritative experiences in the sector of inhalation anaesthesia and regional anaesthesia techniques in obstetrics and delivery assistance are reported. The importance of ensuring the utmost safety for mother and baby is stressed. Disseminated intravascular coagulation is one of the main complications. The final chapters are dedicated to maternal mortality and morbidity, the first measures of basic and advanced resuscitation both in parturients and newborn babies. Lastly, this section deals with some relevant ethical and legal aspects.

Prof. Antonino Gullo
Trieste 16.11.2001

FOCUS ON KEY POINTS ON CRITICAL CARE

One Clinicians Lifetime of Bringing Technology into Medicine and its Impact upon Critical Care Patients

F.M. Bird

The fifty-five year learning curve

As a United States Army Air Corps Pilot during World War II, flying all types of military aircraft, the critical dependence upon supplemental breathing o-xygen during high altitude flight became of paramount importance in terms of survival. I was to learn, in the ensuing years, that there were many parallels in altitude-provoked hypoxia and the typical hypoxia associated with certain cardiopulmonary diseases. With a primary mechanical background leading to the role of a self styled biomedical technologist, I have been a most active student of pathophysiology and the associated basic sciences for well over fifty years. During these years, by osmosis alone, if not by design; I have compounded my basic intelligence with considerable knowledge relative to the interrelationships involved, during the mechanical ventilation of the lung.

Early on, I recognised the "educated hand" of the anaesthesiologist, which to me has remained symbolic of all forms of mechanical ventilation. During my formative years I was "tutored" and assisted in many ways by the Dr. Ralph Waters "Anaesthesia Academic Alumni" who played a major role in providing me with on patient clinical direction.

What started with employing the "Anaesthesia induction room", as a post operative intensive care enclave where we were able to ventilate a compromised cardiopulmonary post surgical patient with an automatic respirator instead of a "hand powered anaesthesia bag", advanced into intensive care. This led to the Institutional development of the modern day "Surgical Intensive Care Unit" (SICU). In 1965 over eighty percent of all the SICU's were directed and staffed by anaesthesiologists. History will reveal why the anaesthesiologist lost control of the SICU to the pulmonologist, who now has almost total control over the SICU's. At this writing, many uniquely qualified anaesthesiologists have been entering into critical care management.

Over the fifty plus years that I have been conceiving and developing mechanical breathing apparatuses, the devices have evolved from innocence and observation toward sophistication, secondary to a lifetime of deductive study and inductive acquisition.

Over these many years, I have created four unique generations of novel cardiopulmonary management systems, which continue to serve my fellow man (in time of need) throughout the world.

When I look back upon the past, review the present and look forward toward the potential future involvement, of what I shall leave behind, I believe my colleagues as well as myself have served to advance the "state of the art" within the specialties dependent upon mechanical cardiopulmonary care. Hopefully, history will reveal how our efforts were contributory in building certain scientific factors into the ensuing aeromedical specialties, dedicated toward the maintenance of cardiopulmonary functions under conditions of stress.

Over the years, as interests within the fields of cardiopulmonary care have materialized, the lack of a common method of communication as the "state of the art" expanded has been a major deterrent toward initiating many of the potentially effective clinical introductions. While modern day mechanical ventilation of the lung is less than sixty years old, few among those presently teaching the subject, have experienced the total evolutionary process.

Without a solid physical understanding of the mechanical concepts involved, as well as the unique patho-physiological aspects of cardiopulmonary care, advances in technique are sequestered by lack of available mass knowledge among those attending. Toward this end, a brief description of each key physical and physiological consideration involved in past, present and future mechanical cardiopulmonary management has been briefly summarized.

Modern day teaching of mechanical cardiopulmonary care involves the rote system, whereby the average student is taught how to attend the 80% plus of the patients that can be effectively ventilated with a pressurised "garden hose" by a knowledgeable clinician. When a patient challenges the competency of the system, by presenting with clinical patho-physiological variables beyond the scope of the functional knowledge possessed by the attending, his or her potential for survival becomes increasingly vague.

As we continue to reach toward new horizons in medicine, we must develop super knowledgeable cardiopulmonary specialists to care for the potential 20% or less of the patients that can not be managed with traditional convective ventilatory techniques, and their common derivatives. To this end, sophisticated diffusive/convective cardiopulmonary management devices are now becoming available.

Above all else, those with limited physical and patho-physiological knowledge, serving in managerial or regulatory positions within the field of mechanical cardiopulmonary care, must not attempt to block clinical introduction of the novel concept, definition and device because of their individual inability and insecurity. It remains, as has always been the case, the primary responsibility of the individual and/or individuals founding a concept to initially determine the most appropriate "descriptive terminology" to best describe the novelty.

The intent of this document is to provide those critical care clinicians who desire to excel in the field of mechanical cardiopulmonary care a source of brief overall understanding, relative to the functional history of mechanical pulmonary ventilation, as the "state of the art" continues to expand the clinicians available armamentarium.

There are certain physical and pathophysiological understandings which serve to determine the unique design concepts as well as operational considerations of dedicated aeromedical ventilatory devices.

Among these are the following:

1. Access to the pulmonary structures through an indwelling airway catheter, in terms of airflow, are determined by the radius of the tube raised to the fourth power divided by the length. Therefore, the smaller and longer the indwelling airway catheter, the greater the resistance to directional airflow, with gas density being a factor of radius (orificial size) and gas viscosity being associated with length.

2. The inspiratory and expiratory resistances to airflow, associated with each unique indwelling airway catheter can serve to determine the required inspiratory and expiratory time constants, as well as flow gradients necessary to provide the desired pulmonary tidal exchange. The smaller and longer the endo-tracheal tube the more critical the pressure/flow relationships.

a. A medical ventilator has ultimate power to overcome the inspiratory resistance within the endo-tracheal tube by increasing the proximal airway delivery pressures, which at a given point can produce barotrauma.

b. The mechanical ventilatory "bottleneck" can be the resistance to passive physiological expiratory flow to ambient, through the confines of the endo-tracheal tube.

3. The required effective minute respiratory exchange during the mechanical ventilation of the lung is more related to the viability of the blood/gas interface, than the actual cyclic tidal volume relationships.

4. The inspiratory/expiratory time relationships (I/E Ratios) play an important role in indexing the mechanically induced dynamic functional residual capacities (D/FRC), during the mechanical ventilation of the lung. D/FRC is defined as the "transient functional residual capacity", when mechanically modified by an apneustic plateau and/or an elevated expiratory baseline.

a. If the expiratory time (E) does not accommodate the emptying of the pulmonary structures, down to the scheduled ambient and/or mechanically maintained baseline, the residual gases within the lungs will be increased beyond physiologically and/or mechanically controlled limits.

5. Intrapulmonary preferential flow relationships, secondary to proximal airway pressure/flow gradient scheduling, during the mechanical ventilation of the lung, can greatly influence baro-traumatic consequence. The greater the sustained inspiratory tidal proximal/distal (P/D) differential, the greater the potential for maldistribution of alveolar gases.

a. The greater the mechanically created inspiratory proximal/distal pressure/flow gradient created at the proximal airway, the greater the pre-selection of airway, favouring the most patent pathways. Therefore, the most dependent lung is potentially hyper-inflated with baro-traumatic potential.

6. Intrapulmonary diffusion, secondary to endo-bronchial mechanical mixing, can preferentially impact upon the diffusion of oxygen across the alveolar capillary membranes.

a. With therapeutic oxygen gradients being most pronounced within the upper airways, increased upper airway "turbulence" can increase "mechanical mixing" within the pulmonary structures, thus facilitating the diffusion of oxygen in a peripheral direction.

7. Intrapulmonary convection, will preferentially impact upon the intrapulmonary "wash out" of carbon dioxide (CO_2).

a. With the intrapulmonary source of carbon dioxide being the periphery, mechanically induced upper airway turbulence will not have the effective diffusive action upon CO_2 mobilization that serves to activate the upper airway O_2 molecule, because of the progressive "fade out" of diffusive mechanical energy as the pulmonary airways are traversed.

8. Cardiac output during the mechanical ventilation of the lung is most influenced by right ventricular filling pressure and the mechanically influenced mean intrathoracic pressures.

9. Necrotising tracheo-bronchitis (NTB) can be created by all known forms of mechanical ventilation, the degree of trauma can be associated with the primary effective perfusion of the involved pulmonary structures, the FIO2 and the sustenance and value of the mechanically induced inflational pressures involved.

10. Pulmonary interstitial emphysema (PIE) as well as pseudo-cystic lung formations, revealed during and/or after the mechanical ventilation of the lung, can be related to the existing condition of the physiological structures, which are secondarily effected by preferential airflows associated with high inspiratory flowrates, capable of generating dissecting proximal airway inflational pressures (PIP's).

a. Inflational pressures must be sustained to produce hyper-inflation and follow on barotrauma. Baro-traumatic potential can be increased secondary to an insufficient expiratory interval, during which time the lung can not passively deflate to a stabilizing nominal FRC and/or the programmed D/FRC (mechanically elevated baseline), before the follow on scheduled re-inflation.

11. Pneumo-thoraces secondary to the mechanical ventilation of the lung, are factored by the existing patho-physiology of the pulmonary structures involved and the sustenance of the applied dissecting inflational pressures.

12. The patency of the pulmonary airways is influenced by diffuse or localized obstructive phenomena such as retained endobronchial secretions, mucosal and submucosal edema, foreign body ingestion or growth and smooth bronchiolar muscle spasm, as well as other considerations.

13. The lower the gross pulmonary compliance (stiffer the pulmonary structures) the more the required inflationary time to obtain "pulmonary conformance" as recruitment pressures are reached, without provoking potential barotrauma.

a. Without absolute inspiratory inflational flowrate control, in the presence of low pulmonary compliance, preferential airway can serve to produce barotrauma.

14. The more restrictive the expiratory airway "bottleneck" (following a given pulmonary inflation) the more positive the scheduled expiratory component of the I/E ratio, required to prevent a progressive mechanical "step ladder". The end result of insufficient expiratory time programming can result in mechanical air trapping and ultimate hyperinflation, leading to potential barotrauma.

15. The larger the mechanically delivered tidal volume the slower the tolerable cycling (phasing) rate. It follows, the smaller the delivered tidal volume the faster the tolerable cycling (phasing) rate. Therefore, with (positive phase) cyclic mechanical ventilation, the smaller the neonate the greater the number of passive baseline returns required per minute, to the programmed baseline, to minimize potential peripheral pulmonary hyperinflation as well as NTB.

16. Intrapulmonary tidal volumes greater than the anatomical dead space have a potentially greater convectional factor than sub tidal volumes less than the anatomical dead space, that are potentially diffusive in nature.

a. PaO_2 is more related to diffusion than convection.

b. $PaCO_2$ is more related to convection than diffusion.

17. At a given right ventricular filling pressure, the longer the mechanically scheduled expiratory (baseline) interval of the I/E ratio, the greater the cyclic reloading potential of the pulmonary circulation.

a. During the cyclic mechanical inspiratory interval, left ventricular filling pressure is increased, as the effective right atrial filling pressure is encroached upon. The net result is a phasic increase in cardiac output during the schedule mechanical inflation of the lungs, at the expense of pulmonary blood volume.
b. During the cyclic mechanical expiratory interval, left ventricular pressure is decreased, as effective right atrial filling pressure is increased. The net result is a preferential reloading of the pulmonary circulation.
c. Without sufficient expiratory interval time (E), to allow a proportionate reloading of the pulmonary circulation, at an ambient or a mechanically governed baseline, a chronic pulmonary hypervolemia can be created during the period of mechanical ventilation.

18. The justification for a positive end expiratory pressure (PEEP) in the apneic patient centres around control over a clinically significant right to left pulmonary shunt. Additionally, PEEP/CPAP can be employed to stabilize pulmonary airways in the presence of a low FRC.

19. A continuous positive airway pressure (CPAP), during spontaneous breathing, can be maintained with a programmable demand flow accelerator, for maintaining a positive expiratory baseline during mechanical end expiration, as well as augmenting spontaneous inspiration; to reduce the work of breathing.

20. PEEP can be maintained during continuous mechanical ventilation (CMV) by scheduling a negative I/E ratio. With a limited passive expiratory flow time (as opposed to Inspiratory Time), breath stacking occurs, causing an expiratory "positive intrapulmonary pressure" creating a mechanically elevated functional residual capacity (D/FRC).

21. A sub ambient expiratory phase can be useful in overcoming the mechanical expiratory resistance within endotracheal tubes which serve as "expiratory time bottlenecks" to passive physiological expiratory flow.

22. If a sub ambient phase is maintained beyond the endotracheal tube, with sufficient amplitude and time, intrapulmonary airway collapse is potentiated.

23. Dynamic positive/sub ambient (push/pull) respirator/ventilators must be pressure limited during both the positive as well as the sub ambient phase.

a. The dynamic expiratory (sub ambient) phase of a ventilator may be time limited to prevent airway "draw down".

24. All medical respirators must be peak pressure limited. For example: 35 cm H_2O for neonates, 50 cm H_2O for paediatrics and 100 cm H_20 for adults.

25. Medical respirator/ventilators can be time cycled, with flow x time determining the tidal volume scheduled, under the selected pressure limit.

26. Inspiratory flowrates can be manually selectable, multi stage with flow

acceleration and/or with deceleration and/or regulated by physiological feed back, through an automatic variable flow "Bernoulli tube" to provide for "pneumatic fluidic clutching".

a. An inspiratory flowrate can be preset.
b. An inspiratory flowrate can be time accelerated or decelerated in stages.
c. An inspiratory flowrate can be physiologically fluid clutched, by employing an ambient gated venturi, in any of the above combinations.

27. Cyclic inspiratory/expiratory interval phasing can be patient triggered by an initial spontaneous inspiratory effort and/or mechanically controlled (assister/controller), depending upon the effective trigger mechanism first activated. With this type of device the Patient is allowed passive spontaneous breathe through.

28. A pressure regulated "post inspiratory apneustic plateau" can be maintained by time, before allowing passive physiological exhalation.

29. Intermittent mandatory ventilation (IMV) employs a mechanical assister/controller respirator/ventilator with programmable PEEP/CPAP, allowing the gradual phase out of mandated (controlled) ventilation during the weaning process.

a. Synchronous inspiratory intermittent mandatory ventilation (SIMV) allows for an assist/control mode to reduce the work of breathing, as a substitute for decreasing the work of spontaneous ventilation with demand CPAP.

30. Volume controlled ventilators employ a selected flowrate until the volume schedule is reached, creating a variable inspiratory time. The selected I/E ratio is then obtained by matching the e component to the variable i time.

31. True volume oriented ventilators employing displacement bellows, time or volume cycling, must employ heated humidification devices which do not add additional gas volume to the system (during calculation), such as could be the case with conventional gas activated nebulizers.

32. Time cycled volume oriented devices, with automatic fluid clutching and expiratory demand CPAP, may employ nebulization for resolution of humidity deficits, as well as to deliver medications and bulk intrapulmonary water.

33. Mechanical respirators may have manual override to control tidal delivery, as well as to pace the expiratory interval.

34. Minute and/or tidal volume controlled ventilators may be augmented with assisting devices to provide pressure support during spontaneous override.

35. Exsufflation devices can provide a patient triggered and/or controlled percussive inspiratory phase (+40 -40 cm H_2O) with or without a sub ambient expiratory phase. These devices were initially employed on polio patients, maintained in mechanical (iron) lungs, to provoke a simulated cough reflex.

36. Insufflation devices deliver a constant and/or cyclic flow of humidified respiratory gases through an indwelling airway catheter, to the area above the carina, for the purpose of reducing anatomical dead space.

37. Mechanical dead space (mechanical re-breathing) can be controlled by the design of the breathing circuit.

38. Physiological dead space is any combination of an embarrassment to alveolar ventilation, diffusion and/or perfusion of the pulmonary structures. A medical respirator/ventilator is capable of reversing certain types of physiological dead space.

39. A full body respirator (iron lung) does not impair cardiac output, when compared to a "trach-positive" device; however, a tank respirator is only about 15% as effective as a trach-positive respirator/ventilator in the presence of decreasing gross pulmonary compliance.

40. Intermittent positive pressure breathing (IPPB) provides a means for the "topical endobronchial delivery" of an airborne alpha/beta type aerosol, within the pulmonary structures, when properly administered. Nebulization can be continuous and/or intermittent.

a. IPPB can, when properly scheduled, re-inflate lungs with diffuse patchy atelectasis.

41. Power nebulization therapy, provides a simple means for an uncomplicated patient, to spontaneously breathe an aerosolized solution of a specific medication.

42. Supplemental free flow humidified oxygen can be delivered with a controlled FIO_2 and flowrate, at the proximal airway through various masks, tubes, etc.

43. Mist inhalation devices can be employed to deliver single doses of medication into the oral passageways, leading to the lungs, with various "mechanical augmentors"; techniques will determine the clinical efficacy.

44. Mechanical expiratory retardation devices can be employed to maintain a graded positive pressure within the physiological expiratory airways, to reduce air trapping in patients with obstructive pulmonary airway disease.

a. Physiological retardation can be accomplished by pursed lips and/or pursing at the level of the chords.

b. Mechanical gating, employing an expiratory orifice, can effectively produce retardation of expiratory flow.

45. Pure high frequency diffusive respiration is provided by a mechanical energy generator (diaphragm) capable of producing airborne shock waves, for delivery within the pulmonary structures. Verification can be obtained with a Pneumo-tachometer positioned at the proximal airway, revealing no net airflow in either direction.

46. A jet insufflator (ventilator) delivers a higher frequency sub tidal volume exchange, through an indwelling insufflation tubing (catheter), positioned above the carina in such a way as to create a minor inspiratory aspiration of upper airway gases, while providing for a physiological airway around the diameter of the tube, to enable a passive exhalation. Peak pressure rise is limited by flowrate and physiological orifice (leak).

47. A combination continuous mechanical ventilation (CMV) and programmed jet insufflation, during the expiratory interval (phase), can be obtained by the slaving of a CMV device with a jet insufflator, employing a multi lumen indwelling airway catheter.

48. Extra-thoracic percussion (chest physiotherapy) can be manually or semi-automatically administered, by the precise positioning of the patient after nebulization (aerosol) therapy, for the enhanced mobilization of endobronchial secretions.

a. The chest vest is a device employed for the mobilization of upper airway secretions. It is capable of "violently shaking the upper torso with an appropriately fitted vest.

49. The rocking bed, provides a means of employing the "abdominal viscera" against the diaphragm, to provoke a phasic tidal exchange in paralytic patients. Additionally, this method has been used in the past with a cyclic Trendelenberg position (18 degrees head down) to facilitate tracheo-bronchial drainage.

50. Partial chest respirators sub ambient (Shell) enhance tidal exchange in paralytic patients with marginal ability to provide adequate physiological tidal exchange.

51. The conceptual development of the Phasitron® (physical physiological interface) with monojet control allowed the precise mixing of traditional convective ventilation with higher frequency percussive techniques. This major development allowed the lungs to be internally percussed, without firing the Hering Breuer reflexes.

a. Additionally, the Phasitron® can be employed to the servo of a unique split phase dynamic diaphragmatic oscillator, capable of generating a closed circuit percussive dynamic (push/pull) oscillation for the slaving of traditional CMV programs.
b. The Phasitron® has served to advance the use of higher frequency diffusive scheduling, during a "diffusive/convective ventilatory programming" at higher frequencies, without the associated inadvertent PEEP, as delivery frequencies are increased.

52. Intrapulmonary percussive ventilation (IPV®) is a combination of a powerful time cycled volume ventilator providing for chest physiotherapy and nebulization. IPV® is directed toward the mobilization of retained endobron-

chial secretions, as well as the resolution of diffuse patchy atelectasis. IPV is administered with a mouthpiece, mask and/or endotracheal tube which can be manually or automatically programmed, at desirable percussive frequencies and amplitudes.

53. The I/E ratio of "pulse generation" is the pulsatile flow/no flow time relationships expressed in milli-second during higher frequency percussive ventilation (IPV®), as opposed to the I/E ratios expressed in seconds during CMV.

54. I/E ratios during high frequency percussive ventilation (HFPV) are employed to express the ratio between the period of percussive inspiratory oscillation and the period at expiratory baseline (whether static or oscillatory). The programmed inspiratory/expiratory interval is expressed as the "Sinusoidal I/E ratio". VDR® is "high frequency percussive ventilation (HFPV)".

55. The pulse generator/mechanical flow interrupter percussionator® can be employed to create a positive higher frequency, amplitude controlled, interruptible wave format, with frequency and band width programmable. Positive phase oscillation can be maintained above an ambient and/or mechanically elevated baseline.

56. Peak to peak pressure monitoring during continuous higher frequency programming is presented as the highest positive pressure reached during oscillation, as well as the peak pressure drop. For example, the highest 50 cm of H_2O, as opposed to the Lowest of -15 cm of H_2O, equals (=) a peak to peak pressure differential of 65 cm of H_2O.

a. Peak to peak pressure monitoring can serve as a valuable clinical guide, during all forms of continuous higher frequency (push-pull) oscillation.

57. A reciprocating device can be employed for dynamic positive/sub ambient (push/pull) oscillation, to provide for continuous neonatal ventilation through a selected CPAP (5 to 25 cm of H_2O), with peak to peak pressure differentials as high as 80 cm of H_2O, at frequencies of over 900 cycles per minute. This can be accomplished, if the I/E transition rate is sufficiently fast for the frequency selected; if not, an undetected persistent systemic CPAP, with peripheral hyperinflation, may be unintentionally programmed.

58. During continuous dynamic neonatal oscillation with certain devices, if the pulmonary recruitment pressure is not reached, with a peak to peak pressure of 30 cm of H_2O, a sinusoidal CPAP may be employed to reduce the potential for barotrauma and the obstruction of central venous return.

59. The concept of volumetric diffusive respiration (VDR®), employs a (low rate) extended convective phasic change in lung volume, while simultaneously delivering higher frequency percussive sub tidal exchanges, resulting in "breath stacking" to the programmed point of oscillatory equilibrium.

a. Continuous sub tidal volume deliveries, during traditional phasic convective tidal changes in lung volume, provide for traditional CO_2 "wash out, during VDR® sinusoidal programming.

60. The unique ability of the ambient gated venturi within the Phasitron® to hold a precise selectable peak pressure limit, during oscillatory equilibrium, allows the lungs to be held in a scheduled post inspiratory percussive apneustic plateau (for increasing intrapulmonary diffusion), before returning to the programmed baseline. Therefore, a mechanical post inspiratory percussive plateau creates a dynamic functional residual capacity (D/FRC), which can be held for a scheduled interval.

61. The concept of traditional time cycled inspiratory flowrate acceleration can be programmed during VDR® scheduling, to allow the lung with low compliance time to conform to a progressive step inflation (to the higher mandated pressures), while reducing tendencies toward barotrauma.

62. The concept of "dynamic volumetric diffusive respiration (DVDR)" is created by slaving a conventional CMV type of ventilation with a dynamic (push/pull) closed circuit, higher frequency (600 to 1000 cycles per minute) diaphragm oscillator. The traditional CMV program is not upset in terms of expected clinical efficacy; however, a percussive diffusive phase is added, to enhance the diffusion of oxygen into, and CO_2 out of, the parenchymal pulmonary structures.

63. The understanding of functional I/E and i/e ratios, as they apply toward the determination of the diffusive/convective components of ventilatory programming, become of increasingly critical importance as the patients cardiopulmonary reserves are encroached upon.

64. Continuous positive (inspiratory) phase higher frequency oscillatory ventilation, must not be employed without appropriate baseline returns, to prevent sustained pulmonary hyperinflation and potential associated barotrauma.

65. Continuous high frequency oscillation, may satisfy PaO_2; however, $PaCO_2$ may overwhelm the patient because of an inadequate convective ventilatory component.

a. If a patient has sufficient spontaneous ventilatory exchange to manage $PaCO_2$, with a low PaO_2, pure high frequency diffusive ventilation could prove effective if properly scheduled.

66. Symbolic of all forms of mechanical pulmonary ventilation is the "hand powered bag of the anaesthetist". The hand can feel changes in physiological airway resistances, thus the term "educated hand". Therefore, the anaesthesiologist can provide full "fluid clutching" for enhancing alveolar distribution by modulating manual servoing pressures during bag compression. By applying

graded expiratory resistances, an "expiratory retard" can be performed in the presence of an obstructive pulmonary disease to decrease FRC.

67. The weaning of respirator dependent patients continues to challenge the clinician, with optioning for the most effective choice of protocol. Essentially, it is frequently much easier to install a patient on a medical respirator than to terminate mechanical respiratory support. The IMV protocol with demand CPAP remains a significant traditional means of weaning from a medical respirator ventilator.

a. The key toward successful weaning is to provide a gradual (over time) increase in the physiological work of breathing as fatigued and/or atrophied respiratory structures are rehabilitated, to provide normal spontaneous respiratory functions. Pressure supported ventilation, as currently defined, is a type of traditional ventilatory assist, native to conventional assister/controller devices.

68. As the use of diffusive/convective ventilatory protocols have become increasingly employed, the cyclic I/E as well as the pulsatile I/E ratios must be carefully scrutinised during the approach to the active weaning process.

a. A typical paradox could involve a neonate who has been steadily improving on an oscillatory protocol with a neutral or negative I/E ratio. As the pulmonary structures become more compliant, the lung volume can be proportionately increased (during the scheduled inspiratory interval) under the existing peak delivery pressure limit, to the point of over-expansion.
b. If the expiratory interval is not sufficiently long (for optimal pulmonary deflation to occur), the potential inspiratory over-expansion of the pulmonary structures can be converted into sustained hyperinflation with a notable increase in D/FRC. The clinican can then be misdirected by the deteriorating clinical presentations of increasing $PaCO_2$.
c. Such a process can justify a typical ventilator reprogramming, consisting in part of an increase in peak delivery pressure to increase tidal exchange, when in fact the expiratory time (time at baseline) should have been increased to cause a decrease in the D/FRC which would serve to increase effective tidal exchange. Thereafter, with improvement, the minute ventilation can be decreased as an active weaning process is undertaken.
d. If the pulsatile i/e ratio during continuous higher frequency neonatal oscillation is not sufficiently positive (1:1.5 etc.) a continuous state of pulmonary hyperinflation can be maintained, with an associated rise in $PaCO_2$.

69. There are various forms of expiratory resistances; among these are physiological as well as mechanical causes and unique combinations thereof. Associated with any expiratory flow restriction is a related intrapulmonary

expiratory pressure sustenance during the initial period of peak expiratory outflow. If sufficient expiratory time is not allowed for deflation down to the existing FRC, mechanically induced air trapping is mandated.

a. A small (cuffed and/or snug) indwelling airway catheter can produce the mechanical expiratory retardation of physiological outflow.
b. A patient with obstructive pulmonary disease can retard physiological expiratory flow by pursing at the level of the chords and/or the lips to decrease FRC. When a large endotracheal tube is passed through the chords, all means of physiological expiratory flow retardation is negated, causing a potential related increase in FRC.
c. Mechanical resistance to physiological expiratory flow within the expiratory limbs of breathing circuits can cause expiratory flow retardation.

70. Expiratory flow retardation differs from PEEP/CPAP in that a retardation of physiological expiratory flow serves to maintain greater airway patency, during the active period of physiological outflow, by providing an orifice within the upper airways to decrease FRC in the presence of lower airway obstructive phenomena, as opposed to PEEP or CPAP, which serves to allow passive exhalation down to a mechanically created end expiratory pressure.

71. The less the mechanical expiratory resistance within a breathing circuit, the more rapid the physiological passive deflation of the pulmonary structures; the faster the FRC is reached, the less expiratory time required, with less expiratory flowtime required to reach the FRC, an increase in minute ventilation and/or a decrease in mean intrapulmonary pressure can be optioned.

72. Without a near instantaneous flow gradient reversal, from the mechanical inspiratory to the expiratory phase, during continuous high frequency oscillatory ventilation, there will be insufficient expiratory time to maintain a normal FRC, causing a mechanically induced D/FRC to be maintained.

73. The measurement of an intrapulmonary tidal exchange, either in or out, can not reveal the effective blood gas interface in terms of bilateral intrapulmonary distribution. A nomogram, based upon a normal perfusion/diffusion, with optimal distribution of the delivered tidal volume, does not reveal the ventilatory schedules required for optimal blood gas interfaces. Cardiopulmonary patients can not be expected to have normal blood gas interfaces; therefore, spirometric means must be backed up by clinical judgement and blood gas profiles.

74. The monitoring of proximal inspiratory airway pressure only determines the potential gradient for proximal/distal intrapulmonary inflow against the prevailing mechanical and physiological resistances.

75. The monitoring of a programmed PEEP/CPAP at the proximal airway reveals the potential for an increase over FRC, by the maintenance of a mechanically induced expiratory D/FRC.

76. The integration of a mean proximal airway pressure can potentially reveal the expected overall ventilatory effect upon cardiac output, secondary to the phasing of proximal airway pressures.

77. Simulated or actual peak to peak proximal airway pressures can serve to reveal the potential transitional pressure gradients (band width) of the pulsatile i/e ratio, during the programmed higher frequency inspiratory and/or continuous oscillatory interval.

78. The measurement of a positive oscillatory band width on a VDR® type oscillator, can only be accomplished accurately with an applicable fast Transducer and appropriate CRT. Most blood pressure type physiological monitoring systems are too slow to measure the true peak pressure rise and do not have an accurate sub ambient pressure measuring capacity.

79. A manometric measuring system for peak to peak pressures can accurately measure the systemic CPAP, peak pressure drop to effective sub ambient values and can be calibrated to simulate proximal airway peak pressure rise.

80. In lieu, or supportive thereof, of the monitoring of a traditional tidal exchange, more recent developments of practical means for determining a simulated arterial O_2 saturation and CO_2 levels, allow the effective indexing of diffusive/convective ventilatory device to each unique patient.

81. The primary method of ventilatory monitoring remains the clinical expertise of the attending in viewing the thorax for the desired level of bilateral ventilation, supported by auscultation, as well as traditional clinical observations.

a. Clinical expertise in cardiopulmonary monitoring, supplemented by blood gas profiles and radiology, continue to be the paramount medium of monitoring mechanical cardiopulmonary management.

82. Physical/physiological airway junctions are employed to interconnect the physiological respiratory airways to the mechanical breathing circuit. Without the proper capturing of the physiological airway, the mechanical ventilatory capacities may be compromised.

a. For those patients with whom the clinician can interrelate, a physiologically sealed airway, consisting of a flanged or circular mouthpiece (sealed by the lips) can be employed for therapeutic protocols. Nasal venting can be resolved by proper introduction without the use of nasal clamps.
b. Masks should only be used as temporary airways, in a patient that is properly positioned to prevent aspiration, if emesis occurs. The maximum possible seal on conventional medical masks would limit peak delivery pressures to well under 35 cm of H_2O.
c. Various appliances for the delivery of free flowing supplemental O_2 can be employed such as vented masks, nasal prongs, insufflation tubes, as well as various combination split and bag type face masks.

d. Indwelling airway catheters can be employed to deliver free flow or pulsatile gases to the carinal levels for anatomical dead space reduction.
e. The most secure mechanical airway, for protection from vomiting and aspiration as well as accommodating peak delivery pressures of over 100 cm of H_2O, is the cuffed endotracheal tube.
f. Cuffed and uncuffed tracheotomy tubes can be employed for long term ventilatory management.
g. Various tracheal fenestration techniques can be employed for the delivery of supplemental O_2 in patients with chronic cardiopulmonary diseases.

83. Intrathoracic vesicular peristalsis effects the bronchial, pulmonary and lymph circulations, within the thoracic cage. Each circulation provides for directional control in a respective direction. Whenever a phasic intrathoracic pressure change with sufficient amplitude occurs, vesicular compression decreases the capacity of the respective circulation; this results in an augmented directional flow of the fluid contents, secondary to the decrease in vesicular calibre.

a. There are two types of vesicular peristalsis: one is created by the physiological intrathoracic pressure changes; the other can be a powerful, mechanically developed intrapulmonary vesicular peristalsis, which is created by intrapulmonary percussive ventilatory (IPV®) scheduling.

84. With the advent of IPV®/VDR®, a powerful means of enhancing physiological cardiopulmonary functions has been advanced. Percussive IPV® serves to effectively increase the "blood gas interfaces", by allowing the clinician to program a balanced mechanical respiration, in terms of endobronchial mechanical mixing, providing for diffusion as well as convection.

a. Generally, by increasing intrapulmonary diffusion, O_2 transport toward the blood gas interface is enhanced; the opposite obtains, as CO_2 is diffused away from the blood gas interface into the peripheral airways, for a convective "wash out".

85. IPV® can produce a powerful augmentive "lymph pump", to decrease the "pulmonary interstitial fluid reservoir", secondary to an increase in retention, caused by left ventricular failure etc. Therefore, the vital capacity, as well as lung compliance, can be facilitated, reducing the potential for barotrauma.

86. Intrapulmonary percussive ventilation (IPV®) provides a method of progressively increasing lung volume, by means of a step inflation, with partially accumulative sub tidal volume deliveries, culminating in an oscillatory equilibrium. Delivery frequencies and pulsatile flowrate selection determine the diffusive/convective balance of endobronchial gas exchange. i/e ratios, delivery frequencies and endobronchial resistances automatically determine the "variable percussive inspiratory flowrates", which in turn determine the automatic CPAP stabilizer, referred to as the "wedge pressure".

a. The IPV® intrapulmonary wedge pressure is an automatic function of cycling rate and inspiratory flowrate (operational pressure) selection, delivering against variable endobronchial resistances.
b. An automatic IPV® Intrapulmonary Wedge pressure is employed to maintain the inspiratory/expiratory competency of the peripherally recruited airways, to prevent their phasic opening and closing, with associated irritation and potential inflammatory processes. Advanced applications of "fluid dynamics" prevail in the novel IPV/VDR concepts.

87. IPV®/VDR® may be summarized by comparison:

In order for PEEP to increase PAO_2 in patients without clinical COPD, the pulmonary artery pressure must be increased by increasing the right to left resistance in preferential pulmonary capillaries, to obtain increased perfusion within other parenchemal structures.

When PEEP is employed on patients with COPD, who have existing alveolar hyperinflation (increasing right to left pulmonary resistances), the pulmonary hypertension and associated right heart failure can be exacerbated.

When PEEP is programmed into a volume oriented CMV ventilatory program, the peak delivery pressures could be expected to be increased to deliver the scheduled tidal volume. This could be a pre-cursor to barotrauma in preferential hyperinflated lung structures.

During the mechanical ventilation of the lung with IPV/VDR programming, partially obstructed peripheral airways are expiratorily supported with a "low pressure wedge", which is maintained in the peripheral airways, by timing the follow on proximal distal tidal wave arrival into the terminal bronchioles, before a post expiratory adhesive airway collapse can occur.

IPV/VDR scheduling near instantaneously drops the post inspiratory injection pressure to ambient at the proximal airway, thus reducing mean intrapulmonary pressures, which expands the peak to peak airway pressure rise and drop within the pulmonary structures; this in turn, serves to enhance pulmonary mechanical vesicular peristalsis facilitating cardiac output (Fig. 1).

During the successive, percussive, sub tidal endo-bronchial deliveries, a repetitive rolling peristaltic pressure wave serves to directionally propel blood within the pulmonary circulation toward the left heart. The acute end inspiratory endobronchial pressure drop between successive tidal waves enhances the reloading of the pulmonary vessels adherent to the conducting pulmonary airways.

The physiological intrathoracic lymph pump is mechanically enhanced, by the phasic compression of the directionally gated lymph vessels within the pulmonary structures, by the percussive phasic inflation and deflation of the pulmonary structures.

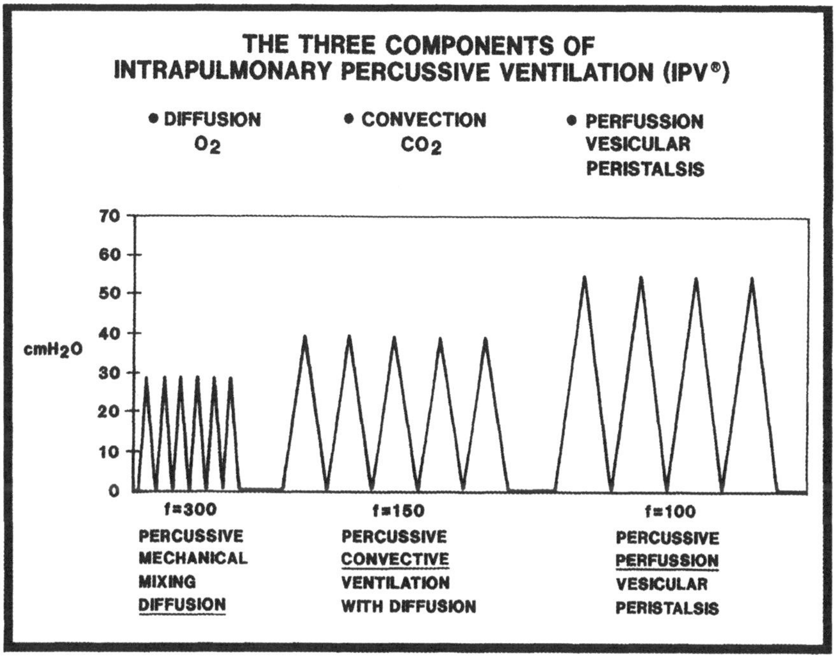

Fig.1. Intrapulmonary percussive ventilation (IPV®)

The repetitive (higher frequency) percussive tidal wave, flow and back flow, through the pulmonary structures, provides for several concomitant functions, namely:

A. Providing for both diffusive and convective intrapulmonary gas exchange.
B. The delivery of topically administered endobronchial vasoconstrictors, dilators and wetting agents, to improve airway calibre.
C. The mobilization and raising of retained endobronchial secretions, by providing an air distal to secretions, for their mobilization and cephalad raising.
D. A mechanical facilitation to the physiological intrathoracic lymph pump, to assist in decongesting the pulmonary interstitial spaces.
E. Depending upon programming, a right to left vesicular peristalsis within the pulmonary circulation directed toward decreasing pulmonary arterial pressure while increasing the peristaltic left ventricular filling pressure.
F. In left congestive failure, depending upon programming, an increase in mean intrathoracic pressure will impair venous return to the right heart, while concomitantly providing a vesicular peristalsis within the pulmonary circulation toward the left heart to reduce the pulmonary blood volume, which will in turn reduce the left ventricular filling pressure, which will then allow the left ventricle to function with more favourable contractile advantages.

Figure 2 reveals the peristaltic effect of higher frequency percussive ventilation, during the ventilation of a patient with a very low pulmonary compliance, secondary to both airway resistance, as well as interstitial congestion. “Alveolar re-setting” during the apneustic plateau reduces potentials for barotrauma.

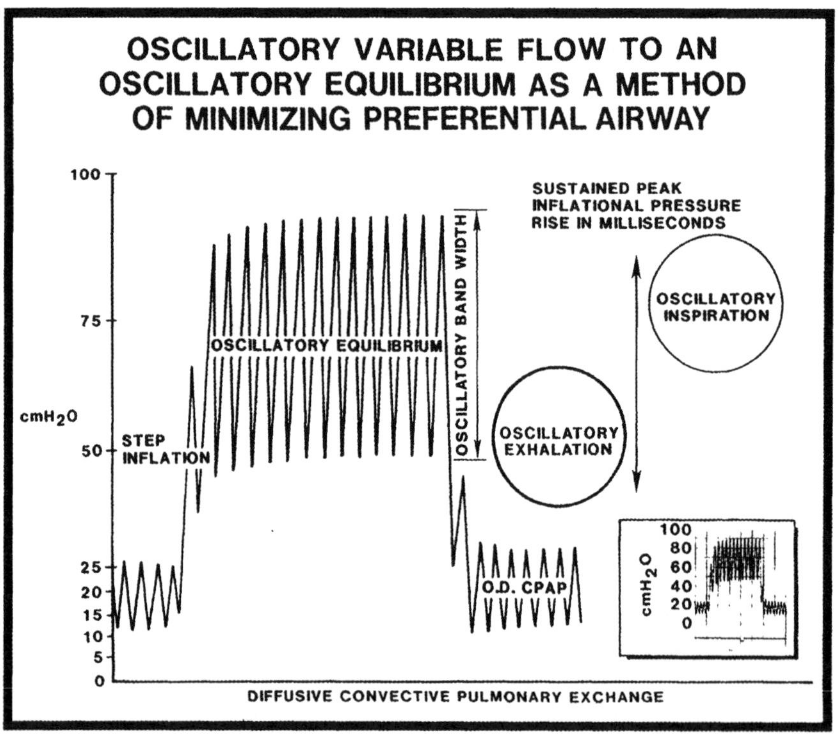

Fig. 2. Oscillatory equilibrium

Monitoring in Acute Brain Injury

E. G. McKEATING

Advances in technology have provided us with an array of monitors that may be used in the intensive care unit (ICU) to monitor patients with acute brain injury (Fig. 1). It is, however, particularly important when considering this topic, to remember that the brain will not function without the support of other body systems, e.g., the cardiovascular and respiratory systems. Proper discussion must therefore start with the basic principles of management and monitoring of the acutely ill patient.

There is a growing understanding of the dangers of secondary brain injury

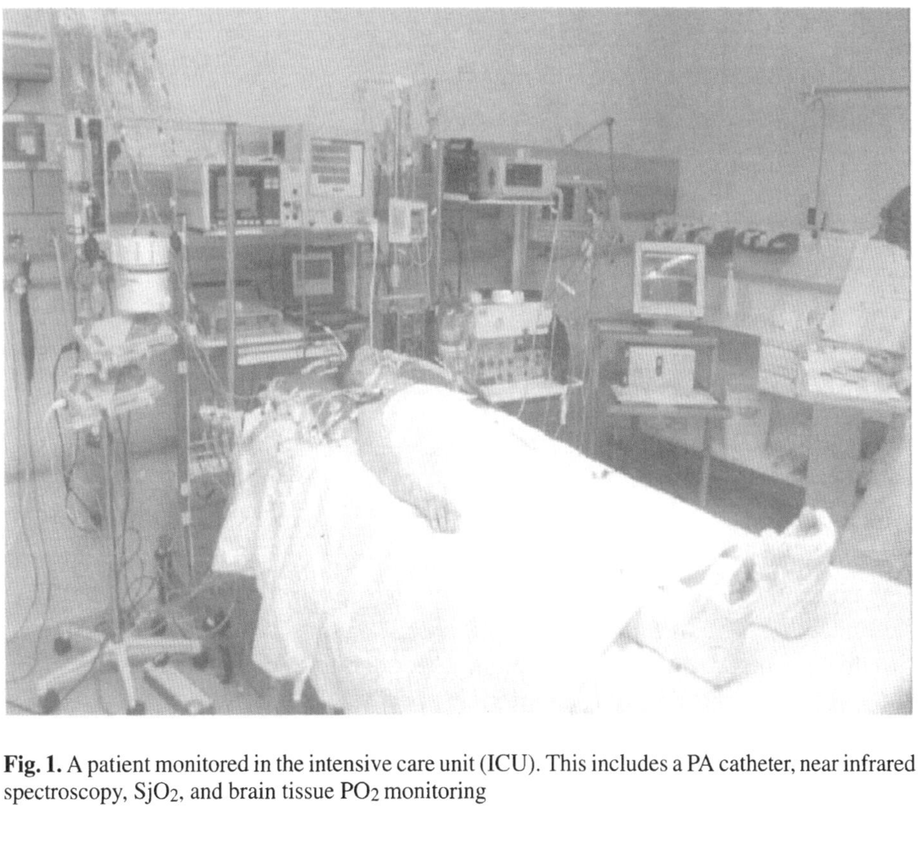

Fig. 1. A patient monitored in the intensive care unit (ICU). This includes a PA catheter, near infrared spectroscopy, SjO_2, and brain tissue PO_2 monitoring

[1, 2] and of secondary insults [3] to the injured brain. Injury to the brain may be divided into two categories – primary and secondary. The primary injury is the damage caused by the initial impact or event, and is generally regarded as irreversible. Secondary injury is neither a direct result, nor an inevitable consequence, of the primary injury, and occurs some time after the initial insult. It may be modified by good or poor pre-, intra-, or inter-hospital patient care. In addition, it has been suggested that the inflammatory processes that lead to secondary injury are accentuated by the occurrence of "secondary insults" that occur after the initial injury. These include systemic hypotension, systemic hypoxia, and pyrexia. Jones et al. [4] showed that in the ICU, comparing survivors with those who had died at 12 months, the most-important predictors of mortality were duration of hypotensive and hypoxic insults, and duration of pyrexia.

It is therefore apparent that what we may classify as "basic" monitoring techniques and equipment will play a vital role in the management of these patients. This will begin in the pre-hospital phase and extend through to the neurological ward after the patient's stay in the ICU.

Initial management

Pre-hospital personnel must use basic clinical monitoring techniques (i.e., look, listen, and feel) to repeatedly assess adequacy of the airway, breathing and circulation. Electronic adjuncts such as electrocardiographic (ECG) monitoring, non-invasive arterial blood pressure (NIBP) monitoring, and pulse oximetry may be available to pre-hospital personnel, depending on location. It is at this stage of patient resuscitation that simple maneuvers, such as clearing the airway, may have a profound effect on neurological outcome. Discovery of a low arterial blood pressure followed by rapid administration of intravenous (IV) fluid may have a similar effect.

On admission to the emergency room, similar management principles apply. Resuscitation should follow ATLS/ALS guidelines (ABCDEs). Clinical monitoring should be supplemented by ECG monitoring, NIBP measurement and pulse oximetry. Decisions regarding further monitoring of the patient will depend on the severity of the brain injury and the environment in which the patient will be managed. Ideally all patients with a mild / moderate injury should be nursed initially in a "high-dependency" environment, where the above basic monitoring may continue. It is of course mandatory that when a patient is monitored with devices such as those listed above, appropriately trained personnel are available to interpret and act upon the data supplied by the device. There is no place for monitoring to be connected to a patient when this support is not available. Patients with more-severe brain injury, or with brain injury together with other pathology, are more likely to be managed in the neuro-intensive care unit (NICU).

After stabilization in the emergency room, either intra- or inter-hospital transfer will be required. These transfers pose a considerable challenge to personnel caring for the patient [5]. It may be necessary to transport a patient with a severe brain injury to a neurosurgical center some distance from the receiving hospital. Guidelines for such transfers have recently been produced in the United Kingdom [6]. Sedation, intubation, and ventilation are mandatory for such transfers. ECG and pulse oximetry must be supplemented by invasive arterial blood pressure (IBP) monitoring. The use of NIBP monitoring in transfer vehicles is not practical. A urinary catheter should be inserted to monitor urine output (UOP). Ideally, the facility for monitoring end-tidal carbon dioxide should also be available. There is increasing interest in the use of intra-cranial pressure (ICP) monitoring at an early stage, and it may be that use of this mode of monitoring increases before and during transfer, although this is uncommon in the United Kingdom at this time.

Monitoring in the NICU

Tables 1 and 2 list the monitoring available for patients in the NICU. The techniques listed in Table 1 will be available to most intensivists working in specialist NICUs. Those listed in Table 2 are currently available often only in larger academic centers.

Table 1. Monitoring commonly used in the neuro-intensive care unit

Pulse oximeter
Core temperature
Electrocardiograph
End-tidal carbon dioxide
Invasive arterial blood pressure
Central venous pressure
Urine output
Pulmonary artery pressures

Table 2. Further advanced monitoring

Intra-cranial pressure
Jugular venous hemoglobin oxygen saturation
Processed cortical electrical activity (CFAM)
Somatosensory evoked potentials
Near-infrared spectroscopy
Trans-cranial Doppler ultrasonography
Direct cerebral blood flow measurement
Laser Doppler flowmetry
Brain tissue PO_2, PCO_2, pH, and temperature
Brain compliance
Brain microdialysis

On admission to the NICU, basic monitoring should be continued. This will include ECG, IBP, pulse oximetry, and UOP. A multi-lumen central venous catheter should be inserted to permit monitoring of central venous pressure and administration of drugs. The internal jugular vein need not be avoided in patients with brain injury, whilst alternative sites include the subclavian and femoral veins. A pulmonary artery (PA) flotation catheter may be indicated in patients with severe cardiac disease or with complications such as neurogenic pulmonary edema. A PA catheter may also be useful if large doses of vasopressor or inotropic drugs are required.

Insertion of an ICP monitoring device should then be considered. There are still some clinicians who believe that monitoring the ICP is not justified [7], given that there are some risks associated with the technique. However, in order to measure the cerebral perfusion pressure (CPP), ICP monitoring is necessary. ICP measurement should therefore be regarded as standard practice in severe acute brain injury. Numerous studies have shown that the technique is generally safe, with an extremely low complication rate [8]. The method used will depend on the type of injury, and appearance of the brain and ventricular system on computed tomography (CT) scanning. In traumatic brain injury (TBI) the ventricles are usually small, therefore fiberoptic solid-state systems, such as those produced by Camino and Codman, are commonly used. After spontaneous subarachnoid hemorrhage, acute hydrocephalus is often seen. In this situation a catheter may be inserted into the ventricular system. This permits drainage of cerebrospinal fluid and permits direct measurement of pressure within the ventricular system. A drawback of this method is the risk of ventriculitis.

The CPP management approach, first advocated by Michael Rosner in the United States, has now been almost universally adopted by neuro-intensivists in the developed countries [9, 10]. The CPP is the arithmetic difference between the mean arterial blood pressure (MAP) and the ICP. Usually autoregulation of cerebral blood flow (CBF) in healthy humans means that CBF is maintained even at a low CPP. This mechanism is often disrupted in acute brain injury, and there is evidence to suggest that CPP should be maintained above at least 60 mmHg in adults who have sustained a TBI [11]. This figure may be as important in gauging effectiveness of treatment as the ICP in isolation. It is obviously a prerequisite that if this approach is to be used, both ICP and IBP are monitored. It is however necessary to state that, as in most areas of neuro-critical care, there is no class one evidence that the use of ICP monitoring results in improved patient outcome.

One of the most-significant advances in bedside monitoring in acute brain injury is the ability to continuously monitor the hemoglobin oxygen saturation in the jugular vein (SjO_2). A fiber-optic catheter is inserted via a narrow sheath, similar to a small PA catheter sheath, which is inserted in a cephalad direction into the dominant internal jugular vein (usually the right) (Fig. 2) [12]. This can be confirmed by compressing the jugular vein on each side of the neck in

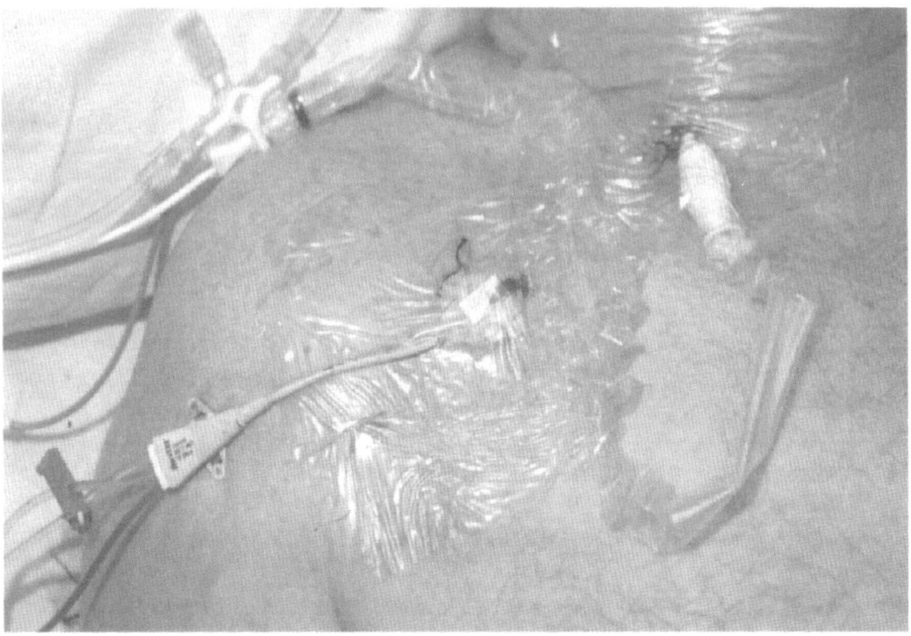

Fig. 2. Right subclavian central venous line together with right internal jugular venous fiberoptic SjO_2 monitoring catheter, which runs via a percutaneous sheath into the jugular bulb

turn, whilst watching the ICP. If the right side is dominant, there will be a higher transient rise in ICP after compression of this vein (and vice versa).

The tip of the catheter sits in the jugular bulb and the SjO_2 is displayed on the monitor screen (as mixed venous SvO_2 data from a pulmonary artery flotation catheter). The normal SjO_2 is 55-75%. Collection of SjO_2 data allows calculation of the cerebral arterio-venous oxygen content difference, and hence gives an indication of CBF and flow-metabolism coupling. It is particularly useful in assisting decisions about the most-appropriate method of treatment when the ICP is raised and the CPP reduced. If the SjO_2 is low, oxygen extraction is high, suggesting either increased brain oxygen demand, or more likely a reduced CBF. If the SjO_2 is high, this suggests that the CBF is higher than that required by the brain (hyperemia) [13].

Processed EEG monitoring using a cerebral function analyzing monitor (CFAM) [14] should be instigated for patients who are receiving muscle relaxants, when seizure activity may go unnoticed. It should also be used in those who are receiving a barbiturate infusion for control of intracranial hypertension, when a "burst suppression" pattern is desirable. These monitors have been available for some years (the first cerebral function monitor was developed in 1967 [15]), and the most-recent model, the CFAM3c (Fig. 3),

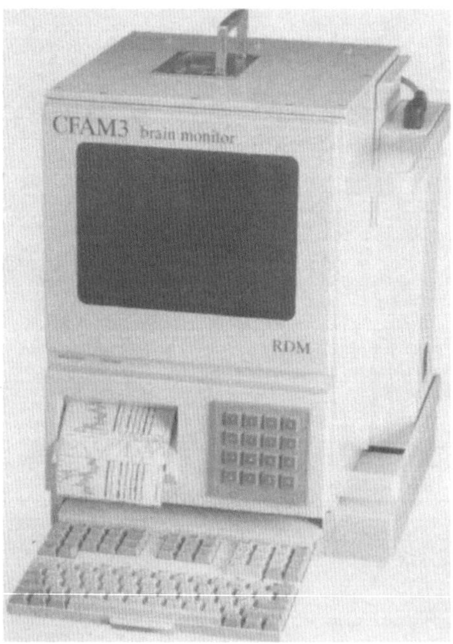

Fig. 3. Cerebral function analyzing monitor (CFAM)

features a multifunction colour display (Fig. 4). It is usual to place five electrodes on to the scalp for a two-channel display. Raw EEG data are displayed at the top of the screen. The left-hand displays show amplitude distribution of the signal for each hemisphere on a logarithmic scale. The bands on the right side display the distribution of frequencies into beta, alpha, theta, and delta bands. There is also a channel to display percentage of time in burst suppression. This monitor is user friendly, and is easily set up on the NICU by nursing staff who have undergone simple training. Nursing staff can also easily interpret the data supplied and may, for example, adjust the dose of barbiturate appropriately. The information supplied by these monitors may be helpful in the future in improving outcome after brain injury [16]. Measurement of somatosensory evoked potentials may also be carried out in the NICU. This technique is particularly useful for predicting those patients in whom there is likely to be a poor neurological outcome.

Trans-cranial Doppler (TCD) sonography of blood flow velocity in the cerebral circulation may yield useful information regarding cerebral hemodynamics [17]. The usual approach is to place a 2-mHz gated probe over

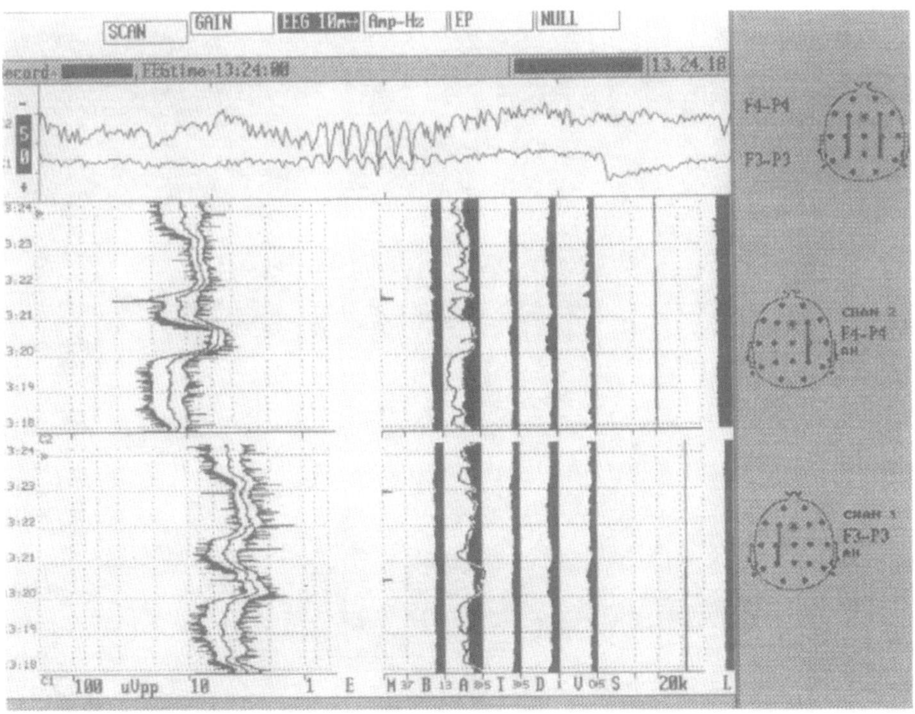

Fig. 4. Screen display from CFAM. Patient is neonate with unilateral subpial hemorrhage

the temporal bony window. The technique is non-invasive and does not measure CBF directly, but measures CBF velocity. One must assume a constant vessel diameter if the device is used to measure CBF trends. Other derived measurements such as the pulsatility index (systolic - diastolic velocity / mean velocity), may assist in distinguishing between arterial vasospasm and cerebral hyperemia. The technique is also useful for defining the lower limit of pressure autoregulation after brain injury [18]. A characteristic appearance of reversed flow in the middle cerebral artery is seen in brain-dead patients (Fig. 5). Training in the technique is required, however, and there are difficulties in keeping the probe in position on a busy ICU. These factors limit the use of TCD in the NICU.

Laser Doppler flowmetry is a development of the above technique [19]. It is based on the detection of the velocity and number of red blood cells in the microcirculation and uses low-power laser light directed at the tissue through an optical fiber. This is placed into brain tissue in a probe placed via a burr hole. Absolute quantification of flow is not possible, and the technique provides a very regional measure. Its use is confined to research centers at present.

Near-infrared spectroscopy (cerebral oximetry) is another non-invasive

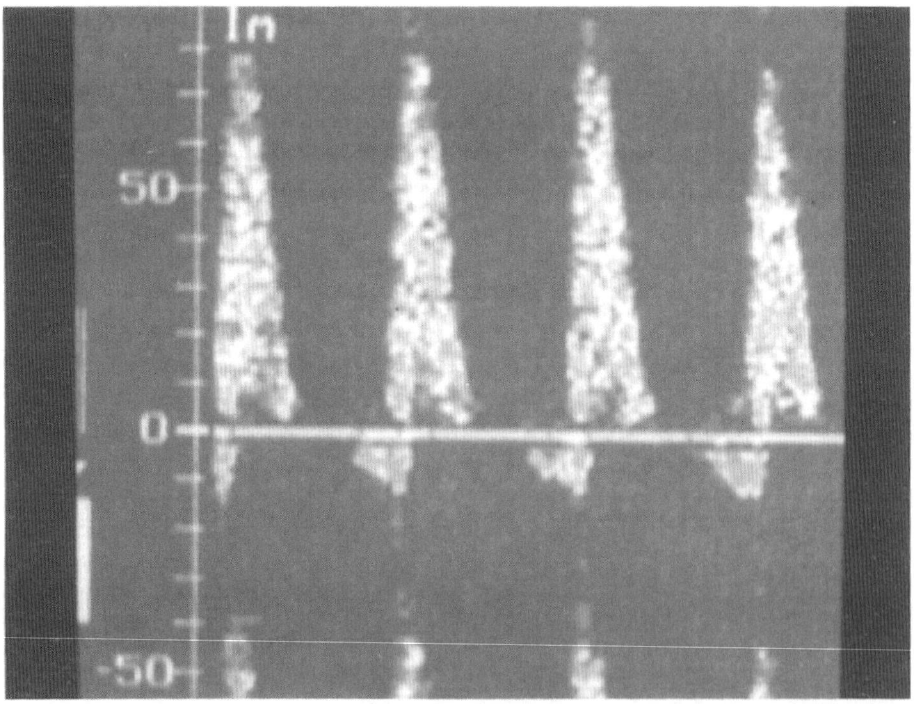

Fig. 5. Characteristic Doppler signal from middle cerebral artery in brain death

technique that can be used to monitor cerebral oxygenation after TBI [20, 21]. The principles are similar to pulse oximetry; several wavelengths of near infrared light are emitted by an optode that is adherent to the patient's forehead (Fig. 6). A detector placed some centimeters from the emitter detects the light reflected back by underlying tissue. A figure for regional hemoglobin oxygen saturation (rSO_2) is derived. There are problems however. It is difficult to ensure that correction for absorption by extra-cranial tissues is accurate, and there are often technical difficulties in the ICU in achieving reliable measurements over time [22]. With further refinement, however, this method may become a useful tool in the ICU.

Direct measurement of CBF

It is possible to measure CBF directly at the bedside. The method is based on the Kety-Schmidt principle which states that the rate of uptake and clearance of an inert diffusible gas is proportional to blood flow [23]. One suitable gas is nitrous oxide, which can be administered in low concentrations via the ventilator tubing and measured directly in serial arterial and jugular venous blood samples. Another method is to administer a trace amount of ^{133}Xe, and measure

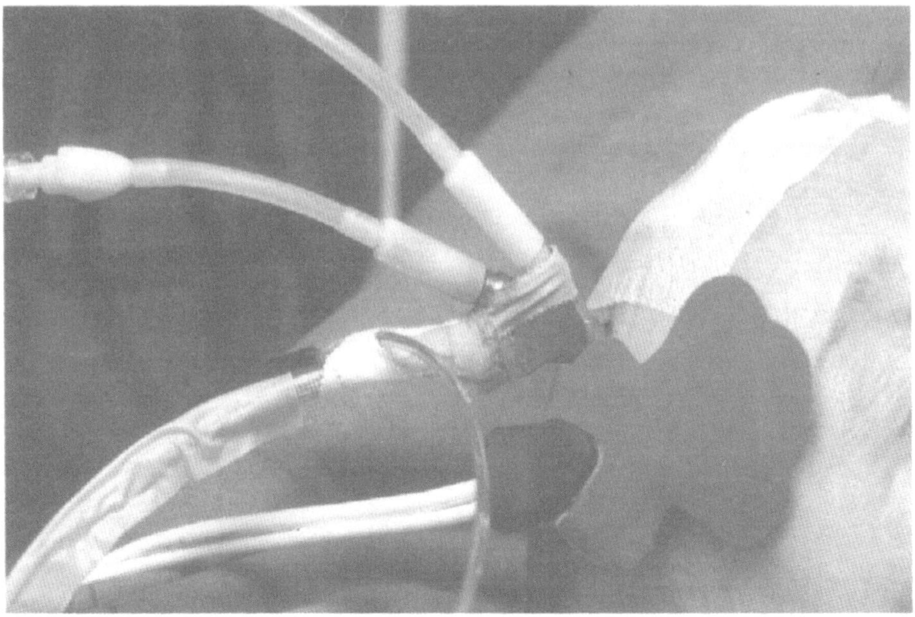

Fig. 6. NIRS optode, together with PO_2, temperature and intra-cranial pressure (ICP) probes

brain concentration with scintillation counters (Fig. 7). A figure for total (or regional CBF with the ^{133}Xe method) can be derived. This method is relatively inexpensive after the initial equipment costs, and can be repeated at regular intervals. It is however complicated, time consuming, and prone to artifacts.

Further direct measurement of CBF requires the patient to be transported to the neuro-radiology department. Here we may use stable Xenon CT scanning [24], single-photon emission tomography [25] (SPECT), or dual-photon emission tomography [26] (PET) to produce flow maps in each slice of brain tissue. Excellent quality images may be produced, but the complexity of these techniques, and their costs, again mean that they are generally confined to research centers. A further disadvantage is that transfer of the patient to the radiology department may result in secondary brain insults.

Recent developments

There has been increasing interest in the direct invasive measurement of regional brain tissue oxygenation using probes inserted trans-cranially. There are two commercially available systems: the first is the LICOX system [27]

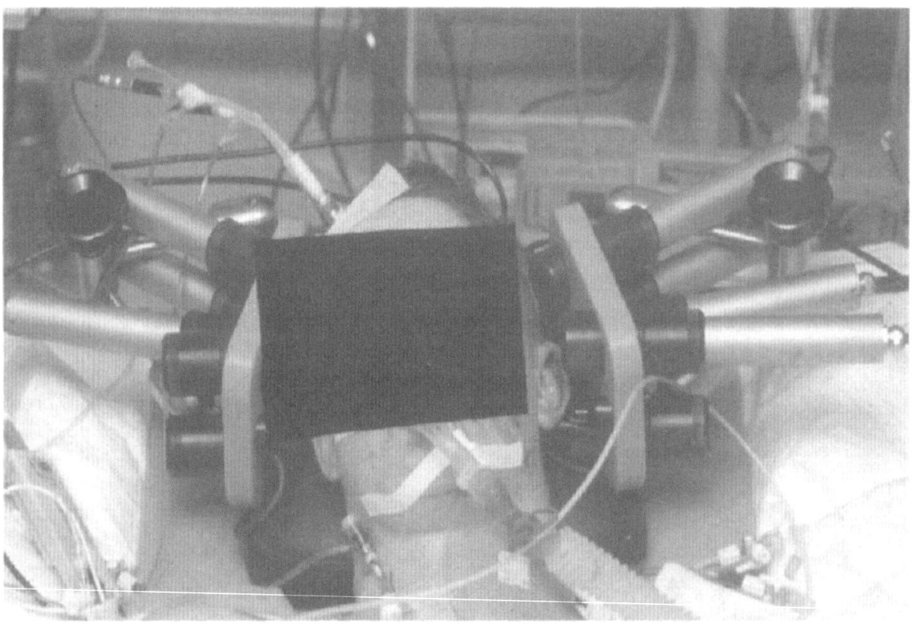

Fig. 7. Scintillation counters surrounding a patient's head during a cerebral blood flow measurement

(GMS, Germany, Fig. 8), which measures brain tissue PO_2 and temperature; the second is the Neurotrend system [28] (Codman, Johnson and Johnson, UK, Fig. 9), which measures PO_2, temperature, PCO_2, and pH. This system was developed from the Paratrend 7 sensor, which was used for continuous monitoring of intra-arterial blood gases.

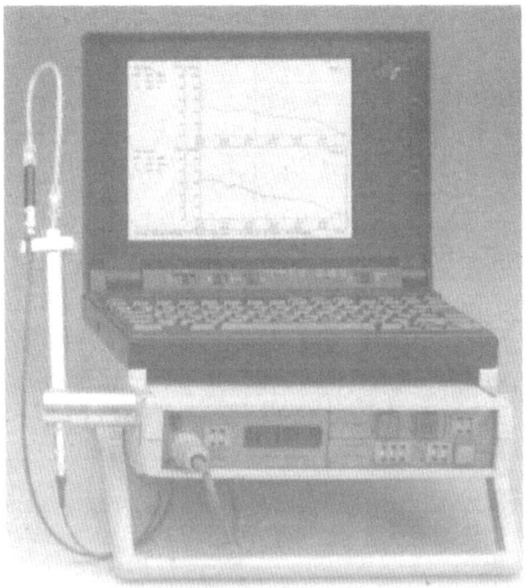

Fig. 8. The Licox monitor (a revised version is now in use)

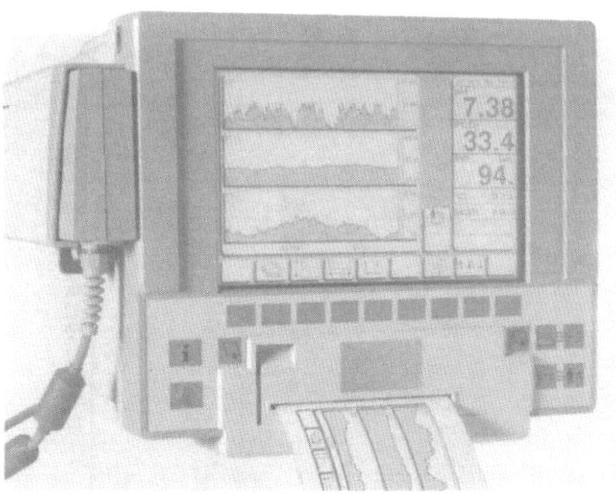

Fig. 9. The Neurotrend monitor

Both systems have the advantage of continuous trend measurements of tissue parameters; however they require a burr hole and deliver a regional measurement only. It is also difficult to interpret the resultant figures. It is possible to greatly increase the measured PO_2 by merely increasing the inspired oxygen concentration, but it is unknown as to whether this is an appropriate therapy. With the increasing use of three-dimensional imaging systems in the neurosurgical operating theater, it is possible to place these probes in particular sites of interest, e.g., the penumbra of a contusion or infarct where tissue is viable, but at particular risk of secondary injury. Therapy may then be targeted towards increasing tissue PO_2. One potential problem with these systems is the significant cost of disposables for each patient. Further research and evaluation is required before these techniques can be recommended.

A recently launched further development of ICP monitoring technology is the Spiegelberg compliance monitor [29] (Fig. 10). This monitor supplies the medical team with information regarding the ICP-volume relationship, and shows the patient's position on this curve (Fig. 11). A small balloon is sited at the end of a probe, which is placed into brain tissue or a ventricle (Fig. 12). A pump adds and removes tiny volumes of gas to and from the balloon, allowing the calculation of ICP and compliance. This is likely to prove to be a useful

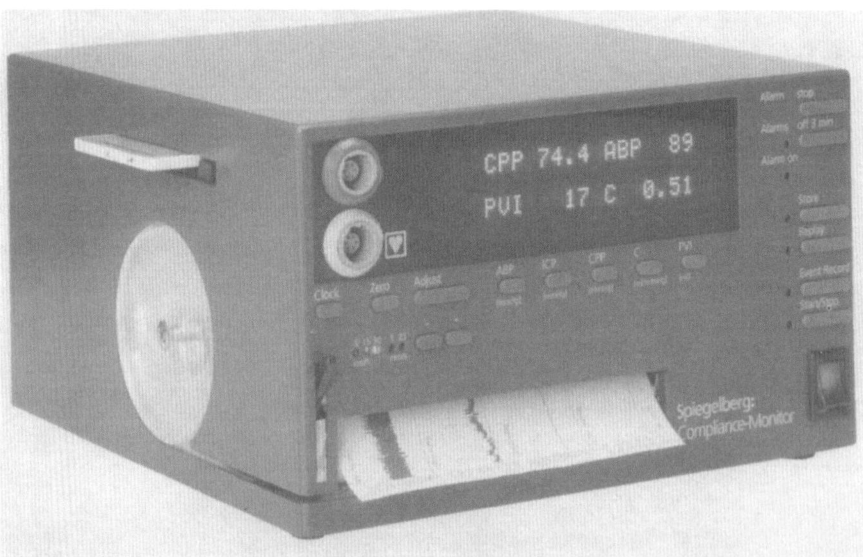

Fig. 10. The Spiegelberg compliance monitor

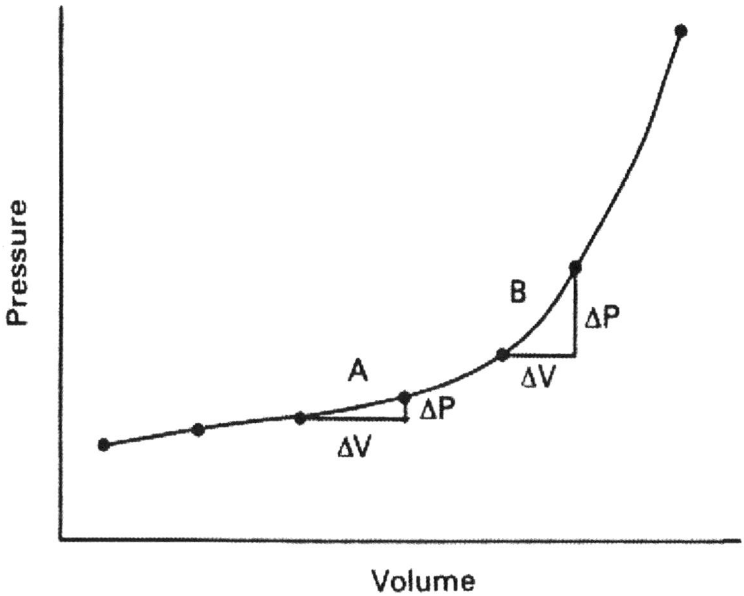

Fig. 11. The intra-cranial-pressure (ICP)-volume relationship

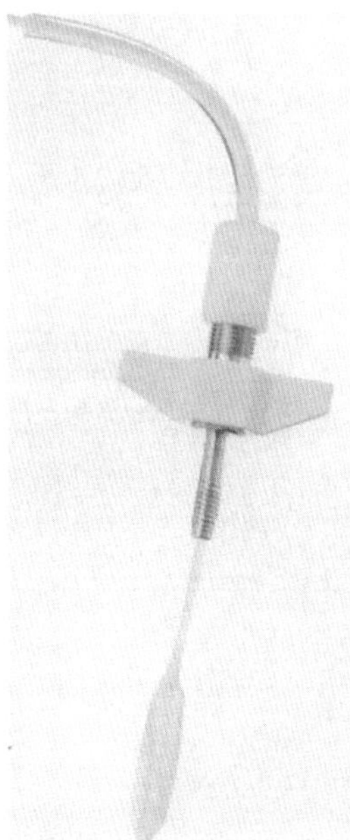

Fig. 12. The Spiegelberg compliance probe

monitor, as it is the patient's position on the pressure-volume curve that is important in planning treatment, rather than just the ICP in isolation [30].

Advances in imaging mean that it is now possible to look at some aspects of brain chemistry using PET scanning and magnetic resonance spectroscopy (MRS). The former will measure regional oxygen consumption and glucose utilization. MRS will give information on regional concentrations of substrates and metabolites, including glutamate, lactate, and creatinine.

One of the most-recent developments in bedside monitoring is direct neurochemical monitoring using cerebral microdialysis [31, 32]. This expensive and labor-intensive technique involves the slow infusion and collection of small-volume fluid samples via microdialysis catheters placed directly into brain tissue. On-line bedside measurement of metabolites such as glucose, pyruvate, lactate and glycerol may be carried out regularly.

Various studies have shown an association between high glutamate and lactate levels and poor outcome [33, 34]. It has been suggested that glycerol is a marker of cell membrane breakdown in ischemia. The lactate/pyruvate ratio has been identified as a useful marker of disturbances in brain metabolism [35]. Currently this technique is confined to research centers within the United Kingdom.

Summary

There has without doubt been an improvement in outcome after acute brain injury in recent decades. Developments in technology mean that there is now a vast array of expensive and theoretically useful monitors available to neuro-intensivists. The introduction of new monitoring technologies may have contributed to this improvement in outcome, but it is very difficult indeed to design trials that will prove that use of a particular device results in benefit to the patient. Probably more important is the increased availability of critical care facilities in which these patients may be managed, together with an increased understanding of the pathophysiology of acute brain injury.

Prevention of secondary brain injury, and secondary brain insults, must be a priority. Several of these monitors will assist in this task. Further evaluation, research, and development will mean that some of these devices will enter routine clinical use within the next 10 years.

References

1. Chesnut RM, Marshall LF, Klauber MR et al. (1993) The role of secondary brain injury in determining outcome from severe head injury. J Trauma 34:216-222
2. Siesjo BK, Siesjo P (1996) Mechanisms of secondary brain injury. Eur J Anaesthes 13:247-268
3. Chesnut RM (1995) Secondary brain insults after head injury: clinical perspectives. New Horiz 3:366-375
4. Jones PA, Andrews PJ, Midgley S, et al (1994) Measuring the burden of secondary insults in head-injured patients during intensive care. J Neurosurg Anesthesiol 6:4-14
5. Andrews PJD, Piper IR, Dearden NM, et al (1990) Secondary insults during intrahospital transport of head-injured patients. Lancet 335:327-330
6. Recommendations for the transfer of patients with acute head injuries to neurosurgical units. (1996) The Neuroanaesthesia Society of Great Britain and Ireland and The Association of Anaesthetists of Great Britain and Ireland
7. Jeevaratnam DR, Menon DK (1996) Survey of intensive care of severely head injured patients in the United Kingdom. BMJ 312:944-947
8. Rossi S, Buzzi F, Paparella A, et al (1998) Complications and safety associated with ICP monitoring: a study of 542 patients. Acta Neurochir [Suppl] (Wien) 71:91-93
9. Rosner MJ, Daughton S (1990) Cerebral perfusion pressure management in head injury. J Trauma 30:933-941
10. Rosner MJ, Rosner SD, Johnson AH (1995) Cerebral perfusion pressure: management protocol and clinical results. J Neurosurg 83:949-962
11. Chan KH, Miller JD, Dearden NM, et al (1992) The effect of changes in cerebral perfusion pressure upon middle cerebral artery blood flow velocity and jugular bulb venous oxygen saturation after severe brain injury. J Neurosurg 77:55-61
12. Souter MJ, Andrews PJD (1996) Validation of the Edslab dual lumen oximetry catheter for continuous monitoring of jugular bulb oxygen saturation after severe head injury. Br J Anaesth 76:744-746
13. Cormio M, Valadka AB, Robertson CS (1999) Elevated jugular venous oxygen saturation after severe head injury. J Neurosurg 90:9-15
14. Sebel PS, Maynard DE, Major E, et al (1983) The cerebral function analysing monitor (CFAM). A new microprocessor- based device for the on-line analysis of the EEG and evoked potentials. Br J Anaesth 55:1265-1270
15. Maynard DE (1967) EEG analysis using an analogue frequency analyser and a digital computer. Electroencephalogr Clin Neurophysiol 23:487
16. Murdoch-Eaton D, Darowski M, Livingston J (2001) Cerebral function monitoring in paediatric intensive care: useful features for predicting outcome. Dev Med Child Neurol 43:91-96
17. Chan KH, Miller JD, Dearden NM (1992) Intracranial blood flow velocity after head injury: relationship to severity of injury, time, neurological status and outcome. J Neurol Neurosurg Psychiatry 55:787-791
18. Chan KH, Dearden NM, Miller JD, et al (1993) Multimodality monitoring as a guide to treatment of intracranial hypertension after severe brain injury. Neurosurgery 32:547-553
19. Fukuda O, Endo S, Kuwayama N, et al (1995) The characteristics of laser-Doppler flowmetry for the measurement of regional cerebral blood flow. Neurosurgery 36:358-364
20. Edwards AD (1994) The clinical role of near infrared spectroscopy. J Perinat Med 22:535-539
21. Kirkpatrick PJ, Smielewski P, Czosnyka M, et al (1995) Near-infrared spectroscopy use in patients with head injury. J Neurosurg 83:963-970
22. McKeating EG, Monjardino JR, Signorini DF, et al (1997) A comparison of the Invos 3100 and the Critikon 2020 near-infrared spectrophotometers as monitors of cerebral oxygenation. Anaesthesia 52:136-140
23. Kety SS (1972) Study of the cerebral circulation by means of inert diffusible tracers. Progr Brain Res 35:375-385

24. Bidabe AM, Gense dB, Gin AM, et al (1990) Measurement of cerebral blood flow by the stable xenon computerized tomography method. J Neuroradiol 17:103-124
25. Wyper DJ (1993) Functional neuroimaging with single photon emission computed tomography (SPECT). Cerebrovasc Brain Metab Rev 5:199-217
26. Herscovitch P (1993) Evaluation of the brain by positron emission tomography. Rheum Dis Clin North Am 19:765-794
27. Filippi R, Reisch R, Mauer D, et al (2000) Brain tissue pO2 related to SjvO2, ICP, and CPP in severe brain injury. Neurosurg Rev 23:94-97
28. Gupta AK, Hutchinson PJ, AlRawi P, et al (1999) Measuring brain tissue oxygenation compared with jugular venous oxygen saturation for monitoring cerebral oxygenation after traumatic brain injury. Anesth Analg 88:549-553
29. Piper I, Spiegelberg A, Whittle I, et al (1999) A comparative study of the Spiegelberg compliance device with a manual volume-injection method: a clinical evaluation in patients with hydrocephalus. Br J Neurosurg 13:581-586
30. Piper I, Dunn L, Contant C, et al (2000) Multi-centre assessment of the Spiegelberg compliance monitor: preliminary results. Acta Neurochir [Suppl] (Wien) 76:491-494
31. Mendelowitsch A (2001) Microdialysis: intraoperative and posttraumatic applications in neurosurgery. Methods 23:73-81
32. Hillered L, Persson L (1999) Neurochemical monitoring of the acutely injured human brain. Scand J Clin Lab Invest 59:9-18
33. Koura SS, Doppenberg EM, Marmarou A, et al (1998) Relationship between excitatory amino acid release and outcome after severe human head injury. Acta Neurochir [Suppl] (Wien) 71:244-246
34. Bullock R, Zauner A, Woodward JJ, et al (1998) Factors affecting excitatory amino acid release following severe human head injury. J Neurosurg 89:507-518
35. Berger C, Annecke A, Aschoff A, et al (1999) Neurochemical monitoring of fatal middle cerebral artery infarction. Stroke 30:460-463

Brain Protection

U.M. Illievich, A.-M. Machata, C.K. Spiss

The brain is critically dependent on a continuous supply of oxygen and glucose. Neuronal function depends almost exclusively on oxidative glucose metabolism and the brain has only limited stores of energy-generating substrates. Reduction of cerebral blood flow below a threshold required for maintaining the integrity compartment of the brain's metabolism results in cerebral ischaemia, the major cause of metabolic brain injury. Cerebral ischaemia can be global or focal, which differ in cause, pathophysiology, localization, and to a certain extent in treatment strategies. Decreased global cerebral blood flow below ischaemic thresholds due to hypotension or insufficient cardiac output usually compromises the entire brain. In animal models of global cerebral ischaemia damage is most likely to occur first in certain vulnerable regions including the pyramidal cells of the CA1 region of the hippocampus (limbic system), Purkinje cells (cerebellum), and layers 3, 5, and 6 of the cortex. This pattern of selective vulnerable neurons has also been observed in humans, and may account for the poor neurologic outcome of survivors of cardiac arrest [1].

In contrast to global ischaemia, the decrease of cerebral blood flow in focal ischaemia leads to a localized lesion that corresponds with the region of maximally reduced cerebral blood flow. Depending on the existence of collateral vessels and local perfusion pressure a penumbra region of still viable neurons surrounds the irreversible damaged neurons in the core. The ischaemic penumbra is characterized by minimal blood flow sufficient for maintenance of the integrity compartment of the brain's metabolism but reduced severely enough to abolish synaptic transmission. Depending on the severity and duration of ischaemia this area may not ultimately undergo infarction. Residual blood flow to the ischaemic area will vary with cerebral perfusion pressure, due to loss of autoregulation. Changes in systemic haemodynamics may influence the outcome from focal ischaemia by increasing or decreasing residual blood flow. Therefore, better outcome after focal cerebral ischaemia may be influenced by changes in haemodynamics. Prevention or amelioration of neuronal damage after global cerebral ischaemia as evidenced by abnormalities in cerebral metabolism, histopathology, or neurologic function is the ultimate measure for neuronal protective strategies. Successful neuronal protection implies improved outcome as evidenced by electro-physiologic, metabolic, histologic or clinical neurologic indices. Depending on the timing of interventions neuroprotection can be achieved as pretreatment (i.e., prevention), or treatment during and after (i.e., resuscitation) a neurologic injury.

Ischaemic cascade

The ischaemic-hypoxic insult triggers a cascade of pathophysiologic processes. Due to the diminished blood flow anaerobic glycolysis occurs, which results in accumulation of lactic acid. This leads to an increased membrane permeability causing cytotoxic cerebral oedema. Anaerobic metabolism is unable to maintain cellular energy stores over a long-period of time leading to adenosine-triphosphate depletion with consecutive failure of the membrane ion pumps. Consecutively terminal membrane depolarization takes place accompanied by excessive release of excitatory neurotransmitters. This results in activation of N-methyl-D-aspartate (NMDA), a-amino-3-hydroxy-5-methyl-4-isoxazolproprionate (AMPA), and voltage-dependant sodium and calcium channels. Intracellular calcium and sodium overload initiate catabolic processes like activation of proteases, phospholipases, and lipidperoxidases, which in turn increase the intracellular concentration of oxygen free radicals and free fatty acids. Parallel activation of caspases (interleukin converting enzyme-like proteins), endonucleases, and translocases triggers structural changes of biological membranes and nucleosomal DNA. All these events lead to membrane degeneration of vascular and cellular structures with the consequences of necrosis or apoptosis (programmed cell death) (Fig. 1).

All therapeutic strategies are aimed to prevent, interrupt or attenuate the above-explained pathophysiologic mechanisms.

Pharmacological therapy, anaesthetic agents

Inhalation anaesthetics

The volatile anaesthetics isoflurane, sevoflurane and desflurane reduce the functional compartment of cerebral metabolic rate in a dose-dependent manner, as evidenced by burst suppression in the electroencephalogram. Additionally they produce a vasodilatory-induced increase in cerebral blood flow (CBF),

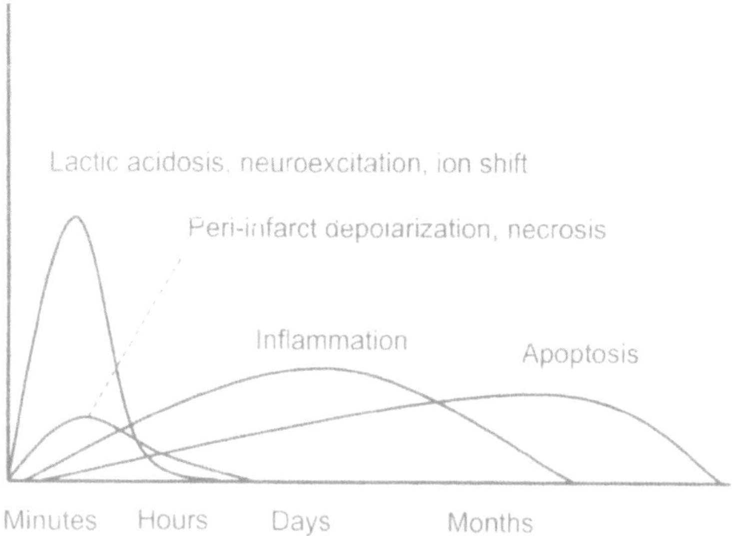

Fig.1. Time profile of an injurious event occuring in response to hypoxic or ischemic injury. Werner C (2000) Pathophysiology of neuronal death: pharmacological interventions. In: Christian K. Spiss(ed) Cerebral protection, resuscitation, and management. Problems in Anesthesia Vol 12 (4). Lippincott Williams & Wilkins, p 444.

resulting in an increase in CBF/CMR ratio. The effect of the reduction in CMR should independently exert a decrease in CBF. This response, however, is effectively blunted by the intrinsic vasodilatatory properties of volatile anaesthetics via nitric oxide related mechanisms. However, laboratory investigations have not been conclusive. In an animal model with focal ischaemia, pretreatment with isoflurane, sevoflurane and desflurane has decreased infarct size and improved neurologic outcome [2, 3]. In a clinical study the critical threshold inducing ischaemic EEG changes during carotid cross clamping was lower in patients anaesthetized with isoflurane compared to enflurane and halothane anaesthesia. The lower CBF tolerated during carotid endarterectomy suggests a greater margin of safety during isoflurane anaesthesia [4]. In contrast, volatile anaesthetics have no neuroprotective properties in the setting of global cerebral ischaemia and when given after the insult. This could be due to the effect, that in those situations CBF is adequate to meet metabolic demand.

In contrast to barbiturates a relatively rapid emergence is possible, thus allowing early neurologic assessment after deep inhalation anaesthesia.

Barbiturates

Barbiturates (oxybarbiturates, e.g., metohexital; thiobarbiturates e.g., thiopental) are some of the most thoroughly investigated drugs with neuroprotective properties, and serve as prototype for anaesthetic protection against ischaemia induced neuronal injury. Besides the well-known reduction of the functional compartment of cerebral metabolic rate, several mechanisms of barbiturate protection have been proposed. These mechanisms include reduction of intracranial pressure, redistribution of cerebral blood flow, suppression of seizures, membrane stabilization, blocking of calcium channels, free radical scavenging, attenuation of free fatty acid accumulation, and loss of thermoregulation.

There is considerable experimental evidence in laboratory animals that barbiturates provide protection from neurologic injury after focal cerebral ischaemia caused by permanent vessel occlusion in stroke models. Fewer experimental studies report an efficacy of barbiturate protection against temporary focal ischaemia. These temporary focal ischaemia models suggest neuronal protection after temporary cerebral vessel clipping which is necessary during carotid endarterectomy and often during aneurysm surgery [5, 6]. The low incidence of morbidity and mortality during cerebral vascular surgery and the multitude of variables (e.g., dose, type of barbiturate, timing, duration, type of vessel occlusion, seizures) possibly influencing clinical outcome during these procedures could contribute to the fact that there are only few clinical studies describing the protective effect [7]. There are no confirmed studies demonstrating neuronal protection by barbiturate administration during or after global cerebral ischaemia. Therefore, the use of barbiturates to ameliorate hypoxic/ischaemic brain damage after cardiac arrest cannot be recommended [8].

Etomidate

Etomidate, a non-barbiturate imidazol derivative, has the advantage of a shorter half-life and produces less cardiovascular depression compared to barbiturates. Similar to barbiturates it produces a dose-related decrease in neuronal function and cerebral metabolic rate. Etomidate is also a direct cerebral vasoconstrictor with the ability to decrease cerebral blood flow and intracranial pressure. Proposed mechanisms of brain protection include decrease of cerebral metabolic rate, reduction of intracranial blood volume and intracranial pressure, and inhibition of free fatty-acid liberation [9]. However, etomidate suppresses the adrenocortical function by affecting the synthesis of cortisol, corticosterone, aldosterone, and 17-alpha-hydroxy-progesterone [10]. This side effect restricts the long term and high-dose application of etomidate.

Propofol

A major disadvantage of high dose barbiturate application is the long half-life, which prolongs postoperative intensive care treatment and impairs neurological assessment. The pharmacokinetic properties of propofol (2, 6 diisopropylphenol) make this drug suitable for both the induction and maintenance of anaesthesia. Human studies have shown that propofol reduces cerebral blood flow and cerebral metabolic rate of oxygen. Even after high doses of propofol early postoperative neurological assessment seems to be possible. High dose propofol causes a maximum reduction of electric cerebral activity, cerebral metabolism and cerebral blood flow, whereas CO_2 reactivity is preserved. Furthermore, high dose propofol application may have cerebroprotective effects, although this possibility remains controversial [11, 12]. Propofol was unable to reduce neurophysiologic deficits after cardiac valve surgery compared with sufentanil [13]. However it significantly reduced increased intracranial pressure (ICP), but neurological outcome did not benefit after head trauma [14].

Ketamine

The dissociative anaesthetic ketamine hydrochloride is a non-competitive N-methyl-D-aspartate (NMDA) antagonist. In an animal model of global cerebral ischaemia pre-treatment with anaesthetic doses of ketamine improved both behavioural and histopathological grading of ischaemic neuronal injury [15]. Decreased plasma catecholamine activity is another mechanism proposed for neuronal protection by ketamine indicated by improved neurologic outcome from incomplete cerebral ischaemia and head injury [16]. However, the increase in cerebral blood flow and intracranial pressure reported in both, normal subjects and patients with intracranial pathology [17] might compromise cerebral perfusion.

Pharmacological therapy, non-anaesthetic agents

Glucose

Numerous studies in a variety of species have demonstrated a detrimental effect of pre-existing hyperglycemia on neurologic injury following episodes of global cerebral ischaemia. Even modest elevations in blood glucose levels markedly worsen neurologic outcome [18] and increase both, the mortality and morbidity, following transient global cerebral ischaemia after cardiac arrest and resuscitation in animals. The adverse effect of increased blood glucose concentration has been demonstrated not only for cerebral ischaemia, but also for neurologic outcome after spinal cord ischaemia [19]. While hyperglycemia in models of global cerebral ischaemia is consistently associated with a worsening of the neurologic injury, the effect of hyperglycemia on neurologic outcome after focal cerebral ischaemia remains unclear. It has been associated with either an increase [20] or decrease [21] in infarct size; however, morbidity and mortality are increased, when hyperglycemia is present after stroke [22]. The mechanism by which glucose affects neuronal injury is not well defined. It is speculated that increased intracellular lactic acidosis and membrane permeability with increased oedema of neurons, neuroglia and endothelial cells may worsen injury.

NMDA-receptor antagonists, excitatory amino acid antagonists

Pharmacological reduction of excitatory amino acid neurotoxicity can be achieved by antagonizing the action of these neurotransmitters on the receptor operated calcium channel. One of the channels allowing a high percentage of Ca2+ influx is the NMDA (N-methyl-D-aspartate) receptor. *Competitive* blockade of this receptor is not only difficult because of the ischaemia induced excitatory neurotransmitter increase, but also because of the poor blood-brain barrier penetration of these usually highly polar compounds. *Non-competitive* antagonists (e.g., ketamine, dextrorphan, dizozilpine) bind to different sites on the receptor or within the receptor channel. They easily cross the blood-brain barrier because of their lipid solubility. However, they have major side effects including impairment of learning, adverse behavioural and psychomimetic properties. Furthermore, it has been suggested that the observed neuroprotection may be the result of coincidental drug-induced hypothermia [16]. Finally, glycine antagonists [23] and drugs inhibiting glutamate release during ischaemia are also being investigated [24].

Calcium entry blocker

Magnesium

Magnesium serves as a cofactor of many enzyme systems and is a physiologic calcium channel blocker. A specific Mg2+ binding site is located within the receptor operated calcium channels. Besides a decrease of the channel opening frequency, Mg2+ induces a voltage dependent block of the activated NMDA receptor associated calcium channel. Mg2+ also blocks the L- and N-type of the voltage sensitive calcium channels, which are major pathways of voltage-gated cellular Ca2+ entry (L-type) and play an important role in the physiological regulation (N-type) of neurotransmitter release. However, besides promising results *in vitro* and *in vivo*, we must consider the poor blood-brain barrier penetration of Mg2+ and less enthusiastic studies reporting worsening of neurologic outcome after pre-ischaemic Mg2+ application [25].

Flunarizine, lidoflacine

Neuroprotective properties of flunarizine and lidoflacine have been investigated in models of global cerebral ischaemia. Proposed mechanisms of cerebroprotection include improvement of post-ischaemic hypoperfusion and Ca2+ entry blockade with prevention of Ca2+ mediated cell death. However, studies performed on these compounds are contradictory [26, 27]. Furthermore flunarizine may cause severe pulmonary oedema. Therefore, the clinical usefulness of these drugs is questionable.

Nimodipine

Nimodipine, a dehydropyridine-type Ca2+ channel blocker, has a highly selective effect on cerebral blood vessels improving cerebral blood flow in models of global and focal ischaemia [28]. Nimodipine is lipophilic with a large distribution volume in the brain, and dilates cerebral vessels at lower concentrations than required for dilatation of peripheral blood vessels. Therefore, nimodipine improves cerebral blood flow at doses not reducing systemic arterial pressure. Beside its well-known effects on the smooth muscles of cerebral blood vessels nimodipine also affects neuronal tissue directly. Nimodipine blocks the L-type of voltage sensitive Ca2+ channels, a binding site represented especially in selectively vulnerable regions of the brain. A neuroprotective effect of nimodipine could be independent of its vasodilating effect by reducing the Ca2+ entry during both the ischaemic and reperfusion periods, or by intracellular Ca2+ antagonism.

Nimodipine has been studied in patients after cardiac arrest and patients with acute stroke. A meta-analysis of nine placebo-controlled trials with acute stroke (3 700 patients) concluded that nimodipine administration appears to be associated with a favourable outcome, if treatment is initiated within the first twelve hours after the onset of the symptoms [29]. However, the most important indication for nimodipine is the treatment of vasospasm after subarachnoid haemorrhage. Although nimodipine has no effect on the severity of vasospasm when determined with cerebral angiography [30], nimodipine treatment of patients with mild or moderate symptoms after subarachnoid haemorrhage results in lower incidence of delayed ischaemic deficits or death, and a better neurologic outcome [31]. This could be confirmed by a meta-analysis of eight placebo-controlled studies with 1 200 patients [32]. Early enthusiasm for nimodipine efficacy in the treatment of traumatic brain injury has diminished [33]. However, the efficacy of nimodipine in severely head-injured patients with traumatic subarachnoid haemorrhage is still under investigation and early treatment of patients with mild or moderate symptoms after subarachnoid haemorrhage caused by aneurysm rupture is recommended [33].

Nicardipine

Nicardipine, another dehydropyridine derivative with cerebral vascular muscle relaxant and neuronal protective properties similar to nimodipine, ameliorates angiographic signs of vasospasm after aneurysmal subarachnoid haemorrhage. However compared to standard management ("triple H therapy"), no improvement in overall outcome was demonstrated. Hypertensive, hypervolemic haemodilution (triple H therapy) is an effective regimen in the prevention of neurologic deficits caused by cerebral vasospasm [34]. Therefore, nicardipine compared with triple H therapy suggests at least similar effectiveness of both regimens.

Free radical scavengers, antioxidants, and inhibitors of lipid peroxidation

Corticosteroids

One important mechanism of neuroprotection by glucocorticoids is the reduction of vasogenic cerebral oedema associated with brain tumors. Additionally, a large clinical trial indicated that methylprednisolone reduces spinal cord injury when administered within eight hours after a trauma (30 mg/kg bodyweight as bolus, 5.4 mg/kg for 48 hours) [35]. Suggested beneficial mechanisms of glucocorticoids include scavenging of free radicals, stabilization of lipid bilayers, and prevention of free fatty acid accumulation by inhibition of lipid peroxydation, reduction of CSF production and increasing the seizure threshold. However, high-dose steroid application in the management of severe head trauma failed to improve intracranial hypertension and neurologic outcome [36]. A recent meta-analysis revealed moderate beneficial and moderate harmful effects in patients with head injury [37]. Furthermore, steroids have numerous side effects, among which are hyperglycemia, gastrointestinal bleeding and immune-suppression. As already mentioned, hyperglycemia can worsen neurologic injury after ischaemia, therefore special attention must focus on blood glucose concentrations in cerebral injured patients treated with steroids.

Lazaroids (21-aminosteroids)

Twenty-one-Aminosteroids lack glucocorticoid activity, but are more effective in (*in vitro*) inhibition of iron-catalyzed lipid peroxidation than glucocorticoid steroids. The antioxidant mechanisms of neuroprotection include scavenging lipid peroxyl and hydroxyl radicals, and stabilizing cellular membranes. Neuroprotective effects are demonstrated in experimental models of traumatic brain injury, but could not be confirmed in head injured patients [38]. More clinically favorable seems to be the use of 21-aminosteroids in patients with subarachnoid haemorrhage [39].

Vitamin E

α-Tocopherol is an important membrane-bound endogenous free radical scavenger acting predominantly as a hydrogen donor under formation of a lower reactive α-tocopherol radical which may be reconverted to α-tocopherol by ascorbic acid. α-Tocopherol, decreases lipid peroxidation, neuronal necrosis, and reactive gliosis *in vitro.* When administered prior to injury, α-tocopherol also exerts neuroprotective properties in experimental models of cerebral ischaemia [40], subarachnoid haemorrhage [41], and traumatic brain injury [42].

Superoxide dismutase, catalase

Superoxide dismutase and catalase are endogenous compounds which enzymatically scavenge superoxide and hydrogen peroxide, respectively. Superoxide dismutase enzymatically converts superoxide radicals to hydrogen peroxide, which in turn is catalyzed to water and oxygen. Conjugation of the enzymes to polyethylene glycol prolongs the circulatory half-life of the native enzymes and enhances their intracellular access. Furthermore, pre-ischaemic application of these compounds reduces infarct volume in focal ischaemia [43].

Mannitol

Mannitol, a 6-carbon sugar, is used as an adjunctive therapy in brain protection primarily by reducing cerebral oedema and/or intracranial pressure. Besides an increase in serum osmolality, mannitol leads to a decrease in blood viscosity, an increase in cerebral blood flow, and may play a role as a free radical scavenger. In a model of transient focal and forebrain ischaemia repetitive administration of mannitol *after* the ischaemic insult significantly reduced the extent of delayed neuronal injury in the neocortex through its action as an osmotic agent in reducing cerebral oedema [44].

Non-pharmacological therapy

Hypothermia and neuronal protection (experimental)

During deep hypothermia, the main neuroprotective mechanism is the decrease in cerebral energy consumption. For mild and moderate hypothermia alternative mechanisms are proposed [45]. Indeed, relatively small variations in brain temperature affect multiple cellular processes in the brain, and may account for the dramatic effects of temperature variations in numerous animal models of brain injury. Mild hypothermia ameliorates, and mild hypothermia worsens ischaemia-induced neuronal injury [46]. Mild and moderate hypothermia inhibits the ischaemia induced excitatory neurotransmitter increase [47], suggesting this effect as one mechanism of neuronal protection [48]. Other mechanisms involved are the effects on ion membrane permeability [49], recovery of post-ischaemic protein synthesis [50], prevention of the ischaemia-induced translocation and subsequent downregulation of protein kinase C [51], reduction of lipid peroxidation products and inhibition of free radical scavenger consumption [52], inhibition of apoptosis [53], and reduction of blood-brain barrier disruption [54].

Neuronal protection (clinical)

a. Head injury

Four controlled randomized clinical studies on the use of therapeutic moderate hypothermia for severe closed head injuries have been published [55-59]. Hypothermia significantly reduced ICP and CBF, and neither parameter showed a significant rebound after patients were rewarmed. The authors concluded, that therapeutic hypothermia (32°C) after severe closed head injury appeared to indicate a good patient tolerance as well as improvement in ICP, cerebral oxygen supply/demand, and outcome. The significantly better GOS in one of the latest publications [57] was challenged by an editorial in the Journal of Neurosurgical Anesthesiology [60], criticizing the statistical analysis and the methodology (less severe CT class in the hypothermia group, hyperthermia up to 38.5°C was allowed in the control group). The North American multicenter trial, sponsored by the National Institute of Health was terminated in May 1998. In this study Clifton et al. enrolled 392 comatose patients (GCS 3 to 8) with closed head injuries. Patients were randomly assigned to treatment with hypothermia (bladder temperature, 33°C), which was initiated within 6 hours after injury and was maintained for 48 hours by means of surface cooling, or normothermia. Poor outcome (defined as severe disability, a vegetative state, or death) was assessed in 57% of the patients in both groups. A mortality rate of 28% was similar in both groups (hypothermia vs. 27% normothermia group, $p=0.79$). However, patients in the hypothermia group had more hospital days with complications than the patients in the normothermia group. Fewer patients in the hypothermia group had high intracranial pressure than in the normothermia group. The authors concluded that treatment with hypothermia, with the body temperature reaching 33°C within eight hours after injury, is not effective in improving outcomes in patients with severe brain injury [59]. However, there were differences in the pattern of body temperature between the subgroups with hypothermia or with normothermia on admission. Among the patients who had hypothermia on admission and were treated with hypothermia, 61% had poor outcomes, as compared with 78% of those with hypothermia on admission who were in the normothermia group. Furthermore, in contrast to European practice of intensive care in head injured patients both groups received sedation with morphine requiring non-depolarizing neuromuscular blockade for treatment of shivering and facilitation of artificial ventilation, respectively.

b. Aneurysm surgery

A survey conducted in 1994 indicates that a large majority of neuroanaesthesiologists use intraoperative mild to moderate hypothermia [61]. Preliminary results about the use of mild hypothermia in aneurysm clipping surgery are encouraging [62] and the American National Institute of Health (NIH) funds a multicenter trial – the "Intraoperative hypothermia for aneurysm surgery trial 2 (IHAST 2)" which started in 2000.

c. Cardiac arrest

The efficacy of hypothermia in preserving neurological function before and during certain no-flow cardiovascular states has been well documented, both clinically and experimentally. Recent clinical investigations regarding the effect of moderate hypothermia induced in the emergency department on patients with anoxic brain injury following out-of-hospital cardiac arrest revealed a significant decrease in the morbidity and mortality in hypothermic patients compared to the normothermic control group [63, 64]. A European multicenter trial on hypothermia and cardiac arrest finished recently after enrolment of 500 patients and the final results are in publication.

Induced hypertension

A precise regulatory system guarantees adequate cerebral blood flow under various conditions. Autoregulation is the response of cerebral blood vessels to the changes in systemic blood pressure independent of flow-to-metabolism coupling. Therefore, induced hypertension may only be effective in situations where autoregulation is not fully intact or mean arterial blood pressure exceeds the range of autoregulation. Besides the use of induced hypertension outside the operating room as an element of the triple H regimen [34], it is used in the operating room to improve collateral blood flow during periods of cerebral vessel occlusion in cerebral aneurysm or cerebral arteriovenous malformation surgery, and during carotid endartectomy. Furthermore autoregulation is impaired in areas of ischaemia, therefore an increase in mean arterial blood pressure increases cerebral perfusion pressure and improves cerebral blood flow. The clinical usefulness of induced hypertension may be limited by risk of cerebral haemorrhage and myocardial infarction.

Hypervolemia and haemodilution

Hypervolemia and haemodilution in combination with hypertension is widely accepted as a therapy and prevention of ischaemic neurologic deficits by cerebral vasospasm [65]. The rationale behind this therapy is based on the impaired autoregulation in ischaemic areas. In these areas cerebral blood flow depends on cerebral perfusion pressure, which in turn is determined by mean arterial blood pressure and intravascular volume. Furthermore, lowering haematocrit by haemodilution results in a decreased blood viscosity. The resulting increase in cerebral blood flow outweighs to a certain extent the decrease in oxygen transport capacity. In a canine model of permanent focal cerebral ischaemia haemodilution to a target haematocrit of 30% reduced infarct volume significantly [66]. Hypervolemic haemodilution may be achieved with crystalloid or colloids and is limited by cardiopulmonary side effects. However, if appropriate monitoring is applied, hypervolemic haemodilution is probably more efficacious than isovolemic haemodilution in improving cerebral blood flow [67, 68].

References

1. Collins RC, Dobkin BH, Choi DW (1989) Selective vulnerability of the brain: new insights into the pathophysiology of stroke. Ann Intern Med 110:992-1000
2. Werner C, Möllenberg O, Kochs E, Schulte am Esch J (1995) Sevoflurane improves neurological outcome after incomplete cerebral ischaemia in rats. Br J Anaesth 75:756-760
3. Engelhard K, Werner C, Reeker W, Lu H, Mollenberg O, Mielke L, Kochs E (1999) Desflurane and isoflurane improve neurological outcome after incomplete cerebral ischaemia in rats. Br J Anaesth 83:415-421
4. Warner DS (1989) Volatile anesthetics and the ischemic brain. Journal of Neurosurgical Anesthesiology 1:290-294
5. Spetzler RF, Martin N, Hadley MN, Thompson RA, Wilkinson E, Raudzens PA (1986) Microsurgical endarterectomy under barbiturate protection: a prospective study. J Neurosurg 65:63-73
6. Belopavlovic M, Buchthal A (1980) Barbiturate therapy in the management of cerebral ischaemia. Anaesthesia 35:271-278
7. Nussmeier NA, Arlund C, Slogoff S (1986) Neuropsychiatric complications after cardiopulmonary bypass: cerebral protection by a barbiturate. Anesthesiology 64:165-170
8. Brain Resuscitation Clinical Trial I Study Group (1986): Randomized clinical study of thiopental loading in comatose survivors of cardiac arrest. N Engl J Med 314:397-403
9. Milde LN, Milde JH, Michenfelder JD (1985) Cerebral functional, metabolic, and hemodynamic effects of etomidate in dogs. Anesthesiology 63:371-377
10. Wagner RL, White PF, Kan PB, Rosenthal MH, Feldman D (1984) Inhibition of adrenal steroidogenesis by the anesthetic etomidate. N Engl J Med 310:1415-1421
11. Ridenour TR, Warner DS, Todd MM, Gionet TX (1992) Comparative effects of propofol and halothane on outcome from temporary middle cerebral artery occlusion in the rat. Anesthesiology 76:807-812
12. Kochs E, Hoffman WE, Werner C, Thomas C, Albrecht RF, Schulte am Esch J (1992) The effects of propofol on brain electrical activity, neurologic outcome, and neuronal damage following incomplete ischemia in rats. Anesthesiology 76:245-252
13. Roach GW, Newman MF, Murkin JM, Martzke J, Ruskin A, Li J, Guo A, Wisniewski A, Mangano DT (1999) Ineffectiveness of burst suppression therapy in mitigating perioperative cerebrovascular dysfunction. Multicenter Study of Perioperative Ischemia (McSPI) Research Group. Anesthesiology 90:1255-1264
14. Kelly DF, Goodale DB, Williams J, Herr DL, Chappell ET, Rosner MJ, Jacobson J, Levy ML, Croce MA, Maniker AH, Fulda GJ, Lovett JV, Mohan O, Narayan RK (1999) Propofol in the treatment of moderate and severe head injury: a randomized, prospective double-blinded pilot trial. J Neurosurg 90:1042-1052
15. Marcoux FW, Goodrich JE, Dominick MA (1988) Ketamine prevents ischemic neuronal injury. Brain Res 452:329-335
16. Hoffman WE, Pelligrino D, Werner C, Kochs E, Albrecht RF, Schulte am Esch J (1992) Ketamine decreases plasma catecholamines and improves outcome from incomplete cerebral ischemia in rats. Anesthesiology 76:755-762
17. Wyte SR, Shapiro HM, Turner P, Harris AB (1972) Ketamine-induced intracranial hypertension. Anesthesiology 36:174-176

18. Lanier WL, Stangland KJ, Scheithauer BW, Milde JH, Michenfelder JD (1987) The effects of dextrose infusion and head position on neurologic outcome after complete cerebral ischemia in primates: examination of a model. Anesthesiology 66:39-48
19. Drummond JC, Moore SS (1989) The influence of dextrose administration on neurologic outcome after temporary spinal cord ischemia in the rabbit. Anesthesiology 70:64-70
20. de Courten-Myers G, Myers RE, Schoolfield L (1988) Hyperglycemia enlarges infarct size in cerebrovascular occlusion in cats. Stroke 19:623-630
21. Zasslow MA, Pearl RG, Shuer LM, Steinberg GK, Lieberson RE, Larson CP, Jr. (1989) Hyperglycemia decreases acute neuronal ischemic changes after middle cerebral artery occlusion in cats. Stroke 20:519-523
22. Woo J, Lam CW, Kay R, Wong AH, Teoh R, Nicholls MG (1990) The influence of hyperglycemia and diabetes mellitus on immediate and 3- month morbidity and mortality after acute stroke. Arch Neurol 47:1174-1177
23. Wood ER, Bussey TJ, Phillips AG (1993) A glycine antagonist 7-chlorokynurenic acid attenuates ischemia-induced learning deficits. Neuroreport 4:151-154
24. Bacher A, Zornow MH (1997) Lamotrigine inhibits extracellular glutamate accumulation during transient global cerebral ischemia in rabbits. Anesthesiology 86:459-463
25. Blair JL, Warner DS, Todd MM (1989) Effects of elevated plasma magnesium versus calcium on cerebral ischemic injury in rats. Stroke 20:507-512
26. Newberg LA, Steen PA, Milde JH, Michenfelder JD (1984) Failure of flunarizine to improve cerebral blood flow or neurologic recovery in a canine model of complete cerebral ischemia. Stroke 15:666-671
27. Vaagenes P, Cantadore R, Safar P, Moossy J, Rao G, Diven W, Alexander H, Stezoski W (1984) Amelioration of brain damage by lidoflazine after prolonged ventricular fibrillation cardiac arrest in dogs. Crit Care Med 12:846-855
28. Milde LN, Milde JH, Michenfelder JD (1986) Delayed treatment with nimodipine improves cerebral blood flow after complete cerebral ischemia in the dog. J Cereb Blood Flow Metab 6:332-337
29. Paci A, Ottaviano P, Trenta A, Iannone G, De Santis L, Lancia G, Moschini E, Carosi M, Amigoni S, Caresia L (1989) Nimodipine in acute ischemic stroke: a double-blind controlled study. Acta Neurol Scand 80:282-286
30. Zabramski J, Spetzler RF, Bonstelle C (1986) Chronic cerebral vasospasm: effect of calcium antagonists. Neurosurgery 18:129-135
31. Robinson MJ, Teasdale GM (1990) Calcium antagonists in the management of subarachnoid haemorrhage. Cerebrovasc Brain Metab Rev 2:205-226
32. Barker FG, 2nd, Ogilvy CS (1996) Efficacy of prophylactic nimodipine for delayed ischemic deficit after subarachnoid hemorrhage: a metaanalysis. J Neurosurg 84:405-414
33. The European Study Group on Nimodipine in Severe Head Injury (1994) A multicenter trial of the efficacy of nimodipine on outcome after severe head injury. J Neurosurg 80:797-804
34. Awad IA, Carter LP, Spetzler RF, Medina M, Williams FC, Jr. (1987) Clinical vasospasm after subarachnoid hemorrhage: response to hypervolemic hemodilution and arterial hypertension. Stroke 18:365-372
35. Bracken MB, Shepard MJ, Collins WF, Holford TR, Young W, Baskin DS, Eisenberg HM, Flamm E, Leo-Summers L, Maroon J et al (1990) A randomized, controlled trial of methylprednisolone or naloxone in the treatment of acute spinal-cord injury. Results of the Second National Acute Spinal Cord Injury Study. N Engl J Med 322:1405-1411
36. Saul TG, Ducker TB, Salcman M, Carro E (1981) Steroids in severe head injury: A prospective randomized clinical trial. J Neurosurg 54:596-600
37. Alderson P, Roberts I (1997) Corticosteroids in acute traumatic brain injury: systematic review of randomized controlled trials. BMJ 314:1855-1859
38. Marshall LF, Maas AI, Marshall SB, Bricolo A, Fearnside M, Iannotti F, Klauber MR, Lagarrigue J, Lobato R, Persson L, Pickard JD, Piek J, Servadei F, Wellis GN, Morris GF, Means ED, Musch

B (1998) A multicenter trial on the efficacy of using tirilazad mesylate in cases of head injury. J Neurosurg 89:519-525
39. Kassell NF, Haley EC, Jr., Apperson-Hansen C, Alves WM (1996) Randomized, double-blind, vehicle-controlled trial of tirilazad mesylate in patients with aneurysmal subarachnoid hemorrhage: a cooperative study in Europe, Australia, and New Zealand. J Neurosurg 84:221-228
40. Yamamoto M, Shima T, Uozumi T, Sogabe T, Yamada K, Kawasaki T (1983) A possible role of lipid peroxidation in cellular damages caused by cerebral ischemia and the protective effect of alpha-tocopherol administration. Stroke 14:977-982
41. Sakaki S, Ohta S, Nakamura H, Takeda S (1988) Free radical reaction and biological defense mechanism in the pathogenesis of prolonged vasospasm in experimental subarachnoid hemorrhage. J Cereb Blood Flow Metab 8:1-8
42. Clifton GL, Lyeth BG, Jenkins LW, Taft WC, DeLorenzo RJ, Hayes RL (1989) Effect of D-alpha-tocopheryl succinate and polyethylene glycol on performance tests after fluid percussion brain injury. J Neurotrauma 6:71-81
43. Liu TH, Beckman JS, Freeman BA, Hogan EL, Hsu CY (1989) Polyethylene glycol-conjugated superoxide dismutase and catalase reduce ischemic brain injury. Am J Physiol 256:H589-593
44. Luvisotto TL, Auer RN, Sutherland GR (1996) The effect of mannitol on experimental cerebral ischemia, revisited. Neurosurgery 38:131-138; discussion 139
45. Michenfelder JD, Theye RA (1970) The effects of anesthesia and hypothermia on canine cerebral ATP and lactate during anoxia produced by decapitation. Anesthesiology 33:430-439
46. Minamisawa H, Nordstrom CH, Smith ML, Siesjo BK (1990) The influence of mild body and brain hypothermia on ischemic brain damage. J Cereb Blood Flow Metab 10:365-374
47. Busto R, Globus MY, Dietrich WD, Martinez E, Valdes I, Ginsberg MD (1989) Effect of mild hypothermia on ischemia-induced release of neurotransmitters and free fatty acids in rat brain. Stroke 20:904-910
48. Illievich UM, Zornow MH, Choi KT, Scheller MS, Strnat MA (1994) Effects of hypothermic metabolic suppression on hippocampal glutamate concentrations after transient global cerebral ischemia. Anesth Analg 78:905-911
49. Katsura K, Minamisawa H, Ekholm A, Folbergrova J, Siesjo BK (1992) Changes of labile metabolites during anoxia in moderately hypo- and hyperthermic rats: correlation to membrane fluxes of K+. Brain Res 590:6-12
50. Widmann R, Miyazawa T, Hossmann KA (1993) Protective effect of hypothermia on hippocampal injury after 30 minutes of forebrain ischemia in rats is mediated by postischemic recovery of protein synthesis. J Neurochem 61:200-209
51. Cardell M, Boris-Moller F, Wieloch T (1991) Hypothermia prevents the ischemia-induced translocation and inhibition of protein kinase C in the rat striatum. J Neurochem 57:1814-1817.
52. Lei B, Tan X, Cai H, Xu Q, Guo Q (1994) Effect of moderate hypothermia on lipid peroxidation in canine brain tissue after cardiac arrest and resuscitation. Stroke 25:147-152
53. Edwards AD, Yue X, Squier MV, Thoresen M, Cady EB, Penrice J, Cooper CE, Wyatt JS, Reynolds EO, Mehmet H (1995) Specific inhibition of apoptosis after cerebral hypoxia-ischaemia by moderate post-insult hypothermia. Biochem Biophys Res Commun 217:1193-1199
54. Jiang JY, Lyeth BG, Kapasi MZ, Jenkins LW, Povlishock JT (1992) Moderate hypothermia reduces blood-brain barrier disruption following traumatic brain injury in the rat. Acta Neuropathol 84:495-500
55. Shiozaki T, Sugimoto H, Taneda M, Yoshida H, Iwai A, Yoshioka T, Sugimoto T (1993) Effect of mild hypothermia on uncontrollable intracranial hypertension after severe head injury. J Neurosurg 79:363-368
56. Marion DW, Obrist WD, Carlier PM, Penrod LE, Darby JM (1993) The use of moderate therapeutic hypothermia for patients with severe head injuries: a preliminary report. J Neurosurg 79:354-362
57. Marion DW, Penrod LE, Kelsey SF, Obrist WD, Kochanek PM, Palmer AM, Wisniewski SR,

DeKosky ST (1997) Treatment of traumatic brain injury with moderate hypothermia. N Engl J Med 336:540-546

58. Clifton GL, Allen S, Barrodale P, Plenger P, Berry J, Koch S, Fletcher J, Hayes RL, Choi SC (1993) A phase II study of moderate hypothermia in severe brain injury. J Neurotrauma 10:263-271
59. Clifton GL, Miller ER, Choi SC, Levin HS, McCauley S, Smith KR, Jr., Muizelaar JP, Wagner FC, Jr., Marion DW, Luerssen TG, Chesnut RM, Schwartz M (2001) Lack of effect of induction of hypothermia after acute brain injury. N Engl J Med 344:556-563
60. Hartung J, Cottrell JE (1998) Statistics and hypothermia. J Neurosurg Anesthesiol 10:1-4
61. Craen RA, Gelb AW, Eliasziw M, Lok P (1994) Current anesthetic practices and use of brain protective therapies for cerebral aneurysm surgery at 41 North American Centers. J Neurosurg Anesthesiol 6:303
62. Hindman BJ, Todd MM, Gelb AW, Loftus CM, Craen RA, Schubert A, Mahla ME, Torner JC (1999) Mild hypothermia as a protective therapy during intracranial aneurysm surgery: a randomized prospective pilot trial. Neurosurgery 44:23-32
63. Bernard SA, Jones BM, Horne MK (1997) Clinical trial of induced hypothermia in comatose survivors of out-of- hospital cardiac arrest. Ann Emerg Med 30:146-153
64. Holzer M, Behringer W, Schorkhuber W, Zeiner A, Sterz F, Laggner AN, Frass M, Siostrozonek P, Ratheiser K, Kaff A (1997) Mild hypothermia and outcome after CPR. Hypothermia for Cardiac Arrest (HACA) Study Group. Acta Anaesthesiol Scand Suppl 111:55-58
65. McGrath BJ, Guy J, Borel CO, Friedman AH, Warner DS (1995) Perioperative management of aneurysmal subarachnoid hemorrhage: Part 2. Postoperative management. Anesth Analg 81:1295-1302
66. Lee SH, Heros RC, Mullan JC, Korosue K (1994) Optimum degree of hemodilution for brain protection in a canine model of focal cerebral ischemia. J Neurosurg 80:469-475
67. Tu YK, Heros RC, Candia G, Hyodo A, Lagree K, Callahan R, Zervas NT, Karacostas D (1988) Isovolemic hemodilution in experimental focal cerebral ischemia. Part 1: Effects on hemodynamics, hemorheology, and intracranial pressure. J Neurosurg 69:72-81
68. Tu YK, Heros RC, Karacostas D, Liszczak T, Hyodo A, Candia G, Zervas NT, Lagree K (1988) Isovolemic hemodilution in experimental focal cerebral ischemia. Part 2: Effects on regional cerebral blood flow and size of infarction. J Neurosurg 69:82-91

Respiratory Effects of Anesthesia

P.R.M. Rocco, W.A. Zin

Anesthesia affects respiration, changing arterial oxygenation in either spontaneous or controlled breathing patients [1-5]. In addition, these respiratory effects are more severe in the elderly [6, 7], the obese [8], and smokers [9]. Anesthesia causes ventilation-perfusion relationship changes, mainly shunt, that correlate closely with the degree of atelectasis [6,10-11]. Furthermore, anesthesia changes respiratory system ventilation, muscle function, and respiratory mechanics. This chapter presents a brief overview of respiratory effects of anesthesia, detailing the changes in ventilation, functional residual capacity (FRC), respiratory mechanics, and pulmonary gas exchange.

Ventilation

Spontaneous ventilation is usually reduced during anesthesia [12]. However, the effect of a given anesthetic on respiratory function depends on the depth of general anesthesia. When the depth of anesthesia is inadequate [less than one minimum alveolar concentration (MAC)], the respiratory pattern may vary from excessive hyperventilation and vocalization to breath-holding. When anesthesia is light (equals one MAC) the irregular respiration progresses to a more regular pattern, which is associated with a larger than normal tidal volume. As anesthesia deepens to moderate levels, respiration becomes faster and more regular but shallower. During deep anesthesia increasing depression of respiration is manifested by even more rapid, shallow breathing. With very deep anesthesia, respiration is jerky or gasping in character and irregular in pattern. This situation results from loss of active intercostal muscle contribution to inspiration [13].

Tidal volume

Tidal volume is reduced during general anesthesia because of: (1) increased airway resistance, (2) decreased lung compliance, and (3) the patients may be less willing to breathe spontaneously during general anesthesia (decreased chemical control of breathing). In addition, a decreased tidal volume may cause hypoxemia because: (1) shallow breathing may promote atelectasis and cause a decrease in FRC [14] and (2) decreased ventilation diminishes the overall ventilation-perfusion relationship of the lung, which decreases paO_2, mainly during moderate to deep levels of anesthesia (in which the chemical control of breathing is significantly altered).

In general, all volatile anesthetics decrease tidal volume. However, the resultant depression of minute ventilation may be partially offset by a concomitant increase in respiratory rate. Early studies demonstrated that isoflurane produced more-profound respiratory depression than did halothane. In contrast to halothane, isoflurane did not progressively increase respiratory frequency. Enflurane, like halothane, dose-dependently reduces tidal volume and minute ventilation with a dose-related tachypnea. The degree of respiratory depression, as shown by increased resting $paCO_2$, lessened with prolonged administration (3-7 h) of halothane or enflurane. The newer inhalation anesthetics desflurane and sevoflurane also exhibit dose-related ventilatory depression, primarily by reducing tidal volume [15]. Unlike isoflurane, sevoflurane and desflurane both cause dose-related increases in respiratory frequency. Thus, desflurane does not significantly reduce minute ventilation until concentrations greater than 1.6 MAC have been achieved. However, at higher concentrations, the reduction of respiratory rate was less than that which occurred with halothane. The relative increases in $paCO_2$ as an index of respiratory depression with volatile anesthetics (<1.24 MAC) are: enflurane > desflurane = isoflurane > sevoflurane = halothane. At higher concentrations the ventilatory depression produced by desflurane is similar to that of enflurane, and sevoflurane is similar to isoflurane. Doi and Ikeda [16] found that with sevoflurane anesthesia, tidal volume decreased and $paCO_2$ increased with increasing depth of anesthesia. Recently, we observed that sevoflurane anesthesia increased tidal volume and diminished breathing frequency, yielding constant minute ventilation during the first 30 min of anesthesia [17].

Respiratory muscles

The effect of an anesthetic on the respiratory muscles is non-uniform. After induction of general anesthesia there is a loss of the inspiratory tone and an appearance of end-expiratory tone in the abdominal expiratory muscles at the end of exhalation. In the supine position, the end-expiratory tone in the abdominal expiratory muscles increases intra-abdominal pressure, forces the diaphragm cephalad, and decreases FRC [18, 19]. At high doses, anesthetics attenuate the activities of all respiratory muscles. However, at moderate depths of anesthesia, anesthetics may produce respiratory depression by altering the distribution and timing of neural drive to respiratory muscles, rather than by producing a global depression of activity [20]. For example, at 1.2 MAC halothane anesthesia depresses activity in some respiratory muscles (such as parasternal intercostals) but actually increases activity in others (such as transversus abdominis) [21]. Thus, respiratory muscle dysfunction is, in some cases, more a matter of a lack of co-ordination than a lack of overall activity leading to hypoventilation. In addition, deformation of the chest wall alters the underlying lung, decreasing FRC and producing atelectasis in dependent lung regions. Chest wall distortion and atelectasis also occur when the respiratory muscles are inactive during mechanical ventilation, and persist even with positive end expiratory pressure.

Functional residual capacity

Anesthesia is accompanied by a reduced FRC or resting lung volume [13]. Possible mechanisms involve a loss of tonic parasternal intercostal muscle activity [22, 23] and development of phasic expiratory activity of respiratory muscles, alteration in diaphragm position (cephalad displacement of diaphragm) [24, 25], or changes in thoracic blood volume (shift of blood from the thorax to the abdomen) [25].

Anesthesia is usually performed with the patient in the supine position. In changing the patient from the upright to the supine position, FRC decreases by 0.5 - 1.0 l because of a 4-cm cephalad displacement of the diaphragm by the abdominal viscera.

The decrement in FRC is higher in the Trendelenburg position, because it allows the abdominal contents to push the diaphragm further cephalad, so that the diaphragm not only must ventilate the lungs, but it also must lift the abdominal contents out of the thorax [26]. Increased pulmonary blood volume and gravitational force on the mediastinal structures are additional factors that may decrease pulmonary compliance and FRC. In the steep Trendelenburg position, most of the lung may be below the left atrium and therefore in a zone 3 or 4 condition. As such, the lung may be susceptible to the development of pulmonary interstitial edema.

In the lateral decubitus position, the dependent lung experiences a moderate decrease in FRC and is predisposed to atelectasis, whereas the nondependent lung may have an increased FRC. The overall result is usually a slight to moderate increase in total lung FRC [27]. The kidney and lithotomy positions also cause small decreases in FRC above that caused by the supine position. The prone position may increase FRC moderately.

Paralysis

In the upright subject, the FRC and the position of the diaphragm are determined by the balance between the lung elastic recoil pulling the diaphragm cephalad and the weight of the abdominal contents pulling it caudad [28]. There is no transdiaphragmatic pressure gradient.

The situation is more complex in the supine position. The diaphragm separates two compartments of markedly different hydrostatic gradients. On the thoracic side, pressure increases by approximately 0.25 cmH_2O/cm of lung height, and on the abdominal side by 1.0 cmH_2O/cm of abdominal height [28]. This means that in horizontal postures, progressively higher transdiaphragmatic pressures must be generated toward dependent parts of the diaphragm to keep the abdominal contents out of the thorax. In the awake spontaneously breathing patient, the active tension in the diaphragm is capable of overcoming the weight of the abdominal contents, and the diaphragm moves the most in the posterior portion (because the posterior diaphragm is stretched higher into the chest, it has the smallest radius of curvature and therefore it contracts most effectively) and least in the anterior portion. This is an adequate circumstance because the greatest amount of ventilation occurs where the perfusion is highest (posteriorly or dependently), and the least amount of ventilation occurs where there is the least perfusion (anteriorly or nondependently).

During muscle paralysis, a shift of the diaphragm to a more-cephalad position occurs [29]. The latter position must express the true balance of forces on the diaphragm, unmodified by any passive or active muscle activity. The magnitude of the change in the diaphragmatic motion pattern with paralysis varies with body position [29, 30]. During paralysis and positive pressure breathing, the passive diaphragm is displaced by positive pressure preferentially in the anterior nondependent portion (where there is the least resistance to diaphragmatic movement) and is displaced minimally in the posterior dependent portion (where there is the most resistance to diaphragmatic movement). Consequently, the greatest amount of ventilation now occurs where there is the least perfusion, and vice-versa.

Respiratory mechanics

There are several studies describing that the respiratory system static compliance (Cst) is reduced during anesthesia [31]. Many reasons explain this decrement in Cst: relaxation of the inspiratory muscles changing chest wall compliance, right shift of the pressure-volume curve but unaltered compliance of the chest wall on induction of anesthesia (reduced expansion pressure), which may contribute to the reduction of FRC [32].

Airway resistance usually increases during general anesthesia. The decreases in FRC caused by the supine position (0.8 l) and the induction of anesthesia (0.4 l) are often sufficient to explain the increased resistance seen in the healthy anesthetized patient [23]. In addition, there are a number of additional special potential sites of increased airway resistance: the endotracheal tube (if present), the upper and lower airway passages, and the external anesthesia apparatus. The increase in resistance associated with commonly used breathing circuits and endotracheal tubes may impose an additional work of breathing [33-35]. Endotracheal intubation reduces the size of the trachea, usually by 30 - 50%. Conversely, the laryngeal mask airway triggers less bronchoconstriction than does the endotracheal tube in paralyzed anesthetized adult patients. This may have implications for maintaining intraoperative pulmonary function and reducing the risk for atelectasis and pulmonary infection [36].

Recently we analyzed the effects of different anesthetic agents in respiratory mechanics: halothane, sevoflurane, and ketamine. Halothane anesthesia acts both at airway as well as at lung tissue levels. In the former, dilation results, whereas lung periphery stiffens. Consequently, these opposite effects account for no apparent change in mechanical properties, when the total behavior is considered, although there are reciprocal changes within the total mechanics found during the use of halothane in normal animals and subjects [37]. Sevoflurane anesthesia also increased pulmonary viscoelastic/inhomogeneous properties and decreased static compliance [17]. These findings were supported by the histological demonstration of increased areas of alveolar collapse and hyperinflation, and the greater amount of airway secretion. The pre-treatment with atropine reduced the amount of central and peripheral airway secretion, thus lessening but not eliminating lung inhomogeneities (Fig. 1). Volatile anesthetics are traditionally considered to be potent bronchodilators and are even used to treat status asthmaticus. However, we observed no functional or histological evidence of bronchodilation in sevoflurane anesthesia in animals with no pre-existing airway tone. The respiratory effects of ketamine [38] are noticeable, mainly because it is believed to yield bronchodilation [39], which was firstly observed in asthmatic patients. Supposedly ketamine relaxes the bronchiolar musculature, and prevents the bronchoconstriction induced by

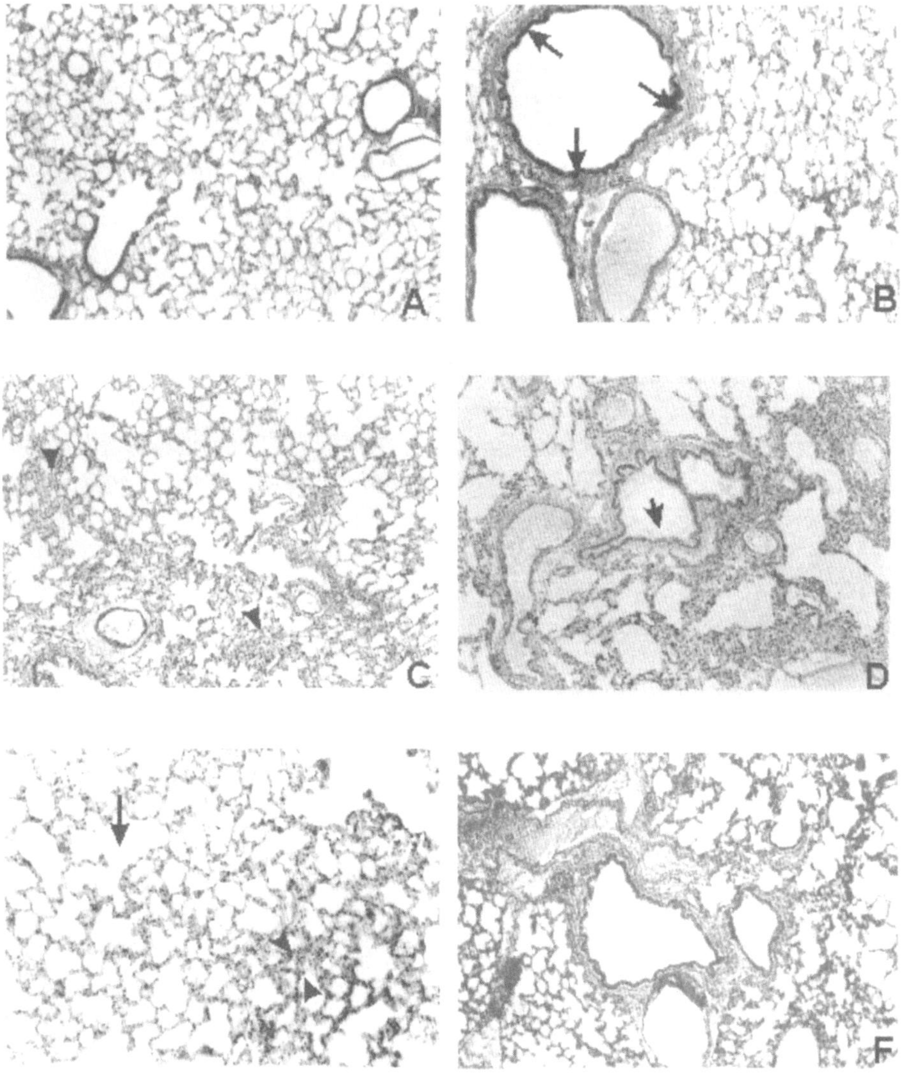

Fig. 1. Representative panel illustrating the histopathological patterns of distal pulmonary parenchyma (A, C and E) and airways (B, D and F) from rats anesthetized with pentobarbital sodium (A and B), sevoflurane (C and D), and anesthetized with sevoflurane but pre-treated with atropine (E and F). In B, *arrows* indicate the absence of airway secretion in the lumen, while in D they indicate the presence of bronchial secretion. *Arrowheads* show regions of atelectasis (C and E). In E, note that lung parenchyma remains altered, with areas of alveolar collapse (*arrowheads*) mixed with hyperinflation (*arrow*). There is no secretion into the airway lumen (F). Hematoxylin-eosin stain; magnification x200 [17]

histamine, which would be an obvious advantage in asthmatic patients. We observed that ketamine [40], in the absence of active smooth muscle tone, did not act at airway level but at lung periphery, increasing mechanical inhomogeneities, which may result from dilation of distal airways and alveolar collapse.

Habre et al. [41] investigated the abilities of halothane, isoflurane, sevoflurane, and desflurane to provide protection against airway constriction induced by methacoline. They observed that isoflurane, sevoflurane, and desflurane are as effective as the widely accepted halothane in protecting against methacholine-induced airway constriction.

Atelectasis

Mead and Collier [42] observed a progressive reduction in lung compliance during anesthesia in either spontaneously breathing or mechanically ventilated dogs. Compliance could be restored to initial values by hyperinflation. Bendixen et al. [43] made similar observations in anesthetized man and found that the decreasing compliance was accompanied by a decreasing paO_2. In their paper they put forward the "concept of atelectasis". They had observed a successive decrease in compliance of the respiratory system and decrease in arterial oxygenation, both in anesthetized humans and in animal experiments. This was assumed to reflect progressive formation of resorption atelectasis. However, other research groups were unable to reproduce their findings, but noticed a more-prompt fall in compliance and paO_2 on induction of anesthesia [2]. Since it has not been possible to demonstrate the occurrence of atelectasis during anesthesia by means of conventional chest radiography, some authors changed their opinion about considering atelectasis as the cause of altered lung mechanics and gas exchange during anesthesia. It took 20 years to make atelectasis an attractive explanation of the shunt during anesthesia. Brismar et al. [44], using computed tomography with transverse exposures of the chest, demonstrated development of atelectasis in dependent regions of both lungs during anesthesia.

Atelectasis appears in almost 90% of all anesthetized patients, it is independent of age, is only loosely related to body configuration, appears during spontaneous breathing and after muscle paralysis, and whether anesthetic is inhalational or intravenous.

General anesthesia is usually administered with an increased FIO_2. The cause of the atelectatic shunting during O_2 breathing is presumably a large increase in O_2 uptake by lung units with low V'A/Q' ratios [45, 46]. A unit that has a low V'A/Q' ratio during air breathing will have a low pAO_2. When an enriched O_2 mixture is inspired, pAO_2 rises, causing the rate at which O_2 moves from the alveolar gas to the capillary blood to increase greatly. The O_2 flux may increase so much that the net flow of gas into the blood exceeds the inspired flow of gas, and the lung unit will become progressively smaller. Collapse is most likely to occur if the FIO_2 is high, the V'A/Q' ratio is low, the time of exposure of the unit with low V'A/Q' to high FIO_2 is long, and the CvO_2 is low [13]. Thus, given the right V'A/Q' ratio and time of administration, an FIO_2 as low as 50% can produce absorption atelectasis [45, 46]. This phenomenon is of considerable significance in the clinical situation for two reasons. Firstly, enriched O_2 mixtures are often used therapeutically, and it is important to know whether this therapy is causing atelectasis. Secondly, the amount of shunt is often estimated during breathing of 100%t O_2, and if this maneuver results in additional shunt, the measurement will be hard to interpret.

Rapid shallow breathing is often a regular feature of anesthesia. Monotonous shallow breathing may cause a decrease in FRC, promote atelectasis, and decrease compliance [43, 47, 48]. These changes with rapid shallow breathing are likely due to progressive increases in surface tension [48].

The atelectasis can be reduced or eliminated by ventilation with positive end-expiratory pressure (PEEP) of 10 cmH_2O, although the shunt is not diminished. This may appear surprising but it is explained by a redistribution of blood flow to dependent regions where atelectasis may still exist. Indeed, PEEP may even increase the shunt in some patients [49]. Moreover, the atelectasis recurs within a minute of the discontinuation of PEEP. In addition, a normal tidal volume, up to airway pressure of 10 cmH_2O, has no effect on the atelectasis, nor a deep sigh to an airway pressure of 20 cmH_2O [50]. A vital capacity maneuver with an airway pressure of 40 cmH_2O is required to reopen all lung tissue completely.

Pulmonary gas exchange

Hypercapnia

Hypoventilation, increased dead space ventilation, increased CO_2 production, and inadvertent switching off of a CO_2 absorber can all cause hypercapnia. Patients spontaneously hypoventilate during anesthesia because it is more difficult to breathe (abnormal surgical position, increased airway resistance, decreased compliance) and they are less willing to breathe (decreased respiratory drive due to anesthetics). As a result, hypoventilation results in hypercapnia.

Hypotension and an increase in airway pressure may augment zone 1 and alveolar dead space ventilation. In addition, pulmonary embolus, thrombosis, and vascular obliteration (kinking, clamping, blocking of pulmonary artery during surgery) may increase the amount of lung that is ventilated but unperfused. Rapid short inspirations may be distributed preferentially to noncompliant (short time constant for inflation) and badly perfused alveoli, while a slow inspiration allows time for gas distribution to more-compliant (long time constant for inflation) and better perfused alveoli. Thus, rapid, short inspirations may have a dead space ventilation effect.

The anesthesia apparatus also increases total dead space (VD/VT) because the apparatus simply increases the anatomical dead space. Inclusion of normal apparatus dead space increases the total VD/VT ratio from 33% to about 46% in intubated patients and to about 64% in patients breathing via a mask [51].

Hyperthermia, shivering, catecholamine release (light anesthesia), hypertension, and thyroid storm cause increased O_2 consumption and CO_2 production. If V'E, total dead space, and V'A/Q' relationships are constant, an increase in CO_2 production will result in hypercapnia.

Many factors, such as patient ventilatory responsiveness to CO_2 accumulation, fresh gas flow, circle system design, and CO_2 production, determine whether hypercapnia will result from accidental switching off or using up of a circle CO_2 absorber. However, high fresh gas flows (5 l/min) minimize the problem with almost all systems for almost all patients.

The maximal stimulant respiratory effect is attained by a $paCO_2$ of about 100 mmHg. With a higher $paCO_2$, stimulation is reduced, and at extremely high levels, respiration is depressed and later ceases altogether. The pCO_2-ventilation response curve is generally displaced to the right, and its slope is reduced by anesthetics and other depressant drugs. With profound anesthesia, the response curve may be flat or even sloping downward, and CO_2 then acts as a respiratory depressant. In patients with ventilatory failure, CO_2 narcosis occurs when the $paCO_2$ rises to more than 90 - 120 mmHg. A 30% CO_2 concentration is sufficient for the production of anesthesia, and this concentration causes total but reversible flattening of the electroencephalogram [52]. As expected, hypercapnia causes bronchodilation in both healthy persons and patients with lung disease [53].

CO_2 exerts two other important effects that influence the oxygenation of the blood. Firstly, if the concentration of nitrogen (or other inert gas) remains constant, the concentration of CO_2 in the alveolar gas can only increase at the expense of O_2, which must be displaced. Thus, pAO_2 and PaO_2 may decrease. Secondly, hypercapnia shifts the oxy-hemoglobin (Hb) curve to the right, facilitating tissue oxygenation.

Hypocapnia

The mechanisms of inducing hypocapnia during general anesthesia are: hyperventilation (spontaneous or controlled ventilation), decreased VD ventilation (change from mask airway to endotracheal tube airway), decreased PEEP, increased Ppa, or decreased rebreathing, and decreased CO_2 production (hypothermia, deep anesthesia, hypotension) [13].

Hypocapnia may cause a decrease in lung perfusion by various mechanisms: (1) hypocapnia can increase intrathoracic pressure, thus decreasing cardiac output, (2) hypocapnia is associated with a withdrawal of sympathetic nervous system activity, and this can decrease the inotropic state of the heart, (3) hypocapnia can increase pH, which can in turn decrease ionized calcium, which may, in turn, decrease the inotropic state of the heart. Hypocapnia with alkalosis also shifts the oxy-Hb curve to the left, which increases the Hb affinity for O_2. Hypocapnia may cause V'A/Q' abnormalities by inhibiting hypoxic pulmonary vasoconstriction or by causing bronchoconstriction and decreased lung compliance. Finally, passive hypocapnia produces apnea.

Hypoxia

There are many causes for hypoxemia during anesthesia: (1) mechanical failure of the O_2 supply system, (2) disconnection of the patient from the O_2 supply system (usually at the juncture of the endotracheal tube and elbow connector), (3) an empty or depleted O_2 cylinder, (4) substitution of a nonoxygen cylinder at the O_2 yoke because of absence or failure of the pin index, (5) an erroneously filled O_2 cylinder, (6) insufficient opening of the O_2 cylinder, (7) failure of gas pressure in a piped O_2 system, (8) faulty locking of the piped O_2 system to the anesthesia machine, (9) inadvertent switching of the Schrader adapters on piped lines, (10) crossing of piped lines during construction, (11) failure of a reducing valve or gas manifold, (12) inadvertent disturbance of the setting of the O_2 flowmeter, (13) employment of the fine O_2 flowmeter instead of the coarse flowmeter, (14) fractured or sticking flowmeters, (15) transposition of rotameter tubes, (16) erroneous filling of a liquid O_2 reservoir with nitrogen, and (17) fresh gas line disconnection from machine to in-line hosing. Monitoring of the inspired O_2 concentration with an in-line FIO_2 analyzer and monitoring of airway pressure should detect most of these causes of failure to deliver O_2 to the patient.

Because the various organs have different blood flow and O_2 consumption rates, the presentation and clinical diagnosis of hypoxia is usually related to symptoms arising from the most-vulnerable organ. This organ is usually the brain in an awake patient and the heart in an anesthetized patient, but in special circumstances it may be the spinal cord (aortic surgery), kidney (acute tubular necrosis), liver (hepatitis), or limb (claudication, gangrene).

The cardiovascular response to hypoxemia [54-56] is a product of both reflex (neural and humoural) and direct effects. The reflex effects occur first and are excitatory and vasoconstrictive. The neuroreflex effects result from aortic and carotid chemoreceptor, baroreceptor, and central cerebral stimulation, and the humoral reflex effects result from catecholamine and renin-angiotensin release. The direct local vascular effects of hypoxia are inhibitory and vasodilatory and occur late. The net response to hypoxia in a subject depends on the severity of the hypoxia, which determines the magnitude of and balance between the inhibitory and excitatory components; the balance may vary according to the type and depth of anesthesia and the degree of pre-existing cardiovascular disease.

The cardiovascular response to hypoxia includes a number of other important effects. Cerebral blood flow increases (even if hypocapnic hyperventilation is present). Ventilation will be stimulated no matter why hypoxia exists. The pulmonary distribution of blood flow is more homogeneous owing to an increased pulmonary artery pressure. Chronic hypoxia causes an increased Hb concentration and a right-shifted oxy-Hb curve (due to either an increase in 2,3-diphosphoglycerate or acidosis), which tends to raise tissue pO_2.

Hyperoxia (oxygen toxicity)

The dangers associated with the inhalation of excessive O_2 are multiple. Exposure to a high O_2 tension clearly causes pulmonary damage in healthy individuals [57, 58]. A dose-time toxicity curve for humans is available from a number of studies [57-59]. Because the lungs of normal human volunteers cannot be directly examined to determine the rate of onset and course of toxicity, indirect measures, such as the onset of symptom formation, have been employed to construct the dose-time toxicity curves. Examination of the curve indicates that 100% O_2 should not be administered for more than 12 h, 80% O_2 should not be administered for more than 24 h, and 60% O_2 should not be administered for more than 36 h [57-59]. No measurable changes in pulmonary function or blood-gas exchange occur in humans during exposures to less than 50% O_2 even for long periods [59]. Nevertheless, it is important to note that in the clinical setting, these dose-time toxicity relationships are often generally obscured [60], owing to its complex multivariable nature.

The dominant symptom of O_2 toxicity in human volunteers is substernal distress, which begins as a mild irritation in the area of the carina and may be accompanied by occasional coughing [61]. As exposure continues, pain becomes more intense, and the urge to cough and to deep breathe also becomes more intense. These symptoms will progress to severe dyspnea, paroxysmal coughing, and decreased vital capacity when the FIO_2 has been 1.0 for longer than 12 h. At this point, recovery of mechanical lung function usually occurs within 12 - 24 h, but it may require more than 24 h in some individuals [59]. As toxicity progresses, other pulmonary function studies such as compliance and blood gases deteriorate. Pathologically, in animals, the lesion progresses from tracheobronchitis (exposure for 12 h to a few days), to involvement of the alveolar septa with pulmonary interstitial edema (exposure for a few days to 1 week), to pulmonary fibrosis of the edema (exposure for more than 1 week) [62].

Ventilatory depression may occur in those patients who, by reason of drugs or disease, have been ventilating in response to a hypoxic drive. By definition, ventilatory depression resulting from removal of a hypoxic drive by increasing the inspired O_2 concentration will cause hypercapnia but does not necessarily produce hypoxia (owing to the increased FIO_2).

The mode of action of O_2 toxicity in tissues is complex, but interference with metabolism seems to be widespread. Most importantly, there is O_2-derived free radical inactivation of many enzymes, particularly those with sulfhydryl groups [60]. Neutrophil recruitment and release of mediators of inflammation occur next and greatly accelerate the extent of endothelial and epithelial damage and impairment of the surfactant systems [60]. The most-acute toxic enzyme effect of O_2 in humans is a convulsive effect, which occurs during exposure to pressures in excess of 2 atm absolute.

Hypoxic pulmonary vasoconstriction

Decreased regional pAO_2 causes regional pulmonary vasoconstriction, which diverts blood flow away from hypoxic regions of the lung to better-ventilated and normoxic regions of the lung. The diversion of blood flow minimizes venous admixture from the underventilated or nonventilated lung regions. Several inhalational anesthetics have been found to inhibit hypoxic pulmonary vasoconstriction (HPV) in isolated lung preparation [63]. Inhibition of regional HPV could impair arterial oxygenation by permitting increased venous admixture from hypoxic or atelectatic areas of the lung. In human studies, the inhalational anesthetics isoflurane and halothane depress HPV by 50% at 2 MAC. However, attenuation of HPV should not impair oxygenation of blood if V'A/Q' match is normal because there would be no functional baseline HPV. Thus there must be an underlying V'A/Q' disturbance if abolition or attenuation of HPV is to affect gas exchange.

Because the pulmonary circulation is poorly endowed with smooth muscle, any condition that increases the pressure against which the vessels must constrict (i.e., the Ppa) will decrease HPV. There are numerous clinical conditions that can increase Ppa and therefore decrease HPV. Mitral stenosis [64], volume overload [64], low (but room air) FIO_2 in nondiseased lung [65], a progressive increase in the amount of diseased lung [65] thromboembolism [65], hypothermia [66], and vasoactive drugs [67] can all increase Ppa. Direct vasodilating drugs (such as isoproterenol, nitroglycerin, and sodium nitroprusside), inhaled anesthetics, and hypocapnia can directly decrease HPV [67]. The application of PEEP to only the nondiseased lung can selectively increase nondiseased lung pulmonary vascular resistance and may divert blood flow back into the diseased lung [68].

Conclusions

Pulmonary effects of anesthesia include alterations in lung volumes related to supine posture and the effects of anesthetic agents, impairment of respiratory muscle function, and altered gas exchange related to changes in lung mechanics and hypoxic pulmonary vasoreactivity. Because most surgery is conducted with the patient supine, the effect of supine posture on lung function is an important consideration. In anesthetized patients, FRC, the resting end-expiratory lung volume at which the forces for chest wall expansion are balanced by those favoring lung contraction, typically falls by 20%. There is a cephalad displacement of the diaphragm after induction of anesthesia and the greater degree of cephalad displacement occurs in the dependent portion of the diaphragm. The resulting decline in FRC is accompanied by a decrease in paO_2 because the resultant atelectasis creates venous admixture and shunting. In addition to effects on respiratory muscle function that alter lung mechanics and volumes, anesthesia may inhibit hypoxic pulmonary vasoconstriction, and lead to increased venous admixture from atelectatic or hypoxic regions of the lung.

References

1. Marshall BE, Wyche MO (1972) Hypoxemia during and after anesthesia. Anesthesiology 37:178-209
2. Nunn JF, Bergman NA, Coleman AJ (1965) Factors influencing the arterial oxygen tension during anaesthesia with artificial ventilation. Br J Anaesth 37:898-914
3. Sykes MK (1970) Mechanics of ventilation. In: Scurr C, Feldman S (eds) Scientific foundations of anesthesia. Davis, Philadelphia, pp 174
4. Nunn JF (1993) Nunn's applied respiratory physiology, 4th edn, Heinemann, Oxford

5. Hedenstierna G (1990) Gas exchange during anaesthesia. Br J Anaesth 64:507-514
6. Gunnarsson L, Tokics L, Gustavsson H, et al (1991) Influence of age on atelectasis formation and gas exchange impairment during general anesthesia. Br J Anaesth 66:423-432
7. Rehder K, Sessler AD, Marsh HM (1975) General anesthesia and the lung. In: Murray JF (ed) Lung disease state of the art. American Lung Association, New York, p 367
8. Vaughan RW, Wise L (1976) Intraoperative arterial oxygenation in obese patients. Ann Surg 184:35-42
9. Dueck R, Young I, Clausen J, et al (1980) Altered distribution of pulmonary ventilation and blood flow following induction of inhalational anesthesia. Anesthesiology 52:113-125
10. Rehder K, Knopp TH, Sessler AD, et al (1979) Ventilation-perfusion relationships in young healthy awake and anesthetized-paralyzed man. J Appl Physiol 47:745-753
11. Tokics L, Hedenstierna G, Strandberg A, et al (1987) Lung collapse and gas exchange during general anesthesia: Effects of spontaneous breathing, muscle paralysis and positive end-expiratory pressure. Anesthesiology 66:157-167
12. Bellville JW, Seed JC (1960) The effect of drugs on the respiratory response to carbon dioxide. Anesthesiology 21:727-741
13. Miller RD (2000) Anesthesia, 5th edn. Churchill Livingstone, Edinburgh
14. Laver MB, Bendixen HH (1966) Atelectasis in the surgical patient. Recent conceptual advances. Prog Surg 5:1-37
15. Lockhart SH, Rampill IJ, Yasuda N, et al (1991) Depression of ventilation by desflurane in humans. Anesthesiology 74:484-488
16. Doi M, Ikeda K (1987) Respiratory effects of sevoflurane. Anesth Analg 66:241-244.
17. Correa FCF, Ciminelli PB, Falcão H, et al (2001) Respiratory mechanics and lung histology in normal rats anesthetized with sevoflurane. J Appl Physiol 91:803-810
18. Don HF, Wahba M, Cuadrado L, et al (1970) The effects of anesthesia and 100 percent oxygen on the functional residual capacity of the lungs. Anesthesiology 32:521-529
19. Freund F, Roos A, Dodd RB (1964) Expiratory activity of the abdominal muscles in man during general anesthesia. J Appl Physiol 19:693-697
20. Warner DO, Weiskopf RB (2000) Preventing postoperative pulmonary complications: the role of the anesthesiologist. Anesthesiology 92:1467-1472
21. Warner DO, Warner MA (1995) Human chest wall function while awake and during halothane anesthesia. Anesthesiology 82:20-31
22. Bergman NA (1963) Distribution of inspired gas during anesthesia and artificial ventilation. J Appl Physiol 18:1085-1089
23. Mead J, Agostoni E (1964) Dynamics of breathing. In: Fenn WO, Rahn H (eds) Handbook of Physiology, section 3. Respiration, vol. 1. Williams and Wilkins, Baltimore, p 411
24. Froese AB, Bryan CH (1974) Effects of anesthesia and paralysis on diaphragmatic mechanics in man. Anesthesiology 41:242-254
25. Hedenstierna G, Strandberg A, Brismar B, et al (1985) Functional residual capacity, thoraco-abdominal dimensions and central blood volume during general anesthesia with muscle paralysis and mechanical ventilation. Anesthesiology 62:247-254
26. Slocum HC, Hoeflich EA, Allen CR (1947) Circulatory and respiratory distress from extreme positions on the operating table. Surg Gynecol Obstet 84:1065-1068
27. Lumb AB, Nunn JF (1991) Respiratory function and ribcage contribution to ventilation in body positions commonly used during anesthesia. Anesth Analg 73:422-426
28. Campbell EJM, Agostini E, David JN (1970) The respiratory muscles: mechanics and neural control, 2nd edn Saunders, Philadelphia
29. Krayer S, Rehder K, Vettermann J (1989) Position and motion of the human diaphragm during anesthesia-paralysis. Anesthesiology 70:891-898
30. Froese AB (1989) Anesthesia-paralysis and the diaphragm: in pursuit of an elusive muscle. Anesthesiology 70:887-890
31. Don H (1977) The mechanical properties of the respiratory system during anesthesia. Int Anesthesiol Clin 15:113-136

32. Westbrook PR, Stubbs SE, Sessler AD, et al (1973) Effects of anesthesia and muscle paralysis on respiratory mechanics in normal man. J Appl Physiol 34:81-86
33. Wright PE, Marini JJ, Bernard GR (1989) In vitro versus in vivo comparison of endotracheal tube airflow resistance. Am Rev Respir Dis 140:10-16
34. Bersten AD, Rutten AJ, Vedig AE, et al (1989) Additional work of breathing imposed by endotracheal tube, breathing circuits and intensive care ventilators. Crit Care Med 17:671-677
35. Rocco PRM, Zin WA (1995) Modeling the mechanical effects of tracheal tubes on normal subjects. Eur Respir J 8: 21-126
36. Berry A, Brimacombe J, Keller C, Verghese C (1999) Pulmonary airway resistance with the endotracheal tube versus laryngeal mask airway in paralyzed anesthetized adult patients. Anesthesiology 90:395-398
37. Reta GS, Riva JA, Piriz H, et al (2000) Effects of halothane on respiratory mechanics and lung histopathology in normal rats. Br J Anaesth 84:372-377
38. Zsigmond EK, Matsuki A, Kotharey SP (1976) Arterial hypoxemia caused by intravenous ketamine. Anesth Analg 55:311-314
39. Corssen G, Gutierrez JJ, Reves JG, et al (1972) Ketamine in the anesthetic management of asthmatic patient. Anesth Analg 51:588-596
40. Alves-Neto O, Tavares P, Rocco PRM, et al (2001) Respiratory mechanics and morphometric changes during anesthesia with ketamine in normal rats. Braz J Med Biol Res (in press)
41. Habre W, Petak F, Sly PD, et al (2001) Protective effects of volatile agents against methacoline-induced bronchoconstriction in rats. Anesthesiology 94:348-353
42. Mead J, Collier C (1959) Relation of volume history of lungs to respiratory mechanics in anesthetized dogs. J Appl Physiol 14:669-678
43. Bendixen HH, Hedley-Whyte J, Laver MB (1963) Impaired oxygenation in surgical patients during general anesthesia with controlled ventilation: a concept of atelectasis. N Engl J Med 269:991-996
44. Brismar B, Hedenstierna G, Lindqvist H, et al (1985) Pulmonary densities during anesthesia with muscular relaxation: a proposal of atelectasis. Anesthesiology 62: 422-428
45. Wagner PD, Laravuso RB, Uhl RR, et al (1974) Continuous distributions of ventilation-perfusion ratios in normal subjects breathing air and 100% O_2. J Clin Invest 54: 54-68
46. Briscoe WA, Cree EM, Filler, et al (1960) Lung volume, alveolar ventilation and perfusion interrelationships in chronic pulmonary emphysema. J Appl Physiol 15:785-792
47. Laver MB, Bendixen HH (1966) Atelectasis in the surgical patient. Recent conceptual advances. Prog Surg.5:1-37
48. Huang YC, Weinmann GG, Mitzner W (1988) Effect of tidal volume and frequency on the temporal fall in lung compliance. J Appl Physiol 65:2040-2045
49. Hewlett AM, Hulands GH, Nunn JF, et al (1974) Functional residual capacity during anaesthesia. Br J Anaesth 46:495-503
50. Rothen HU, Sporre B, Engberg G, et al (1993) Reexpansion of atelectasis during general anesthesia: a computed tomography study. Br J Anaesth 71:788-795
51. Kain ML, Panday J, Nunn JF (1969) The effect of intubation on the dead space during halothane anaesthesia. Br J Anaesth 41:94-103
52. Clowes GHA, Hopkins AL, Simeone FA (1955) A comparison of the physiological effects of hypercapnia and hypoxia in the production of cardiac arrest. Ann Surg 142:446-451
53. Parsons PE, Grunstein MM, Fernandez E (1989) The effects of acute hypoxia and hypercapnia on pulmonary mechanics in normal subjects and patients with chronic pulmonary disease. Chest 96:96-101
54. Heistad DD, Abboud FM (1980) Circulatory adjustments to hypoxia: Dickinson W. Richards Lecture. Circulation 61:463-470
55. Roberts JG (1980) The effect of hypoxia on the systemic circulation during anaesthesia. In: Prys-Roberts E (ed) The circulation in anaesthesia: applied physiology and pharmacology. Blackwell Scientific Publications, Oxford, pp 311

56. Rothe CF, Flanagan AD, Maass-Moreno R (1990) Reflex control of vascular capacitance during hypoxia, hypercapnia, or hypoxic hypercapnia. Can J Physiol Pharmacol 68:384-391
57. Winter PM, Smith G (1972) The toxicity of oxygen. Anesthesiology 37:210-241
58. Lambertsen CJ (1965) Effects of oxygen at high partial pressure. In: Fenn WO, Rahn H (eds) Handbook of physiology, section 3. Respiration, vol. 2. Williams and Wilkins, Baltimore, p 1027
59. Clark JM (1988) Pulmonary limits of oxygen tolerance in man. Exp Lung Res 14:897- 910
60. Klein J (1990) Normobaric pulmonary oxygen toxicity. Anesth Analg 70:195-207
61. Montgomery AB, Luce JM, Murray JF (1989) Retrosternal pain is an early indicator of oxygen toxicity. Am Rev Respir Dis 139:1548-1550
62. Nash G, Blennerhasset JB, Pontoppidan H (1967) Pulmonary lesions associated with oxygen therapy and artificial ventilation. N Engl J Med 276:368-374
63. Sykes MK, Loh L, Seed RF, et al (1972) The effect of inhalational anaesthetics on hypoxic pulmonary vascular resistance in the perfused lung of the dog and cat. Br J Anaesth 44:776-788
64. Benumof JL, Wahrenbrock EA (1975) Blunted hypoxic pulmonary vasoconstriction by increased lung vascular pressures. J Appl Physiol 38:846-850
65. Scanlon TS, Benumof JL, Wahrenbrock EA, et al (1978) Hypoxic pulmonary vasoconstriction and the ratio of hypoxic lung to perfused normoxic lung. Anesthesiology 49:177-181
66. Benumof JL, Wahrenbrock EA (1977) Dependency of hypoxic pulmonary vasoconstriction on temperature. J Appl Physiol 42:56-58
67. Benumof JL (1987) Anesthesia for thoracic surgery. Saunders, Philadelphia
68. Benumof JL (1982) One lung ventilation: which lung should be PEEPed? Anesthesiology 56:161-163

Aspiration of Airway Dead Space: a New Method to Enhance CO_2 Elimination

E. De Robertis, B. Jonson, R. Tufano

Mechanical ventilation is a life-saving therapeutic modality in the treatment of critical diseases such as the acute respiratory injury (ALI) and the acute respiratory distress syndrome (ARDS). However, it can contribute to the progression of pulmonary disease by generating a "ventilatory-induced lung injury" (VILI) [1, 2]. VILI may contribute to morbidity and mortality in ARDS with multiple mechanisms. Trauma resulting from high airway pressure and over-distension may lead to air leakage [3]. Repeated lung collapse and re-expansion leads to important shear forces [4].

It has been suggested that, during mechanical ventilation tidal excursion should be contained within the linear part of the elastic pressure volume curve (Pel/V) of the respiratory system, [i.e., between the lower inflection point (LIP) and the upper inflection point (UIP), respectively]. Thereby the risks connected with repeated collapse and reopening at volumes below the LIP and over-distension at volumes above UIP would be reduced [5].

If we assume that ventilation should be performed above the volume of the LIP, and are aware about that this may imply a risk of overinflation if tidal volume is not reduced, a concept of lung protection emerges. It has been proposed that reduction of pressure-volume swings should be based upon modes of ventilation resulting in the smallest possible pressure amplitude.

The maintenance of an expanded lung during an inspiration that recruits the lung and the prevention of lung units collapse during a short expiration may be achieved by inverse inspiratory:expiratory (I:E) ratio ventilation [6]. In 1982 Jonson [7] suggested that "...a respiratory pattern should open up closed units and maintain aeration and stability throughout the respiratory cycle...". However, prolongation of inspiratory time, by increasing the mean airway pressure, led to negative cardiocirculatory consequences, as well as reduced oxygen transport [8]. Efficient ventilation should be characterized by an "early and sustained insufflation" at a precisely controlled airway pressure and by a proper frequency [9]. Notably, an increase in frequency, by shortening the expiratory time to a suitable extend, will lead to results similar to those of inverse I:E ratio ventilation. This concept may be expanded by drastically increasing frequency. Accordingly, re-aeration and stabilization of collapsed lung units can be obtained with high frequency ventilation (HFV). In HFV, the lungs may be recruited with one or more large insufflations, and are maintained open by sustaining the airway pressure above the closing pressure [10]. This is achieved with minimal alveolar pressure swings. The positive effects are probably based on auto-PEEP developing when frequency is substantially increased [11]. However, since HFV is strongly affected by the patient status and minor changes in the delivery system, great attention has to be paid to the monitoring and a competent supervision is needed [12].

Application of a sufficient positive end expiratory pressure (PEEP) level may reduce lung lesions induced by repeated shear stress of distal lung units. However, any beneficial effect of PEEP may be offset by the overinflation of distensible areas, depending on the magnitude of the tidal volume and the homogeneity of ventilation distribution [13]. PEEP levels from quite low to very high have been studied for years without conclusive results. Routine measurements of a Pel/V curve may offer the best tool to determine the smallest PEEP level needed to keep the lung open and to observe how the lung recruits.

In the last years, others strategies for lung protective ventilation have been proposed, which are based upon substantially reduced tidal volumes. The resulting low alveolar ventilation leads to CO_2 retention, which may either be left untreated, as during permissive hypercapnia [14] or treated by extracorporeal support using a membrane lung [15]. Flushing of the trachea during expiration with fresh gas, or tracheal gas insufflation (TGI) is another principle that may compensate for reduced tidal volumes [16-18]. The potential benefits of extracorporeal CO_2 removal and permissive hypercapnia are hindered by the invasivity of the former and the problems connected with the accumulation of CO_2 latter on.

During TGI-aided ventilation, CO_2 elimination is enhanced by delivering fresh gas into the trachea that can dilute dead space CO_2-rich gas if the TGI is given during expiration or by-pass dead space if given during inspiration. However, TGI is also associated with some recognized drawbacks such as induction or amplification of dynamic hyperinflation, drying of airway secretion, and the risk of damaging the airway mucosa [19].

We have hypothesized that to eliminate the drawbacks of TGI, an alternative would be to aspirate dead space gas from the trachea (ASPIDS) and simultaneously replace it with new gas through ordinary inspiratory tubing. Thus, gas in the ventilator tubing, Y-piece, filter and in the tracheal tube may, during the late part of the expiration, be aspirated from the tip of the tracheal tube and be replaced with fresh gas. The reduction of the airway dead space gas volume that returns to the alveoli during inspiration will increase effective alveolar ventilation and thereby allowing lower tidal volumes and airway pressures.

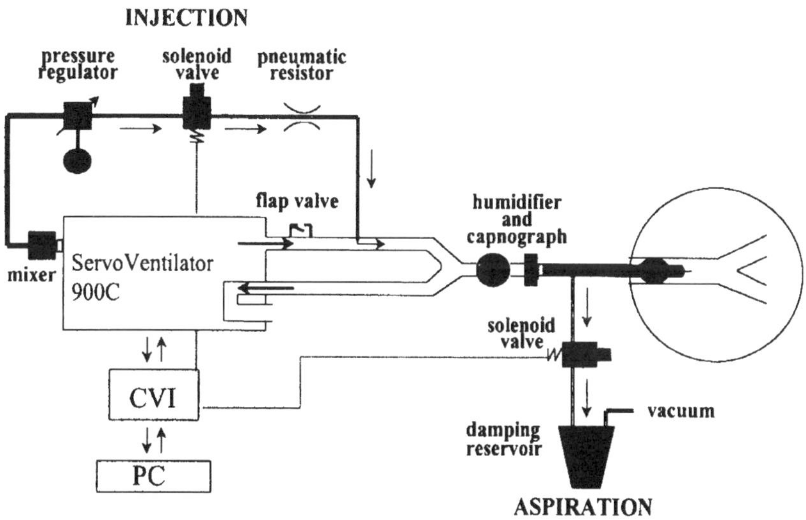

Fig. 1. ASPIDS equipment. When the solenoids valves for aspiration and injection open under the control of the personal computer (PC) and the computer/ventilator interface (CVI) ASPIDS is performed as described in the text.

ASPIDS circuit

The aspirate dead space (ASPIDS) system was constructed and programmed at the Department of Clinical Physiology, University of Lund, Sweden. It has been subjected to a stepwise development. One of the most advanced system is described in Figure 1.

A Servo Ventilator, connected to an IBM compatible personal computer through a ventilator/computer interface (CVI) [20-25], has been used to control the ASPIDS valves, to monitor patients, and to record respiratory mechanics.

Aspiration is performed through a polyethylene end-hole catheter (ID 2 mm; OD 3 mm) inserted into the tracheal tube through a swivel adapter connecting the tube to the ventilator circuit. The tip of the catheter is positioned 2 cm proximal to the tip of the tracheal tube. When activated by the computer through the solenoid valve in the inspiration line, the aspiration catheter is connected to a 3 liter damping reservoir coupled to the central hospital vacuum source. In order to achieve a suitable flow rate of aspirated gas, the degree of negative atmospheric pressure in the reservoir is adjusted by a leakage valve.

The injected fresh gas is delivered directly from the mixer of the ventilator. The injection line comprises of a computer controlled solenoid valve, a variable resistor valve and a tube connected to the inspiratory line of the ventilator circuit. The compensatory flow rate is adjusted with the resistor valve.

A flap valve in the inspiratory line serves as a safety measure against accidental development of a negative pressure in the circuit. The ASPIDS valves can only be opened during expiration and, importantly, all alarm functions of the ventilator are continuously operating during treatment.

Experimental evidences

The ability of ASPIDS to clear the volume of the connecting tubes from CO_2 was first tested in 6 pigs [26]. The intention was to decrease tidal volume (VT) while keeping $PaCO_2$ constant. VT was reduced of the estimated volume of tubing dead space (≅0.90 ml) by decreasing the minute ventilation in two steps, 1.8 and 2.2 L/min, respectively, and by increasing respiratory rate (RR). At ASPIDS, peak airway pressure (Paw_{peak}) was reduced by 35 % when minute ventilation was reduced ($p<0.001$), and by 20% when RR was increased ($p<0.01$). $PaCO_2$ was maintained or reduced at ASPIDS.

Similar results were obtained when ASPIDS was applied in 7 patients with normal lungs [27]. With ASPIDS a basal RR of 12.6 breaths/min, caused a decrease in VT from 602 to 456 ml, as well as a decrease in airway pressures to a corresponding degree. $PaCO_2$ and PaO_2 showed no significant changes. With ASPIDS at a frequency of 20 breaths/min, further reduced VT to 305 ml (50 % compared to the basal VT at the lower frequency) without changing $PaCO_2$.

Finally, in 7 ARDS patients a comprehensive evaluation of respiratory mechanics demonstrated that ASPIDS may be used as a tool for protective ventilation [28]. A preliminary mechanics study indicated that patients required a higher PEEP. Accordingly, with the use of ASPIDS, PEEP was increased from 8.9 to 12.6 cmH_2O and VT significantly reduced from 11 ml/kg to 8.9 at a RR of 14 breaths/min and to 6.9 at a RR of 20 breaths/min. A significant decrease in Paw_{peak} (36.7 *vs* 32 at RR 14 and 28.7 at RR 20, $p<0.001$) and plateau airway pressure (29.9 *vs* 27.3 at RR 14 and 24.1 at RR 20, $p<0.01$) were observed. $PaCO_2$ remained stable.

During ASPIDS-aided ventilation all animals and patients remained haemodynamically stable throughout the experimental period. No side effects of ASPIDS were noticed.

Figure 2 shows the pressure and flow patterns of a typical pig at baseline ventilation and at ASPIDS-aided ventilation. During pressure tracings trivial oscillations were observed at the moments when ASPIDS was switched on and off. The PEEP level set on the ventilator was maintained. PEEP did not develop during ASPIDS, not even at a high respiratory rate. Similar patterns were observed in patients.

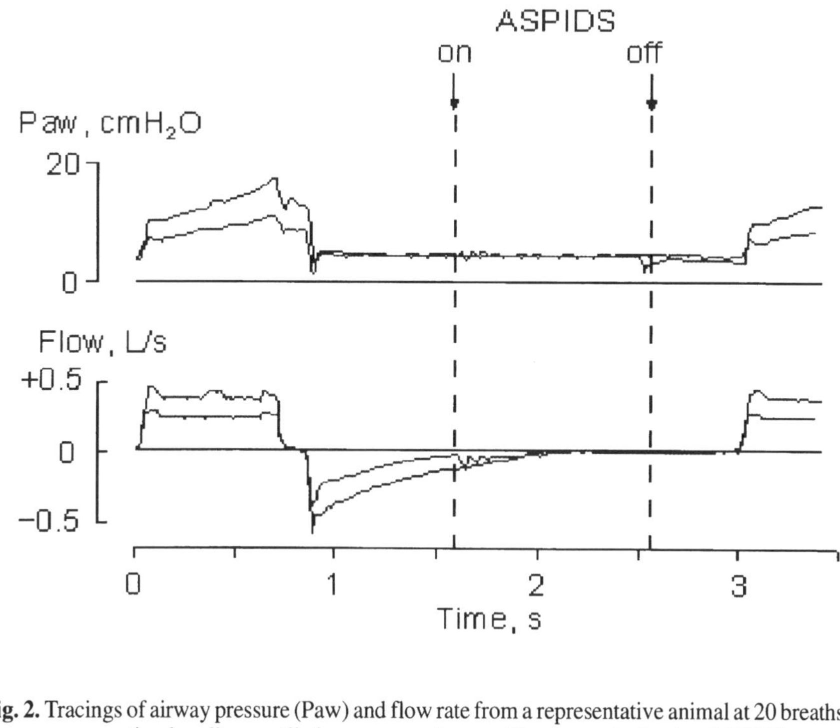

Fig. 2. Tracings of airway pressure (Paw) and flow rate from a representative animal at 20 breaths/min. Curves representing baseline ventilation are superimposed by those obtained at ASPIDS at a minute ventilation reduced by 2.2 L/min. The aspiration and injection valves open (on) and close (off)

Considerations on ASPIDS-aided ventilation

Several methods have been proposed in order to reduce hypercapnia which is induced by low tidal volume ventilation. Methods such as extracorporeal CO_2 removal, high frequency ventilation, and tracheal gas insufflation have only partly solved the problem but have not shown to be clinically beneficial.

TGI may enhance CO_2 elimination in different ways depending on when the gas is insufflated during the breathing cycle [16, 18, 19]. TGI during expiration will lead to a wash out of CO_2 contained in the dead space. ASPIDS may be regarded as a development of the latter principle with the aim to reduce or eliminate problems associated with TGI. Such problems are induction or amplification of dynamic hyperinflation, resulting in the drying of airway secretion. The effect is also poor in patients with an expiratory flow continuing until the end of expiration [19]. During ASPIDS-aided ventilation, in the late part of the expiration, gas in ventilator tubing, y-piece, filter and the tracheal tube is aspirated from the tip of the tracheal tube and replaced with fresh gas through the ordinary inspiratory line of the ventilator. Consequently, by reducing the volume of dead space gas that returns to the alveoli during inspiration, ASPIDS augments alveolar ventilation, allowing a decrease in tidal volume and airway pressure. Our hypothesis that ASPIDS allows a substantial reduction of tidal volumes and airway pressures under maintained isocapnia was confirmed. The use of a particularly low tidal volume at a high respiratory rate combined with ASPIDS was also verified [26, 27].

Since ASPIDS primarily reduces airway dead space, a similar result could be achieved, for instance, by eliminating the heat and moisture exchangers. Such an approach could be useful in dramatic conditions but it is not validated due to the suggested utility of the latest generation of heat and moisture exchangers [29]. The reasons for the use of the exchangers are the ability to easily obtain proper humidification and to a reduce contamination of microorganism in the ventilator circuit.

The respiratory mechanics and CT scan in animal models [24, 25] and in ARDS patients [20, 30, 31] have shown a wide distribution in pressure at which lung units close and reopen. Recently a "protective ventilatory strategy" with a PEEP of 2-3 cmH_2O above the LIP, combined with low a VT, was shown to attenuate cytokine response induced by mechanical ventilation [32] and to reduce mortality in ARDS [33, 34]. These observations indicated that at least part of the benefits from ASPIDS should be used to increase PEEP without risking over-distension and/or hypercapnia. In ARDS patients our hypothesis that isocapnia could be maintained at a higher PEEP and at lower distending pressures was confirmed [28]. Accordingly, ASPIDS gives room for a pattern of ventilation that may reduce VILI. How exactly this room should be utilized remains an open question. If benefits of a low VT should preferably be used to increase lung inflation by a high PEEP or to decrease peak and plateau pressures is unknown. However, a comprehensive evaluation of the underlying disease, achieved with a bedside recording of Pel/V curves appears to convey information of fundamental importance in the set up of lung protective ventilation, may it be in the form of ASPIDS or any other method.

The step wise-development of a computer/ventilator system that allows continuous monitoring as well as recording of pressure and flow rate has lead to a system for ASPIDS that may be clinically applied. The safety level of the system achieved by the combination of the internal safety system of the ventilator and the continuous automated control of the function of the complete system, together with the 100% oxygen safe valves permits it to be used in critically ill patients. However, the present system should still be regarded as experimental and it should be used under surveillance of a well-informed operator. A system for routine clinical use needs to be modified. A measurement for tracheal pressure distal to the site of aspiration in the tracheal should also be considered. When the tracheal pressure inappropriately deviates from the pressure measured in the ventilator the ASPIDS system should automatically be switched off. The safety flap valve, which in the present system makes patient triggering impossible, would be void.

References

1. Dreyfuss D, Saumon G (1993) Role of tidal volume, FRC, and end-inspiratory volume in the development of pulmonary oedema following mechanical ventilation. Am Rev Respir Dis 148: 1194-1203
2. Dreyfuss D, Saumon G (1998) Ventilator-induced lung injury. Lesson from experimental studies. Am J Respir Crit Care Med 157: 294-323
3. Dreyfuss D, Soler P, Basset G, Saumon G (1985) High inflation pressure pulmonary edema. Respective effects of high airway pressure, high tidal volume, and positive end expiratory pressure. Am Rev Respir Dis 132: 880-4
4. Mead J, Takishima T, Leith D (1970) Stress distribution in lungs: a model of pulmonary elasticity. J Appl Physiol 28: 596-608
5. Roupie E, Dambrosio M, Servillo G et al (1995) Titration of tidal volume and induced hypercapnia in acute respiratory distress syndrome. Am J Respir Crit Care Med 152: 121-128
6. Reynolds EOR (1971) Effect of alteration in mechanical ventilator settings on pulmonary gas excahnge in hyaline membrane disease. Arch Dis Child 46: 152-159
7. Jonson B (1982) Positive Airway Pressure: Some physical and biological effects. In: Prakash O (ed) Applied physiology in clinical respiratory care. Martinus Nijhoff, The Hague, pp 125-139
8. Lachmann B, Danzmann E, Haendly B, Jonson B (1982) Ventilator settings and gas exchange in respiratory distress syndrome. In: A Prakash O (ed) Applied physiology in clinical respiratory care. Martinus Nijhoff, The Hague, pp141-176
9. Lachmann B, Jonson B, Lindroth M, Robertson B (1982) Modes of artificial ventilation in severe respiratory distress syndrome. Crit Care Med 10 (11): 724-732
10. Wagner PD (1989) HFV and pulmonary physiology. Acta Anaesthesiol Scand 33 (S 90): 172-175
11. Jonson B (1989) Clinical aspects of HFV. Acta Anaesthesiol Scand 33 (S 90): 177-178
12. Jonson B, Lachmann B, Fletcher R (1989) Monitoring of physiological parameters during high frequency ventilation (HFV). Acta Anaesthesiol Scand 33 (S 90): 165-169
13. Dambrosio M, Roupie E, Mollet JJ et al (1997) Effects of PEEP and different tidal volumes on alveolar recruitment and hyperinflation. Anesthesiology 87: 495-503
14. Hickling KG (1998) The pressure-volume curve is greatly modified by recruitment. A mathematical model of ARDS lungs. Am J Respir Crit Care Med 158: 194-202

15. Gattinoni L, Pesenti A, Mascheroni D et al (1986) Low frequency positive pressure ventilation with extracorporeal CO_2 removal in severe acute respiratory failure. JAMA 256: 881-886
16. Jonson B, Similowski T, Levy P et al (1990) Expiratory flushing of airways: a method to reduce dead space ventilation. Eur Respir J 3: 1202-1205
17. Nahum A, Burke WC, Ravenscraft SA et al (1992) Lung mechanics and gas exchange during pressure controlled ventilation in dogs: augmentation of CO_2 elimination by an intratracheal catheter. Am Rev Respir Dis 146: 965-973
18. Ravenscraft SA, Burke WC, Nahum A et al (1993) Tracheal gas insufflation augments CO_2 clearance during mechanical ventilation. Am Rev Respir Dis 148: 345-351
19. Marini JJ (1996) Adjunctive ventilation with tracheal gas insufflation- Good vibrations? Crit Care Med 24(3): 375-377
20. Servillo G, Svantesson C, Beydon L et al (1997) Pressure-volume curves in acute respiratory failure. Automated low flow inflation versus occlusion. Am J Respir and Crit Care Med 155: 1629-1636
21. Svantesson C, Drefeldt B, Jonson B (1997) The static pressure-volume relationship of the respiratory system determined with a computer-controlled ventilator. Clinical Physiology 17: 419-430
22. Svantesson C, Drefeldt B, Sigurdsson S et al (1999) A single computer-controlled mechanical insufflation allows determination of the pressure-volume relationship of the respiratory system. J Clin Monit 15: 9-16
23. Servillo G, De Robertis E, Coppola M et al (2000) Application of a computerised method to measure static pressure volume curve in acute respiratory distress syndrome. Int Care Med 26: 11-14
24. Liu JM, De Robertis E, Blomquist S et al (1999) Elastic pressure-volume curves of the respiratory system reveal a high tendency to lung collapse in young pigs. Int Care Med 25: 1140-1146
25. De Robertis E, Liu JM, Blomquist S et al (2001) Elastic properties of the lung and chest wall in young and adult healthy pigs. Eur Respir J 17: 703-711
26. De Robertis E, Sigurdsson SE, Drefeldt B, Jonson B (1999) Aspiration of airway dead space: a new method to enhance CO_2 elimination. Am J Respir and Crit Care Med 159: 728-732
27. De Robertis E, Servillo G, Jonson B, Tufano R (1999) Aspiration of dead space allows normocapnic ventilation at low tidal volumes in man. Int Care Med 25: 674-679
28. De Robertis E, Servillo G, Tufano R, Jonson B (2001) Aspiration of Dead Space Allows Isocapnic Low Tidal Volume Ventilation in Acute Lung Injury. Relationships to Gas Exchange and Mechanics. Int Care Med in press
29. Boots RJ, Howe S, George N et al (1997) Clinical utility of hygroscopic heat and moisture exchangers in intensive care patients. Crit Care Med 25: 1707-1712
30. Jonson B, Richard JC, Straus C et al (1999) Pressure-volume curves in acute lung injury. Evidence of recruitment above the lower inflection point. Am J Respir Crit Care Med 159: 1172-1178
31. Gattinoni L, Pesenti A, Bombino M, et al (1988) A Relationships between lung computed tomographic density, gas exchange, and PEEP in acute respiratory failure. Anesthesiology 69: 824-832
32. Ranieri VM, Suter PM, Tortorella C et al (1999) Effect of mechanical ventilation on inflammatory mediators in patients with acute respiratory distress syndrome. A randomized Controlled Trial. JAMA 282 (1): 54-61
33. Amato MBP, Barbas CSV, Medeiros DM et al (1998) Effect of a protective-ventilation strategy on mortality in the acute respiratory distress syndrome. N Engl J Med 338 : 347-354
34. Ventilation with lower tidal volumes as compared with traditional tidal volumes for acute lung injury and the acute respiratory distress syndrome. The Acute Respiratory Distress Syndrome Network (2000). N Engl J Med 342 : 1301-1308

Myocardial Preservation during Cardiopulmonary Resuscitation

T. PELLIS, W. TANG

Sudden cardiac death accounts for 300,000 to 400,000 deaths annually in the United States, it is the most common and often first manifestation of coronary heart disease and is responsible for approximately 50% of mortality for cardiovascular diseases in the United States and other developed countries [1-2]. Sudden cardiac death describes the unexpected natural death from a cardiac cause within a short period, generally ≤ 1 h our from onset of symptoms, in a person without any prior condition that would appear fatal [1]. Cardiopulmonary resuscitation (CPR) effectively restores haemodynamic stability and return to spontaneous circulation (ROSC) in 40% to 60% of arrests. Prolonged survival is significantly lower because of an underlying illness and postresuscitation syndrome, specifically central nervous system injury and left ventricular stunning after resuscitation [3].

Therefore despite the initial success of CPR a majority of victims die within 72 hours, primarily due to heart failure or recurrent ventricular fibrillation, yielding to a functional survival rate of only 1.4% to 5% [4-9]. After successful resuscitation from cardiac arrest myocardial function appears substantially impaired. Normal contractile and haemodynamic functions are restored to pre-arrest values over an interval of hours or days. Accordingly, global ischaemic injury has been demonstrated to reverse spontaneously in what has been termed *postresuscitation myocardial dysfunction* [10, 11].

Postresuscitation myocardial dysfunction with low postresuscitation survival

Postresuscitation myocardial dysfunction and its fatal outcome correspondingly have been documented, in part, in human patients. In the Brain Resuscitation Clinical Trial I [12], which included 12 hospitals in nine countries, 262 patients were resuscitated successfully. Approximately 70% died within the first 72 hours. During the first 8 hours after resuscitation, 117 (45%) patients manifested arterial hypotension, 68 (26%) patients experienced supraventricular and ventricular arrhythmias, and 66 (25%) had recurrent cardiac arrest as a primary event. In the Brain Resuscitation Clinical Trial II, which involved 24 hospitals in eight countries [5], 516 patients were resuscitated and 62% of the patients died within the first week. During the first 24 hours, 335 (65%) patients had systemic hypotension.

In studies of high-dose epinephrine six emergency centres enrolled 1280 victims of out-of-hospital cardiac arrests, and 407 (32%) patients were resuscitated [7]. Although 126 (10%) of these patients died prior to admission to the hospitals, 43% of the 281 remaining victims died during the first 72 hours. Arterial hypotension and fatal ventricular arrhythmias were identified as predominant causes. Only 57 (4.5%) were discharged from the hospitals. In a second multicentre study on high-dose epinephrine, 650 victims of cardiac arrests were enrolled. Spontaneous circulation was restored initially in 132 (21%) patients; however, a majority died within the first 48 hours and only 26 (4%) were discharged from the hospitals [8].

Cray et al. [13] reviewed 185 incidents of out-of-hospital cardiac arrest in their emergency department over a 19 month period. Only 16 patients (9%) were resuscitated successfully but none survived hospitalisation. For the 16 initial survivors, death was attributed to refractory hypotension in seven, fatal arrhythmias in five, and neurologic causes in the remaining four victims.

Initially, studies on postresuscitation myocardial dysfunction were performed on isolated, perfused hearts harvested from Sprague-Dawley rats. Progressive reductions in contractile function (dP/dtmax) were documented together with decreases in myocardial compliance and increases in the slope of the diastolic pressure-volume relationship after a 4-minute duration of ventricular fibrillation and successful resuscitation [10]. Subsequently, investigations were performed in domestic pigs. After a 4 minute interval of untreated ventricular fibrillation and an additional 8 minutes of precordial compression, the pigs were resuscitated successfully. Pressure volume loops of the left ventricle, which served as indicators of myocardial contractility, were strikingly reduced. Stroke volume was reduced to approximately 70% of pre-arrest values and ejection fraction decreased from 41% to 20% [11].

More recently, we confirmed the evidence of two discrete dysfunctions, namely *mechanical dysfunction* characterised by decreased systolic and diastolic function with or without hypotension and *electrical dysfunction* characterised by potentially fatal ectopic ventricular rhythms [14]. Both porcine and murine studies indicated an increase in the severity of both mechanical and electrical dysfunctions with increasing duration of untreated cardiac arrest. The severity also increased after administration of b-adrenergic agonists including epinephrine, during resuscitation, in settings of increasing myocardial hypercarbic acidosis, and after high energy electric defibrillations [15-17].

Clinical observations of patients are consistent with the experimental findings in animals. In three patients who were resuscitated from ventricular fibrillation after approximately 3, 10, and 30 minutes of cardiac arrest, transthoracic echocardiograms demonstrated decreased ejection fractions [18]. Myocardial function was near normal after 2 weeks and such victims typically had long term survival. Lewis et al. [19] reported that of the 248 patients who were discharged from the hospital, 77% survived for more than one year, with negligible deficits. Accordingly, there is substantial evidence that prevention of recurrent cardiac arrest associated with postresuscitation myocardial dysfunction would have a likelihood of improving meaningful survival.

For practical purposes, we also distinguish between two stages of CPR. The first stage is that of initial resuscitation for re-establishing an effective rhythm and spontaneous circulation. The second is that of reversing postresuscitation myocardial failure and ectopic ventricular rhythms and therefore the risk of recurrent cardiac arrest. The intent is to define mechanisms and ultimately interventions that prevent or reverse postresuscitation myocardial dysfunction such that the *ultimate* outcome of CPR may be improved. An increase in postresuscitation functional survival from the current 5% to as little as 10% would serve to rescue more than 50,000 lives each year, a number that conservatively exceeds the annual total of U.S. automobile fatalities of 43,000 in 1994 [20].

Mechanisms of postresuscitation myocardial dysfunction

Postischaemic myocardial dysfunction was initially attributed to the depletion of high energy phosphate stores [21] but the evidence has not fully sustained this hypothesis. The evidence that intracellular ATP is quantitatively predictive of contractile function and cellular viability is controversial [22, 23]. When nucleotide precursors of ATPase were administered by intracoronary infusion, myocardial function was *not* enhanced [24]. Moreover, myocardial contractility was increased after inotropic interventions even when ATP was reduced significantly [25-27]. Accordingly, postresuscitation myocardial dysfunction is more likely to be due to impaired energy usage than to a reduction in the energy supply.

The second and newer hypothesis, derived from studies on regional ischaemia, is that myocardial dysfunction represents a disturbance in Ca^{2+} homeostasis in the cardiomyocyte. Under normal conditions, intracellular Ca^{2+} is maintained at very low levels (<100 nM) by the ATP-dependent Ca^{2+} pump, which moves Ca^{2+} ions back to storage sites in the sarcoplasmic reticulum. In addition, there is electrogenic Na^+-Ca^{2+} exchange on the cell membrane. The action potential that prompts Ca^{2+} release from Ca^{2+} stores in the sarcoplasmic reticulum activates actin and myosin, resulting in contraction of myofibers. During ischaemia, the tissue pH is decreased by lactate production, degradation of high energy phosphate, and reduced removal of CO_2. In addition, free radicals are released by ischaemic tissue, resulting in injury to cell membranes and reduced Na^+-Ca^{2+} exchange. Sarcoplasmic reticulum at the same time fails to sequester Ca^{2+} such that cytosolic calcium concentration is increased. The consequent "calcium overload" reduces the capability of actin-myosin bridging. This is an explanation for reduced Ca^{2+}-triggered myocardial contractility in ischaemic or "stunned" myocardium [28, 29].

This hypothesis is supported in part by studies on the prophylactic use of calcium channel blockers in settings of regional myocardial ischaemia and their effects on postischaemic myocardial dysfunction [30, 31]. Calcium channel blockade minimizes postischaemic myocardial dysfunction. Although it also increases myocardial blood flow, decreases afterload by peripheral arterial vasodilation, and may have anti-inotropic actions, this evidence of calcium channel blocking benefit is not necessarily persuasive of a single action [32]. It is also apparent that calcium channel blockers act on voltage-gated calcium channels. They may not directly affect transport of calcium in the mitochondrial and sarcoplasmic reticulum [33, 34]. Moreover, the voltage-gated calcium channels fail to prevent significant influx of Ca^{2+} during the ischaemic interval, and therefore calcium channel blockers may be effective only if administered prior to the ischaemic insult [35].

The concept of ischaemic preconditioning was developed by Reimer et al. [36] in the course of their investigations on the relationship between high energy phosphate depletion during tissue ischaemia and accumulation of catabolites for explaining cell death. In a dog model, they occluded circumflex coronary blood flow for 5 minutes and then reperfused this artery for 5 minutes. When four of the 5-minute occlusion/reperfusion cycles were completed, the investigators occluded the left circumflex coronary artery of such "preconditioned" animals for 40 minutes. The magnitude of infarction in such "preconditioned" animals was only 25% of that of unpreconditioned controls [37]. An initial decline in ATP was observed, but successive ischaemic challenges failed to further reduce the ATP content of the myocardium. This suggested that myocytes adapted to repetitive ischaemic insults such that they were protected against more severe ischaemic insults that produced cell death. This was the genesis of the term "ischaemic preconditioning". The myocardial protective effect of ischaemic preconditioning in which infarct size was reduced was demonstrated subsequently in pigs [38], rabbits [39], and in rats [40]. Ischaemic preconditioning not only ameliorated myocardial contractile dysfunction [41], but also ischaemia-related ventricular dysrhythmias in isolated rat hearts [42], intact rats [43], rabbits [44], pigs [45], and, most significantly, in human patients [46, 47].

Ischaemic preconditioning was induced subsequently by hypoxic insults. Mei and Gross [48] demonstrated in dogs that perfusion of the left anterior descending coronary artery with blood in which PO_2 was reduced to between 30 and 40 mm Hg for an interval of 5 minutes significantly reduced infarct size after the same artery was occluded for a duration of 60 minutes. This protective effect was blocked by a KATP channel antagonist, glibenclamide. Rapid ventricular pacing of a 30-minute duration also minimised myocardial infarction in pigs, although such protection persisted for only 15 minutes. This protective effect again was abolished by glibenclamide [49]. The duration of the protective effect of following more conventional "ischaemic preconditioning" interventions is typically 1 hour [50-53]. Accordingly, the protective effect is dissipated when the interval between preconditioning and the actual ischaemic insult exceeds these time limits.

The role of KATP channel activation

Adenosine was initially suspected as the primary mediator of ischaemic preconditioning. Studies were performed by Liu et al. [54] on rabbits. Intracoronary infusion of adenosine or the A, receptor agonist R-PIA evoked preconditioning. The adenosine receptor antagonist PD 1151199 ablated the myocardial protective effects of ischaemic preconditioning. Adenosine itself decreased myocardial oxygen consumption comparable to that observed after preconditioning.

The adenosine hypothesis postulated coupling of adenosine receptors to G proteins [55]. G proteins activate protein kinase C through phospholipase C and the second messenger diacyl glycerol. The translocation of protein kinase C from cytosol to the cell membrane during ischaemia then may be implicated as a mechanism accounting for ischaemic preconditioning. At the time of this writing, the key role of protein kinase C is sustained but it is linked more directly to KATP channels through the important work of Gross et al. [56, 57]. Their findings prompted our interest in ischaemic preconditioning and its relationship to KATP channel function in settings of cardiac resuscitation.

In isolated perfused rat hearts, Behling et al. [58] investigated the effect of KATP channel activator, cromakalin, on intracellular Ca^{2+} during ischaemia and reperfusion using ^{19}F-NMR. These investigators demonstrated that the cytosolic Ca^{2+} concentration in control hearts increased from a pre-ischaemia level of 310 ± 40 nM to 1000 ± 130 nM after 25 minutes of global myocardial ischaemia. It was followed by partial recovery to 530 ± 100 nM during reperfusion. In contrast, the cytosolic Ca^{2+} concentration in hearts treated with cromakalin decreased from pre-ischaemia level of 240 ± 20 nM to 170 ± 30 nM after the same insult and returned to pre-ischaemia levels following reperfusion. KATP channel activator therefore prevented cytosolic Ca^{2+} overload in isolated, perfused hearts.

The myocardial protective effects of KATP channel activator have been demonstrated in several species. In guinea pigs, cromakalin significantly shortened the myocardial action potential duration to 59% of the baseline value. Improved post-ischaemic myocardial function was measured with a right ventricular force transducer. Only mild reductions in developed force of 20% were observed in cromakalin-treated isolated perfused guinea pig hearts after 20 minutes of ischaemia. This finding contrasted with results from perfused control hearts in which the contractile function was decreased by 66% of baseline values after the same duration of ischaemia and in the absence of KATP channel activation [59]. In isolated rat hearts, the KATP channel activator, nicorandil, significantly improved postischemic myocardial contractility and compliance after 45 minutes of global myocardial ischaemia [41]. Comparable observations have been reported in dogs [60], pigs [49], rabbits [61], and human myocardium [62].

This led to our current understanding that a brief ischaemic insult followed by reperfusion produces endogenous adenosine, which activates adenosine receptors. The activated adenosine receptors then couple with G proteins followed by activation of protein kinase C. This opens KATP channels to allow an efflux of potassium from cells during repolarisation [63]. Increases in extracellular potassium reduce the duration of the myocardial action potential and the time available for voltage-dependent calcium influx [59]. Intracellular Ca^{2+} therefore is maintained closer to physiologic levels, even though other Ca^{2+} extrusion mechanisms, including Ca^{2+} pumps are impaired when intracellular ATP is reduced. Myocardial oxygen consumption is reduced, myocardial ATP is preserved, and myocardial contraction during ischaemia is better sustained. More recent studies further demonstrated that opening KATP channels improves myocardial blood flow by selectively augmenting b_1-adrenoceptor-mediated coronary vasodilation [64]. Evidence supports the hypothesis that KATP channel activators provide myocardial protection both during ischaemia and reperfusion. KATP channel activators therefore may be appropriate alternatives to calcium channel blocking agents for preserving myocardial function both in settings of regional ischaemia and, we anticipate, in settings of global ischaemia of cardiac arrest and resuscitation

.

Nevertheless, the KATP channel activation hypothesis was challenged recently by Vegh et al. [65] and Parratt et al. [66], who reasoned that activation of the KATP channel would be proarrhythmic rather than antiarrhythmic. The powerful antiarrhythmic effect of ischaemic preconditioning therefore would remain unexplained. This group of investigators further postulated that the antiarrhythmic effect of ischaemic preconditioning stems from bradykinin (3_2 receptors that activate both L-arginine nitric oxide and cyclooxygenase pathways to produce nitric oxide and prostacyclin.

Although the bradykinin hypothesis is not excluded, activation of KATP channels remains the most likely mechanism that accounts for the myocardial protective effects of ischaemic preconditioning. The KATP channel mechanism complies with the criteria most recently proposed by Gross et al. [67] to explain ischaemic preconditioning, namely 1) pharmacological blocking of KATP channels with agents such as glibenclamide, which completely blocks the myocardial protective effects of ischaemic preconditioning; 2) pharmacological activation of KATP channels through cromakalin, which mimics the effects of ischaemic preconditioning; 3) mediators, which induce the ischaemic preconditioning-like effect, including adenosine, acetylcholine and bradykinin, which are blocked by KATP channel antagonists; 4) the time-course ("memory") of protection produced by the activators of KATP channels, which is comparable to that of ischaemic preconditioning; and 5) these conditions apply universally to mammalian species exclusive of rats. These criteria are convincing for us, explaining mechanisms of ischaemic preconditioning and indicating KATP channel function as it applies to myocardial ischaemic injury, and also suggesting the potential implications of KATP channel activators with respect to management of postresuscitation myocardial dysfunction.

Most recently, we have investigated the role of the KATP channel activator in settings of cardiac arrest and resuscitation in the rat model. The KATP channel activator cromakalin was injected into the right atrium of 500-g rats during untreated ventricular fibrillation. After successful resuscitation, the severity of postresuscitation myocardial dysfunction was reduced significantly compared with saline placebo. This agent also was associated with significantly increased postresuscitation duration of survival [68]. Moreover we investigated the effects of ischaemic preconditioning and activation of KATP channels on post resuscitation myocardial function. After 4 min of untreated ventricular fibrillation and 6 min of CPR defibrillation was attempted in Sprague-Dawley rats. Post resuscitation myocardial function and duration of survival, was significantly improved in both preconditioned and KATP channel opener-treated animals. KATP channel blocker administered 45 min before induction of ischaemic preconditioning completely abolished the myocardial protective effects of preconditioning [69]. We therefore confirmed the myocardial protective effects of KATP channel activator in settings of cardiac arrest and CPR; this may provide an option for improving postresuscitation myocardial dysfunction.

Conclusion

Despite the universal acceptance and implementation of modern CPR, the science of cardiac resuscitation is in its infancy. Myocardial preservation during CPR addresses a problem in which approximately 40% of cardiac arrest victims who are initially resuscitated but as few as 2% to 5% of these leave the hospital and are able to function. The magnitude of this issue deserves more comprehensive research.

References

1. Zipes DP, Wellens HJJ (1998) Sudden cardiac death. Circulation 98:2334-2351
2. American Heart Association (1991) Heart and Stroke Facts. Dallas: American Heart Association
3. Thel MC, O'Connor CM, Durham (1999) Cardiopulmonary resuscitation: Historical prespective to recent investigations. Am Heart J 137:39-48

4. Liberthson RR, Nagel EL, Hirschman JC (1974) Prehospital ventricular fibrillation. Prognosis and follow-up course. N Engl J Med 291:317-321
5. Brain Resuscitation Clinical Trial II Study Group (1991) A randomized clinical study of a calcium-entry blocker (lidoflazine) in the treatment of comatose survivors of cardiac arrest. N Engl J Med 324:1125-1231
6. Becker LB, Ostrander MP, Barrett J et al (1991) CPR Chicago: outcome of cardiopulmonary resuscitation in a large metropolitan area-where are the survivors? Ann Emerg Med 20:355-361
7. Brown CG, Martin DR, Pepe PE (1992) A comparison of standard-dose and high-dose epinephrine in cardiac arrest outside the hospital. N Engl JMed 327:1051-1055
8. Stiell IG, Herbert PC, Weitzman BN (1992) High-dose epinephrine in adult cardiac arres.t N Engl J Med 327:1045-1050
9. Lombardi G, Gallagher J, Gennis P (1994) Outcome of out-of-hospital cardiac arrest in New York city: the Pre-hospital Arrest Survival Evaluation (PHASE) study. JAMA 271:678-683
10. Tang W, Weil MH, Sun S et al (1993) Progressive myocardial dysfunction after cardiac resuscitation. Crit Care Med 21:1046-1050
11. Gazmuri RJ, Weil MH, Bisera J et al (1996) Myocardial dysfunction after successful resuscitation from cardiac arrest Crit Care Med 24:992-1000
12. Brain Resuscitation Clinical Trial I Study Group (1986) A randomized clinical study of thiopental loading in comatose survivors of cardiac arrest. N Engl J Med 314:397-403
13. Gray WA, Capone RJ, Most AS (1991) Unsuccessful emergency medical resuscitation-are continued efforts in the emergency department justified? N Engl J Med 325:1393-1398
14. Tang Z, Weil MH, Sun S et al (1997) High energy countershocks increase ventricular ectopy after successful CPR [abstract]. Crit Care Med 25:A57
15. Tang W, Weil MH, Sun S et al (1995) Epinephrine increases the severity of post-resuscitation myocardial dysfunction. Circulation 92:3089-3093
16. Sun SJ, Weil MH, Tang W et al (1996) Effects of buffer agents on post-resuscitation myocardial dysfunction. Crit Care Med 24:2035-2041
17. Xie J, Weil MH, Sun SJ et al (1997) High power defibrillation increases the severity of post-resuscitation myocardial dysfunction. Circulation 96:683-688
18. DeAntonio HJ, Kaul S, Lerman BB (1990) Reversible myocardial depression survivors of cardiac arrest. Pacing Clin Electrophysiol 13:982-985
19. Lewes SJ, Holmberg S, Quinn E (1993) Out-of-hospital resuscitation in EastSussex: 1981-1989. Br Heart J 70:568-573
20. United States Statistical Abstract 116th Edition, 1994
21. Steenbergen C, Murphy E, Watts JA et al (1990) Correlation between cytosolic free calcium, contracture, ATP, and irreversible ischemic injury in perfused rat heart. Circ Res 66:135-146
22. Murry CE, Richard VJ, Jennings RB et al (1991) Myocardial protection is lost before contractile function recovers from preconditioning. Am J Physiol 260:H796-H804
23. Johnson BA, Weil MH, Tang W et al (1995) Mechanisms of myocardial acidosis during arrest J Appl Physiol 78:1579-1584
24. Hoffmeister HM, Mauser M, Schaper W (1985) Effects of adenosine and AICAR on ATP content and regional contractile function in reperfused canine myocardium. Basic Res Cardiol 80:445-458
25. Kusuoka H, Porterfield JK, Weisman HF et al (1987) Pathophysiology and pathogenesis of stunned myocardium: depressed Ca^{2+} activation overload in ferret hearts. J Clin Invest 79:950-961
26. Schafer S, Heusch G (1990) Recruitment of a time-dependent inotropic reserve by postextrasystolic potentiation in normal and reperfused myocardium. Basic Res Cardiol 85:257-269
27. Kida M, Fujiwara H, Uegaito T et al (1993) Dobutamine prevents both myocardial stunning and phosphocreatine overshoot without affecting ATP level. J Mol Cell Cardiol 25:875-8135
28. Marban E (1991) Myocardial stunning and hibernation. The physiology behind the colloquialisms. Circulation 83:681-688

29. Li XY, McCay PB, Zughaib M et al (1993) Demonstration of free radical generation in the "stunned" myocardial in the conscious dog and identification of major differences between conscious and open-chest dogs. J Clin Invest 92:1025-1041
30. Ehring T, Bohm M, Heusch G (1992) The calcium antagonist shows the functional recovery of reperfused myocardium only when given before ischemia. J Cardiovasc Pharmacol 20:63-74
31. Du Toit EF, Opie LH (1992) Modulation of severity of reperfusion stunning in the isolated rat heart by agents altering calcium flux at the onset of reperfusion. Circ Res 70:960-967
32. Ehring T, Heusch G (1995) Stunned myocardium and the attenuation of stunning by calcium antagonists. Am J Cardiol 75:61E-67E
33. Schwartz A (1992) Molecular and cellular aspects of calcium channel antagonism. Am J Cardiol 70(suppl):6F-8F
34. Ferrari R, Visioli O (1994) How do calcium antagonists differ in clinical practice? Cardiovasc Drug Ther 8:565-575
35. Tanskela JS, Shoubridge EA (1996) Intercellular calcium dynamics and cellular energetics in ischemic cells studied by concurrent and doublequantum filtered spectroscopy. J Neurochem 66:266-276
36. Reimer KA, Murry CE, Yamasawa I et al (1986) Four brief periods of ischemia cause no cumulative ATP loss or necrosis. Am J Physiol 251:H1306-H1305
37. Murry CE, Jennings RB, Reimer KA (1986) Preconditioning with ischemia: a delay of lethal cell injury in ischemic myocardium. Circulation 74:1124-1136
38. Schott RJ, Rohmann S, Braun ER et al(1990) Ischemic preconditioning reduces infarct size in swine myocardium. Circ Res 66:1133-1142
39. Iwamoto T, Miura T, Adachi T et al (1991) Myocardial infarct size-limiting effect if ischemic preconditioning was not attenuated by oxygen free-radical scavengers in the rabbit. Circulation 83:1015-1022
40. Yellon DM, Alkhulaifi AM, Browne EE et al (1992) Ischemic preconditioning limits infarct size in the rat heart. Cardiovasc Res 26:983-987
41. Menasche P, Kevelaitis E, Mouuas C et al (1995) Preconditioning with potassium channel openers: a new concept for enhancing cardioplegic protection? J Thorac Cardiovasc Surg 110:1606-1614
42. Takeda S, Satoh T, Osada M et al (1995) Protective effect of pacing on reperfusion-induced ventricular arrhythmias in isolated rat hearts. Can J Cardiol 11:573-579
43. Shiki K, Hearse DJ (1987) Preconditioning of ischemic myocardium: reperfusion-induced arrhythmias. Am J Physiol 253:H1470-H1476
44. Cohen MV, Liu GS, Downey JM (1991) Preconditioning causes improved wall motion as well as smaller infarcts after transient coronary occlusion in rabbits. Circulation 84:341-349
45. Sun JZ, Tang XL, Park SW et al (1996) Evidence for an essential role of reactive oxygen species in the genesis of late preconditioning against myocardial stunning in conscious pigs. J Clin Invest 97:562-576
46. Xu C, Chen Y, Lu M (1995) A clinical study on limitation of infarct size ischemic preconditioning in 100 cases of acute myocardial infraction. Chung Hua Nei Ko Tsa Chih 34:16-18
47. Pasceri V, Lanza GA, Patti G (1996) Preconditioning by transient myocardial ischemia confers protection against ischemia-induced ventricular arrhythmias in variant angina. Circulation 94:1850-1856
48. Mei DA, Gross GJ (1995) Evidence for the involvement of the ATP-sensitive potassium channel in a novel model of hypoxic preconditioning in dogs. Cardiovasc Res 30:222-230
49. Koning MM, Gho BC, van Klaarwater E et al (1996) Rapid ventricular pacing produces myocardial protection by nonischemic activation of KATP channels. Circulation 93:178-186
50. Murphy E, Penman M, London RE et al (1991) Amiloride delays the ischemic-induced rise in cytosolic free calcium. Circ Res 68:1250-1258
51. Van Winkle DM, Thornton RB, Downey JM (1991) Cardioprotection from ischemic preconditioning is lost following prolonged reperfusion in the rabbit. Coron Artery Dis 2:613-619

52. Li YW, Whittaker P, Kloner RA (1992) The transient nature of the effect of ischemic preconditioning on myocardial infarct size and ventricular arrhythmia. Am Heart J 123:346-353
53. Simkhovich BA, Whittaker P, Przyklenk K et al (1995) Transient preischemic acidosis protects the isolated rabbit heart subject to 30 minutes, but not 60 minutes, of global ischemia. Basic Res Cardiol 90:397-403
54. Liu GS, Thornton J, Van Win et al (1991) Protection against infarction afforded by preconditioning is mediated by A1, adenosine receptors in the rabbit heart. Circulation 84:350-356
55. Thornton JD, Liu GS, Downey JM (1993) Pretreatment with pertussis toxin blocks the protective effects of preconditioning: evidence for a Gprotein mechanism. J Mol Cell Cardiol 25:311-320
56. Gross GJ, Auchampach JA (1992) Blockade of ATP-sensitive potassium channels prevents myocardial preconditioning in dogs. Circ Res 70:223-233
57. Auchampach JA, Grover GJ, Gross GJ (1992) Blockade of ischemic preconditioning in dogs by the novel ATP dependent potassium channel antagonist sodium 5-hydroxydecanoate. Cardiovasc Res 26:1054-1062
58. Behling RW, Malone HJ (1995) KATP-channel openers protect against increased cytosolic calcium during ischemia and reperfusion. J Mol Cell Cardiol 27:1809-1817
59. Shigematsu S, Sato T, Abe T (1995) Pharmacological evidence for the persistent activation of ATP-sensitive K^+ channels in early phase of reperfusion and its protective role against myocardial stunning. Circulation 92:2266-2275
60. Mizumura T, Nithipatikom K, Gross GJ (1995) Bimakalin, an ATP-sensitive potassium channel opener, mimics the effects of ischemic preconditioning to reduce infarct size, adenosine release, and neutrophil function in dogs. Circulation 92:1236-1245
61. Lawton JS, Sepic JD, Allen CT et al (1996) Myocardial protection with potassium-channel openers is as effective as St Thomas' solution in the rabbit heart. Ann Thorac Surg 61:31-38
62. Cleveland JC, Meldrum DR, Rowland RT et al (1997) Adenosine preconditioning of human myocardium is dependent upon the ATP-sensitive K channel. J Mol Cell Cardiol 29:175-182
63. Liu Y, Gao WD, O'Rourke B (1996) Synergistic modulation of ATP-sensitive K^+ currents by protein kinase C and adenosine. Implications for ischemic preconditioning. Circ Res 78:443-454
64. Katsuda Y, Egashira K, Ueno H et al (1996) ATP-sensitive K^+ channel opener pinacidil augments b_1-adrenoceptor-induced coronary vasodilation in dogs. Am J Physiol 270:H2210-H2215
65. Vegh A, Papp JG, Parratt J (1994) Attenuation of the antiarrhythmic effects of ischemic preconditioning by blockage of bradykinin Bs receptors. Br J Pharmacol 113:1167-1172
66. Parratt J, Vegh A, Papp JG (1995) Pronounced antiarrhythmic effects of ischemic preconditioning-are there possibilities for pharmacological exploitation? Pharmacol Res 31:225-234
67. Gross GJ, Mei DA, Schultz JJ (1996) Criteria for a mediator or effector of myocardial preconditioning: do KATP channels meet the requirements? Basic Res Cardiol 91:31-34
68. Tang W, Weil MH, Sun SJ (1997) KATP channel activation improves post resuscitation myocardial function [abstract]. Circulation 96:1366
69. Tang W, Weil MH, Sun S et al (2000) K(ATP) channel activation reduces the severity of post resuscitation myocardial dysfunction. Am J Physiol Heart Circ Physiol 279: H1609-H1615

Reduced Post-Resuscitation Myocardial Dysfunction after Low-energy Biphasic Waveform Defibrillation

T. Pellis, W. Tang

Approximately one half of the 2 million deaths that occur each year in the United States are due to cardiovascular disease. Of these, approximately one-third or 350,000 occur suddenly and outside of the hospital. Each minute in the United States one person is the victim of "sudden (cardiac) death" and almost one half of the victims are under 65 years of age [1]. Though the initial success of cardiopulmonary resuscitation (CPR) is approximately 39% (range 13 to 59%), a majority of these victims die within 72 hours, primarily due to heart failure and/or recurrent ventricular fibrillation. CPR itself therefore yields a functional survival rate of only 1.4 to 5% [2,3]. After successful resuscitation from cardiac arrest myocardial function is substantially impaired such that normal contractile and haemodynamic function are restored over an interval of hours or days. Accordingly, there is evidence that the global ischaemic injury is spontaneously reversed. This has been termed "post-resuscitation myocardial dysfunction" (PRMD), which was initially observed during controlled studies in both pigs and rats [4,5].

Characteristics of PRMD

Initial studies on PRMD were performed on both rat and pig models of cardiac arrest and resuscitation. In rats, after successful resuscitation from a 4 minute duration of VF, progressive reductions in contractile function were documented together with decreases in myocardial compliance and increases in the slope of the diastolic pressure-volume relationship [4]. In pigs, after a 4 minute interval of untreated VF and an additional 8 minutes of precordial compression, pressure volume loops of the left ventricle were strikingly reduced. Stroke volume was reduced to approximately 70% of pre-arrest values and ejection fraction from 41 to 20% [5].

More recently, two discrete dysfunctions were confirmed, namely mechanical dysfunction characterised by decreased systolic and diastolic function and electrical dysfunction characterised by potentially fatal ectopic ventricular rhythms [6]. Both porcine and murine studies indicated that the severity of both mechanical and electrical dysfunctions were increased with increasing duration of untreated cardiac arrest. The severity was also increased after administration of ß-adrenergic agonists, including epinephrine during resuscitation, in settings of increasing myocardial hypercarbic acidosis, and after high energy electrical defibrillations [6-9].

High energy defibrillation increases the severity of PRMD

After direct current transthoracic defibrillation was introduced for the treatment of VF, both the magnitude and duration of the transthoracic electrical shock utilized for defibrillation from VF were suspects of causes of myocardial injury. In isolated tissue cultures of myocardial cells, irregularities of contraction followed a single shock with a peak intensity of either 80 or 200 V/cm [10]. Synchronized shocks with an energy of 35 joules applied directly to the fibrillating canine ventricle significantly decreased cardiac output [11]. After cardiac arrest in dogs, a transthoracic 400 joule countershock produced both histological and metabolic impairment of myocardial cells [12]. After successful defibrillation of patients who sustained cardiac arrest, post-resuscitation hypotension and decreased post-resuscitation survival were documented [13].

More recent studies have implicated the total electrical energy delivered during defibrillation attempts as a correlation of the severity of PRMD and survival. After 4 minutes of untreated VF and 6 additional minutes of precordial compression, a single 2, 10, 20 J countershock restored spontaneous circulation. The severity of PRMD in this rat model increased in close relationship to the increases of the electrical energy delivered. The duration of post-resuscitation survival was inversely related to the total energy delivered. Animals survived for more than 24 hours after 2 J of energy, decreasing to 15 and 5 hours after 10 and 20 J, respectively. We therefore anticipated lesser PRMD and improved survival with low-energy shocks provided that the energy delivered was adequate for successful defibrillation [8].

Low-energy biphasic waveform defibrillation

Currently available defibrillators utilize two waveform morphologies. Biphasic waveforms deliver both positive and negative current with evidence of successful defibrillation utilizing significant lower energy levels. During the past two decades, biphasic waveform defibrillation has been examined in experimental and clinical settings of VF. Lower biphasic waveform defibrillation energy requirements have been demonstrated in short-duration VF in both animals and humans [13-15]. More recently, in victims of out-of-hospital settings of prolonged VF (6-9 min), there were a greater number of successful defibrillations with 150 J impedance-compensating biphasic waveform shocks when compared with conventional monophasic waveform [15-17], validating the potential benefits of lower defibrillation energies.

In a randomized clinical study, the effects of fixed, low-energy biphasic waveform defibrillation on the initial success of defibrillation, on the likelihood of restoration of spontaneous circulation, on the incidence of hospital admission, and on the number of victims discharged from the hospital were compared with conventional escalating monophasic waveform defibrillation [18]. Biphasic defibrillation waveform with a fixed energy of 150 J significantly improved the efficacy of successful defibrillation (98% vs 67%, p.<0001) when compared with conventional monophasic defibrillation. This was associated with a significantly greater rate of restoration of spontaneous circulation (76% vs 55%, p.<02).

In an isolated rat heart model, Gazmuri et al. [19] demonstrated that repetitive low-energy electrical shocks do not accentuate PRMD. In our porcine model of cardiac arrest and resuscitation, the effects of low-energy biphasic wave defibrillation and conventional escalating energy monophasic defibrillation on post-resuscitation myocardial function were compared [20]. Fixed low-energy biphasic waveform defibrillation significantly reduced the severity of post-resuscitation myocardial systolic and diastolic dysfunction when compared with escalating high energy conventional monophasic waveform defibrillation after either short (4 minutes), intermediate (7 minutes), or prolonged (10 minutes) duration of cardiac arrest. Our results are consistent with those observed on human patients during implantation of cardioverter-defibrillator. Reddy RK et al [21] found a significantly greater elevation of ST-segment after 200 J monophasic waveform defibrillation when compared with 115 or 130 J biphasic waveform defibrillation.

Both experimental and clinical data confirm that biphasic waveform shocks with a fixed energy of 150 joules were at least as effective as conventional sequential monophasic waveform with progressive energy levels of 200, 300, and 360 joules for successful defibrillation following prolonged cardiac arrest. However the low-energy biphasic waveform shocks significantly decreased the severity of PRMD. The low-energy biphasic waveform defibrillation is therefore likely to be the future direction of transthoracic defibrillation in settings of cardiopulmonary resuscitation.

References

1. Becker LB, Ostrander MP, Barrett J et al (1991) CPR Chicago: outcome of cardiopulmonary resuscitation in a large metropolitan area - where are the survivors? Ann Emerg Med 20:355-361
2. Brown CG, Martin DR, Pepe PE (1992) A comparison of standard-dose and high-dose epinephrine in cardiac arrest outside the hospital. N Engl J Med 327:1051-1055
3. Lombardi G, Gallagher J, Gennis P (1994) Outcome of out-of-hospital cardiac arrest in New York City: the Pre-hospital Arrest Survival Evaluation (PHASE) study. JAMA 271(9):678-683
4. Tang W, Weil MH, Sun S et al (1993) Progressive myocardial dysfunction after cardiac resuscitation. Crit Care Med 21: 1046-1050
5. Gazmuri RJ, Weil MH, Bisera J et al (1996) Myocardial dysfunction after successful resuscitation from cardiac arrest. Crit Care Med 24:992-1000
6. Tang W, Weil MH, Sun S et al (1995) Epinephrine increases the severity of post-resuscitation myocardial dysfunction. Circulation 92:3089-3093
7. Sun SJ, Weil MH, Tang W et al (1996) Effects of buffer agents on post- resuscitation myocardial dysfunction. Crit Care Med 24:2035-2041
1. Xie J, Weil MH, Sun S et al (1997) High energy defibrillation increases the severity of post-resuscitation myocardial dysfunction. Circulation 96:683-688
8. Jones JL, Proskauer CC, Paull WK et al (1980) Ultrastructural injury to chick myocardial cells in vitro following "electric countershock". Circ Res 46:387-394
9. Gazmuri RJ (2000) Effects of repetitive electrical shocks on post-resuscitation myocardial dysfunction. Crit Care Med 28:N228-N232
10. Osswald S, Trouton TG, O'Nunain SS et al (1994) Relation between shock-related myocardial injury and defibrillation efficacy of monophasic and biphasic shocks in a canine model. Circulation 90:2501-2509
11. Niemann JT, Adomian GE, Garner D et al (1985) Endocardial and transcutaneous cardiac pacing, calcium chloride, and epinephrine in postcountershock asystole and bradycardias. Crit Care Med 13:699-704
12. Weaver WD, Cobb LA, Copass MK et al (1982) Ventricular fibrillation-A comparative trial using 175-J and 320-J shocks. N Engl J Med 307:1101-1106
13. Jones J, Swartz J, Jones R et al (1990) Increasing fibrillation duration enhances relative asymmetrical biphasic versus monophasic defibrillation waveform efficacy. Circ Res 67:376-84
14. Bardy G, Marchlinski F, Sharma A (1996) Multicenter comparison of truncated biphasic shocks and standard damped sine wave monophasic shocks for transthoracic ventricular defibrillation. Circulation 94:2507-2514
15. Gliner BE, Jorgenson DB, Poole JE (1998) Treatment of out-of-hospital cardiac arrest with a low-energy impedance-compensating biphasic Waveform automatic external defibrillator. Biomedical Instrumentation & Technology. 32:631-644
16. White RD (1997) Early out-of-hospital experience with an impedance compensating low-energy biphasic waveform automatic external defibrillator. J Intervent Card electrophysiol 1:203-208

17. Poole JE, White RD, Kanz KG (1997) Low-energy impedance compensating biphasic waveforms terminate ventricular fibrillation at high rates in victims of out-of-hospital cardiac arrest. J Cardiovasc Electrophysiol 8:1375-85
18. Schneider T, Martens Ppaschen HR, Wolcke B et al (1999) Prospective, randomized trial demonstrating improved defibrillation and post-shock neurologic status after use of 150J biphasic waveforms on cardiac arrest victims. Circulation 100:I315
19. Gazmuri RJ, Deshmukh S, Shah PR (2000) Myocardial effects of repeated electrical defibrillation in isolated fibrillating rat heart. Crit Care Med 28: 2690-2696
20. Tang W, Weil MH, Sun SJ et al (1999) The effects of biphasic and conventional monophasic defibrillation on post-resuscitation myocardial function. J Am Coll Cardiol 34:815-822
21. Reddy RK, Gleva MJ, Gliner BE et al (1997) Biphasic transthoracic defibrillation causes fewer ECG ST-segment changes after shock. Ann Emerg Med 30:127-134

Myocardial Dysfunction in the Perioperative Period

O. F. Boyd

Perioperative myocardial dysfunction is an important cause of post-operative mortality and morbidity, due to myocardial infarction and sudden death and also due to changes in vital organ perfusion caused by myocardial failure. This contribution will describe methods of pre-operative risk stratification that can be used to identify patients at risk of post-operative myocardial dysfunction and will describe what goes wrong with myocardial function during the perioperative period. Furthermore it will discuss techniques and treatment that can be employed to prevent post-operative myocardial dysfunction, and the consequences of this.

Preoperative risk stratification

There are a number of tests that can be used to pre-operatively stratify patients for risk of post-operative myocardial dysfunction. These can be divide into general tests and scores, and those specific for myocardial problems, specifically post-operative myocardial infarction and sudden cardiac death.

General preoperative risk stratification

Two well known cardiac risk indices are the Goldman index and the Detsky index. The Goldman index gives scores for a number of cardiac conditions, the higher the overall score the greater the risk of cardiac events [1]. The second index was developed by Detsky and colleagues with similar results [2]. However it is well known that other factors influence outcome, for example in abdominal aortic aneurysm repair renal and lung function are more important than age [3]. The situation is also complicated by the fact that intra and post-operative factors also influence the outcome of surgical procedures [4], and therefore no pre-operative system will be completely accurate. The established cardiac risk indexes increase accuracy by having odds ratios of 0.642

confidence interval (CI), 0.588 to 0.695) for the Goldman index, 0.601 (CI, 0.544 to 0.657) for the modified Detsky index, and 0.654 (0.601 to 0.708) for the Canadian Cardiovascular Society index [5].

Because myocardial dysfunction can account for other poor outcomes as well as poor cardiac outcomes, more general outcome scoring systems can also be used. One of these that is widely used in perioperative patients is the POSSUM score [6]. This is generally accepted to be a good scoring system for routine use [7], and is better than the APACHE system for a general surgical group of patients [8]. However, POSSUM scoring may not be universally applicable. In ruptured abdominal aortic aneurysms the POSSUM scoring was not a good predictor of outcome and the APACHE scoring was better [9]. However the APACHE score, while being better for the group of patients, was not good at discrimination between those that survived and those that died [9]. Other variations of POSSUM scoring have been suggested and may work better in gastrointestinal [10] and vascular surgery [11]. Furthermore, in one study the POSSUM scoring has been used as part of a risk stratification analysis to identify patients who might benefit from post-surgical high dependency or Intensive care unit (ICU) care [12].

A slightly different approach has been taken by Older and colleagues who have performed preoperative cardiopulmonary testing to define an anaerobic threshold in patients in the pre-operative period [13, 14]. In an initial study of 187 patients, there were 55 patients in whom the anaerobic threshold was less than 11 ml/min/kg and of these, 10 died (mortality rate of 18 %). There were 132 patients with an anaerobic threshold greater than 11 ml/min/kg and of these, 1 patient died (mortality rate of 0.8%). Low anaerobic threshold associated with preoperative ischaemia on the ECG resulted in the death of 8 out of 19 patients (mortality rate of 42%). When the ischaemia was associated with the higher anaerobic threshold, then 1 patient out of 25 died (mortality rate of 4 %) [13]. This work has been taken further, by describing different treatment paths for the high and low anaerobic threshold groups, and although this is not a randomized trial, the results show that greater degrees of intervention in the low anaerobic threshold group reduce mortality [14].

Preoperative risk stratification for myocardial events

There are many methods to investigate cardiac function and coronary artery perfusion, and it is hardly surprising that many have been investigated for their ability to risk stratify surgical patients. It is disappointing that while many of these can clearly identify different risks, there is very little information that the outcome is improved by knowing the risk. This is because there are very few studies assessing the utility of different treatment regimens in high risk patients.

A recent study has confirmed that exercise stress testing can be a useful method of risk stratification. Gauss and colleagues showed that a ST-segment depression of 0.1 mV or more in the exercise electrocardiogram (ECG) had an odds ratio of 5.2 (95% CI, 1.5 18.5; P = 0.01) of predicting a myocardial infarction or post-operative myocardial cell injury in non-cardiac surgery patients [15]. A combination of clinical variables and exercise electrocardiography improved preoperative risk stratification.

Other studies have used echocardiography and stress echocardiography to risk stratify surgical patients. A study of 570 patients undergoing non-cardiac surgery showed that left ventricular hypertrophy, mitral regurgitation and a significant aortic valve gradient were all predictors of major post-operative cardiac events [16]. However, an earlier study had found that adding echocardiographic information to established predictive models containing known clinical risk factors did not alter sensitivity, specificity, or predictive values in a clinically important way [17].

Adding stress to the cardiac image produced by the echocardiography might accentuate potential abnormalities. Dobutamine stress echocardiography related hypotension has been found to be predictive of perioperative cardiac events [18]. In another study dobutamine stress echocardiography had incremental value over clinical, electrocardiographic and rest echocardiographic variables for identifying patients at low, intermediate and high-risk for postoperative cardiac events, with ischaemia occurring at less than 60% of age-predicted maximal heart rate in identified patients at highest-risk [19]. Wall motion abnormalities on dobutamine stress echocardiography provide useful prognostic information that is enhanced by also considering rest-wall motion, stress ECG response, and dobutamine induced ejection fraction changes [20]. There might potentially be many patients who could enter groups requiring screening by stress echocardiography. A recent study investigated the additional predictive value of dobutamine stress echocardiography and found it to be limited in clinically low-risk patients receiving β-blockers [21]. The authors concluded that in clinical practice, dobutamine stress echocardiography may be avoided in a large number of patients who can proceed safely for surgery without delay. In clinically intermediate and high-risk patients receiving β-blockers, dobutamine stress echocardiography may help identify those in whom surgery can still be performed and those in whom cardiac revascularization should be considered [21].

Other stress echocardiographic techniques such as dipyridamole echocardiography have also been used. The relative risk of having a cardiac event if dipyridamole echocardiography was abnormal was 78 (95% CI, 11 to 564; $p < 0.0001$) in one study [22]. In a comparison of exercise and pharmacological stress echocardiography, for a group of 136 at risk patients with a predominance of one-vessel coronary artery disease, the overall diagnostic accuracy of stress echocardiography tests was higher for exercise than for dobutamine or dipyridamole [23]. Furthermore echocardiography may be superior to the routine use of dipyridamole thallium-201 scintigraphy for screening of intermediate-risk patients [24], although future information may provide an independent additional risk assessment [25].

What goes wrong with myocardial function perioperatively?

The two main pathological processes that inhibit cardiac function during the perioperative period are ischaemia and "pump failure" which is caused by inadequate pre-load and myocardial cell dysfunction. Traditionally the emphasis has been on ischaemia as the major influence in post-operative cardiac problems. This is probably because the pathological changes, such as myocardial infarction, could be relatively easily identified and also because monitoring for ischaemic events was thought to be effective with the use of a perioperative ECG recording and the development of a continuous ST-segment analysis. More recently the importance of inadequate cardiac filling and inflammation as important causes of perioperative myocardial dysfunction have been recognized. By understanding the importance of these influences therapy can be directed in a rational way. Good perioperative cardiac function is vital to maintain tissue perfusion in the perioperative time.

Ischaemia

Recent studies have confirmed the hypothesis that ischaemia is a major cause of cardiac dysfunction. Studying 1,023 patients undergoing cardiac surgery, Slogoff and Keats [26] showed that ECG ischaemia occurred in 36.9% of patients, and that post-operative myocardial infarction was almost three times as frequent in patients with ischaemia (6.9% vs. 2.5%) and was independent when ischaemia occurred. They also showed that this was significant to tachycardia but not hypertension nor hypotension. These findings have been confirmed in non-cardiac surgery patients with ischaemia being common during the perioperative period, occurring in up to 42% of patients at risk of coronary artery disease [27]. The ischaemic events can occur up to a week after the operation and are often associated with tachycardia [28]. Ischaemic events have been reported in various types of surgery such as cataract surgery where patients have a 31% ischaemia rate, with general anaesthesia slightly worse than local anaesthesia [29], and carotid surgery where a 20% ischaemia rate has been reported, again with general anaesthesia having a worse rate than local anaesthesia, although the clinical consequences were not significantly different [30]. Patients undergoing transurethral resection of the prostate have an 18% incidence of myocardial ischaemia, the degree of ischaemia being related to the amount of prostate tissue resected and greater blood loss [31]. Other studies show no relationship with local or general anaesthesia but show that ischaemia is related to blood pressure and heart rate excursions [32].

However, the issue is not as clear as would be expected because the link between perioperative ischaemia and post-operative clinical outcome, in terms of post-operative myocardial infarction, has not been confirmed. For example in vascular surgery patients 40% showed ST-segment changes but no relationship could be found between troponin T release, used as a marker of myocardial damage, and the magnitude of ST-depression or the number of ST-depression episodes [33]. Furthermore, postoperative exercise stress tests performed in patients who have significant ST-segment changes in the perioperative period are not necessarily positive, indicating that many patients may not have significant coronary artery disease, and that the ST-segment changes may be caused by other factors [34].

Another perioperative risk factor is tachycardia, which is closely related to ischaemia. Studies have shown this to be a poor risk factor, but it is unclear whether tachycardia carries the risk or whether tachycardia occurs as a result of other factors, such as inadequate fluid replacement therapy. Rao and colleagues showed that tachycardia was a particularly poor risk factor if accompanied by hypertension [35]. Other work has showed that tachycardia is common, when associated with ischaemic episodes (57%) [27, 28].

As mentioned above the cause of tachycardia may be important in its own right. Rosenberg and colleagues showed that post-operative hypoxaemia appeared to be related to cardiac dysrhythmias [36]. Recently, a study of 100 unselected patients has shown that postoperative oxygen therapy increased arterial oxygen saturation and decreased heart rate after uncomplicated abdominal surgery in a consecutive unselected group of patients who received routine postoperative care [37].

Pump failure

Further to the already discussed causes of myocardial dysfunction there are other negative influences on myocardial function less easy to define. When considering an individual patient there are frequent multi-factorial effects and the importance of these depends on the pre-existing myocardial function and the physiological reserve of the patient. For purposes of discussion these can be divided into dysfunction of the cardiac muscle, abnormalities of cardiac pre-load (ventricular filling), and alterations in cardiac after-load (vascular resistance).

There are numerous problems with cardiac muscle function that can occur during the perioperative period. These include dysrhythmias, the myocardial depressant effects of drugs, particularly anaesthetic agents, and metabolic effects. The metabolic effects can be caused by underlying problems requiring the surgery, such as vomiting resulting in a low serum potassium, or may occur after the surgery, such as increased fluid and electrolyte losses from upper gastrointestinal fistulae. Dysrhythmias can occur for a multitude of reasons, in the perioperative period these might be related to electrolyte disturbances or variations in cardiac perfusion due to changes in blood volume. Various drugs used during the perioperative period can have myocardial depressant effects. These can be direct depressant effects of the drugs themselves, for example many of the anaesthetic agents, or may be related to vasodilatation and reduction of intrinsic sympathetic tone. Vasodilatation is also caused by many anaesthetic drugs and this may result in a drop in blood pressure which may in turn impair myocardial perfusion in cases of increased myocardial wall tension of the failing ventricle, or in cases of significant coronary arterial disease. There are also rare but important causes of myocardial dysfunction such as allergic reactions which, in conjunction with vasodilatation, will include direct myocardial depression effects. Frequently a many of these problems enumerated above will link to others and form a vicious circle.

As the physiological reserve of the myocardium is impaired by age, pre-existing disease or various myocardial muscle problems discussed, the maintenance of an adequate cardiac output will rely on appropriate filling and dilatation of the cardiac chambers. Starlings Law of the Heart describes the relationship between the stretch of the myocardial fibrils and the development of contraction power. In the perioperative patient numerous factors converge to effect the relative fluid status of the body. The ritual of surgical preparation with pre-operative starvation and bowel preparation renders patients relatively hypovolaemic. Then the disease process requiring surgery may have additional effects, particularly in cases of haemorrhage, vomiting, diarrhoea and bowel obstruction.

At the time of surgery, anaesthetic drugs cause vasodilatation and relative dehydration, and this may be exaggerated by the vasodilatation of the epidural or spinal anaesthesia. Positive pressure ventilation results in increases in intrathoracic pressure which impairs cardiac compliance and reduces venous return. In all these instances an increase in intravascular volume is required as an appropriate compensatory mechanism. In the post-operative period there may be hidden fluid losses as a result of fluid redistribution into the extra-vascular space, as well as hidden haemorrhage. And there may be overt losses due to haemorrhage, gastrointestinal loss and pyrexia.

In the perioperative period there are also changes in cardiac after-load, both increases and decreases can be seen. Increases in after-load can result from thromboembolism, excessive vasoconstriction, or surgical procedures such as aortic cross-clamping. Decreases in after-load have been eluded to the above and result from excessive vasodilatation, as seen in sepsis or anaesthetic agents.

On a more theoretical basis, it has become increasingly recognized that inflammatory mediators, particularly cytokines are involved in cardiac dysfunction [38, 39]. It is also well known that surgery and the perioperative period is a potent stimulator of inflammatory cytokines [40, 41]. It is worthwhile to consider the role inflammatory products in myocardial depression during the perioperative period.

Strategies of preventing perioperative myocardial dysfunction

Avoidance of ischaemia

There are two small trials which investigated the use of β-blockade in surgical patients. Mangano and colleagues gave atenolol in a randomized trial of 100 patients [42], which showed a late effect on mortality reaching significance at 6 months. Poldermans and colleagues, used perioperative bisoprolol in a randomized trial of 59 patients [43]. Despite the small size of the earlier trial the American College of Cardiology formally recommended that β-blockade should be used in surgical patients at risk of ischaemic events [44]. This author considers this recommendation to be premature due to outstanding issues not addressed and the small size of the trials. Others have come to the same conclusion [45], particularly in patients at low or intermediate risk, questioning issues of β-blockade in emergency surgery, particularly with hypovolaemia, sepsis and haemorrhage, and pointing out that there is no information on the interaction of β-blockade and epidural anaesthesia for post-operative pain relief [45]. Even at a theoretical level the presumed link between perioperative tachycardia, ischaemia and post-operative myocardial infarction is not clear [46, 47]. Moreover there are a number of safety issues regarding the perioperative use of β-blockade. Both Mangano [42] and Poldermans [43] report a very low incidence of side-effects, much lower than other studies using β-blockers albeit in differing contexts [48]. A further complicating issue is found in the study of Mangano relating to the delayed reduction in mortality at 6 months

[42]. Fleisher [46] has pointed out that the placebo group in Mangano's study [42] had a higher incidence of coronary artery disease than the treatment group and a significantly lower incidence of pre-operative β-blocker therapy, which continued in the post-operative period. This suggests that the survival benefit found by Mangano [42] could be demonstrating the benefit of the long term β-blockade in patients with established coronary artery disease. Furthermore, β-blockade is known to have effects on platelet [49] and immune function [50], in surgical patients. Even though it is clear that β-blockade during the perioperative period might be of importance in reducing surgical mortality, little is known and further studies are needed.

Perioperative optimization of cardiac function

An alternative approach has attempted to optimize cardiac function and tissue perfusion using a whole body approach and realized that it is not just coronary artery blood flow that might be impaired during the perioperative period. It has been known for many years that patients undergoing surgery are more likely to die and have serious complications if they have limited cardiovascular reserve [51, 52]. As described above, this relationship between cardiac reserve and outcome has been used as the basis for scoring systems to predict patient outcome [1]. While developing even more powerful scoring systems further studies showed that patients who survived major surgery had higher cardiac index and lower systemic vascular resistance [53, 54]. Furthermore, it was found that the commonly monitored vital signs, heart rate, temperature, central venous pressure and haemoglobin were the poorest predictors of mortality, while perfusion related variables, such as cardiac output and total body oxygen delivery, were the best [55, 56]. Recent studies assessing the impact of oxygen transport variables on postoperative mortality and morbidity show similar trends [57-59].

New therapeutic options and monitoring techniques that became available in the 1970's, particularly the introduction on the pulmonary artery flow directed catheter [60], opened up the possibility of measuring and manipulating an individual's cardiovascular system. It was hypothesized that targeting treatment in all patients to the values manifested by the survivors of surgery would improve the outcome in these patients [61]. An important principle of this manipulation was an augmentation of cardiac output and blood flow with an implied or measured increase in tissue perfusion above baseline levels. Underlying the principle of this approach is the need to monitor cardiac function and tissue perfusion by some suitable method and to consider very accurate fluid management as a fundamental basic requirement to maintain optimal cardiac function. In addition some investigators have used inotropes and vasodilators to give additional supplementation to cardiac function [62-77].

Since the 1970's a number of randomized clinical trials have been performed in patients during the perioperative period which have investigated this issue. However, the trials have different characteristics, namely: 1) differing patient groups with differing co-morbidities and anticipated mortality rates; 2) different techniques have been used to influence DO_2; 3) the studies are not blinded, which lowers their statistical impact; 4) some studies have limited statistical power due to low baseline mortality rates; 5) different endpoints for initial treatment as well as the use of continuing treatment; 6) two different approaches of measuring cardiac output have been used, either right heart catheterization or Doppler studies, 7) the variation in control for co-intervention. Despite this a number of reviews have attempted to group identified studies together to draw general conclusions [78-83]. However, these reviews identify differing studies and have not taken into consideration the rigorous techniques for searching, examination and analysis that are required by, for example, the Cochrane collaboration [84, 85].

It has been almost 30 years since initial uncontrolled data was presented suggesting that perioperative augmentation of the cardiovascular system might improve outcome in higher risk surgical patients [86]. Subsequently randomized trials have been performed and published, and preliminary reviews tend to indicate an improvement in outcome [78-83]. However, risks attached to the techniques, the time required and costs in terms of space, equipment and expertise have limited the widespread adoption of this policy.

Conclusion

An understanding of which patients are at risk of perioperative myocardial dysfunction and of the multifactorial causes of myocardial dysfunction, allow the various logical therapeutic regimens to be instituted. Although there is some doubt about the universal adoption of perioperative β–blockade, management techniques aimed at improving and maintaining optimal myocardial function and tissue perfusion have been shown to reduce post-operative morbidity and mortality.

References

1. Goldman L, Caldera DL, Nussbaum SR et al (1977) Multifactorial index of risk in noncardiac surgical procedures. N Eng J Med 297: 845-850.

2. Detsky AS, Abrams HB, Forbath N et al (1986) Cardiac assessment for patients undergoing noncardiac surgery. A multifactorial clinical risk index. Arch Intern Med 146(11): 2131-4.
3. Brady AR, Fowkes FG, Greenhalgh RM et al (2000) Risk factors for postoperative death following elective surgical repair of abdominal aortic aneurysm: results from the UK Small Aneurysm Trial. On behalf of the UK Small Aneurysm Trial participants. Br J Surg 87(6): 742-9.
4. Becquemin JP, Chemla E, Chatellier G et al (2000) Peroperative factors influencing the outcome of elective abdominal aorta aneurysm repair. Eur J Vasc Endovasc Surg 20(1): 84-9.
5. Gilbert K, Larocque BJ, Patrick LT (2000) Prospective evaluation of cardiac risk indices for patients undergoing noncardiac surgery. Ann Intern Med 133(5): 356-9.
6. Copeland GP, Jones D, Walters M (1991) POSSUM: a scoring system for surgical audit. Br J Surg 78(3): 355-360.
7. Jones HJ, de Cossart L (1999) Risk scoring in surgical patients. Br J Surg 86(2): 149-57.
8. Jones DR, Copeland GP, de Cossart L (1992) Comparison of POSSUM with APACHE II for prediction of outcome from a surgical high-dependency unit. Br J Surg 79: 1293-1296.
9. Lazarides MK, Arvanitis DP, Drista H et al (1997) POSSUM and APACHE II scores do not predict the outcome of ruptured infrarenal aortic aneurysms. Ann Vasc Surg 11(2): 155-8.
10. Tekkis PP, Kocher HM, Bentley AJ et al (2000) Operative mortality rates among surgeons: comparison of POSSUM and p-POSSUM scoring systems in gastrointestinal surgery. Dis Colon Rectum 43(11): 1528-32, discusssion 1532-4.
11. Midwinter MJ, Tytherleigh M, Ashley S, (1999) Estimation of mortality and morbidity risk in vascular surgery using POSSUM and the Portsmouth predictor equation. Br J Surg 86(4): 471-4.
12. Curran JE, Grounds RM (1998) Ward versus intensive care management of high-risk surgical patients. Br J Surg 85(7): 956-61.
13. Older P, Smith R, Courtney P et al (1993) Preoperative evaluation of cardiac failure and ischemia in elderly patients by cardiopulmonary exercise testing. Chest 104(3): 701-4.
14. Older P, Hall A, Hader R (1999) Cardiopulmonary Exercise Testing as a Screening Test for Perioperative Management of Major Surgery in the Elderly. Chest 116: 355-362.
15. Gauss A, Rohm HJ, Schauffelen A et al (2001) Electrocardiographic exercise stress testing for cardiac risk assessment in patients undergoing noncardiac surgery. Anesthesiology 94(1): 38-46.
16. Rohde LE, Polanczyk CA, Goldman L et al (2001) Usefulness of transthoracic echocardiography as a tool for risk stratification of patients undergoing major noncardiac surgery. Am J Cardiol 87(5): 505-9.
17. Halm EA, Browner WS, Tubau JF et al (1996) Echocardiography for assessing cardiac risk in patients having noncardiac surgery. Study of Perioperative Ischemia Research Group. Ann Intern Med 125(6): 433-41.
18. Day SM, Younger JG, Karavite D et al (2000) Usefulness of hypotension during dobutamine echocardiography in predicting perioperative cardiac events. Am J Cardiol 85(4): 478-83.
19. Das MK, Pellikka PA, Mahoney DW et al (2000) Assessment of cardiac risk before nonvascular surgery: dobutamine stress echocardiography in 530 patients. J Am Coll Cardiol 35(6): 1647-53.
20. Krivokapich J, Child JS, Walter DO et al (1999) Prognostic value of dobutamine stress echocardiography in predicting cardiac events in patients with known or suspected coronary artery disease. J Am Coll Cardiol 33(3): 708-16.
21. Boersma E, Poldermans D, Bax JJ et al (2001) Predictors of cardiac events after major vascular surgery: Role of clinical characteristics, dobutamine echocardiography, and beta-blocker therapy. Jama 285(14): 1865-73.
22. Tischler MD, Lee TH, Hirsch AT et al (1991) Prediction of major cardiac events after peripheral vascular surgery using dipyridamole echocardiography. Am J Cardiol 68(6): 593-7.
23. Beleslin BD, Ostojic M, Stepanovic J et al (1994) Stress echocardiography in the detection of myocardial ischemia. Head-to-head comparison of exercise, dobutamine, and dipyridamole tests. Circulation 90(3): 1168-76.
24. Roghi A, Palmieri B, Crivellaro W et al (1999) Preoperative assessment of cardiac risk in noncardiac major vascular surgery. Am J Cardiol 83(2): 169-74.

25. Takase B, Younis LT, Byers SL et al (1993) Comparative prognostic value of clinical risk indexes, resting two-dimensional echocardiography, and dipyridamole stress thallium-201 myocardial imaging for perioperative cardiac events in major nonvascular surgery patients. Am Heart J 126(5): 1099-106.
26. Slogoff S, Keats AS (1985) Does perioperative myocardial ischemia lead to postoperative myocardial infarction? Anesthesiology 62(2): 107-14.
27. Mangano DT, Hollenberg M, Fegert G et al (1991) Perioperative myocardial ischemia in patients undergoing noncardiac surgery--I: Incidence and severity during the 4 day perioperative period. The Study of Perioperative Ischemia (SPI) Research Group. J Am Coll Cardiol 17(4): 843-50.
28. Mangano DT, Wong MG, London MJ et al (1991) Perioperative myocardial ischemia in patients undergoing noncardiac surgery--II: Incidence and severity during the 1st week after surgery. The Study of Perioperative Ischemia (SPI) Research Group. J Am Coll Cardiol 17(4): 851-7.
29. Glantz L, Drenger B, Gozal Y (2000) Perioperative myocardial ischemia in cataract surgery patients: general versus local anesthesia. Anesth Analg 91(6): 1415-9.
30. Sbarigia E, DarioVizza C, Antonini M et al (1999) Locoregional versus general anesthesia in carotid surgery: is there an impact on perioperative myocardial ischemia? Results of a prospective monocentric randomized trial. J Vasc Surg 30(1): 131-8.
31. Wong DH, Hagar JM, Mootz J et al (1996) Incidence of perioperative myocardial ischemia in TURP patients. J Clin Anesth 8(8): 627-30.
32. Christopherson R, Glavan NJ, Norris EJ et al (1996) Control of blood pressure and heart rate in patients randomized to epidural or general anesthesia for lower extremity vascular surgery. Perioperative Ischemia Randomized Anesthesia Trial (PIRAT) Study Group. J Clin Anesth 8(7): 578-84.
33. Rapp HJ, Rabethge S, Luiz T et al (1999) Perioperative ST-segment depression and troponin T release. Identification of patients with highest risk for myocardial damage. Acta Anaesthesiol Scand 43(2): 124-9.
34. Fleisher LA, Zielski MM, Schulman SP (1997) Perioperative ST-segment depression is rare and may not indicate myocardial ischemia in moderate-risk patients undergoing noncardiac surgery. J Cardiothorac Vasc Anesth 11(2): 155-9.
35. Rao TLK, Jacobs KH, El-Etr AA (1983) Reinfarction following anesthesia in patients with myocardial infarction. Anesth 59: 499-505.
36. Rosenberg J, Dirkes WE, Kehlet H (1989) Episodic arterial oxygen desaturation and heart rate variations following major abdominal surgery. Br J Anaesth 63(6): 651-4.
37. Rosenberg-Adamsen S, Lie C, Bernhard A et al (1999) Effect of oxygen treatment on heart rate after abdominal surgery. Anesthesiology 90(2): 380-4.
38. Haque R, Kan H, Finkel MS (1998) Effects of cytokines and nitric oxide on myocardial E-C coupling. Basic Res Cardiol 93(Suppl 1): 86-94.
39. Kan H, Finkel MS (2001) Interactions between cytokines and neurohormonal systems in the failing heart. Heart Fail Rev 6(2): 119-27.
40. Hill GE, Whitten CW (1998) Proinflammatory mediator release after total hip arthroplasty. Anesthesiology 88(5): 1407-8.
41. Hill GE (1998) Cardiopulmonary bypass-induced inflammation: is it important? J Cardiothorac Vasc Anesth 12(2 Suppl 1): 21-5.
42. Mangano DT, Layug EL, Wallace A et al (1996) Effect of atenolol on mortality and cardiovascular morbidity after noncardiac surgery. Multicenter Study of Perioperative Iscemia Research Group. N Eng J Med 335: 1713-1720.
43. Poldermans D, Boersma E, Bax JJ et al (1999) The effect of bisoprolol on perioperative mortality and myocardial infarction in high-risk patients undergoing vascular surgery. Dutch Echocardiographic Cardiac Risk Evaluation Applying Stress Echocardiography Study Group. N Engl J Med 341(24): 1789-94.
44. ACC/AHA task force report (1996) Special report: guidelines for perioperative cardiovascular evaluation for noncardiac surgery. Report of the American College of Cardiology/American

Heart Association Task Force on practice guidelines (Committee on Perioperative Cardiovascular Evaluation for Noncardiac Surgery). J Cardiothorac Vasc Anesth 10(4): 540-52.
45. Howell SJ, Sear JW, Foex P (2001) Peri-operative beta-blockade: a useful treatment that should be greeted with cautious enthusiasm. Br J Anaesth 86: 161-164.
46. Fleisher LA (1999) Con: beta-blockers should not be used in all patients undergoing vascular surgery. J Cardiothorac Vasc Anesth 13(4): 496-7.
47. Dawood MM, Gutpa DK, Southern J et al (1996) Pathology of fatal perioperative myocardial infarction: implications regarding pathophysiology and prevention. Int J Cardiol 57(1): 37-44.
48. UK Prospective Diabetes Study Group, (1998) Efficacy of atenolol and captopril in reducing risk of macrovascular and microvascular complications in type 2 diabetes: UKPDS 39. Br Med J 317: 713-20.
49. Winther K, Willich SN (1991) Beta 1-blockade and acute coronary ischemia. Possible role of platelets. Circulation 84(6 Suppl): VI68-71.
50. Katafuchi T, Take S, Hori T (1993) Roles of sympathetic nervous system in the suppression of cytotoxicity of splenic natural killer cells in the rat. J Physiol 465: 343-57.
51. Boyd AR, Tremblay RE, Spencer FC et al (1959) Estimation of cardiac output soon after cardiac surgery with cardiopulmonary bypass. Ann Surg 150: 613-625.
52. Clowes GHA, Jr., Del Guercio LRM (1960) Circulatory response to trauma of surgical operations. Metabolism 9(1): 67-81.
53. Shoemaker WC (1972) Cardiorespiratory patterns of surviving and non-surviving postoperative surgical patients. Surg Gynecol Obstet 134(5): 810-814.
54. Shoemaker WC, Montgomery ES, Kaplan E et al (1973) Physiologic patterns in surviving and non-surviving shock patients. Use of sequential cardiorespiratory parameters in defining criteria for therapeutic goals and early warning of death. Arch Surg 106(5): 630-636.
55. Shoemaker WC, Czer LSC (1979) Evaluation of the biologic importance of various haemodynamic and oxygen transport variables. Crit Care Med 7(9): 424-429.
56. Shoemaker WC, Appel PL, Kram HB (1993) Hemodynamic and oxygen transport responses in survivors and non-survivors of high-risk surgery. Crit Care Med 21: 977-990.
57. Kusano C, Baba M, Takao S et al (1997) Oxygen delivery as a factor in the development of fatal postoperative complications after oesophagectomy. Br J Surg 84(2): 252-7.
58. Peerless JR, Alexander JJ, Pinchak AC et al (1998) Oxygen delivery is an important predictor of outcome in patients with ruptured abdominal aortic aneurysms [In Process Citation]. Ann Surg 227(5): 726-34.
59. Polonen P, Hippelainen M, Takala R et al (1997) Relationship between intra- and postoperative oxygen transport and prolonged intensive care after cardiac surgery: a prospective study. Acta Anaesthesiol Scand 41(7): 810-7.
60. Ganz W (1971) A new technique for measurement of cardiac output by thermodilution in man. Am J Cardiol 27(4): 392-396.
61. Bland RD, Shoemaker WC, Shabot MM (1978) Physiologic monitoring goals for the critically ill patient. Surg Gynecol Obstet 147(6): 833-841.
62. Schultz RJ, Whitfield GF, LaMura JJ et al (1985) The role of physiologic monitoring in patients with fractures of the hip. J Trauma 25: 309-316.
63. Shoemaker WC, Appel PL, Kram HB et al (1988) Prospective trial of supranormal values of survivors as therapeutic goals in high-risk surgical patients. Chest 94(6): 1176-86.
64. Berlauk JF, Abrams JH, Gilmour IJ et al (1991) Preoperative optimization of cardiovascular hemodynamics improves outcome in peripheral vascular surgery. Ann Surg 214(3): 289-297.
65. Fleming A, Bishop M, Shoemaker W et al (1992) Prospective trial of supranormal values as goals of resuscitation in severe trauma. Arch Surg 127(10): 1175-9; discussion 1179-81.
66. Boyd O, Grounds RM, Bennett ED (1993) A randomized clinical trial of the effect of deliberate perioperative increase of oxygen delivery on mortality in high-risk surgical patients. JAMA 270: 2699-2707.
67. Bishop MH, Shoemaker WC, Appel PL et al (1995) Prospective, randomized trial of survivor

values of cardiac index, oxygen delivery, and oxygen consumption as resuscitation endpoints in severe trauma [see comments]. J Trauma 38(5): 780-7.

68. Mythen MG, Webb AR (1994) Intra-operative gut mucosal hypoperfusion is associated with increased post-operative complications and cost. Int Care Med 20: 99-104.
69. Durham RM, Neunaber K, Mazuski JE et al (1996) The use of oxygen consumption and delivery as endpoints for resuscitation in critically ill patients. J Trauma 41(1): 32-9; discussion 39-40.
70. Ziegler DW, Wright JG, Choban PS et al (1997) A prospective randomized trial of preoperative "optimization" of cardiac function in patients undergoing elective peripheral vascular surgery. Surgery 122(3): 584-92.
71. Bender JS, Smith-Meek MA, Jones CE (1997) Routine pulmonary artery catheterization does not reduce morbidity and mortality of elective vascular surgery: results of a prospective, randomized trial. Ann Surg 226(3): 229-36; discussion 236-7.
72. Sinclair S, James S, Singer M (1997) Intraoperative intravascular volume optimization and length of hospital stay after repair of proximal femoral fracture: randomized controlled trial. Br Med J 315: 909-912.
73. Ueno S, Tanabe G, Yamada H et al (1998) Response of patients with cirrhosis who have undergone partial hepatectomy to treatment aimed at achieving supranormal oxygen delivery and consumption. Surgery 123(3): 278-86.
74. Valentine RJ, Duke ML, Inman MH et al (1998) Effectiveness of pulmonary artery catheters in aortic surgery: a randomized trial. J Vasc Surg 27(2): 203-11; discussion 211-2.
75. Wilson J, Woods I, Fawcett J et al (1999) Reducing the risk of major elective surgery: randomized controlled trial of preoperative optimization of oxygen delivery. Br Med J 318: 1099-1103.
76. Polonen P, Ruokonen E, Hippelainen M et al (2000) A prospective, randomized study of goal-oriented hemodynamic therapy in cardiac surgical patients. Anesth Analg 90(5): 1052-9.
77. Lobo SM, Salgado PF, Castillo VG et al (2000) Effects of maximizing oxygen delivery on morbidity and mortality in high-risk surgical patients. Crit Care Med 28(10): 3396-404.
78. Boyd O, Bennett ED (1996) Enhancement of perioperative tissue perfusion as a therapeutic strategy for major surgery. New Horiz 4(4): 453-65.
79. Forst H (1997) Maximierung des O_2-Transports beim kritisch Kranken, Ein rationales Therapie-konzept? Anaesthetist 46: 46-52.
80. Ivanov RI, Allen J, Sandham JD et al (1997) Pulmonary artery catheterization: a narrative and systematic critique of randomized controlled trials and recommendations for the future. New Horiz 5(3): 268-76.
81. Heyland DK, Cook DJ, King D et al (1996) Maximizing oxygen delivery in critically ill patients: a methodologic appraisal of the evidence [see comments]. Crit Care Med 24(3): 517-24.
82. Leibowitz AB, Beilin Y (1997) Pulmonary artery catheters and outcome in the perioperative period. New Horiz 5(3): 214-21.
83. Boyd O, Hayes M (1999) The oxygen trail - the goal. Br Med Bull 55(1): 125-139.
84. Bennett D, Boyd O (2000) Oxygen delivery in surgical patients--doesn't work, or does it? Crit Care Med 28(10): 3564-5.
85. Boyd O, Bennett ED (2000) The right heart catheter: leaner, fitter patient management. Crit Care Med 28(3): 881-2.
86. Shoemaker WC, Appel PL, Waxman K et al (1982) Clinical trial of survivors cardiorespiratory patterns as therapeutic goals in critically ill postoperative patients. Crit Care Med 10(6): 398-403.

Trauma Resuscitation

L. J. KAPLAN

Not only has the optimal solution for resuscitation after traumatic injury been hotly contested, so too has the concept of resuscitation at all prior to definitive hemorrhage control [1]. The ideal resuscitation strategy following penetrating or blunt trauma associated with hypoperfusion to provide maximal survival remains to be defined. Currently, there is a trend towards limited volume resuscitation instead of aggressive crystalloid volume expansion. Vitally related to these controversies are the debated endpoints of resuscitation – physiological and metabolic markers of the adequacy of resuscitation [2]. Ideally, these markers should reflect changes in both systemic and microcirculatory flow. Increasingly evidence suggests that this is not the case. Moreover, the immunomodulatory effects of resuscitation and resuscitation fluids have influenced the casual selection of fluid type and amount for plasma volume expansion. This paper will explore the current state of trauma resuscitation ,with a particular focus on the acid-base sequelae of resuscitation, the impact of these sequelae, and their interpretation on the endpoints of resuscitation, potentially useful strategies to aid in resuscitation, and future areas of investigation.

Current paradigm

The standard United States trauma resuscitation guidelines derive from the Advance Trauma Life Support (ATLS) manual developed by the American College of Surgeons Committee on Trauma (ASCOT). These guidelines promote an initial 2,000 ml crystalloid fluid bolus for the severely injured patient as an initial resuscitation strategy. Ongoing hypotension is met with an additional fluid challenge, as well as packed red blood cells, based on the assumption that hypovolemic shock is the operative phenomenon. Diagnostic and therapeutic interventions may occur concomitantly. The underlying concept is the restoration of the stressed volume [3] to treat cellular hypoxia, and improve organ and organism viability. Although ATLS was originally developed as a guide to aid the physician who would initially treat and resuscitate a trauma patient at an outlying facility, its tenets have been nearly universally adopted at community and level 1 trauma center alike.

An aggressive fluid resuscitation posture as espoused by ATLS has been challenged in the last decade. The concept of limiting fluid resuscitation to preserve organism viability, but not restore normal perfusion pressures, until definitive hemorrhage control could be obtained arose from the well-quoted and equally well-criticized work of Bickell et al. [4]. The notion of limited fluid resuscitation was then frequently confused with "no resuscitation", as an unintended consequence.

Accordingly, a number of animal models, and recently, a large human trial have addressed the value of lesser volume and lower pressure resuscitation in comparison with larger volume, higher pressure strategies (R. Dutton, unpublished data; [5]). Improved survival in both animal models and human trials has been associated with the low-volume and low pressure strategy. In fact, worse survival was obtained in a high-lethality splenic injury animal model where large volume normotonic saline or hypertonic saline resuscitation was undertaken, compared with no resuscitation at all [5]. The mechanism underlying increased mortality in the high-volume high-pressure groups was accelerated hemorrhage compared with the lower-volume and lower-pressure groups. The human data suggest that trauma patients with hypovolemic shock, regardless of mechanism of injury, achieve improved outcomes (as measured by gross survival) with a pre-hemorrhage control target of a mean blood pressure (MAP) of 50-60 mmHg (R. Dutton, unpublished data). Furthermore, this MAP is sustainable without untoward sequelae for up to 1 h. Longer periods of relative hypotension lead to poorer outcomes by comparison. This observation certainly supports the "golden hour" concept so entrenched in trauma resuscitation. Once hemorrhage control is achieved, fluid resuscitation with management of oxygen delivery and utilization using blood products, electrolytes, and metabolic fuel proceeds quite aggressively. A key endpoint for trauma resuscitation then becomes the time course of lactic acidemia [6].

The role and value of lactic acid

Lactic acid is a normal metabolic endproduct of glucose metabolism. Immediately following traumatic injury, an elevated lactic acid level almost always represents lactic acidemia that is associated with hypoperfusion and anaerobic metabolism, due to impaired oxygen delivery, oxygen utilization, or both. The time dependence of the clearance of lactate as a prognostic indicator has been previously identified with enhanced survival, associated with more-rapid clearance rates [6]. Recently, the concept of "occult hypoperfusion" has been intensely investigated [7].

Occult hypoperfusion is defined as an elevated lactic acid level in a patient who is thought to be well resuscitated, who has seemingly normal vital signs and other physiological indicators, such as heart rate, blood pressure, and urine output. Increased percentage and risk of infections were associated with the presence of occult hypoperfusion, and improved outcome (decreased mortality) followed in the wake of successful resolution of the elevated lactic acid level [8]. The intervention to "clear the lactate" was increased fluid resuscitation (crystalloid). While seemingly attractive, and supportive of the notion of microcirculatory resuscitation as well as systemic resuscitation, there are a few unexplored aspects to these studies.

Recall that a normal epinephrine level is 15-100 pg/ml, and that trauma may increase circulating levels to 4,000 pg/ml [9]. Furthermore, it has been observed that an increased epinephrine concentration may persist after trauma for as long as 2 weeks, at levels that exceed 2,000 pg/ml. Importantly, epinephrine increases glycolytic flux and activates ATPases that generate pyruvate as well as lactate, giving rise to a normal pyruvate:lactate ratio. Increased epinephrine levels (in a resuscitated patient) will increase both pyruvate and lactate in equal proportion, thus preserving the normal ratio. It would be of interest to learn whether the increased lactate values in the "occult hypoperfusion" studies were truly representative of hyperlactatemia (i.e., elevated lactate, but normal pH) with a normal pyruvate:lactate ratio, instead of under-resuscitation of the microcirculation. Unfortunately, the accompanying pH values were not reported, which weakens the conclusions of the studies. Functionally, these observations further buttress the existing paradigm of aggressive resuscitation, and increasing amounts of fluid loading in critically ill patients. The selection of fluids for large-volume plasma volume expansion is absolutely critical in the critically ill, especially with regard to the impact of the resuscitation fluid on acid-base balance.

The endpoints of resuscitation

Many markers have been proposed as the ideal indicators of either the success of (or targets for) a resuscitative effort, or harbingers of mortality in discrete patient populations. Markers that have been rejected as good indicators of either include vital signs, urine output, and hyperdynamic cardiac performance. Controversy surrounds the utility of gastric tonometry in trauma resuscitations, with pH_i values being discarded in favor of the more-solid $pgCO_2$ gap [10, 11]. Markers associated with poor outcomes include low presentation pH [12], large base deficit (or excess) [13], elevated lactate [6], low cardiac index (<2.0 l/min per m^2) [14], large volume requirement [15], coagulopathy [16] (exclusive of traumatic brain injury), and hypothermia (core temperature < 34°C) [16]. Of this latter group, lactate surfaces as the marker with the greatest utility and correlation with survival across diverse patient groups.

Newer markers of the adequacy of resuscitation, such as near-infrared spectroscopic evaluation of skeletal muscle tissue oxygen saturation [17] or sublingual capnometry [18], may provide early and more-sensitive indicators of the adequacy of resuscitation than the conventional markers. The importance of these latter two techniques is that they are a valuable step towards regional evaluation of tissue perfusion (much like the touted value of gastric tonometry), instead of relying on the currently available data that groups systemic variables in an unknown, and potentially changeable, proportion. Non-invasive (or less -invasive) hemodynamic monitoring tools are increasingly common and include the Fick principle-dependent PICCO (peripherally inserted continuous cardiac output) catheter system, as well as the various permutations of transesophageal Doppler probes that assess aortic flow or pulse-gated volumetric changes in diameter. While one of the derived indices of the PICCO system, intra-thoracic blood volume, has been favorably compared with the Parkland formula and pulmonary artery (PA) catheter-guided resuscitation, the utility of these newer tools in guiding trauma resuscitation remains undefined [19]. Conventional wisdom incorporates the clinical response to therapy with acid-base balance and lactate metabolism with or without objective hemodynamic monitoring tools to develop a coherent management plan with regard to ongoing resuscitation. It is in this aspect of patient management that the Stewart method of evaluation of acid-base balance, based on strong ion physiology, may have its greatest impact on patient care.

Stewartian acid-base physiology

The strong ion difference apparent (SIDa), strong ion difference effective (SIDe), and the strong ion gap (SIG) have been described in detail in an earlier article by Kellum [20]. The power of this methodology is that it allows one to understand the mechanisms behind acid-base disturbances, as well as the expected sequelae of an intervention. Moreover, the technique allows one to understand the importance of protein concentration and charge to pH maintenance. Lastly, and perhaps most importantly, the Stewart methodology accurately and reliably identifies unmeasured ions that are not accounted for by the anion gap or the corrected anion gap. The seemingly "new" discovery of hyperchloremic metabolic acidemia as a sequelae of large volume crystalloid [principally 0.9% normal saline solution (NSS)] resuscitation is a prime example of physiology that is both predicted and explained by strong ion principles.

In an animal model of hemorrhagic shock [21], an adult model of resuscitation from elective surgery [22], and a pediatric intensive care unit (ICU) model of critically ill patients [23], aggressive resuscitation with large volumes of NSS [especially when compared with lactated Ringer's (LR)] resulted in a predictable decrease in plasma positive charge (principally from markedly increased Cl^- levels), a narrowed SIDa, and a hyperchloremic metabolic acidemia that occurred in an almost dose-dependent fashion. The dose-dependent nature of this phenomenon has been confirmed in an ex vivo whole-blood model of escalating Cl^- levels with 0.9% NSS as well as 3% NSS [24]. These data question the merit, and underscore the risks, associated with injudicious fluid prescriptions that administer large volumes of Cl^- as part of a resuscitation regimen. Especially during the early phase of resuscitation, when lactic acidemia is likely to be present, an added acidosis from hyperchloremia may significantly lower pH to an unacceptable level (i.e., pH < 7.25). The impact upon multiple organ systems may be profound.

Hyperchloremia has been long identified as an undesirable physiological state. Increased Cl^- is associated with independent decreases in glomerular filtration rate, urine flow, and creatinine clearance [25]. Moreover, even healthy volunteers who were volume loaded with either NSS or LR at equivalent rates and volumes took longer to urinate and had increased discomfort when they received the Cl^--rich fluid [26]. Similar data have been reported in elderly patients undergoing planned major general surgery. Patients resuscitated with Cl^- -rich solutions had a much greater incidence of hyperchloremic metabolic acidemia, lower urine volumes the operating room (OR), longer times to recovery of gastrointestinal function, and higher pain scores [27]. The importance of recognizing that the induced acidemia is out of proportion to changes in lactate or the anion gap cannot be overstated, as therapeutic interventions frequently hinge on pH values in the critically ill [28, 29]. A complete understanding of pH in a given setting must also incorporate unmeasured ions into the equation.

The role and importance of unmeasured ions

The Stewart methodology also precisely identifies unmeasured ions as part of the evaluation of plasma charge difference between the SIDa and SIDe in light of the observed pH; this is known as the strong ion gap. Unmeasured ions have been documented to accompany critical illness as part of severe hepatic insufficiency, renal failure, as well as traumatic injury. Early increases in unmeasured ions in patients with major vascular injury were strongly predictive of outcome [as was initial pH, base deficit (BD), lactate, and SIDa] [30]. In comparison, the anion gap was poorly predictive in this patient population, being normal in 42% of nonsurvivors on presentation to the emergency department. Relatedly, in a mixed group of trauma patients, a strong ion gap > 7 strongly correlated with uniform mortality at 72 h [31]. These data are comparable to those obtained in the liver failure population, where an unmeasured ion load > 5 is strongly predictive of mortality. In the ex vivo hyperchloremia experiments cited above, the progressive increases in Cl^- were also associated with an increasing and linearly developed SIG, the source of which remains unclear [24]. It is unknown whether the SIG developed from white cells, platelets, or red blood cells. Development of the SIG was an unexpected observation whose meaning may be linked to either apoptotic signaling (preprogrammed cell death), or the development of a pro-inflammatory state following a simulated plasma volume expansion. In this series of experiments, hydroxyethyl starch solutions (HES in LR or NSS) failed to initiate such a process, and were not associated with hyperchloremia (given in volumes identical to the 3% NSS). The significance of these observations lies in the selection of a resuscitation fluid prescription that minimally disturbs acid-base balance, and does not initiate untoward biochemical or molecular events.

Resuscitation fluid prescription

It is clear from the preceding papers and the above discussion that iatrogenically increasing Cl^- out of proportion to Na^+ predictably leads to hyperchloremic metabolic acidosis. Therefore, in patients who require large volume resuscitation, regardless of timing (pre or post definitive hemorrhage control), avoiding hyperchloremia is an intelligent aspect of planning a resuscitation fluid prescription. A Cl^--rich solution, such as 0.9% NSS, is a poor choice as a primary large volume resuscitation fluid, as it will predictably induce acidemia. LR solution (or its related formulations available outside of the United States) are less rich in Cl^- than 0.9% NSS and will induce less hyperchloremia (and less acidosis) on an equivolume basis compared with 0.9% NSS. It is these two fluids that are principally used in the United States for trauma resuscitation. Hypertonic saline is used in limited amounts in the United States for acute volume management in patients with traumatic brain injury, as well as post craniotomy, when cerebral edema is a prominent feature and is accompanied by intra-cranial hypertension. In comparison, colloids are more liberally utilized for resuscitation throughout the rest of the industrialized world.

Despite the intense debate that has surrounded the meta-analyses of albumin resuscitation in a variety of disease states [32-34], colloids as part of a resuscitation strategy may have their most-valuable role in trauma resuscitation based on that which they lack-Cl^-. Colloids currently available in the United States are albumin (5% or 25%), HES (6% HES; 670/0.75) in either 0.9% NSS (Hespan) or LR (Hextend), or fresh-frozen plasma (FFP). A wider variety of colloid solutions is marketed elsewhere, and includes gelatins, HES in hypertonic saline (Hyper-HES), HES of different molecular weights and degrees of substitution (e.g., 130/0.4) in 0.9% NSS or LR, as well as hypertonic saline-dextran combinations (HSD; Rescue-Flow). Combination colloid resuscitation (crystalloid + colloid ± blood products) creates an intelligently designed fluid prescription strategy, as it achieves the stated goals of resuscitation rapidly and effectively. Moreover, it takes into account acid-base impact, in that the colloid component reduces the total volume of required plasma expander due to greater retention in the vascular space than crystalloids. The reduced volume translates into reduced Cl^-, less hyperchloremia, and an improved acid-base profile.

Impact of resuscitation volume and pH on damage control procedures

Major abdominal trauma may create injury complexes that require massive resuscitation and a total operative time greater than that which the patient can tolerate in the first few hours post injury. Improved survival following hepatic trauma was noted using the technique of "abbreviated laparotomy" [35]. This technique enumerated three goals: (1) hemorrhage control (including packing for temporary tamponade of microvascular hemorrhage), (2) source control of peritoneal contamination from gastrointestinal tract injury, and (3) rapid transit from the OR to the ICU for metabolic resuscitation, rewarming, and correction of coagulopathy and acidosis [36]. The amount of time that has been computer modeled for optimal outcome using this technique is 60-90 min of surgery [37]. This strategy is currently termed "damage control", and is typically terminated using a temporary abdominal wall closure technique to permit rapid and easy re-entry into the peritoneal space, as well as avoid intra-abdominal hypertension and the abdominal compartment syndrome. Avoiding the abdominal compartment syndrome is essential in re-establishing and maintaining organ perfusion and viability [38]. Despite such measures, a post-operative compartment syndrome is estimated to complicate up to 20% of damage control laparotomies performed for trauma, even when the abdomen was reconstructed using a temporary closure method that provided an expanded peritoneal space.

The overwhelming majority of papers describing post-operative abdominal compartment syndrome have utilized crystalloid plus blood product resuscitation strategies. Importantly, not all of the papers have identified the compartment syndrome as a result of hemorrhage. Rather, a number of the authors cite bowel wall and organ edema as the etiology of the compartment syndrome [35, 38]. One must question whether the syndrome would have developed if the volume required for resuscitation had been reduced using colloids as part of the resuscitation fluid prescription. Some early work has suggested that organ edema following major resuscitation can be reduced by avoiding a normotonic crystalloid resuscitation strategy; this model used a hypertonic solution, although a colloid could presumably been used to an identical effect [39].

Coagulopathy: relationship to acidemia and colloids

Conventional wisdom dictates that massive volume resuscitation dilutes plasma clotting factors, and will do so in a more-rapid fashion when there is concomitant hemorrhage as well as resuscitation with packed red blood cells without FFP. A variety of studies documented that FFP was not warranted until definitive hemorrhage control could be achieved. The sole exception to this observation was the massively injured patient who required a massive transfusion protocol for volume resuscitation; increased survival has been identified in these significantly injured patients using such a transfusion strategy [40].

The coagulopathy that accompanies massive resuscitation has been variously (and often dubiously) ascribed to dilution, calcium chelation, FFP and other clotting factor consumption, hypothermia, elevated tissue thromboplastin release (brain injury), acute hepatic failure, and under-resuscitation [16]; it has earned the appellation of "the bloody viscious cycle" due to its self-sustaining nature and the mortality that exceeds that of multi-system organ failure. It is curious that little work has addressed the impact of acidemia on the function of the clotting cascade and the interaction of the arachidonic acid pathway with platelets and the fibrinolytic cascade. The reader should recall that clotting factors are serine proteases, and as such, have a pH-dependent activity profile. Unsurprisingly, clotting factor enzyme kinetics are maximal at or near physiological pH. The enzyme kinetics that so readily explain the deleterious impact of hypothermia have been blithely ignored with regard to proton concentration.

It is not surprising that this has received little attention, given the limited choices for fluid resuscitation in the United States. Experience in the 1970's and 1980's with HES preparations mixed in 0.9% NSS identified coagulopathy as a consequence of volume infusion that exceeded approximately 20-25 ml/kg body weight per day. Thus, little choice remained besides NSS, LR, or blood products. Whole blood all but disappeared after the Korean military experience, and the subsequent years witnessed the ascendancy of blood component banking and selective transfusion of desired components. With such a limited array of solutions, the impact of those solutions was not a priority except with regard to perfusion restoration. Currently, there are more choices and an altered resuscitation posture, leading to intensified investigation into the sequelae of resuscitation fluids.

An ex vivo model addressed the impact of deliberate increases in Cl^- concentration on readily available measures of clotting, prothrombin time (PT) and activated partial thromboplastin time (aPTT) [24]. As Cl^- concentration increased, and pH deceased, clotting times became prolonged. Since clotting times were prolonged with both 0.9% NSS and 3% NSS, the abnormal times cannot be ascribed to dilution of clotting factors, since the 3% NSS volume increased the whole blood volume less than 1%. Interestingly, HES given in the same volume as the 3% NSS failed to alter the coagulation profile, calling into question the mechanism that underpinned the earlier identified coagulopathy associated with administration of > 20-25 ml HES/kg body weight per day. The explanation may lie not with the starch, but with the diluent.

The prior observations were made using high molecular weight and highly substituted starch in a 0.9% NSS diluent. Since it has been established that: (1) large-volume NSS delivery will lead to hyperchloremic acidosis and (2) hyperchloremic acidemia can induce a coagulopathy, it is reasonable to postulate that the coagulopathy may have occurred on the basis of an acid-base effect of resuscitation fluid, rather than an effect of HES. Current human data support this contention.

A large human trial evaluating the impact of HES resuscitation of patients with traumatic brain injury documented the safety of volumes up to 70 ml/kg body weight per day using HES 130/0.4 [40]. Additional data using the same preparation documented similar results at lower volumes per day over several days, in patients with ischemic stroke [41]. A United States retrospective evaluation of patients resuscitated using the higher molecular weight HES (670/0.75) product Hextend (Abbott) demonstrated resuscitation efficacy, lactate clearance and virtually no coagulopathy (6% of patients with an increase in PT or aPTT) in a mixed group of trauma patients admitted to the ICU [42]. A worsened coagulation profile was noted in patients in three distinct groups:

traumatic brain injury (TBI), severe hepatic injury, or a pre-existing coagulopathy. It is important to note that these study patients received approximately 35 ml/kg body weight per day for resuscitation - well above the accepted "limit" for HES solution. Improved coagulation profiles were noted in the remainder (94%) of the trauma patients (26% were on a massive transfusion protocol). The absence of a worsened coagulation profile using a HES resuscitation strategy is supported by thromboelastography data obtained in a swine model of hemorrhagic shock and resuscitation where changes in platelet counts, fibrinogen level, and maximal amplitude were ascribed to dilution rather than the starch [43].

Impact on endpoint of resuscitation interpretation

From the preceding discussion of the Stewart approach, it should be apparent that one of the more-common indicators of acid-base balance, and the adequacy of resuscitation, BD (or excess) varies with changes in perfusion, but also changes with a given patient's Cl^- profile. Thus, the utility of the BD after resuscitation with large volumes of fluid (and thus Cl^-) must be viewed with some degree of circumspection. No changes in BD interpretation on presentation need be made, and the interpretation of BD as an indicator of mortality immediately after trauma remains valid [13]. By way of example, a patient sustaining multicavity blunt injury with a pulmonary contusion, liver fracture and pelvic crush with retroperitoneal hemorrhage may present with a BD of –13, a lactate of 11 mmol/l, a pH of 7.25 at a PCO2 of 32 torr, a hemoglobin of 8 mg%, and an expected mortality of close to 50% with a SIG of approximately 7. With a 24-h resuscitation of 10L of LR, 2L of NSS, 8 U of packed red blood cells, and 16 U of FFP, the following values might be observed: pH of 7.29, PCO2 of 32 torr, BD of –7, but a persistent SIG of 7.3. While the BD had improved and the lactate was almost normal, there was a small increase in pH due to the induced hyperchloremic metabolic acidosis, but no change in the SIG. Clearly, such a scenario changes the value of bicarbonate as an endpoint of resuscitation. Instead, the data indicate bicarbonate to be dependent variable whose value is set by CO_2, A_{TOT}, and the SIDa. Moreover, the standard paradigm would administer additional fluid to correct the lactic acid level, worsening the hyperchloremia, and unintentionally further decreasing the pH. Instead, recognizing that this is the expected consequence, one might design a different fluid regimen.

It is similarly important to recognize when an elevated lactate level represents hyperlactatemia instead of lactic acidemia. Hypermetabolism can clearly accompany trauma resuscitation, especially following the first 24 h post injury. Patients with acute lung injury may have accelerated lactate flux and release into the systemic circulation [44]. Treating hyperlactatemia with additional volume expansion may not be efficacious, nor beneficial. Increased Cl^- concentration, worsened peripheral and organ edema, as well as unintended immunomodulatory effects of fluid administration may accompany such a treatment plan. Instead, when one identifies an increased lactate level, and an inappropriately high pH relative to the PCO_2, one must determine if the pH reflects hyperlactatemia, or a concomitant metabolic alkalemia. The Stewart approach allows one to interpret the serum chemistry in the light of the existing protein concentration and electrochemical gradients. If the SIDa is nearly normal as is the albumin and phosphate concentration, then the pH reflects hyperlactatemia. If instead, the SIDa is larger than normal with a normal albumin and phosphate, then there is a concomitant metabolic alkalemia, and the lactate likely represents anaerobic metabolism. A third scheme arises if the SIDa is narrow and the albumin and phosphate are low as well (the common scenario). Only the Stewart approach allows one to precisely understand the resultant plasma charge and the net effect on H^+ concentration to accurately determine the presence or absence of metabolic alkalemia to correctly interpret the lactic acid level.

The development of metabolic acidemia following traumatic injury has been proposed as a strong indicator of the risk for subsequent acute lung injury (ALI) [45]. Patients with an ISS16 were evaluated in the emergency department and ICU for acid-base markers, total fluids, and the development of ALI/acute respiratory distress syndrome. The authors reported (not surprisingly) that the patients with the lowest pH values were also the ones with the greatest amount of administered (required?) fluid, and thus, delivered Cl^-. Relatedly, the patients with low pH and large volume resuscitation were more likely to develop ALI than their counterparts. One must question whether the ALI arose as a result of larger volumes of fluids as an independent mechanism that had nothing to do with acid-base balance, but had more to do with the immunomodulatory (pro-inflammatory) effects of crystalloid resuscitation. Moreover, since the large-volume group received more Cl^-, one questions whether the lower pH simply reflects hyperchloremic metabolic acidosis from the resuscitation regimen; no relationship to cellular perfusion needs be created nor assumed. Unfortunately, such data are unavailable.

Combination fluid therapy - the concept of balanced fluids

Resuscitation wisdom holds that only "normotonic" fluids are given during the early phase of resuscitation, based on the known distribution of crystalloid fluids principally into the extravascular space (25% intravascular, 75% extravascular). This observation is the principle mechanism responsible for edema formation during massive volume resuscitation. Given the relatively low efficiency of this process, hypotonic fluids have been avoided, as much greater volumes would be required for equivalent circulating volume expansion. Also, solutions containing dextrose have not been used during the first 24 h of care, in an effort to avoid overwhelming the k_m of the kidney for glucose transport (180 mg/dl). Such an event may lead to an artificially elevated urine flow and the incorrect assumption that the patient's circulating volume was adequately repleted. Thus, the vast majority of critically injured and ill patients develop hyperchloremia by the 24-h post-injury mark.

In an effort to avoid the deleterious effects of an injudicious amount of Cl^- administration, one might change the paradigm of "balanced fluid" to "balanced fluids". By way of example, the first 2,000 ml of fluid a patient receives (rapidly or slowly) may be crystalloid. Ongoing hypotension or hypoperfusion may be treated with a "low" Cl^- regimen (lower Cl^- than NSS; lower than the total amount of Cl^- delivered using only crystalloid), such as LR or a colloid such as HES in LR (Hextend), in addition to component blood product transfusion. Once hemorrhage control has been achieved (definitive or temporary), resuscitation can proceed with the same low Cl^- regimen. One should note that quite large volumes of LR will also lead to hyperchloremic metabolic acidosis, but not as rapidly as would NSS. Alternatively, the LR could be omitted, and only the HES in LR solution utilized, as this will decrease the total Cl^- load relative to crystalloid infusion.

Concomitantly, "maintenance" fluids should also be administered by the start of the second 24-h period. Maintenance fluids serve multiple purposes in the massively resuscitated patient. First, and least importantly, a minimal amount of calories in the form of dextrose are provided to support glycolysis and ATP production. By 24 h, the reversible blockade of pyruvate dehydrogenase should be ameliorated, allowing glucose metabolic byproduct entry into the Krebs cycle. Second, since the majority of patients will have hyperchloremia, by understanding the impact of the hyperchloremia (i.e., a narrowed SIDa), one may design a "maintenance" fluid that helps restore electrochemical balance. By way of example, a common fluid prescription in the author's ICU for this circumstance is D_5W + 150 mEq $NaHCO_3$/l at a rate appropriate for body weight calculated for 100% maintenance. The dextrose amount is not overwhelming, as the fluid is not bolused or used for resuscitation. The delivered Na^+ is in a Cl^--free milieu. Thus, the Na^+ will rise only slightly or not at all, but the Cl^- will fall significantly; only pre-existing severe hypernatremia limits this prescription, and lesser concentrations of $NaHCO_3$ may be prescribed instead. The result of broadening the SIDa is to decrease $[H^+]$ and thus raise pH.

Immunomodulatory effects of resuscitation fluid regimens

Increasing evidence suggests that the effects of a specific fluid extend beyond expansion of a fluid compartment, myocardial performance, and organ or cellular perfusion. Much like the recently discovered immune-modulating effects of certain dietary components, the impact of fluids on immune effector cells and immune system responsiveness has been intensely investigated. It should be recognized that the impact on patient outcome as a result of the identified immunomodulatory effects remains unknown. However, certain observations merit discussion.

In an ex-vivo model, different solutions were added to human blood and assessed for polymorphonuclear leukocyte oxidative burst and CD18 expression as measures of cellular inflammation [46]. Crystalloids (0.9% NSS and LR) and HES (in 0.9% NSS) initiated the greatest oxidative burst, while dextran and HES resulted in the most-intense CD 18 expression. It should be noted that albumin (5% or 25%) was relatively non-reactive in either assay. Relatedly, T-cells may be recruited by hypertonic NSS, as manifested by protein tyrosine kinase and pk38 activation; activation of these subcellular signaling pathways may be one mechanism to restore depressed T-cell function in trauma patients [47]. Additionally, T-cell activation potential and mitogenic responsiveness was not depressed by gelatin or HES resuscitation fluids, confirming that these two colloids did not depress systemic immune responsiveness by impeding T-cell activity [48]. The clinical relevance of these findings, however, remains to be clarified.

Future directions

The future of trauma resuscitation in the United States may be different from the future in other countries; certain generalities, however, will likely apply to both. As our understanding of specific injury states (or non-traumatic disease states) increases, we may design specific fluid prescriptions and fluid delivery rates that optimize outcome for each unique disease state. Monitoring techniques (likely ultrasonography based) may be applied in the field to guide resuscitation to targeted organ perfusion, instead of gross systemic measures.

On-line acid-base marker evaluation in a continuous fashion may also guide the extent of resuscitation. At the most recent United States Military Combat Fluid Resuscitation conference, the expert consensus recommendation was to initiate field resuscitation of injured military personnel using a HES-based regimen. This represents a major departure from United States trauma resuscitation dogma concerning crystalloid resuscitation, but has taken an important and forward-thinking step into designing the fluid prescription(s) of the future. Two additional areas of research in trauma resuscitation also merit attention.

Resuscitation of the patient in extremis is rarely successful. Two techniques that may enable salvage of the otherwise currently unsalvageable are: (1) suspended animation using hypothermic circulatory arrest and (2) acellular hemoglobin carrying solutions. The concept of suspended animation has been most notably advanced by the group in Pittsburgh at the Safar Resuscitation Research Center. Using severe hemodilution, as well as metabolic supplementation strategies and a novel antioxidant (Tempol), they were able to recover dogs from up to 1 h of hypothermic (10°C) circulatory arrest with normal neurological outcome and brain histology [49]. The challenge lies in garnering the time to allow the necessary support systems and machinery to be brought on-line with appropriate vascular access. One novel solution is ice-cold lavage using LR that is delivered via an aortic catheter inserted into the femoral artery. In a dog model, this technique affords approximately 30 min of arrest, with good neurological recovery following profound hypothermic circulatory arrest for up to 2 h [49, 50]. The role of antioxidants in such a strategy cannot be underestimated, with regard to the expected reperfusion injury and high-energy phosphate metabolism derangements that follow in the wake of oxygenated reperfusion of the macro- and microcirculation.

Microcirculatory support may rely on oxygen delivery techniques that bypass cellular transport mechanisms. Despite the recent failure of a major trial of hemoglobin resuscitation solution, new advances in hemoglobin technology have designed polymerized hemoglobin solutions as well as pegylated solutions that demonstrate improved pharmacodynamics and pharmacokinetics. In a porcine controled hemorrhagic shock model, a polymerized bovine hemoglobin -based oxygen-carrying solution was used as a resuscitation fluid. This novel fluid enabled reversal of anaerobic metabolism despite a low mean arterial pressure target (60 mmHg) and a relatively low cardiac index; metabolic markers such as lactate were normalized despite the global indices of hypoperfusion [51]. Resuscitation to a target MAP of 50 mmHg demonstrated reduced survival. These data are in agreement with the human data provided by Dutton (personal communication from the R. Adams Cowley Shock Center, Baltimore, Md., USA). The additional importance of this study is that it underscores the importance of strategies other than simple fluid resuscitation to improve outcome, and that some of our traditionally accepted markers of the adequacy of resuscitation (cardiac performance) may not be as powerful as we would like to believe. It is likely that future trauma resuscitation strategies will also incorporate acellular hemoglobin-based oxygen-carrying solutions.

References

1. Dries DJ (1996) Hypotensive resuscitation. Shock 6:317-318
2. Durham RM, Neunaber K, Mazuski JE, et al (1996) The use of oxygen consumption and delivery as endpoints for resuscitation in critically ill patients. J Trauma 41:32-39
3. Mager S, De Varenes (1998) Clinical death and the measurement of stressed vascular volume. Crit Care Med 26:1061-1064
4. Bickell W, Wall MJ, Pepe PE, et al (1994) Immediate versus delayed fluid resuscitation for hypotensive patients with penetrating torso injuries. N Engl J Med 331:1105-1109
5. Solomonov E, Hirsh M, Yahiya A, et al (2000) The effect of vigorous fluid resuscitation in uncontrolled hemorrhagic shock after massive splenic injury. Crit Care Med 28:749-754
6. Abramson D, Scalea TM, Hitchcock R, et al (1993) Lactate clearance and survival following injury. J Trauma 35:584-589
7. Blow O, Magliore L, Claridge JA, et al (1999) The golden hour and the silver day: detection and correction of occult hypoperfusion within 24 hours improves outcomes from major trauma. J Trauma 47:964-969
8. Claridge JA, Crabtree TD, Pelletier SJ, et al (2000) Persistent occult hypoperfusion is associated with a significant increase in infection rate and mortality in major trauma patients. J Trauma 48:8-14
9. James JH, Luchette FA, McCarter FD, et al (1999) Lactate is an unreliable indicator of tissue hypoxia in injury or sepsis. Lancet 354:505-508
10. Gomersall CD, Joynt GM, Freebairn RC et al (2000) Resuscitation of critically ill patients based on the results of gastric tonometry: a prospective, randomized, controlled trial. Crit Care Med 28:607-614
11. Kellum JA, Rico P, Garuba AK, et al (2000) Accuracy of mucosal pH and mucosal-arterial carbon dioxide tension for detecting mesenteric hypoperfusion in acute canine endotoxemia. Crit Care Med 28:462-466
12. Millham FH, Malone M, Blansfield J, et al (1995) Predictive accuracy of the TRISS survival statistic is improved by a modification that includes admission pH. Arch Surg 130:307-311
13. Rutherford EJ, Morris JA, Reed GW, et al (1992) Base deficit stratifies mortality and determines therapy. J Trauma 33:417-422
14. Chang MC, Meredith JW (1997) Cardiac preload, splanchnic perfusion, and their relationship during resuscitation in trauma patients. J Trauma 42:577-584
15. Henry S, Scalea TM (1999) Resuscitation in the new millennium. Surg Clin North Am 79:1259-1267
16. Cosgriff N, Moore EE, Sauaia A, et al (1997) Predicting life-threatening coagulopathy in the massively transfused trauma patient: hypothermia and acidosis revisited. J Trauma 42:857-862
17. McKinley BA, Marvin RG, Cocanour CS, et al (2000) Tissue hemoglobin O_2 saturation during resuscitation of traumatic shock monitored using near infrared spectroscopy. J Trauma 48:637-642
18. Weil MH, Nakagawa Y, Tang W, et al (1999) Sublingual capnometry: a new noninvasive measurement tool for diagnosis and quantification of severity of circulatory shock. Crit Care Med 27:1225-1229

19. Holm C, Melcer B, Harbrand F, et al (2000) Intrathoracic blood volume as an endpoint in resuscitation of the severely burned: an observational study of 24 patients. J Trauma 48:728-734
20. Kellum JA (1998) Metabolic acidosis in the critically ill: lessons learned from physical chemistry. Kidney Int 53 [Suppl 66]:S81-S86
21. Healey MA, Davis RE, Liu FC, et al (1998) Lactated ringer's is superior to normal saline in a model of massive hemorrhage and resuscitation. J Trauma 45:894-899.
22. Scheingraber S, Rehm M, Semisch C, et al(1999) Rapid saline infusion produces hyperchloremic acidosis in patients undergoing gynecologic surgery. Anesthiology 90:1265-1270
23. PICU CM article
24. Patterson T, Bailey H, Kaplan LJ (2000) Hyperchloremia induces acidosis, increases the strong ion gap, and impairs coagulation. Crit Care Med 28:A118
25. Wilcox CS (1983) Regulation of renal blood flow by plasma chloride. J Clin Invest 71:726-735
26. Williams EL, Hildebrand KL, McCormick SA, et al (1999) The effect of intravenous lactated ringer's solution versus 0.9% sodium chloride solution on serum osmolality in human volunteers. Anesth Analg 88:999-1003
27. Wilkes N, Woolf R, Stephens R, et al (2001) The effects of balanced versus saline based intravenous solutions on acid-base status and gastric mucosal perfusion in elderly surgical patients. Anesth Analg (in press)
28. Prough DS, Bidani A (1999) Hyperchloremic metabolic acidosis is a predictable consequence of intraoperative infusion of 0.9% saline. Anesthiology 90:1247-1249
29. Waters JH, Miller LR, Clack S, et al (1999) Cause of metabolic acidosis in prolonged surgery. Crit Care Med 27:2142-2146
30. Kaplan LJ, Bailey H, Kozar R, et al (1999) Initial pH, base deficit, lactate, strong ion difference and gap, but not anion gap predict outcome from major vascular injury. Crit Care Med 27:A174
31. Kaplan LJ, Bailey H, Klein A, et al (1999) Strong ion gap: a predictor of early mortality following blunt or penetrating trauma. Crit Care Med 27:A42
32. Schierhout G, Roberts I (1998) Fluid resuscitation with colloid or crystalloid solutions in critically ill patients: a systematic review of randomized trials. BMJ 316:961-964
33. Alderson P, Hawkins V (2000) Colloid solutions for fluid resuscitation. Cochrane Database of Systematic Reviews (computer file). 2:CD001319
34. Wilkes MM, Navickis RJ (2001) No evidence of excess mortality in patients receiving human albumin: a meta-analysis of randomized controlled trials. Crit Care 5[Suppl 1]:S54
35. Burch JM (1997) New concepts in trauma. Am J Surg 173:44-46
36. Garrison JR, Richardson JD, Hilakos AS, et al (1996) Predicting the need to pack early for severe intra-abdominal hemorrhage. J Trauma 40:923-929
37. Hirshberg A, Sheffer N, Barnea O (1999) Computer simulation of hypothermia during "damage control" laparotomy. World J Surg 23:960-965
38. Moore EE (1996) Staged laparotomy for the hypothermia, acidosis, and coagulopathy syndrome. Am J Surg 172:405-410
39. Kinsky MP, Milner SM, Button B, et al (2000) Resuscitation of severe thermal injury with hypertonic saline dextran: effects on peripheral and visceral edema in sheep. J Trauma 49:844-853
40. Cinat ME, Wallace WC, Nastanski F, et al (1999) Improved survival following massive transfusion in patients who have undergone trauma. Arch Surg 134:964-970.
41. Neff T, Jungheinrich C, Doelberg M, et al (2001) Advantages of 6% hydroxyethyl starch 130/0.4 (Voluven) at repetitive high dose levels in patients with severe cranio-cerebral trauma. Crit Care 5[Suppl 1]:S53
42. Grauer MT, Baus D, Woessner, et al (2001) Effects on general safety and coagulation after long-term, high-dose volume therapy with 6% hydroxyethyl starch 130/0.4 in patients with acute ischemic stroke. Results of a randomized, placebo controlled, double-blind study. Crit Care 5[Suppl 1]:S53-54.
43. Via D, Kauffman C, Anderson D, et al (2001) Effect of hydroxyethyl starch on coagulopathy in a swine model of hemorrhagic shock and resuscitation. J Trauma 50:1076-1082

44. Kellum JA, Kramer DJ, Lee K, et al (1997) Release of lactate by the lung in acute lung injury. Chest 111:1301-1305
45. Eberhard LW, Morabito DJ, Mathay MA, et al (2000) Initial severity of metabolic acidosis predicts the development of acute lung injury in severely traumatized patients. Crit Care Med 28:125-131
46. Rhee P, Wang D, Ruff P, et al (2000) Human neutrophil activation and increased adhesion by various resuscitation fluids. Crit Care Med 28:74-78
47. Junger WG, Hoyt DB, Hamreus M, et al (1997) Hypertonic saline activates protein kinases and mitogen-activated protein kinase p38 in T-cells. J Trauma 42:437-443
48. Sillett HK, Whicher JT, Trejdosiewicz LK (1998) Effects of resuscitation fluids on T cell immune responses. Br J Anaesth 81:242-243
49. Safar P, Tisherman SA, Behringer W, et al (2000) Suspended animation for delayed resuscitation from prolonged cardiac arrest that is unresuscitable by standard cardiopulmonary-cerebral resuscitation. Crit Care Med 28[11 Suppl]:N214-218
50. Behringer W, Prueckner S, Kentner R, et al (2000) Rapid hypothermic aortic flush can achieve survival without brain damage after 30 minutes cardiac arrest in dogs. Anesthiology 93:1491-1499
51. McNeil JD, Smith DL, Jenkins DH, et al (2001) Hypotensive resuscitation using a polymerized bovine hemoglobin-based oxygen-carrying solution (HBOC-21) leads to a reversal of anaerobic metabolism. J Trauma 50:1063-1075

Monitoring of Intra-Abdominal Pressure and Clinical Challenges in Intensive Care Unit Patients

P. PELOSI, P. CAIRONI, L. GATTINONI

Increased intra-abdominal pressure (IAP) may occur in a number of different situations encountered by intensivists, such as tense ascites, abdominal hemorrhage, use of military antishock trousers, abdominal obstruction, during laparoscopy, large abdominal tumors, and peritoneal dialysis [1-7]. Both clinical and experimental evidence support the hypothesis that an increase in IAP may affect cardiac, renal, respiratory, and metabolic functions [1-12], as traditionally believed by most surgeons and intensivists. Nevertheless, increased IAP is rarely recognized and treated in intensive care unit (ICU) settings. This may be due to two different reasons: on the one hand the physiological consequences and the clinical importance of increased IAP are not well known to most physicians; on the other, the easy and precise measurement of IAP has not been well documented. Furthermore, the limits of increased IAP, above which it is necessary to intervene, are not well established.

Here, we will briefly report: (1) definitions of normal and pathological values of IAP; (2) the different methods proposed to evaluate IAP in ICU; (3) the physiological consequences of increased IAP; and (4) the current clinical evidence about the real effect and clinical relevance of increased IAP in patients admitted to the ICU.

Definitions

In spontaneously breathing subjects, IAP is normally equal to 0 mmHg or slightly subatmospheric (negative). In mechanically ventilated and paralyzed patients, it is slightly positive (9.0 ± 2.4 cmH_2O) [13], due to the transmission of positive intrathoracic pressure across the diaphragm [14].

From a clinical point of view, it is possible to identify a syndrome characterized by an increased value of IAP, the "abdominal compartment syndrome." Generally, it is defined as the occurrence of at least one of the following signs:

(1) abdominal distention; (2) increased IAP; (3) oliguria unsolved by volume administration; (4) increased peak inspiratory pressure; (5) hypercarbia; (6) hypoxemia refractory to increasing FiO2 and positive end-expiratory pressure (PEEP); (7) refractory metabolic acidosis; and (8) increased intracranial pressure.

The exact level of IAP above which it is possible to consider the intra-abdominal compartment syndrome is still debatable. Some authors suggest 25 mmHg as the critical value, while others suggest that even levels of IAP as low as 10 mmHg can determine organ dysfunction [15-20]. Recently, the use of the abdominal perfusion pressure (the difference between mean arterial pressure and IAP) has been suggested, instead of IAP, as a clinically more-useful endpoint and a more-effective predictor of patient survival during treatment for abdominal compartment syndrome [21].

IAP and its measurement

IAP can be measured either by direct or indirect methods. However, it is evident that direct methods can only be used as referral methods; they are not routinely applicable due to their invasiveness.

Direct method

Direct measurements through the use of an intraperitoneal catheter connected to a pressure transducer have been used as referral methods in several experimental studies [1, 10, 12, 22]. In some cases, an inflatable bag was placed into the abdominal cavity to produce and measure elevated pressure [23, 24].

Indirect methods

Two main indirect methods of estimating IAP have been proposed: (1) bladder pressure measurement and (2) gastric pressure measurement.

Bladder pressure

The estimate of IAP value through the measurement of bladder pressure was initially introduced in 1984 by Kron et al. [25], after small animal studies. Subsequently, several experimental studies were performed, to better understand the exact value of this technique, and in the last few years some authors have tried to validate the technique in patients [26].

Physiologically, the pressure in the bladder increases linearly within a range of 50 - 400 ml of infusion (0.5 cmH_2O /ml). It is extremely important to take into account this range, above all in obtaining reproducible and comparable data when subsequent measurements are performed. Probably different results achieved by several authors can be related to a different infusion volume used for bladder pressure measurement.

Briefly, 100 - 250 ml of sterile saline is injected into an empty bladder through a Foley catheter. The tubing of the drainage bag is then clamped distal to the sampling aspiration port and connected to the catheter. The clamp is released to allow the proximal drainage tubing to fill with saline from the bladder and then reapplied. A 16-gauge needle is inserted through the sampling aspiration port of the catheter and it is connected to a water manometer or a pressure transducer. Alternatively, a three-way stopcock can be added between the catheter and the drainage bag. With the patient in the supine position, the zero reference point is computed at the pubis level and the height of the water column above this level represents the IAP as measured in centimeters of water.

It has been reported, in experimental conditions [22], that bladder pressure is equal to IAP, as measured by peritoneal catheter within a range of 5 - 70 mmHg. Recently, some researchers have tested the validity of this technique in patients. Johna et al. [26], comparing the simultaneous direct measurement of bladder and abdominal pressure in a prospective study of surgical patients, reported an inequality between the absolute values of bladder and abdominal pressure, but they observed high positive correlation coefficients between these two variables, suggesting a good relationship between the variation of both. Moreover, they observed a higher baseline pressure of urinary bladder compared with abdomen pressure in each patient studied, attributing this inequality to the intrinsic detrusor muscle activity stimulated by the infusion volume. In another study, Fusco et al. [27] observed a close relationship between intravesicular and IAP; furthermore, they suggested an infusion volume of 50 ml to improve the accuracy of the bladder pressure in measuring elevated IAP.

Further studies are needed to define the exact accuracy of bladder pressure in estimating IAP, better characterizing different clinical conditions, the effects of different volumes of infusion, and other variables that can influence this relationship.

Gastric pressure

The accuracy and precision of IAP measurement by means of gastric pressure is controversial. Some authors did not find a good correlation between direct measurement of IAP and gastric pressure [28]. Others suggest that gastric pressure measured by nasogastric tube or gastric tonometer can appropriately estimate IAP [15, 29]. Gastric pressure is determined through the infusion of

50 - 100 ml of water into a nasogastric tube, positioned in the lumen of the stomach. The proximal end of the open tube is held perpendicular to the floor. The distance from the water level to the midaxillary line is taken as IAP in centimeters of water. Pressure obtained with this system has been correlated with bladder pressure [29]. Gastric pressure can even be measured using a gastric tonometer balloon, instilled with 2.5 - 3 ml of air [15].

IAP variations and physiological effects

The effects of IAP on physiological function of different organs may appear with an increased IAP of only 10 mmHg or more, and these have been evaluated both in animal and human studies.

Pulmonary effects

The pulmonary effects of increased IAP have been recognized for many years [3, 30-33]. IAP is transmitted to the thorax both directly and through cephalic deviation of the diaphragm. The elevation of the diaphragm likely increases the intrathoracic pressure, resulting in an extrinsic compression of the pulmonary parenchyma and the development of pulmonary dysfunction [1, 3]. The IAP can deeply affect gas exchange, respiratory mechanics, or work of breathing [1, 30, 32, 33].

Parenchymal compression results in alveolar atelectasis intrapulmonary shunt. With computed tomography analysis of lung images, we recently found, in an experimental model in supine pigs [34], that even a relatively low level of IAP (15 mmHg) can produce extensive atelectasis, especially at pulmonary base level, with a one third reduction of the total lung volume. In normal subjects undergoing increased abdominal pressure (15 mmHg) for laparoscopic surgery [35], we observed a more-limited reduction in lung volume and oxygenation, with marked alteration in lung and chest wall mechanics (reduction in compliance and increase in both "ohmic" and viscoelastic resistances). However, these patients were studied in the anti-Trendelenburg position, thus likely minimizing the effects of increased IAP on lung volume. Similar findings were reported in obese patients, who are characterized by increased IAP compared with normal subjects (18 ± 7.8 vs. 9.0 ± 2.4 cmH_2O) [13]. We found that the increase in IAP accounted for the reduction in lung volume (by one-third), oxygenation and respiratory compliance.

In patients with acute lung injury / acute respiratory distress syndrome (ALI / ARDS), during sedation and paralysis, several authors [36, 37] demonstrated that: (1) ALI / ARDS patients could be different in terms of lung and chest wall mechanics; (2) underlying etiologies and co-morbidities are important in explaining such differences; (3) the values of upper and lower inflection points of the pressure volume curve of the respiratory system can be unreliable; (4) IAP can affect chest wall mechanics; and (5) abdominal decompression may sometimes have a beneficial effect on respiratory mechanics and oxygenation. Malbrain [38] found a good correlation between the lower inflection point of the respiratory system and IAP, especially in patients with extra-pulmonary ALI / ARDS.

The IAP may also affect the respiratory function during assisted and/or spontaneous breathing. It has been clearly shown that lung volume and oxygenation are decreased, and work of breathing is increased, in the postoperative period, especially in obese patients [39].

All these findings have important clinical implications in the interpretation of respiratory mechanics and ventilatory management of patients. In the presence of increased IAP it follows that: (1) the static pressures of the respiratory system do not correctly represent the real transpulmonary pressure; (2) the recruitment pressures and the level of PEEP need to be titrated to higher; (3) the lung protective strategy suggested by the literature [40] may be difficult to apply; (4) the weaning phase can be more difficult than expected.

Cardiovascular effects

The increase in IAP, raising the intrathoracic pressure, generally results in diminished cardiac output [10, 24, 30-32]. Moreover, increased IAP may cause direct cardiac compression, reducing ventricular compliance and contractility [31], even if there is some recent evidence that the decrease in cardiac output is unlikely due to a significant decrease in cardiac contractility, but rather due to an increase in systemic vascular resistance [41]. Mean arterial pressure is usually unaffected by an increase in systemic vascular resistance (compression of both aorta and systemic and pulmonary vasculature), but it may decrease in patients with marginal cardiac contractility or inadequate vascular volume [10, 24, 30, 32].

Intracardiac pressures [i.e., wedge pressure (WP) and central venous pressure, (CVP)] usually increase with the increase of IAP [10, 12, 24, 31, 32, 42]. However, the rise in these pressures should be measured relative to the intrathoracic pressure. Consequently, increased IAP may affect interpretation of hemodynamics. Normal parameters of preload (WP and CVP) are unreliable. Moreover, it is likely that the requirement for vasoactive drugs in patients with abnormal IAP may be increased. Finally, increased IAP reduces the venous return from the lower extremities, thus promoting the formation of peripheral edema and the possible development of deep venous thrombosis.

Renal effects

Several studies showed a reduction in renal blood flow and function with increased IAP [23, 30, 32]. Different mechanisms have been proposed: (1) direct renal compression with consequent ischemia and failure [43, 44], with the histological evidence of parenchymal damage [45], and (2) compression of renal veins [30, 46]. Increase in IAP decreases glomerular filtration, with a consequent increase in blood urea nitrogen and serum creatinine clearance [23, 30, 32]. Thus, in patients with increased IAP, a renal protection, such as maintenance of generous urine output, should be warranted.

Gastrointestinal effects

The gut and the liver are considered the abdominal organs most sensitive to the increase in IAP. From a physiological point of view, IAP represents one of the most-important factors in determining mesenteric flow, especially in hypovolemic patients. The reduction in mesenteric flow and the loss of intestinal barrier function may facilitate bacterial translocation and the consequent development of multiple organ failure [47 – 49]. Thus, in patients with increased IAP, it is important to consider that: (1) selective decontamination can be useful; (2) vasoactive drugs with major negative effects on visceral perfusion (dopamine and adrenaline) should be used cautiously; (3) a mild hypovolemic status is always preferable; (4) the use of a gastric motility prokinetic (metoclopramide, cisapride, or erythromicin) can be useful.

Usually, in the presence of intra-abdominal hypertension or "abdominal compartment syndrome", the operative decompression of the abdominal cavity has been proposed as the "standard of care" [50, 51]. We think that the use of this approach should not be determined by intravescical pressure threshold per se but, rather, by the physiological consequences of increased IAP.

Central nervous system effects

Cerebral perfusion and intracranial pressure (ICP) are directly affected by increased IAP [52 – 56]. The mechanisms by which IAP increases ICP can be different: (1) decreased lumbar venous plexus blood flow with a consequent increase in cerebrospinal fluid pressure; (2) alteration in ventilation perfusion ratio, with a consequent increased in $paCO_2$, and (3) decreased cerebral blood outflow. Recently, we showed [57] that patients with neurosurgical problems (either traumatic or not) show higher levels of IAP compared with normal subjects after few days of mechanical ventilation. In another recent study performed in head trauma patients, Citerio et al. [58] reported a significant rise in ICP due to a rapid increase in IAP by positioning a soft water bag on the patients' abdomen. According to the authors, this effect seemed to be the result of an increase in intrathoracic pressure, with a consequent functional obstruction to cerebral venous outflow.

Thus, it follows that, in these patients, it is important to clinically consider: (1) a reduction of the central sympathetic output; (2) an increase in gastric motility with prokinetic drugs; (3) maintenance of a semi-supine position, and (4) a careful titration of dopamine, opioids, and sedatives, which can negatively affect gut perfusion.

Clinical data

Most of the data relative to IAP are obtained from anecdotal reports, animal studies, or small prospective studies, especially in the surgical literature. Very few data are from large multicenter trials in general ICUs. Two large prospective, observational studies were recently performed [38, 59]. Malbrain [38] enrolled 405 patients in a prospective pilot study performed in Belgium in a single unit. They found that the prevalence of IAP greater than 12 mmHg in the whole population was 17.2%, with a mean IAP value of 15.8±3.6 mmHg. The prevalence of IAP greater than 12 mmHg was 39.4% in emergency surgery patients, 19.8% in medical patients, and 6.1% in scheduled surgical patients. They also found that IAP was significantly higher in patients who died in ICU (13.2±5.2 vs. 7.0±3.6 mmHg), as well as in patients who died in hospital (11.5±5.3 vs. 6.9±3.6 mmHg). Multivariate analysis showed that IAP was an independent risk factor for ICU and hospital mortality, with an adjusted odds ratio of 1.5 (1.3 - 1.6) for ICU mortality, and 1.4 (1.2 - 1.5) for hospital mortality. Moreover, an IAP value greater than 12 mmHg was also predictive for the need for and the duration of mechanical ventilation, the occurrence of renal failure, and the need for renal replacement therapy, the cost of ICU and hospital stay, and the length of ICU stay. The authors concluded that the prevalence of a IAP value greater than 12 mmHg in the general population is quite high, the presence of only a slight rise of IAP can cause significant organ dysfunction, and it is an independent predictor of mortality and morbidity.

More recently, we performed a prospective observational multicenter study on IAP in a group of critically ill patients [59]. The study was performed in four different ICUs (Ospedale di Circolo – Varese, Italy; Ospedale Maggiore Policlinico – Milan, Italy; Ospedale S. Giovanni di Dio – Florence, Italy; Ospedale Civico – Lugano, Switzerland) for a period of 2 months.

All patients admitted to the ICU during the study period and staying in the ICU for at least 48 h were enrolled in the study. IAP was measured by bladder measurement each day in the first 5 days, and subsequently every 5 days up to the 1st month. Patient categories were defined according to Knaus et al. [60], while organ dysfunction was classified according to Bone et al. [61]. We enrolled 90 patients (61 males / 29 females, aged 52±28 years, SAPS 34.2±13.6) equally distributed into surgical (53.3%) and medical (46.7%) categories. The prevalence of patients treated with abdominal surgery in the surgical patient group was 32.2%. A control group of 25 patients undergoing general anesthesia for elective surgery not involving the abdomen was also evaluated. The mean IAP value in the 1st day was significantly higher in the study group than in the control group (13.1±7.13 vs. 6.1±2.4 mmHg, $P<0.01$). In the study group, the frequency distribution of IAP followed a Gaussian distribution (IAP $\leq$ 10 mmHg, 27.3%; 10<IAP$\leq$20 mmHg, 57.2%; 20<IAP$\leq$30 mmHg, 11.5%; IAP >30 mmHg, 3.9%). The average value and the distribution of IAP did not change significantly with time, being 13.4±7.0 mmHg at the end of the 1st week and 15.1±7.1 mmHg at the end of the 2nd week. Interestingly, we did not find significant differences in IAP values between surgical and medical patients (13.1±6.2 vs. 15.2±6.7 mmHg, respectively). However, IAP markedly differed within surgical and medical categories. In the medical patient group, IAP was higher ($P<0.01$) in patients with abdominal non-surgical problems (19.3±5.7 mmHg) compared with patients with cardiological, neurological or respiratory problems (10.0±6.1, 11.2±7.4, 19.8±6.9 mmHg, respectively). In surgical patients, IAP was higher ($P<0.01$) in neurosurgical and cardiosurgical patients (18.7±4.3 and 17.6±4.9 mmHg, respectively) compared with thoracic and abdominal surgical patients (11.1±2.1 and 13.4±1.7 mmHg, respectively). The effects of IAP on organ function are summarized in Table 1.

IAP was different between intubated and non-intubated patients (15±6 vs. 12±7 mmHg, respectively; $P<0.05$). Moreover, PEEP and peak pressure increased, while paO_2 / FiO_2 decreased with increased IAP. However, $paCO_2$ was not influenced by IAP. The increased IAP was also associated with a decrease in mean arterial pressure and a marked increase in the use of vasoactive drugs, being 83% of the patients treated with IAP 20 mmHg. Conversely, the IAP values in the group of patients treated with vasoactive drugs were higher than in the group of untreated patients (15±6 vs. 12±7 mmHg, respectively, $P<0.01$). Similarly, diuresis decreased and blood urea increased with increased IAP. However, these effects were more pronounced in patients using diuretics

Table 1. Effects of intra-abdominal pressure (IAP) (mmHg) on organ function. Data are expressed as mean (± SD)

	IAP ≤ 10	10 IAP ≤ 20	IAP >20
PEEP (cmH_2O)	7.1 ± 4.2	8.2 ± 5.1	10.3 ± 6.2*
Peak (cmH_2O)	24.9 ± 7.4	25.6 ± 6.3	28.4 ± 7.7*
PaO_2 / FiO_2	308 ± 144	284 ± 136	248 ± 120*
$PaCO_2$ (mmHg)	42.9 ± 8.7	40.0 ± 8.6	42.9 ± 9.0
MAP (mmHg)	90 ± 16	91 ± 16	83 ± 14*
Vasoactive drugs (%)	24	54	83*
Diuresis (ml/day)	2,636 ± 1139	2,645 ± 1,316	1,902 ± 1,627*
Blood urea (mg/dl)	61 ± 50	60 ± 54	80 ± 69*

*(ANOVA: P <0.001)

compared with those not using diuretics. No significant difference was found in IAP between ICU survivors and non-survivors (13.6±7.3 vs. 14.0±6.3 mmHg, respectively), even though IAP values were linearly associated (r = 0.58, P<0.01) with sepsis-related organ failure assessment (SOFA) score [62].

Conclusions

Considering overall the physiological data from animal and human studies, and the findings of the two large studies reported above, we can conclude that:

1) the majority of critically ill patients show an IAP between 10 and 20 mmHg and increased values compared with normal subjects;
2) IAP is different among different categories of patients, and its increase is not limited to surgical patients only;
3) the increase in IAP appears to influence the respiratory system, hemodynamic status and renal function;
4) IAP seems to be correlated with severity scores, but its relation to mortality is controversial.

Future trials are warranted to evaluate both the influence of routine IAP measurement in the management of critically ill patients and the mechanical and pharmacological methods to reduce IAP.

References

1. Richardson JD, Trinkle JK (1976) Hemodynamic and respiratory alterations with increased intra-abdominal pressure. J Surg 20:401-404
2. Lynch FP, Ochi T, Scully JM, et al (1974) Cardiovascular effects of increased intra-abdominal pressure in newborn piglets. J Pediatr Surg 9:621-626
3. Barnes GE, Laine GA, Giam PY, et al (1985) Cardiovascular responses to elevation of intra-abdominal hydrostatic pressure. Am J Physiol 248:208-213
4. Robotham JL, Wise RA, Bromberger-Barnea B (1985) Effects of changes in abdominal pressure on left ventricular performance and regional blood flow. Crit Care Med 13:803-809
5. Burchard KW, Ciombor DM, McLeod MK, et al (1985) Positive end expiratory pressure with increased intra-abdominal pressure. Surg Gynecol Obstet 161:313-318
6. Celoria G, Steingrub J, Dawson JA, et al (1987) Oliguria from high intra-abdominal pressure secondary to ovarian mass. Crit Care Med 15:78-79
7. Schurig R, Gahl GM, Becker H, et al (1979) Hemodynamic studies in long-term peritoneal dialysis patients. Trans Am Soc Artif Intern Organs 3:215-218
8. Ivankovich AD, Miletich DJ, Albrecht RF, et al (1975) Cardiovascular effects of intraperitoneal insufflation with carbon dioxide and nitrous oxide in the dog. Anesthesiology 42:281-287
9. Le Roith D, Bark H, Nyska M, et al (1982) The effect of abdominal pressure on plasma antidiuretic hormone levels in the dog. J Surg 32:65-69
10. Kashtan J, Green JF, Parsons EQ, et al (1981) Hemodynamic effects of increased abdominal pressure. J Surg 30:249-255
11. Burchard KW, Slotman GJ, Jed E, et al (1985) Positive pressure respirations and pneumatic antishock garment application – hemodynamic response. J Trauma 25:83-89
12. Diamant M, Benumof JL, Saidman LJ (1978) Hemodynamics of increased intra-abdominal pressure: interaction with hypovolemia and halothane anesthesia. Anesthesiology 48:23-27
13. Pelosi P, Ravagnan I, Giurati G, et al (1999) Positive end-expiratory pressure improves respiratory function in obese but not in normal subjects during anesthesia and paralysis. Anesthesiology 91:1221-1231
14. Schein M, Wittman DH, Aprahamian CC, et al (1995) The abdominal compartment syndrome: the physiological and clinical consequences of elevated intra-abdominal pressure. J Am Coll Surg180:745-753
15. Sugrue M, Buist MD, Lee A, et al (1994) Intra-abdominal pressure measurement using a modified nasogastric tube: description and validation of a new technique. Intensive Care Med 20:588-590
16. Schein M, Ivatury R (1998) Intra-abdominal hypertension and abdominal compartment syndrome. Br J Surg 85:1027-1028
17. Ivatury RR, Diebel L, Porter JM, et al (1997) Intra-abdominal hypertension and the abdominal compartment syndrome. Surg Clin North Am 77:783-799
18. Kron IL, Harman PK, Nolan SP (1984) The measurement of intra-abdominal pressure as a criterion for abdominal re-exploration. Ann Surg 199:28-30
19. Sugrue M, Jones F, Janjua KJ, et al (1998) Temporary abdominal closure: a prospective evaluation of its effects on renal and respiratory physiology. J Trauma 45:914-921
20. Meldrum DR, Moore FA, Moore EE, et al (1997) Prospective characterization and selective management of the abdominal compartment syndrome. Am J Surg 174:667-673
21. Cheatham ML, White MW, Sagraves SG, et al (2000) Abdominal perfusion pressure: a superior parameter in the assessment of intra-abdominal hypertension. J Trauma 49:621-626
22. Iberti TJ, Kelly KM, Gentili DR, et al (1987) A simple technique to accurately determine intra-abdominal pressure. Crit Care Med 15:1140-1142
23. Harman PK, Kron IL, McLachlan HD, et al (1982) Elevated intra-abdominal pressure and renal function. Ann Surg 196:594-597
24. Caldwell CB, Ricotta JJ (1987) Changes in visceral blood flow with elevated intraabdominal pressure. J Surg 43:14-20

25. Kron IL, Harman PK, Nolan SP (1984) The measurement of intra-abdominal pressure as a criterion of abdominal re-exploration. Ann Surg 199:28-30
26. Johna S, Taylor E, Brown C, et al (1999) Abdominal compartment syndrome: does intra-cystic pressure reflect actual intra-abdominal pressure ? A prospective study in surgical patients. Crit Care 3:135-138
27. Fusco MA, Martin RS, Chang MC (2001) Estimation of intra-abdominal pressure by bladder pressure measurement: validity and methodology. J Trauma 50:297-302
28. Lacey SR, Bruce J, Brooks SP, et al (2000) The relative merits of various methods of indirect measurement of intraabdominal pressure as a guide to closure of abdominal wall defects. J Pediatr Surg 22:1207-1211
29. Collee GG, Lomax DM, Ferguson C, et al (1993) Bedside measurement of intra-abdominal pressure (IAP) via an indwelling naso-gastric tube: clinical validation of the technique. Intensive Care Med 19: 478-480
30. Shenasky JH, Gillenwater JY (1972) The renal hemodynamic and functional effects of external counterpressure. Surg Gynecol Obstet 134:253-258
31. Cullen DJ, Coyle JP, Teplich R, et al (1989) Cardiovascular, pulmonary, and renal effects of massively increased intra-abdominal pressure in critically ill patients. Crit Care Med 17:118-121
32. Iberti TJ, Lieber CE, Benjamin E (1989) Determination of intra-abdominal pressure using a transuretheral bladder catheter: clinical validation of the technique. Anesthesiology 70:47-50
33. Fietsam R, Villalba M, Glover JL, et al (1989) Intra-abdominal compartment syndrome as a complication of ruptured abdominal aortic aneurysm repair. Am Surg 56:396-402
34. Luecke T, Hezzman P, Caironi P, et al (2001) Oleic acid and intra-abdominal pressure effects on lung morphology in an experimental animal model. Proceedings 9th ESA Annual Meeting.
35. Pelosi P, Foti G, Cereda M, et al (1996) Effects of carbon dioxide insufflation for laparoscopic cholecystectomy on the respiratory system. Anaesthesia 51:744-749
36. Gattinoni L, Pelosi P, Suter PM, et al (1998) Acute respiratory distress syndrome caused by pulmonary and extrapulmonary disease. Different syndromes ? Am J Respir Crit Care 158:3-11
37. Ranieri VM, Brienza N, Santostasi S, et al (1997) Impairment of lung and chest wall mechanics in patients with acute respiratory distress syndrome: role of abdominal distention. Am J Respir Crit Care 156:1082-1091
38. Malbrain MLNG (1999) Abdominal pressure in the critically ill: measurement and clinical relevance. Intensive Care Med 25:1453-1458
39. Pelosi P, Croci M, Ravagnan I, et al (1996) Total respiratory system, lung, and chest wall mechanics in sedated-paralyzed postoperative morbidly obese patients. Chest 109:144-151
40. Amato MBP, Barbas CSV, Medeiros DM, et al (1998) Effect of a protective-ventilation strategy on mortality in the acute respiratory distress syndrome. N Engl J Med 338:347-354
41. Kaklamanos IG, Condos S, Merrell RC (2000) Time-related changes in hemodynamic parameters and pressure-derived indices of left ventricular function in a porcine model of prolonged pneumoperitoneum. Surg Endosc 14:834-838
42. Bendahan J, Coetzee CJ, Papagianopoulos C et, al (1995) Abdominal compartment syndrome. J Trauma 38:152-153
43. Watson RA, Howdieshell TR (1998) Abdominal compartment syndrome. South Med J 91:326-332
44. Stone HH, Fulenwider TJ (1977) Renal decapsulation in the prevention of post-ischemic oliguria. Ann Surg 35:11-18
45. Altintas F, Tunali Y, Bozkurt P, et al (2001) An experimental study on the relationship of intra-abdominal pressure and renal ischemia. Middle East J Anesthesiol 16:55-56
46. Richards WO, Scovill W, Shin B, et al (1983) Acute renal failure associated with increased intra-abdominal pressure. Ann Surg 197:183-187
47. Diebel LN, Myers T, Dulchavsky S (1997) Effects of increasing airway pressure and PEEP on the assessment of cardiac preload. J Trauma 42:585-591
48. Diebel LN, Dulchavsky SA, Brown WJ (1997) Splanchnic ischemia and bacterial translocation in the abdominal compartment syndrome. J Trauma 43:852-855

49. Gargiulo NJ3, Simon RJ, Leon W, et al (1998) Hemorrhage exacerbates bacterial translocation at low levels of intra-abdominal pressure. Arch Surg 133:1351-1355
50. Sherck J, Seiver A, Shatney C, et al (1998) Covering the "open abdomen": a better technique. Am Surg 64:854-857
51. Brock WB, Barker DE, Burns RP (1995) Temporary closure of open abdominal wounds: the vacuum pack. Am Surg 61:30-35
52. Bloomfield GL, Ridings PC, Blocher CR, et al (1996) Effects of increased intra-abdominal pressure upon intracranial and cerebral perfusion pressure before and after volume expansion. J Trauma 40:936-943
53. Bloomfield GL, Blocher CR, Fakhry IF, et al (1997) Elevated intra-abdominal pressure increased plasma renin activity and aldosterone levels. J Trauma 42:997-1004
54. Luce JM, Huseby JS, Kirk W, et al (1982) Mechanism by which positive end-expiratory pressure increases cerebrospinal fluid pressure in dogs. J Appl Physiol 52:231-235
55. Josephs LG, Este-McDonald JR, Birkett DH, et al (1994) Diagnostic laparoscopy increases intracranial pressure. J Trauma 36:815-819
56. Burchiel KJ, Steege TD, Wyler AR (1981) Intracranial pressure changes in brain-injured patients requiring positive end-expiratory pressure ventilation. Neurosurgery 8:443-449
57. Pelosi P, Colombo G, Gamberoni C, et al (2000) Effects of positive end-expiratory pressure on respiratory function in head injured patients. Intensive Care Med 26:S329
58. Citerio G, Vascotto E, Villa F, et al (2001) Induced abdominal compartment syndrome increases intracranial pressure in neurotrauma patients: a prospective study. Crit Care Med 29:1466-1471
59. Pelosi P, Malacrida R, Oggioni M, et al (2001) Intra-abdominal pressure in critically ill patients: a prospective, observational, multicentre study. Proceedings 9th ESA Annual Meeting.
60. Knaus WA, Wagner DP, Draper EA, et al (1991) The APACHE III prognostic system. Risk prediction of hospital mortality for critically ill hospitalized adults. Chest 100:1619-1636
61. Bone RC, Fisher CJ, Clemmer TP, et al (1987) A controlled clinical trial of high dose methylprednisolone in the treatment of severe sepsis and septic shock. N Engl J Med 317:653-658
62. Vincent JL, Moreno R, Takala J, et al (1996) The SOFA (sepsis-related organ failure assessment) score to describe organ dysfunction/failure. Intensive Care Med 22:707-710

Experimenting on Your Fellow Humans in 2001. Update of the Declaration of Helsinki and Progress from the International Conference on Harmonization

J. H. SILVERSTEIN

We are all the beneficiaries of a culture sufficiently developed that we can expect to prescribe drugs that are effective. We expect that the side effect profile of an approved drug is well enough understood, such that there is agreement that the benefits outweigh the risks of taking the drug. We also universally believe that, in the process of developing drugs, subjects of research should not be abused. On the other hand, we would not think that every country would require completely different types of information in order to make such decisions. Nonetheless, this has been the case for many years. In general, it was easier to introduce a new drug in Europe than in the United States even though there is little reason to suspect that the risk:benefit ratio would be different on one side of the Atlantic versus the other. Furthermore, the information used to bring a drug to market in Europe and the United States had little value when seeking regulatory approval from Japanese authorities. Therefore, a number of international efforts to develop and support international standards have developed. These developing frameworks of global perspective on pharmaceuticals and human subject protections have both seen recent updates.

Declaration of Helsinki

The Declaration of Helsinki is an international document declaring standard for human subjects protections. It is issued by the World Medical Association (WMA). The document has neither the force of law nor treaty. This years updated declaration seeks to advance the level of protection afforded research subjects, one of which, the elimination of most placebo controls, has been the subject of some controversy.

In August of 1947, the Nazi doctors trial concluded with the conviction of

15 of 23 defendants charged with murder, torture, and other atrocities committed in the name of medical science. In their judgement, the judges included a set of standards by which they deliberated. What has become known as the Nuremberg Code stated that:

- The informed consent of volunteers must be obtained without coercion in any form.
- Human experiments should be based upon prior animal experimentation.
- Anticipated scientific results should justify the experiment
- Only qualified scientists should conduct medical research
- Physical and mental suffering and injury should be avoided
- There should be no expectation of death or disabling injury from the experiment

Although it represents the beginning of the modern era of human subject protection, the Nuremberg Code was crafted by judges, as opposed to individuals involved in human research. After nearly 10 years of deliberation, the World Medical Association issued the Declaration of Helsinki in 1964. This statement of ethical principles defined rules for therapeutic and non-therapeuticly research. It has been amended five times, most recently at the 52nd WMA General Assembly held in Edinburgh, Scotland in October of 2000. The current revision has attempted to strengthen human subject protection. In doing so, the current Declaration has made two recommendations that are fairly controversial.

The revised declaration states that new treatments should be tested against the "best current" treatment, not a placebo, unless no proven treatment exists. The interpretation and practical implications of such a sweeping statement are not clear. The United States Food and Drug Administration (FDA) argues that placebo-controlled studies should remain the gold standard for evaluating any new drug. Even for new pain drugs, the FDA frequently requires a placebo control. Although in recent years with the acceptance of morphine sparing as an end point, placebo controls have become less onerous for patients. Others argue that it may be justified to test a new treatment against both a placebo and the best current treatment. This type of study design may be particularly appealing when currently commonly used treatments have limited efficacy or have been proven in substantially different populations than the proposed study. A strict interpretation of the revised declaration prohibits such three-armed studies, although many study design experts support their use.

The term "best current therapy" is also controversial. For researchers conducting trials outside the European Economic Community, particularly in developing countries, does it mean the best care available in the European Union, or the best available locally? Important examples of the dilemma were raised by recent AIDs/HIV studies in Africa. Complicated triple drug regimens that are the standard of care in developed countries require exact timing of drug consumption and vigilance for side effects. Some investigators have argued that using a complicated three-drug regimen in impoverished countries, where there is no medical infrastructure and frequently no running water, is actually dangerous for the participants. However, patients' rights advocates respond that this is precisely the intent of the Declaration. They argue that the best proven universal therapy must be provided and point out that the Declaration of Helsinki is a scientific standard, not an economic one.

Using the same example, another controversial aspect of the revised Declaration reads "At the conclusion of the study, every patient entered into the study should be assured of access to the best proven prophylactic, diagnostic and therapeutic methods identified by the study." Who or what group is supposed to make the therapies available is not contained in the document. The Declaration does not define, nor even suggest, the circumstances by which they should be made available. Frequently the results of a study are not available for months following completion of data collection. So, when should participants expect follow-up medication? Should the governments of developing nations pay for the treatments, even though developing nations generally spend relatively few dollars on health care? The pharmaceutical industry is unlikely to provide drugs free of charge to large numbers of study participants.

The Declaration of Helsinki is not the only international standard that might be applied to human subject protection. The Council of Europe has issued a statement entitled Convention on Human Rights and Biomedicine that is referred to as the Bioconvention. The International Conference on Harmonization (ICH), an international consortium of drug regulatory agencies indicates that if no harm comes to the patient, a placebo is allowable. The World Health Organization (WHO) and the United Nations Educational, Scientific, and Cultural Organization (UNESCO) are also involved in global research ethics.

The latest rendition of the Declaration of Helsinki contains a number of other new issues. An important suggestion is a call to publish negative studies that do not support a treatment's effectiveness. The WMA stated that the importance of negative information has long been ignored, particularly by journal editors.

The International Conference on Harmonization

The International Conference on Harmonisation (ICH) of Technical Requirements for Registration of Pharmaceuticals for Human Use began in 1990 by bringing together members of the pharmaceutical community with regulatory authorities from the European Union, Japan, and the United States.

The ICH seeks to provide a coherent set of rules for drug development, manufacture, and marketing across multiple nations. The evolution of the European Economic Community and increased access to information about drugs in various countries has provided a backdrop for this attempt to provide a rational environment for drug development. An example of a goal of the ICH is a system in which a series of clinical trials would be adequate for submission for regulatory clearance in three regions (Europe, US, Japan), as opposed to requiring separate and distinct clinical trials for each country in which a pharmaceutical might be marketed.

There are six parties directly involved as well as observers and the International Federation of Pharmaceutical Manufacturers Association (I-FPMA). The original six parties include: The European Commission - European Union; European Federation of Pharmaceutical Industries and Associations (EFPIA); Ministry of Health, Labor and Welfare, Japan (MHLW); Japan Pharmaceutical Manufacturers Association (JPMA); the FDA; Pharmaceutical Research and Manufacturers of America (PhRMA). Since ICH was initiated, in 1990, there have been observers associated with the process, to act as a link with non-ICH countries and regions. The Observers to ICH are: WHO, The European Free Trade Area (EFTA), represented at ICH by Switzerland, and Canada.

The Fifth ICH (ICH5) took place in San Diego, 9-11 November, 2000 marking the tenth anniversary of this important harmonization activity. The Conference followed the meeting of the ICH Steering Committee and Expert Working Groups earlier in the week at which a final harmonized Common Technical Document (CTD) was completed. The CTD is an important step towards standardizing regulatory submissions across regions. The electronic version of this document (eCTD) is nearing completion.

In addition to the CTD, a large number of technical documents were presented at ICH5. Guidelines on Good Manufacturing Practices for Active Pharmaceutical Ingredients (Q7A), Safety Pharmacology (S7), Revision of the Stability Guideline (Q1A), and Revision of Toxicokinetics/Pharmacokinetics Guideline (S5/M3) were finalized. The Sixth International Conference on Harmonization (ICH6) will take place in Japan in fall 2003.

Practising physicians may engage in research activities or administer to patients who are asked to participate in research projects. The Declaration of Helsinki represents an international standard that seeks to protect the rights of human subjects, an evolving field that is not without controversy. Few practising physicians will even come into direct contact with the processes of the

ICH, but should be aware of attempts for global standardization of drug development and regulation.

For further information of the Declaration of Helsinki see:
http://www.wma.net/e/approvedhelsinki.html

For further information on the International Conference on Harmonization see:
http://www.ifpma.org

Ethical, Legal, Practical and Scientific Challenges in Perioperative Medicine

P.D. LUMB

Cost-effective, safe, timely, and socially responsible are the watchwords of accountable, outcome-dependent twenty-first century medical care and its delivery. Requisite physician and allied professional behavioral changes necessary to accommodate new performance standards are most noted in the acute interventional and perioperative specialties because immediacy is associated not only with advanced technology, but also with obvious outcome accountability. Anaesthesiologists, critical care physicians and surgeons are equally accountable in the new paradigm, and the likely direction of change may be predicted in the new publication from the Institute of Medicine, Crossing the Quality Chasm: A New Health System for the 21st Century. This is the sequel to the report To Err is Human published in November 1999, and it focuses attention in different but equally difficult areas to change. William Richardson, (President W.K. Kellogg Foundation and Chair, Committee on Health Care in America) preceded the introduction of the report with a widely publicised opening statement and executive summary. He prefaced his remarks noting the "U.S. health care system is in need of fundamental change. Americans ought to be able to count on receiving care that is safe and uses the best scientific knowledge. But there is strong evidence that this is not the case. Health care today harms too frequently, and fails to deliver its potential benefits routinely. ... Between the care we have and the care we could have lies not just a gap, but a wide chasm" [1].

The committee presented both a strategy and implementation plan that seeks to address specific concerns and eliminate public mistrust of the health care rendered. The report concentrates on the following agenda items:

1. Care should be safe. Patients should not be harmed by the care that is intended to help them.
2. Care should be effective, that is, based on sound scientific knowledge.
3. Care should be patient-centered. It should be respectful and responsive to individual preferences, needs, and values.

4. Care should be timely. Unnecessary waits and sometimes harmful delays should be reduced.
5. Care should be efficient, not wasteful of equipment, supplies, ideas, or energy.
6. Care should be equitable. Care should not vary in quality because of patient characteristics, such as ethnicity or geographic location [1].

The committee also presented the following ten rules to underscore the patient-physician relationship in the new century:

1. Care should be based on continuous healing relationships. The health care system should be responsive at all times, and access to care should be provided over the Internet, by telephone, and by other means in addition to face-to-face visits.
2. Care should be customized based on patient needs and values. The system of care should be designed to meet the most-common types of needs, but have the capability to respond to individual patient choices and preferences.
3. Control should reside with the patient. Patients should be given the necessary information and the opportunity to exercise the degree of control they choose over health care decisions that affect them.
4. Knowledge and information should be shared with the patient. Patients should have unfettered access to their own medical information and to clinical knowledge.
5. Clinical decisions should be evidence based, that is, patients should receive care based on the best scientific evidence.
6. The care system should be safe. Patients should not have to worry about injury.
7. The health system should be more transparent and make information available to patients and their families that allows them to make informed decisions when selecting a health plan, hospital, or clinical practice, or when choosing among alternative treatments.
8. The health system should anticipate patient needs rather than simply reacting to events.
9. The health system should not waste resources or patient time.
10. There should be more co-operation among clinicians to ensure an appropriate exchange of information and co-ordination of care [1].

In the intensive care unit (ICU), some of these responsibilities will be delegated to family members, but overall the sweeping changes implied in these initiatives can not be ignored and, indeed, must be embraced by the acute care community. The real question is not when the change must occur, rather, supplemental instruction in strategic planning and mechanisms of change are becoming as prevalent as basic and clinical science electives in medical school and residency programs. Many private practice groups are requiring that new partners be instructed in and conform to the business practices of the organization. Utilization of restricted formularies is common, not only to control excess cost, but also to insure quality and safety. Physician autonomy, once thought to be sacrosanct, is becoming more myth than reality.

Linked to and equally important to medical practice is the increased and legitimate public oversight placed on medical research and human subject protection by Institutional Revue Boards (IRB). Headlines in the Los Angeles Times on July 22 read "Death Halts Human tests at University" [2]. The article relates the unfortunate death of a young human research volunteer at a well--respected research university and the apparent lack of appropriate oversight by the institution's human subject's review board. Subsequently, testing was resumed, but the public scrutiny and concern over the event will linger legitimately.

In this environment, it is not surprising that the familiar subjects of scientific publication (results of controlled clinical trials, multi-center reviews, results of new drug formulations, or medical techniques, etc.) are joined by discussions of ethical and quality improvement issues seasoned with administrative techniques that target cost-effective and socially responsible practice. Although these discussions have always been a part of ethical practice, the new reality includes a greater public sophistication and interest in the outcome of the medical process. In the United States, legal interest in medical outcome has long been a part of medical practice, and it is apparent that this interest has been globalized in the past few years. A recent report prepared for the Agency for Healthcare and Quality, Making Health Care Safer: A Critical Analysis of Patient Safety Practices [3] notes in its introduction: "Patient safety has become a major concern of the general public and of policymakers at the State and Federal levels. This interest has been fuelled, in part, by news coverage of individuals who were the victims of serious medical errors and by the publication in 1999 of the Institute of Medicine's (IOM's) report To Err is Human: Building a Safer Health System. In its report, the IOM highlighted the risks of medical care in the United States and shocked the sensibilities of many Americans, in large part through its estimates of the magnitude of medical-errors-related deaths (44,000 to 98,000 deaths per year) and other serious adverse events." Subsequently, the report notes, "Three months after publication of the IOM report, an interagency Federal government group, the Quality Interagency Coordination Task Force (QuIC), released its response, Doing What Counts for Patient Safety: Federal Actions to Reduce Medical Errors and Their Impact. That report, prepared at the President's request, both inventoried ongoing Federal actions to reduce medical errors and listed more than 100 action items to be undertaken by Federal agencies." It was noted that "an action promised by the Agency for Healthcare Research and Quality (AHRQ), the Federal agency leading efforts to research and promote patient safety, was "the development and dissemination of evidence-based, best safety practices to provider organizations." [3] It is this promise and inclusion of federal regulation that should interest practitioners and forewarn of the significant changes in personal prerogative that these changes portend.

In a publicly accessible informational page hosted by the Institute of Medicine and referring to the report Crossing the Quality Chasm, the following statement appears: "Without substantial changes in the way health care is delivered, problems resulting from the growing complexity of medical science and technologies will only increase. To illustrate some of the serious problems facing patients and clinicians today, the report provides a *case study* – a composite based on the real experiences of many patients – describing the delays in care and frustrations faced by a woman who is eventually diagnosed with breast cancer. Revamping health care services and incorporating new technologies could improve the *care of such a patient* dramatically in the future. To spur an overhaul, Congress should create an "innovation fund" of U.S.$1 billion for use during the next 3 - 5 years to help subsidise promising projects and communicate the need for rapid and significant change throughout the health system. The report offers examples of projects that might be supported through such a fund, including *using information technology* to improve a hospital emergency department, *forming a partnership* to improve care for people with chronic diseases, and *reorganising staff* for patient-centred primary care" [4]. The web browser availability of such information increases the likelihood of public awareness of and interest in the newer medical technologies. Patients are encouraged to research rare illnesses, and it is increasingly common for patients to arrive for a medical appointment armed with the latest research information relating to their condition. In some cases, this may be embarrassing for the under-prepared physician; in many, it may lead to false expectation and legitimate disappointment. This situation alone has required a change in the management style of many practitioners.

Perhaps of more interest to anesthesiologists and critical care physicians is a recent *JAMA* article questioning the use of the pulmonary artery catheter in patients undergoing non-cardiac surgery [5]. The conclusion states, "No evidence was found of reduction in complication rates associated with use of perioperative RHC (right heart catheterisation) in this population. Because of the morbidity and the high costs associated with RHC, the impact of this intervention in perioperative care should be evaluated in randomised trials." The study is companioned by an editorial in which the use of the pulmonary artery catheter (PAC) is criticized in the following manner: "Despite its widespread use, the efficacy and safety of the PAC remains uncertain. It is clear that the PAC provides haemodynamic data that are used to make therapeutic decisions. The critical question is whether these therapeutic decisions improve outcomes. Some studies suggested that use of the PAC may actually worsen outcomes" [6]. The reason this study is important for anesthesiologists is that it compares outcomes in matched patients undergoing major non-cardiac surgery at a tertiary care teaching hospital. The results suggest that there is no evidence to support improved outcome secondary to PAC placement and use, and that the converse may be true. Dalen continues, "In the final analysis, diagnostic tests and monitoring devices do not determine clinical outcomes–treatment does. If the PAC does not alter treatment decisions, it can have no effect on the clinical outcome other than that attributed to the potential complications of PAC itself (<5%). To benefit patients, the PAC must provide information that is not otherwise available, and that information must be necessary to select a treatment plan that has proven clinical benefit" [6]. The study is interesting because it pits clinical intuition against hemodynamic monitoring, and intuition appears to be the victor. This is at variance with the popular beliefs that have supported the development of many critical initiatives developed over the past several years. Also, it is important to note that "because 91% of patients (182/100) who underwent abdominal aortic aneurysm repair also had RHC, patients undergoing this procedure were excluded from the analysis." This is of specific interest to anesthesiologists who, although providing data to the study, appear not to have been involved in the study design or management. It is imperative that the anesthesiology and critical care communities collaborate on prospective studies to determine whether it is possible to establish management protocols for defined surgical populations in which invasive monitoring decisions are based on outcome determinants rather than on personal bias, institutional custom or fiscal considerations.

Similarly, anesthesiologists in the United States are challenged today by "economic and social pressures (on workers) to place production, not safety, as their primary priority" [7]. This issue of the *Anesthesia Patient Safety Newsletter* quotes a study of California anesthesiologists in which "overt external production pressure was noted from surgeons, administrators, and policies of managed care organizations." This is an interesting situation because it is one in which anesthesiologists are defining themselves as patient advocates despite a financial disincentive to delay or otherwise interfere with surgical case volume. In part, this situation may have developed because of the exposure anesthesiologists face for an immediate poor outcome following surgical procedures. Certainly, public expectation is high, and it is interesting to note that South African plastic surgeons are now participating in "scalpel safaris", package tours designed for a combination plastic surgery remake and a traditional South African safari [8]. Obviously, the public has little awareness of surgical morbidity, yet recent reports have raised concerns about the safety of liposuction procedures under some outpatient conditions. In an introduction to this issue, Morrell and Prielipp note "if you still remain skeptical, then remember, too, that you cannot 'prove' that dragons do not exist" [9].

Change will not be without cost, and the recent controversy surrounding the National Institute of Health's reports have prompted medical scientists to conclude that significant government investment will be required to provide the intellectual, scientific and information systems architecture necessary to spur the necessary research and development to initiate and study change. In addition to the previously suggested innovation fund [4], additional investment is likely to come from partnerships between medical institutions and private corporations. It will be important to prevent financial conflict of interest in these relationships, and corporate and professional integrity must be preserved, especially in the face of increased public scrutiny. The situation has been exacerbated in the United States by market forces that are reducing and/or delaying payments to hospitals and physicians. The situation will be exacerbated by government-mandated investments in new computer technology necessary to comply with the Health Insurance Portability and Accountability Act of 1996 (HIPAA); in California alone the investment is expected to be approximately U.S. $2.5 billion. [10] Although the report concentrates on a number of problems unique to this state, including special building programs necessary to insure earthquake integrity, nonetheless, most of the issues are relevant to institutions world-wide. Increasing sophistication in pharmaceuticals and technology comes at an increased cost, increasingly resented by government, private and public payers alike. Indeed, a recent article underscores this trend by reporting that, "For nearly a century, every time the American economy boomed, it left an enduring legacy of vast new public works and bold private initiatives that were intended to benefit all. But as the nation comes off the expansion of the 1990s, the longest in its history, it has few similar accomplishments to show for the good times. Americans are twice as likely to own a personal computer as they were when the growth began. But they're also more likely to run short of the power needed to operate it. *They can purchase the most technologically advanced health care on Earth but face a rising risk of being unable to find an emergency room or a variety of basic drugs. They can buy Perrier but can't always get clean tap water.* The chief reason: The prosperity of the last decade has been a peculiarly private affair" [11]. The implications should be of significant concern to all individuals involved in health care delivery from individual patient concerns (the sharp end), to the systems approach necessary to insure the public good. This will all occur under new public awareness and scrutiny, with heightened interest in outcome and accountability. This is not to imply that prior activities were somehow lacking; rather, the environment has changed and expectations have accelerated. Also, the likely consequences of public and governmental misbehaviors are more likely to engender public outrage.

Occasionally, public activities for profit organizations defy logic, and a recent initiative in which Philip Morris attempted to influence politicians in the Czech Republic was based on the "indirect positive effects of smoking" that reflected "5.23 years of life lost for the average smoker" that helped ease the much higher costs of smoking. "In 1999, those costs included U.S. $296 million in additional health care for smokers and U.S. $29.6 million in additional health care for people sickened by second-hand smoke". The report accepted that "22,000 deaths due to tobacco smoking occurred in the Czech Republic in 1999" [12]. This is a macabre manner in which to advocate curtailment of healthcare costs, and there can be little sympathy for initiatives of this nature. However, physicians involved in the daily treatment of the critically ill can not remain ignorant of the greater public and private sector pressures that impact daily on therapeutic prerogatives and treatment options. Medicine is clearly in the public eye and it will be interesting to see how changes accrue in the next decade. It is certain that outcome accountability will become the watchword, and international collaboration through improvements in communications technology and data transmission are likely to be at the forefront of these initiatives. Physicians and their organizations must be prepared to educate themselves to be in a position to influence and lead these activities. The alternative that leaves medical care and its allocation devoid of medical jurisdiction is unacceptable.

As anesthesiologists and intensive care professionals, we share an interesting footnote in one of the most unpredictable stories of medical discovery, the use of anesthesia. "Ironically, the 'discovery' was really no discovery at all: Ether and nitrous oxide had been known for more than forty years to cause insensitivity to pain, yet with names like 'laughing gas', they were used almost solely for entertainment. Meanwhile, patients still underwent operations during which they saw, heard and felt every cut the surgeon made. ... With hope of relief seemingly long gone, the breakthrough finally came about by means of a combination of coincidence and character, as a cunning Boston dentist crossed paths with an inventive colleague from Hartford and a brilliant Harvard trained physician. William Morton, Horace Wells and Charles Jackson: a con man, a dreamer and an intellectual. Though Wells was crushed by derision when he tried to introduce anaesthetics, Morton prevailed, with help from Jackson. The result was Ether Day, October 16, 1846, celebrated around the world. By that point, though, no honour was enough. Ether Day was not only the dawn of modern surgery, *but the beginning of commercialized medicine as well, as Morton patented the discovery."* [13, author italics] Malcolm Gladwell in The Tipping Point underscores the importance of understanding that ideas may disseminate in similar fashion to a familiar medical epidemic, flu or measles. "Three characteristics – one, contagiousness; two, the fact that little causes can have big effects; and three, that change happens not gradually but at one dramatic moment" define dissemination of ideas and practice. "Of the three, the third trait – the idea that epidemics can rise or fall in one dramatic moment – is the most important, because it is the principle that makes sense of the first two and permits the greatest insight into why modern change happens the way it does. The name given to that one dramatic moment in an epidemic when everything can change all at once is the Tipping Point" [14].

It is interesting to note international medical trends through general editorial selection and interpretation, rather than the usual concentration on specialty medical journals. "Recently I asked an orthopedic surgeon how we could make the BMJ more useful for him." I've no idea," he answered, "I never read it. You must understand that I'm interested only in elbows." If my elbow were smashed to pieces I might be grateful to be treated by such a surgeon, but generally I feel that there is more to me than my elbows. "It would be a tragic loss," writes Prince Charles "if traditional human caring had to move to the domain of complementary medicine, leaving orthodox medicine with just the technical management of disease" [15]. Smith continues in another edition to note that the fundamental requirement for all physicians is to understand change.

"Change is a bugger. People often don't want to change even if they are unhappy with their lot. Nobody has described this better than Giuseppe Tomasi di Lampedusa in The Leopard, the story of the Sicilian Prince of Salina threatened with change by the arrival of Garibaldi in 1860. "The Sicilians," says the Prince, "never want to improve for the simple reason they think themselves perfect; their vanity is stronger than their misery." Moslem imams, King Roger's knights, Swabian scribes, Angevin barons, Catholic Kings, Spanish viceroys, and Charles III's reforming functionaries all tried to reform Sicily. Yet "Sicily went to sleep in spite of their invocations; for why should she listen to them if she herself is rich, if she's wise, if she's civilised, if she's honest, if she's admired and envied by all, if, in a word, she's perfect." Yet talk of change has never been more strident. No modern politician, no matter how conservative could declare the status quo to be the way forward. ... Health care, argues Jane Smith in an editorial, needs radical change redesign even (p *1257*). "Health care systems fail to provide treatments that are known to work, persist in using treatments that don't work, enforce delays, and tolerate high levels of error." She describes attempts on both sides of the Atlantic to change health care as fundamentally as the car industry was changed a decade or so ago. The people she has talked to are far from Sicilian: change is energising them [16]. Other issues have focused on error, fatigue and neglected aspects of medical practice such as appropriate management of pain and its sequelae. Ultimately, the challenge will be for all physicians to determine the code of a new practice that is evolving not only in the public eye but also in the arena of enhanced and at times, exaggerated expectation. This is demonstrated in passage of Patients' Rights Legislation in the United States, and despite recent political maneuvering, the discussions may benchmark future legislation and health care policy for the next generation. However, the cost is not to be underestimated. "It will raise costs of health insurance and employer health plans – and ultimately force individual employees to directly pay more of the cost of their health insurance and medical care. That's the reality, say economists, physicians, investment analysts, hospital administrators, and executives of health care companies. ... Perhaps by legislative change, we are moving towards a model in which consumers take more interest in the costs of their health care [17]. Perhaps, but in this instance, the education of the investing public, i.e., patients, is potentially inadequate to meet the responsibility of individual choice. The difficulty for interventional and critical care specialists will be to help educate the patient and his/her family in differentiating between therapeutic options, that may include withdrawal of service, in the most emotionally charged classroom imaginable. Physicians are ill equipped for this additional role, and in future may find it increasingly difficult to be absent from allegations of conflict of interest and provision of inappropriate care.

This discussion focuses on a number of issues that increasingly influence medical care for a number of reasons that are usually absent from the common medical school curriculum and residency training programs. However, increased public and professional interest and expected medical accountability is reflected in the references from the daily news, medical journals, and best-selling books from the lay press. Also, the enhanced visibility of the medical profession, especially as it relates to popular television, has led to an unanticipated accountability for unrealistic results and resources. When couched in terms of science fiction, the resources and achieved results are incredible, but when less clearly defined as imaginative fiction, they become the yardstick against which public opinion judges a health system's outcomes. The surgical, interventional, and critical care specialties are in the sights of this challenge. It will be up to these disciplines to anticipate demand, regulate treatment, and educate layman and professional alike in the therapeutic paradigms of the new millennium.

References

1. Richardson W (2001) Crossing the quality chasm: a new health system for the 21st century; Institute of Medicine, Public Briefing. March 1 2001
2. Zitner Aaron (Times Staff Writer) (2001) Death halts human tests at university. Los Angeles Times, July 22 2001
3. *www.ahrq.gov/clinic/ptsafety*
4. www4.nas.edu/onpi/webextra.nsf/web/chasm?OpenDocument
5. Polanczyk CA, Rohde LE, Goldman L, et al (2001) Right heart catheterization and cardiac complications in patients undergoing noncardiac surgery; an observational study. JAMA 286:309-314
6. Dalen JE (2001) The pulmonary artery catheter-friend, foe or accomplice? JAMA 286:348-350
7. Gaba DM (2001) Patient safety and production pressure: anesthesia practice issues. APSF Newslett 16:4-5 *www.apsf.org*
8. Simmons AM (Time staff writer) (2001) In South Africa, surgery tours offer beauty and the beasts. Los Angeles Times July 29, A1,A8
9. Morrell RC, Prielipp RC (2001) Production pressure: does the pressure to do more, faster, with less endanger patients? APSF Newslett 16:1 www.apsf.org
10. Haugh R Seeing red in the golden state; market forces and outside pressures are rocking California. *www.hhnmag.com/asp/ArticleDisplay.asp?PubId=1&articleID=13868*
11. Gosselin PG (2001) The 90's: private boom stingy on public good. Los Angeles Times, 5 August, A1:22
12. Holley D (2001) Philip Morris angers Czechs with tobacco toll report. Los Angeles Times, 5 August, A1:9
13. Fenster JM (2001) Ether day; the strange tale of America's greatest medical discovery and the haunted men who made it. Harper Collins
14. Gladwell M (2000) The tipping point; how little things can make a big difference. Little Brown
15. Smith R (2001) Restoring the soul of medicine. BMJ 322:
16. Smith R (2001) Change: both desired and resisted. BMJ 322:
17. Flanigan J (2001) Patients' rights and health-care costs are expanding together. Los Angeles Times, 4 August, C1:16

The World Health Organization and Cancer Pain

V. VENTAFRIDDA

Since 1980, except for a few experts involved with the issue, cancer pain has been a neglected public health problem. The World Health Organization (WHO) served as a catalyst to develop policies and advance treatment *strategies* to benefit patients with cancer and pain.

A distinctive character of the WHO's global program is its public health approach, based upon the principle of putting science into practice to reach the maximum number of patients, to educate health professionals about the need for pain control and palliative care, to sensitize patients and their *families* to the clear policies, and to ensure availability *of drugs*, particularly *morphine*.

The chronology of the major steps in the establishment of the WHO program are:

1982, Pomerio, Italy. A group of consultants brought together by WHO and Floriani Foundation produces an initial draft of the WHO *Guidelines for Cancer Pain Relief.*

1984, Geneva. A WHO meeting of experts in cancer pain, drug regulation, public health, pharmacology, and nursing, produces the monograph *Cancer Pain Relief* that has since become the standard reference worldwide.

This method called the *three-step ladder* is based on the use of drugs orally, like aspirin, codeine, and morphine, according to the intensity of the pain. The administration should be given hourly and individualized for any single patient.

When used correctly, the WHO method for the relief of cancer pain according to the validation studies [1-3] is capable of controlling pain in 80%-90% of patients. It is scientifically valid and can be adopted at the level of the family/community. The monograph has been translated into 28 languages, with a total press run of over 500,000 copies to date. We may summarize, according to the WHO in 13 points, the principles of this ladder [4].

1. Cancer pain can, and should, be treated.
2. Evaluation and treatment of cancer pain are best achieved by a team approach.
3. The first steps are to take a detailed history, and to examine the patient carefully, to determine if the pain is:

caused by the cancer, related to the cancer, caused by anticancer treatment, or caused by another disorder;
part of a specific syndrome;
nociceptive, neuropathic, or mixed nociceptive and neuropathic.

4. Treatment begins with an explanation and combines physical and psychological approaches, using both non-drug and drug treatments.
5. It is useful to have a sequence of specific aims, such as:
   to increase the hours of pain-free sleep;
   to relieve the pain when the patient is at rest;
   to relieve pain when the patient is standing or active.
6. Drugs alone usually give adequate relief from pain caused by cancer, provided that the right drug is administered in the right dose at the right time intervals.
7. "By mouth": the oral route is the preferred route for analgesics, including morphine.
8. "By the clock": for persistent pain, drugs should be taken at regular time intervals and not "as needed".
9. "By the ladder":
   Unless the patient is in severe pain, begin by prescribing a non-opioid drug and adjust the dose, if necessary, to the maximum recommended dose.
   If or when the non-opioid no longer adequately relieves the pain, an opioid drug should be prescribed in addition to the non-opioid.
   If or when an opioid for mild to moderate pain (e.g., codeine) no longer adequately relieves the pain, it should be replaced by an opioid for moderate to severe pain (e.g., morphine).
10. "For the individual": the right dose of an analgesic is the dose that relieves the pain. The dose of oral morphine may range from as little as 5 mg to more than 1,000 mg.
11. Adjuvant drugs should be prescribed as indicated.
12. For neuropathic pain, a tricyclic antidepressant or an anticonvulsant is the analgesic of choice.
13. "Attention to detail": it is essential to monitor the patient's response to the treatment to ensure that the patient obtains maximum benefit with as few adverse effects as possible.

Further steps on the WHO program are:

1988, Geneva. All drugs included in the WHO essential drug list [5].

1989, Geneva. WHO and the International Narcotics Control Board (INCB, Vienna) addresses the need of cancer patients for *opioids* [6].

1989, Geneva *Guidelines for Cancer Pain Relief* are updated and the draft on opioid availability is approved for later publication [7].

1993, Gargonza, Italy. WHO-International Association for the Study of Pain (IASP) group of experts meet to begin drafting guidelines for the relief of cancer pain in children.
1995, Geneva. The handbook *National Cancer Control Programs: Priorities and Managerial Guidelines* is published. Over 60 countries have adopted cancer pain and palliative care as a priority as part of their national cancer control program [8].

Further publications:
1996, 1998. *Symptom Relief in Terminal Illness, Cancer Pain Relief and Palliative Care in Children.* These manuals and monographs express a consensus reached by world authorities in keeping with WHO's commitment to simple technology.

Palliative care stands a chance of making an impact provided that three specific measures are ensured:

1. the mainstay of cancer pain relief and to implement the WHO three-step pain ladder: a governmental policy;
2. *education* of health professionals, their patients, and families;
3. drug availability.

It is crucial that palliative care be included as part of *total care* at the time the cancer is diagnosed.

A growing number of governments are recognizing the importance of pain relief and palliative care. Many ministers of health have adopted a *national policy* on cancer control as part of the country's health priorities. Eventually, every country should develop a national cancer control program that includes pain relief and palliative care.

In 1989, the Expert Committee endorsed guidelines on teaching and training of health care professionals in cancer pain relief [6].

Pain control and palliative care should not belong strictly to pain control specialists. It is time for pain control/palliative care to be incorporated into existing systems of care and for physicians most likely to see chronically ill patients in the first line of duty (general practitioners, oncologists) to make pain control and palliative a part of their routine clinical practice [9].

Seven collaborating centers have been set up by the WHO to support its program in cancer pain relief and palliative care. The centers cover quality of life (Amsterdam, The Netherlands), cancer pain and palliative care (Milan, Italy), palliative care (Oxford, United Kingdom), *cancer symptom* evaluation (Madison, Wisconsin, USA), quality of life in cancer care (Winnipeg, Canada), and cancer pain relief and *quality of life* (Saitama, Japan).

The WHO Cancer and Palliative Care Unit has designated as "*Focal Points*" individuals who can provide strong and effective leadership. These are generally individuals who make a difference and who can serve as models, or reference points for others.

Pain relief has been used as the model to reach the greatest number of *patients*. This approach is valid not only for cancer but for other diseases, and ultimately for the majority of the 5 million people who die every year worldwide.

The need for palliative care will increase due to a combination of factors, including the ageing of the world population, increases in cancer deaths related to tobacco use, and acquired immunodeficiency syndrome (AIDS).

Just as important as research in the purely medical aspects of pain and palliative care are the social, economic, and cultural attitudes toward pain, suffering, and the terminally ill. This is especially true as the proportion of care-givers declines relative to the growing number of patients who need care.

In order to improve the attention to the pain problem the WHO suggests three major issues that are strictly correlated, as we mentioned above:

1. education directed toward the public, including patients and families and health care professionals (doctors, nurses, pharmacist), and to the other health care policy makers, administrators, and drug regulators.
2. drug availability; pain control can not be achieved without the use of opioids for adequate control of severe pain. It is important to act in order to provide the changes in health care regulations-legislation to improve drug availability, specially opioids, facilitate the prescription, distribution and administration of drugs.
3. the principal issue is governmental policy; according to the WHO we can not improve pain control without a national or state policy that emphasizes the need to alleviate chronic cancer pain though education, drug availability, and governmental support/endorsement. Such policy can stand alone, be part of national-state cancer control program, be part of an overall policy care of the terminal ill, which means the recognition of palliative care in the health program in academic education, and finally such a program could be part of a policy on chronic intractable pain.

The WHO also gives some examples of policies that could be applied in order to improve pain control and palliative care, recrue political commitment and leadership to implement palliative care, integrate palliative care as a part of routine health care, insure access to opioids, apply palliative care early in the course of illness, believe the patient, involve the family to ensure that the largest number of terminal ill patients receive palliative care, and include pain control in palliative care in the standard curriculum of physicians an nurses.

Approval of the WHO recommendation by government is very important to measure the outcomes of such a policy. The WHO suggests an open dialogue between health professionals and government representatives to achieve better pain care. This allows a demonstration of inexpensive methods to control cancer pain and formulation of a national policy emphasizing the need to alleviate chronic cancer pain.

This should include:

linking palliative care to previously existing resources,

involving *oncology* and primary care in palliative care,

creating curricula in palliative care,

showing increases in the number of terminally ill patients covered,

showing reduction in pain prevalence,

respecting cross-cultural differences, and testing approaches for cross-cultural validity.

The WHO Programme on Cancer Control has estimated that by the year 2020, approximately 70% of the annual 20 million new cancer cases will occur in developing countries [4], where most patients are diagnosed when the disease is already in the late stages. Pain is prevalent in cancer, but especially in the late stages, near the end of life.

The opioid analgesics, such as codeine and morphine, are absolutely necessary for the management of pain due to cancer. When cancer pain is moderate to severe, there is no substitute for opioids in the therapeutic group of morphine [5].

Opioids are classified as narcotic drugs because they have a potential for abuse. As a consequence, they are regulated by international treaties and national drug control policies. The INCB, the WHO, and national governments report that opioids are not sufficiently available for medical purposes. There are a number of reasons, including the low priority for pain management in health care systems, greatly exaggerated fears of addiction, overly restrictive national drug control policies, and problems in procurement, manufacture, and distribution of opioids.

In some countries, governments and health care professionals have been working together to improve cancer pain management and palliative care; some have begun to identify and correct overly restrictive regulatory control over the medical use of opioid analgesics. Other countries have yet to address these matters. These guidelines can be used by governments to determine whether their national drug control policies have established the legal and administrative framework to ensure the medical availability of opioid analgesics, according to international treaties and the recommendations of the INCB and the WHO.

Pain is prevalent among people who have cancer. Cancer patients may need pain relief at every stage of the disease. More than two-thirds of patients with advanced cancer will experience pain, often severe [7]. For these patients, pain relief should be part of their overall treatment. For patients who have late-stage cancer, the management of pain and other symptoms should be the primary aim of national cancer control programmes.

In 1996, the WHO Expert Committee on Cancer Pain Relief and Active *Supportive Care* [7] stated:

"In most parts of the world, the majority of cancer patients present with advanced disease. For them, the only realistic treatment option is pain relief and palliative care" (p v).

Surveys suggest that more than 50% of cancer patients suffer unrelieved pain [10]. Unrelieved pain can impair all aspects of a person's life, including appetite, mood, self-esteem, relationships with others, and even the ability to move. In some countries, it has been reported that unrelieved pain can lead to the wish for death and inquiries about euthanasia and assisted suicide. Relief of pain has been demonstrated to improve quality of life.

In 1986, the participants of the WHO Meeting on the Comprehensive Management of Cancer Pain [10] declared that:

"In patients with severe pain, morphine -- a strong opioid -- is the drug of choice" (p 18).

Morphine and opioids in the therapeutic group of morphine are considered essential when pain is moderate or severe [7, 10, 11]. Health care professionals have been encouraged to use the proven three-step Analgesic Method that was developed by the WHO as an effective method to treat pain.

The WHO Expert Committee on Cancer Pain Relief and Active Supportive Care [11] stated in 1990 that:

"Freedom from pain should be seen as a right of every cancer patient and access to pain therapy as a measure of respect for this right" (p 10).

Relief of severe cancer pain depends on the availability and use of opioids in the therapeutic group of morphine. These opioids do not have an "analgesic ceiling" (i.e., a pharmacological characteristic of a drug when an increased dose provides no additional analgesia). They can be administered safely in increasing doses until the pain is relieved, as long as side effects are tolerated [7]. There is no standard treatment dose for these opioids. The appropriate dose to relieve the pain should be determined by the individual needs of the patient.

Morphine and one or more other opioid pain medications, as well as other drugs used for pain and symptom management, must be available in adequate amounts, when patients need them, and in the places where patients are living [11].

In 1986, participants of the WHO Meeting on the Comprehensive Management of Cancer Pain [10] stated:

"Of 22 drugs commonly used for cancer pain relief, eight are covered by the 1961 Single Convention on Narcotic Drugs and one by the 1971 Convention on Psychotropic Substances..." (p 27).

The WHO Expert Committee on Essential Drugs [5] has for many years designated morphine, codeine, and other opioids as "essential drugs," defined as:

"those that satisfy the health care needs of the majority of the population; they should therefore be available at all times in adequate amounts and in the appropriate dosage forms..." (p 2).

The total global consumption of morphine increased significantly as some national governments and health professionals adopted the WHO Analgesic Method for cancer pain relief. However, the majority of the increasing consumption of morphine occurred in a small number of developed countries that represent a small part of the world's population [12]. More recently, morphine consumption has begun to increase in other countries, including in a number of developing countries. The statistical data from the INCB for the period from 1990 to 1997 show that substantial increases have occurred in both developed and developing countries, while consumption in other countries has remained stable or even decreased. Most countries use very little morphine.

The consumption of a wider range of opioids stated in the form of defined daily dose per million, and expressed as a 5-year average (Annex 4) allows for the comparison of the consumption of a number of opioids (n) and between countries. In many countries, consumption remains extremely low in comparison to the medical need, and many national governments have yet to address this important deficit [12].

The publication of the WHO three-step Analgesic Method for cancer pain relief in 1986 contributed to the increased consumption of morphine throughout the world. Prior to the early 1980s, morphine consumption was low and stable (Fig. 1).

In 1993, the WHO Expert Committee on Drug Dependence [13] recognized:

"... that there was a great need to ensure, in seeking to reduce the non-me-

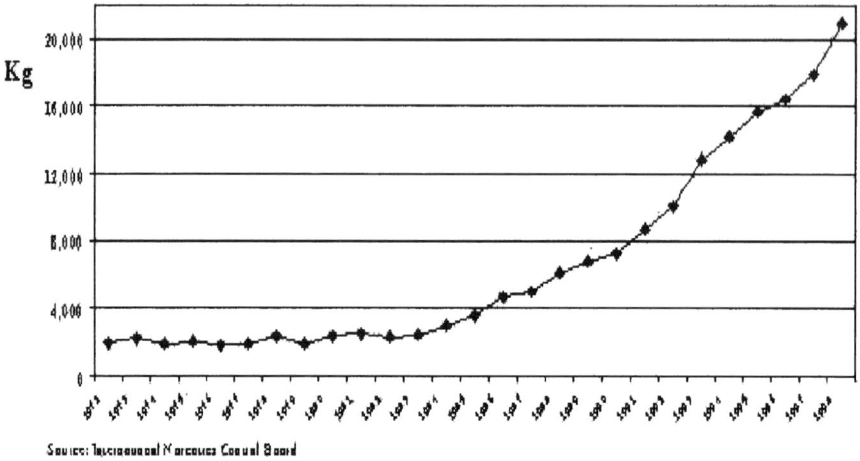

Fig. 1. Global consumption of morphine (1972-1998)

dical use of therapeutic psychoactive drugs, *that patients with legitimate medical needs are not prevented from being treated with adequate amounts of appropriate medications. Evidence suggests that* medical needs for opioids *are not being fully satisfied, particularly among patients with cancer, who may require large doses of opioids to obtain optimal pain relief" (p 20).*

According to a 1995 survey of governments by the INCB [12], the injectable forms of morphine are still more available than the oral form recommended by the WHO. Although 60% of governments surveyed had endorsed the WHO Analgesic Method, approximately one-half of governments that responded to the survey reported that morphine is not available in all hospitals with cancer programs. Success in implementing the WHO Analgesic Method has been limited by the lack of opioid analgesics; future success will depend on governmental efforts to identify and address impediments in their health care and regulatory systems.

There are three levels of barriers to adequate pain management: economic, *medical, and regulatory*. Economic and medical barriers play major roles in the inadequate treatment of pain. For example, in some countries, for economic reasons, health care professionals are encouraged to use more-expensive and less-effective pharmaceutical products. This may exacerbate inadequate *availability*, both for the health care system in general, and for the individual patient.

In some countries, scarce medical resources are spent on expensive curative treatments that are futile for patients with late-stage cancer. Such policies preclude the provision of palliative care. Finally, medical education that does not address pain management contributes to inadequate pain management.

As far as concerns the impediments to opioid availability, the INCB and the WHO have called attention to the inadequate treatment of pain and have concluded that this is due, in part, to overly restrictive laws and regulations that impede the adequate availability and medical use of opioids [6, 7, 11, 12, 14, 15].

As early as 1986, the participants of the WHO Meeting on the Comprehensive Management of Cancer Pain [10] recognized the need to update national drug regulatory systems to respond to changing medical needs:

"Systems regulating the distribution and prescription of opioid drugs were designed before the value of the oral use of opioid drugs for cancer pain management was recognized. These systems were developed to prevent the social misuse of strong opioids; there was no intention to prevent the use of opioids for pain relief in cancer" (p 27).

We now have a new WHO publication aimed at improving availability of opioid analgesics in the world, titled *Achieving Balance in National Opioids Control Policy: Guidelines for Assessment* [16].

This document provides 16 guidelines that can be used by governments and health professionals to assess the national opioid control policies of any country, to determine if they contain the provisions, procedures, and cooperation that are necessary to ensure the availability of opioid analgesics that are essential for the relief of pain. This principle, which is carefully and extensively documented, asserts that governments not only have an obligation to prevent drug abuse, but also to ensure the availability of opioid analgesics for medical purposes, and further, that efforts to prevent drug abuse and diversion must not interfere with the adequate availability of opioid analgesics for patients' pain relief.

References

1. Ventafridda V, Caraceni A, Gamba A () Field testing of the WHO guidelines for cancer pain relief: summary report of demonstration projects. In: Bonica J, Foley KM, Ventafridda V (eds)
2. Ventafridda V, Tamburini M, Caraceni A et al (1987) Cancer pain relief 1986 which allow to achieve pain control in 80% of patients A validation study of the WHO method for cancer pain relief. Cancer 15:850-856
3. Zech DFL, Grond S, Lynch J et al (1995) Validation of WHO guidelines for cancer pain relief: a 10 year prospective study. Pain 68:65-76
4. World Health Organization Programme on Cancer Control (1998) Developing a global strategy for cancer. Sikora K (ed)
5. World Health Organization (1998) The use of essential drugs: Report of a WHO Expert Committee (Technical Report Series 882). WHO, Geneva, Switzerland
6. International Narcotics Control Board (1989) Demand for and supply of opiates for medical and scientific needs. In: Report of the International Narcotics Control Board for 1989. UN, New York
7. World Health Organization (1996) Cancer pain relief with a guide to opioid availability, 2nd edn. WHO, Geneva, Switzerland
8. World Health Organization Cancer Control Programme (1994) Introducing the national cancer control programmes. Cancer Care 1:1-5
9. Stjernsward J, Colleau SM, Ventafridda V (1996) The World Health Organization Cancer Pain and Palliative Care Program. Past, present, and future. J Pain Symptom Manage 12:65-72
10. World Health Organization (1986) Cancer pain relief. WHO, Geneva, Switzerland
11. World Health Organization (1990) Cancer pain relief and palliative care: Report of a WHO expert committee (Technical Report Series 804). WHO, Geneva, Switzerland
12. International Narcotics Control Board (1996) Availability of opiates for medical needs. In: Report of the International Narcotics Control Board for 1995. UN, New York
13. World Health Organization (1993) WHO Expert Committee on Drug Dependence. Twenty eighth report. (Technical Report Series 836). WHO, Geneva, Switzerland
14. Joranson DE (1993) Availability of opioids for cancer pain: Recent trends, assessment of system barriers, new World Health Organization guidelines, and the risk of diversion. J Pain Symptom Manage 8:353-360
15. Joranson DE (1996) New international efforts to ensure availability of opioids for medical purposes. J Pain Symptom Manage 12:85-86
16. Narcotic and Psychotropic drugs. Achieving balance in natinal opioids control policy. Guidelines for assessment. WHO/EDM/QSM/2000.4

High Frequency Percussive Ventilation

U. Lucangelo, L. Fontanesi, F. Bird

High frequency percussive ventilation (HFPV) is a method of ventilation that was introduced at the beginning of the 1980s. While it was initially destined for the treatment of lung injuries produced by smoke inhalation and burning, later on it was used in pathologies characterized by a serious alteration of gas exchange, where conventional ventilation methods were not decisive. HFPV was introduced in Europe in the second half of the 1990s. In Italy we were the first to use this technique in critical patients. Preliminary results will be presented at the end of this chapter.

Functioning principles

A percussive ventilator can be defined as a time-cycled controlled-pressure system, combined with a device that allows the passage of gases coming from the pneumatic generator to which it is connected (Fig. 1). This device called "phasitron" is the key element of percussive ventilation and the interface between patient and machine [1]. The functioning of phasitron is based on Venturi's principle: for each part of gas coming form the pneumatic system, the piston inside the phasitron can draw up to 5 parts of ambient air mixed with nebulized particles. The small volume of air in the phasitron is then pushed into progressively smaller pipes, so as to increase its speed and decrease its pressure. The increase of airway pressure is accompanied by a decrease in the quantity of air drawn from outside. The phasitron functions can be summarized as follows:

1. Insufflating the volume of gas into the airways with a set pressure.
2. Increasing this volume up to 5 times by using ambient air.
3. Automatically adapting to the variation of lung resistance by converting the flow into pressure and vice versa with Venturi's principle. Flow control makes it possible to increase distribution into the airways, thus avoiding preferential ventilation and the risk of baro-volutrauma.

4. Providing a perfect synchronization of inspiratory/expiratory intervals with the minimum piston inertial delay.
5. Keeping a constant communication with the external environment, thereby ensuring the utmost safety.
6. Ensuring the continuous monitoring of airways.
7. Guaranteeing humidification and administration of aerosol drugs.
8. Ensuring the administration of a number of small volumes until the desired pressure is reached, and therefore keeping the lung on an oscillatory plateau.

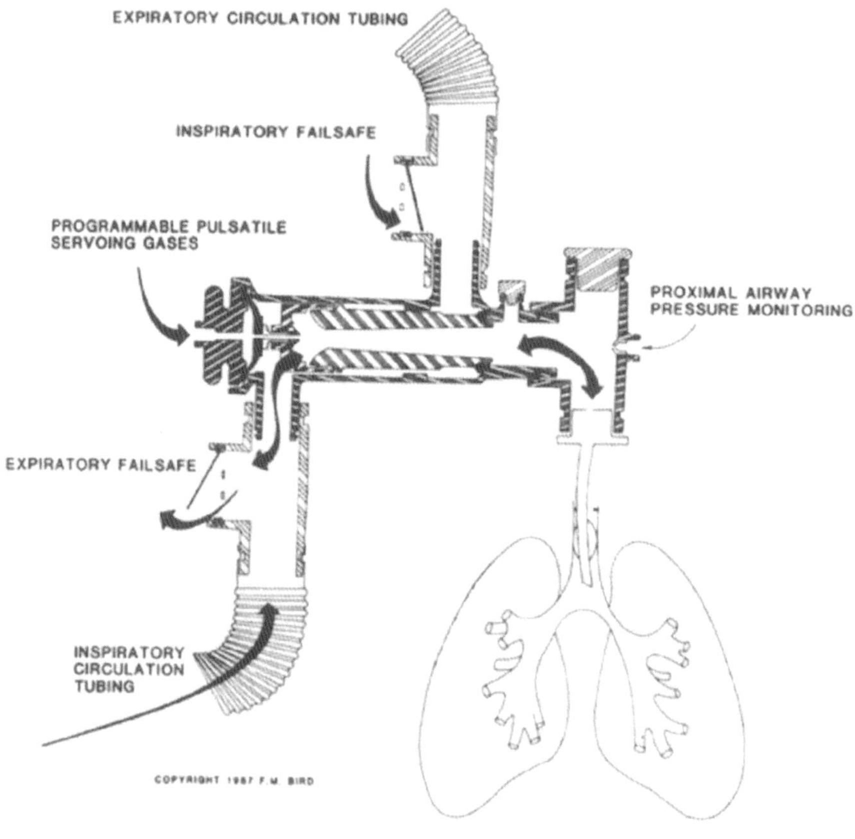

Fig. 1. Entrance, exit, and safety systems of the respiratory circuit

Figure 2 demonstrates what was said in (2). The values of the airway pressure (in cm of water) are plotted on the abscissa and the ratio of gas from source to gas from outside on the ordinate.

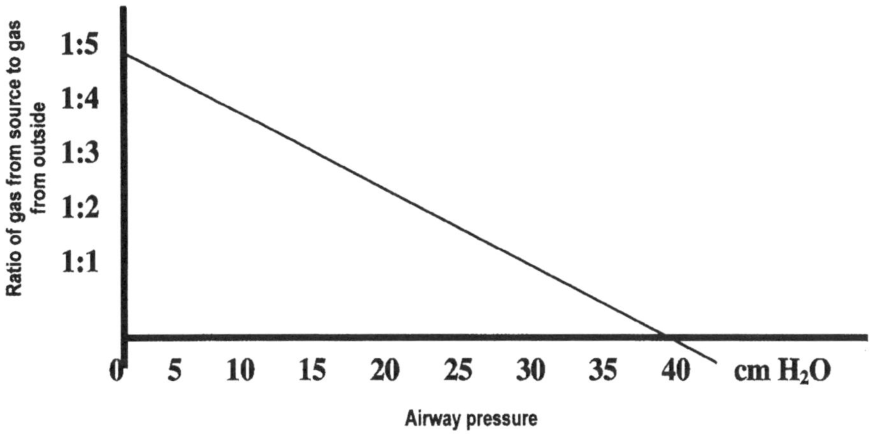

Fig. 2. Ratio of gas from source to gas from outside plotted against airway pressure

The distribution in succession of small current volumes with a frequency ranging from 200 to 900 cycles/min, superimposed on a normal inspiratory/expiratory cycle, at controlled pressure, makes it possible to administer the current volume. The programmable parameters are peak inspiratory pressure (PIP), inspiratory time (T_I), expiratory time (T_E), positive end-expiration pressure (PEEP), CPAP, and percussive frequency.

During inspiration, the progressive accumulation of microvolumes makes it possible to increase pressure and total volume in the airways gradually, avoiding preferential ventilation of unobstructed alveoli and therefore fostering their recruitment. The net result is the gradual decrease of peak pressure, while there is an increase of the average pressure. In addition, the high frequency ensures the fluidification of secretions, improving bronchial cleansing. During expiration the flow is interrupted, airway pressure returns to its base value and air trapping is avoided. It is interesting to note that expiration is not totally passive, as for conventional ventilation, because the expiratory volume can be fractioned, facilitating the upward movement of secretions.

The nebulizer is placed in series in the circuit (Fig. 3) and ensures the humidification (up to 100%) of circulating air, and the administration of bronchodilators and other drugs to reduce adhesion and cohesion of stagnating secretions.

The movement of secretions is mainly due to three factors:

1. The succession of pressure peaks causes a vibration of the bronchial mucosa and secretions.
2. The variation of percussive frequency creates turbulences in the airways.
3. The high flow combined with pressure fosters mucus-ciliary clearance.

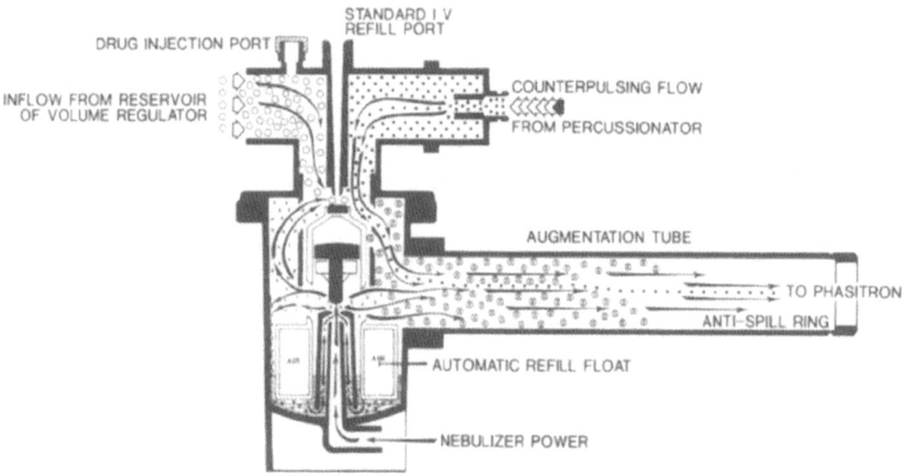

Fig. 3. Nebulizer for the administration of aerosol drugs

Draining and the recruitment of atelectatic lung areas is ensured by three essential factors:

1. High-flow aerosol coupled with percussion provides an effective therapy and guarantees an adequate humidification of airways.
2. The CPAP effect makes it possible to keep atelectatic lung areas open.
3. Microvolume high-flow percussions make it possible to overcome mucous blocks and, due to alveolar elastic return forces, guarantee their upward movement.

Finally, the improvement of gas exchange is due to both the high flow (approximately 40 l/min) and an increase of Brownian motion at the alveolar level, which ensures the diffusion of O_2 towards the capillary bed.

On the other hand, the elimination of CO_2 does not require higher pressures, as with the other high-frequency ventilation methods. With HFPV, the elimination of CO_2 is strictly connected with the inspiratory percussive duration and frequency. In this respect, percussive ventilation has another distinctive feature compared with both other high-frequency and conventional ventilation methods.

Main applications

Percussive ventilation was initially used for the treatment of airway injuries caused by burning and gas inhalation [2-8]. Owing to the good results obtained, this method was applied more generally to chronic obstructive bronchus and lung pathologies, and was designed so as to be managed by paramedics. Later, its use was generalized as first admission treatment, not only in relapsed chronic obstructive pulmonary disease (COPD) patients, but also in other pathologies, for which conventional mechanic ventilation, although necessary to maintain vital functions, could cause iatrogenic damage [4, 9]. The significant improvement of gas exchanges [10, 11], together with a lower incidence of complications connected, for example, to peak pressures and too high O_2 inspiration fractions, and the reduction of injuries caused by a scarce humidification of the gas mixture delivered, make HFPV clearly indicated in acute respiratory distress syndrome (ARDS) patients [12-14], restrictive pathologies, pulmonary injuries caused by burning, thoracic trauma [15], and what is known as "hyaline membrane disease" in new-born babies [16, 17]. The data reported in the literature are often the result of a comparison between HFPV and the other ventilation methods [11, 18, 19]. Apart from the above-mentioned advantages, no negative effects were noted on the patients' hemodynamic situation. In addition, HFPV can be used in both patients with spontaneous respiratory activity and sedated patients to whom curare has been administered. The only absolute contraindication to the use HFPV is non-drained pneumothorax. Lyell's syndrome and pulmonary pathologies with risk of hemorrhage are relative contraindications, although the utmost caution is necessary in the use of HVPV.

Preliminary experience

Our sample, including 23 patients (average age 58.6±20.6 years, 16 males), in intensive care for acute respiratory insufficiency, had been subjected to conventional ventilation for at least 48 h. The average value of the PaO2/FiO2 ratio achieved was 197.96±57.4, with a range included between 84 and 300. Subsequently, owing to the poor response to ventilation or a worsening of the gas exchanges, treatment with percussive ventilation was started, keeping the same PEEP and FiO2 values, while the value of peak pressure was two-thirds of that obtained with conventional mechanical ventilation.

The blood gas levels (expressed as average and standard deviation) obtained with conventional ventilation and after treatment with HFPV are reported in Table 1.

Table 1. Blood gas levels with conventional ventilation and high-frequency percussive ventilation

	Conventional ventilation	High-frequency percussive ventilation
PaO_2/FiO_2	197.96± 57.4	270.7± 84*
$PaCO_2$	35.19± 4.83	33.65± 3.74
pH	7.47± 0.05	7.48± 0.04

* Value statistically significant compared with conventional ventilation
($P < 0.001$) calculated with Student's ± - test for dependent samples

Although the population examined includes a heterogeneous group of patients (15 cases of acute respiratory failure, 3 of ARDS, 5 of COPD), the increase of the PaO_2/FiO_2 ratio occurred in each of the categories treated. The good response in terms of oxygenation made it possible to reduce the O_2 inspiratory fraction in all patients. Another element to highlight is the very high efficiency of the CO_2 elimination obtained during HFPV. In order to avoid an undesired decrease of $PaCO_2$, on the basis of the blood gas level, respiratory frequency was reduced during the treatment.

In particular, patients in whom the highest quantity of secretions was removed benefited from HFPV. This preliminary experience shows that the improvement of gas exchange was more marked 12 h after the treatment, irrespective of the basic respiratory pathology.

Figure 4 shows the pressure curve obtained during the treatment with percussive ventilation. Notice how the pressure peak reached is similar to the results normally obtained with conventional ventilation.

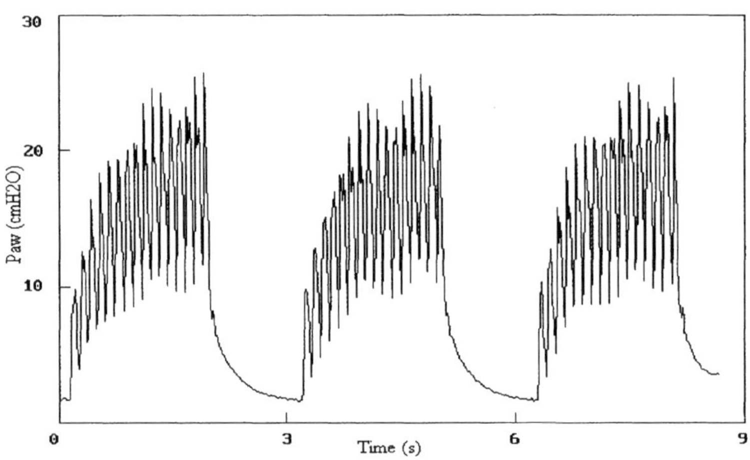

Fig. 4. Pressure curve obtained with high-frequency percussive ventilation

Conclusions

Accordance with the data reported in the literature, HFPV appears to be a valid alternative to conventional ventilation both in relapsed chronic respiratory disorders requiring ventilation (e.g., COPD) and in traumatic thorax pathologies, in which the cyclic movement necessarily imposed on the pulmonary parenchyma can, in itself, be the cause of further damage [14, 15].

In addition, the use of this method is advisable when the gas exchange is seriously compromised and, at the same time, the patient's hemodynamic situation is heavily influenced by mechanical ventilation, as in ARDS.

It has to be stressed that optimal use of HFPV needs more-constant and attentive instrumental monitoring. On-line $EtCO_2$ surveys and hourly monitoring of the blood gas level in the initial phase of the treatment are necessary. As was demonstrated for our patients, with the same ventilation per minute, there is a vigorous elimination of CO_2 compared with the conventional treatment. In addition, the repeated elimination and quantification of secretions is another important parameter for the assessment of the effectiveness of the treatment.

The components of the system are easy to assemble and can be sterilized repeatedly with all conventional systems. This means, of course, a significant reduction of management costs.

The mechanisms producing a better oxygenation and more-effective elimination of CO_2 are not yet completely clear. Many theories have been suggested (convective transport, dispersive transport, higher molecular diffusion in the alveolar membrane, due to a higher kinetic energy of the O_2 molecules) [1]. In our experience, considering the whole sample, a highly statistically significant improvement was achieved of the paO_2/FiO_2 ratio.

The respiratory system compliance did not vary in a statistically significant way between the beginning and the end of the treatment with HFPV. During the treatment, however, there was a progressive increase of Vt, accompanied by a simultaneous decrease of peak pressure. As reported in the literature [20], the average airway pressure did not vary, despite the application of constant CPAP plus PEEP. In our experience, only a moderate increase with scarce clinical significance was noted compared with the basic condition (2–4 cm H_2O). For a correct evaluation of this increase, auto-PEEP was calculated before the beginning and at the end of the treatment by using the Puritan-Bennet 7200 ventilator. The curve obtained was further processed by least square fitting.

The resistances did not vary in a statistically significant way, although we noticed some decrease during the treatment, probably due to the effective removal of the secretions and the relative increase of the system compliance [21, 22].

No significant variation was noted in arterial pressure. This was carefully confirmed in patients with Swan-Ganz catheter and in patients with cranial trauma, with a device for the measurement of intra-cranial pressure. In contrast, a more-effective elimination of CO_2 was a useful aid to protect the cerebral parenchyma in the first hours after the trauma [23, 24].

Weaning from ventilation is one of the most-frequent problems for intensive care therapists. Although no retrospective analysis was carried out regarding the average duration of ventilation in patients who normally have this problem (e.g., COPD), the use HFPV as first admission treatment may lead to a more rapid recovery of the patient's autonomy, since this method of ventilation can have both the primary assistance role and the rehabilitative role proper. In this respect, HFPV is superior to every other method used for weaning.

In the light of what has been said, it seems possible that future applications of HFPV may include its use in surgery. The problems regarding ventilation in laparoscopic surgery (e.g., biliary tract) i.e., the increase of endoabdominal pressure and moving the patient in Trendelemburg's position, can often cause significant rises of the airway pressure, even in healthy individuals. In these circumstances, HFPV could help achieve and maintain an adequate maximum pressure, ensuring the gas exchange and avoiding, at the same time, the formation of microatelectasis, a frequent occurrence during general sedation.

The most-evident results, however, are expected in thoracic surgery. It is known that a serious ventilation imbalance ensues from laying the patient on his side. Mioresolution, the opening of the thorax, the movement of abdominal organs, and, lastly, single-lung ventilation, further complicate this situation. The problem was partly solved, in the past, with differential ventilation, applying a positive end-expiration pressure in the lung exposed to gravity and a CPAP in the other lung. The use of HFPV in the lung not exposed to gravity, with high percussive frequencies, low peak-pressure, and minimum respiratory frequency with inverted inspiration/expiration ratio, may guarantee an optimal expansion of the parenchyma, while keeping the right exchanges, without compromising the hemodynamic situation of the patient and interfering with surgery. In addition, the easy movement of secretion, fosters an immediate post operative recovery.

References

1. Product information (1997) Percussionaire Corporation, Sandpoint, Idaho
2. Reper P, Dankaert R, van Hille F, et al (1998) The usefulness of combined high frequency percussive ventilation during acute respiratory failure after smoke inhalation. Burns 24:34-38
3. Rodeberg DA, Housinger TA, Warden GD (1994) Improved ventilation function in burn patients using volumetric diffuse ventilation. J Am Coll Surg 179:518-522

4. Rodeberg DA, Maschinot NE, Housinger TA (1992) Decreased pulmonary barotrauma with the use of volumetric diffuse ventilation in pediatric patients with burns. J Burn Care Rehabil 13:506-511
5. Mlcak RP (1996) Ventilation strategies for smoke inhalation. J Respir Care Pract 103-106
6. Loring WR III, Cioffi WG, Mason AD, et al (1993) Improved survival of burned patients with inhalation injury. Arch Surg 128:772-780
7. Lentz CW, Peterson HD (1996) Smoke inhalation is a multilevel insult to the pulmonary system. Curr Opin Crit Care 2:230-235
8. Barillo DJ, Dickerson EE, Cioffi WG, et al (1997) Pressure controlled ventilation for the long range aeromedical transport of patients with burns. J Burn Care Rehabil 18:200-205
9. Birnkrant DJ, Pope JF, Stegmaler J, Besunder JB (1996) Persistent pulmonary consolidation treated with intrapulmonary percussive ventilation: a preliminary report. Pediatr Pulmonol 21:246-249
10. Kaiser KG, Davies NJH, Rodriguez-Roisin R, et al (1985) Efficacy of high-frequency ventilation in presence of extensive ventilation-perfusion mismatch. J Appl Phisiol 58:996-1004
11. Hurst JM, Branson RD, Kenneth Davis Jr, et al (1990) Comparison of conventional mechanical ventilation and high-frequency percussive ventilation. Ann Surg 211:486-491
12. Baird JS, Johnson JL, Escudero J, Powars DR (1994) Combined pressure control/high frequency ventilation in adult distress respiratory syndrome and sickle cell anemia. Chest 106:1913-1916
13. Velmahos GC, Chan LS, Tatevossian R, et al (1999) High-frequency percussive ventilation improves oxygenation in patients with ARDS. Chest 116:440-446
14. Borg UR, Stoklosa JC, Siegel JH, et al (1989) Prospective evaluation of combined high frequency ventilation in post traumatic patients with adult respiratory distress syndrome refractory to optimized conventional ventilatory management. Crit Care Med 17:1129-1141
15. Hurst JM, Branson RD, De Haven CB (1987) The role of high-frequency ventilation in post-traumatic respiratory insufficiency. J Trauma 27:236-241
16. Pfenninger J, Minder C (1988) Pressure-volume curves, static compliance and gas exchange in hyaline membrane disease during conventional mechanical and high frequency ventilation. Intensive Care Med 14:364-372
17. Gaylord MS, Quissel BJ, Lair ME (1987) High frequency ventilation in the treatment of infants weighing less than 1500 grams with pulmonary interstitial emphysema: a pilot study. Pediatrics 79:915-921
18. Gallagher JT, Boysen PG, Davidson DD, et al (1989) High frequency percussive ventilation compared with mechanichal ventilation. Crit Care Med 17:364-366
19. Shinozaki T, Deane RS, Perkins FM, et al (1985) Comparison of high frequency ventilation with mechanical lung ventilation. J Thorac Cardiovasc Surg 89:269-274
20. Simon BA, Weinmann GG, Mitzner W (1984) Mean airway pressure and alveolar pressure during high frequency ventilation. J Appl Physiol 57:1064-1078
21. Landau LI, Phelan PD (1973) Evaluation of two techniques for measurement of respiratory resistance by forced oscillation. Thorax 28:136-141
22. Mlcak R, Cortiella J, Desai M, Herndon D (1997) Lung compliance, airway resistance, and work of breathing in children after inhalation injury. J Burn Care Rehabil 18:531-534
23. Hurst JM, Branson RD, Davis K Jr (1988) High frequency percussive ventilation in the management of elevated intracranial pressure. J Trauma 28:1363-1367
24. Barrette RR, Hurst JM, Branson RD, Davis K Jr (1987) A comparison of conventional mechanical hyperventilation with two forms of high frequency ventilation for the control of intracranial pressure in closed head injury. Respir Care 32:733-740

LUNG

Experimental Models of Acute Lung Injury

P. R.M. Rocco, W.A. Zin

The first descriptions of acute respiratory distress syndrome appeared in 1967, when Ashbaugh et al. described 12 patients with acute respiratory distress, cyanosis refractory to oxygen therapy, decreased lung compliance, and diffuse infiltrates evident on the chest radiograph [1] . It is not defined by a specific pathogenesis, but reflects the lung's nonselective response to numerous insults and precipitating factors. Although the term acute respiratory distress syndrome (ARDS) is often used interchangeably with acute lung injury (ALI), by strict criteria ARDS should be reserved for the most severe end of the spectrum (Table 1) [2].

Table 1. Recommended criteria for acute lung injury (ALI) and acute respiratory distress syndrome (ARDS) [2]

	Timing	Oxygenation	Chest radiograph	Pulmonary artery wedge pressure
ALI criteria	Acute onset	$PaO_2/FIO_2 \leq 300$ (regardless of PEEP level)	Bilateral infiltrates seen on frontal chest radiograph	≤18 mmHg when measured or no clinical evidence of left atrial hypertension
ARDS criteria	Acute onset	$PaO_2/FIO_2 \leq 200$ (regardless of PEEP level)	Bilateral infiltrates seen on frontal chest radiograph	≤18 mmHg when measured or no clinical evidence of left atrial hypertension

Despite recent advances in intensive care, mortality rates persist at between 50-70%. Events triggering ALI are numerous, as are the animal models used to study this syndrome. Because so many etiologies of ALI exist, it is useful to separate the causes into two categories: the direct effect of an insult on the lung parenchyma and the indirect result of an acute systemic inflammatory response (Table 2) [3]. Sepsis, usually from gram-negative infections, is the most prevalent and lethal cause of ARDS (50%). Much of the scientific research in ALI has centered on sepsis and lung injury [4]. Pulmonary aspiration and trauma account for a further 25%. Drug overdose, pancreatitis, smoke inhalation, lung contusion, and other factors comprise the remaining risk factors.

Table 2. Major categories of acute lung injury risk

Direct lung injury	Indirect lung injury
Common causes	*Common causes*
Pneumonia (bacterial, fungal, viral, atypical)	Sepsis syndrome
Aspiration of gastric contents	Severe non-thoracic trauma with shock and multiple transfusions (multiple long bone fractures, hypovolemic shock)
Less common causes	*Less common causes*
Severe thoracic trauma (pulmonary contusion)	Cardiopulmonary bypass
Fat emboli	Hypertransfusion of blood products for emergency resuscitation
Near-drowning	Drug overdose (opiates, paraldehyde, thiazides, paraquat)
Inhalation injury (smoke, oxygen, chorine, phosgene)	Acute pancreatitis
Reperfusion pulmonary oedema after lung transplantation or pulmonary embolectomy	Disseminated intravascular coagulation

ALI can be divided into an exudative phase and a proliferative phase. In the exudative phase, alveoli contain proteinaceous fluid, red blood cells, neutrophils, and macrophages. Oedema and neutrophils accumulate in the interstitium, and alveolar ducts contain hyaline membranes. Microatelectasis is present. Endothelial cells are swollen, and focal destruction of endothelial and type I epithelial cells occurs. The proliferative phase is characterized by type II epithelial cell hyperplasia and accumulation of fibroblasts and numerous monocytes in the interstitium. Normal acinar architecture is destroyed and replaced by thick layers of fibrotic tissue that obliterates the alveolar spaces and alveolar ducts.

There are many causes that trigger ALI, but determination of its precise pathophysiology needs to be clarified. Extensive animal studies have examined the inflammatory cascades initiated by infection, trauma, burns, and haemorrhage [5]. These studies have demonstrated the complexity and multiplicity of pathways involved in these pathophysiologic processes, and they indicate that differences in the initial insult, combined with underlying conditions, can result in the activation of different inflammatory mechanisms. Understanding the range of pathways that lead to pulmonary dysfunction, it may be possible to assess several novel treatments to specific areas of the pathologic cascade in an attempt to modify lung injury.

This chapter presents a brief overview of different experimental models of acute lung injury, detailing what we have learned from animal studies, and indicates how they led to the development of a new generation of pharmacological agents and ventilatory therapies that may in the future allow clinicians to interfere and reverse the acute lung injury process. In addition, we describe how to develop four different models of acute lung injury induced by paraquat, oleic acid, saline lavage, and endotoxin.

Experimental models

There is an enormous variety of animal species available for biological research. The use of experimental animals to reproduce ALI began in the 1960's [6]. The most employed are haemorrhagic hypotension, tissue injury, or sepsis in efforts to recapitulate the antecedents most frequently recognized clinical presentation in humans [7-10]. These models presented various physiologic changes and abnormalities of surfactant, but structural changes in the lung were either incompletely described or not described at all. Lung histology showed patchy congestion, oedema, and atelectasis without hyaline membrane.

A conference on acute respiratory failure sponsored by the National Institutes of Health (1976) reviewed possible mechanisms that might cause acute alveolar injury and the known structural and functional responses to such injury [11]. Noting the lack of a valid experimental model as a major difficulty to progress, the conference included among its recommendations for future efforts the development of such models. Since then information derived from several models has provided critical insights into possible mechanisms of human ALI and the structural and metabolic consequences thereof.

How to select an animal model?

The selection of the animal model is based on multiple considerations: a) local availability, b) financial cost, c) public opinion regarding the use of animal research (rodent experiments do not engender the same emotive feeling as experiments on dogs or primates; in addition, if survival is considered as the study endpoint and large numbers of animals are required to achieve statistical power, rodent studies provide an ideal option), d) studies requiring invasive physiologic monitoring with multiple blood sampling (large animals such as sheep or swine have easier anatomic access and large blood volume), e) correlation between model and clinical syndrome (the closer the species is to humans phylogenetically, the better the clinical correlation), f) direct versus indirect insult to the lung, and g) isolated perfused lung preparations (*in vitro*) or study of intact animals (*in vivo*) (*in* vitro experiments permit accurate control over the experimental environment, but whole animal studies, although often more difficult to interpret due to uncontrolled variables, clearly provide closer clinical correlates) [12].

In order to be clearly relevant to human ALI, an animal model must not only recapitulate its histological evolution; it must also share a common pathogenesis. Because their only index of relevance to the human injury is their structural similarity, such models must closely reproduce human injury at least in its major characteristics, that is, they must be acute and diffuse, feature necrosis and regeneration of alveolar epithelial cells, and follow the temporal evolution of the human process. The aetiology and pathogenesis of ALI are not yet clearly understood, and the multiple models of acute lung injury testify that none is perfect. Care must be exercised not to draw false conclusions because of an inappropriate animal model.

Two important limitations of the use of experimental models to understand the pathogenesis and pathophysiology of ALI are: species variability and the differences in the intensity and temporal evolution of the lesion between the experimental and human studies [13].

Contribution of experimental models to the understanding of ALI

Ashbaugh et al. (1967) reasoned that ARDS might result from defective surfactant synthesis, similarly to the pathogenesis of infant respiratory distress [1]. Four years later, Staub et al. observed changes in alveolar capillary membrane permeability, using the lung lymph flow preparation in awaken sheep [14]. Brigham et al. (1974) in order to demonstrate that *Pseudomonas* bacteremia predictably causes increased pulmonary vascular permeability to protein, that the lung lymphatics have a large capacity to pump excess filtered fluid and protein, and that the lung lymphatic system is very sensitive to increases in fluid filtration, have described a good model for experimental studies of vascular permeability in the lung [15]. Craddock et al. (1977), noted that during the initiation of haemodialysis, patients developed transient pulmonary dysfunction in concert with complement-mediated neutropenia and increased neutrophil sequestration within the lung [16]. Hammerschmidt et al. (1980) suggested that aggregation of polymorphonuclear granulocytes (PMN), in response to activated complement, might contribute to the genesis of the ARDS, aggregating PMN causing pulmonary dysfunction by becoming lodged in the lung as leucoemboli [17] . They developed the complement theory of ARDS pathogenesis. A series of animal experiments provided further support for this hypothesis. Varying degrees of lung injury could be induced by the infusion of activated complement fragments in sheep [16], the intravascular activation of complement in rats [18], and the infusion of C5a into rabbits [19]. In the rabbit model, although neutrophils were retained within the lung microvasculature in response to the infusion of C5a, pulmonary vascular permeability did not increase unless the animal was exposed to a second insult. By contrast, in mice specifically deficient in C5, lung injury induced by pneumococcal sepsis, burns and hyperoxia was significantly attenuated [20]. The administration of antibodies to C5a decreased mortality in baboons with gram-negative sepsis [21] and pretreatment with CR1 abrogated lung injury in rats with gram-negative infections [22]. In addition, Dehring et al. (1987) and Flick et al. (1986) showed only moderate improvement and no improvement, respectively, in lung injury sustained in porcine and sheep models of sepsis-induced ALI after interventional complement depletion using cobra venom factor [23, 24]. These studies suggested that complement activation was an important component of the inflammatory process, which leads to the development of ARDS. However, they also suggested that other mediators of inflammation needed to be identified and considered.

Thus, studies indicated that eicosanoids play an important role in the pathogenesis of ALI. Arachidonic acid serves as a substrate for generation of a large number of biologically active metabolites comprising the eicosanoids. Arachidonic acid is metabolized to leukotrienes via the lipoxygenase pathway and to thromboxane (TX) and prostaglandin (PGE2, prostacyclin, and other prostaglandin) via the cyclooxygenase pathway. Animal studies showed that endotoxin administration causes a rapid increase in the production of cyclooxygenase-derived lipid mediators of inflammation. In a sheep model of ALI, thromboxane stimulates aggregation of both platelets and neutrophils and also increases the adhesiveness of neutrophil [25]. In addition, TX stimulates the constriction of both the vasculature and airways, and may also cause increased permeability, contributing to the development of pulmonary hypertension, hypoxemia, and increased airway resistance observed in ALI [26]. Injured lung also releases both TX and prostacyclin. Prostacyclin and PGE2 present modulating effects on the pathophysiology of ALI. Prostacyclin is a potent pulmonary vasodilator, and PGE2 can inhibit release of pro-inflammatory cytokines from macrophages and other inflammatory cells. There are several reasons to suspect that lipooxygenase products of arachidonic acid may play an important role in the pathogenesis of ALI (e.g., nonsteroidal, anti-inflammatory drugs, such as a cyclooxygenase inhibitor (ibuprofen) changed eicosanoic response and the evolution of sepsis and lung injury [27-28]). Leukotriene (LTB4) is a potent activator of neutrophils and plays a major role in lung injury: inducing lung oedema by increasing vascular permeability, enhancing chemotaxism and migration of PMN cells, and participating in the development of pulmonary arterial hypertension by its vasoconstrictive action [29, 30]. These effects are enhanced by platelet-aggregating factor (PAF), a cell membrane-derived ether lipid produced, not only by inflammatory cells such as macrophages, but also by endothelial and epithelial cells, and fibroblasts. Even small amounts of PAF can induce an ALI-like lung injury in rats when given in combination with lipopolysaccharide (LPS), while it is insufficient to induce any inflammation by itself [31]. In summary, animal models led to the conclusion that these compounds may have adverse effects in the lung during ALI because they promote neutrophil chemotaxis and adhesion, bronchoconstriction, increased vascular permeability, and platelet aggregation.

In parallel with discoveries regarding the role on inflammatory mediators in ALI, it was realized that neutrophils are intimately associated with the syndrome. The focus on the role of the neutrophil in ALI aroused from early observations in lung histology that neutrophils accumulate in the air spaces and interstitium of the lung [32], the appearance of neutrophils in lavage fluids and development of acute peripheral neutropenia in numerous animal models of sepsis induced ALI. Neutrophils have been shown to accumulate in the lung within 30 min of intravenous endotoxin in several species, including sheep and rabbits, and precede structural evidence of endothelial injury [33]. In certain animal models of ALI, neutrophils depletion or inhibition of neutrophils products ameliorates the lung injury [34]. Neutrophils are capable of producing an impressive array of toxic products (reactive oxygen radicals and proteases) that are principally available to destroy invading microorganisms [35]. The addition of inhibitors of toxic products produced by neutrophils attenuated ALI [36]. Although there was an initial excitement surrounding neutrophils and ALI, subsequent evidences have shown that ALI occurs in models in which animals were neutropenic [37]. Thus, intrapulmonary accumulation of neutrophils does not prove a causal relationship with lung injury. Lessons learned from animal studies suggest neutrophils may be instrumental in recruiting monocytes, initiating repair, or stimulating antioxidant protection. In addition, neutrophils are now viewed as a critical, but not essential factor in the development of ALI.

In the early 1980's, tumour necrosis factor alpha (TNF-α) was discovered and the explanation of the pathophysiology of ALI changed [38]. TNF-α appears early in circulation after intravenous injection of LPS, with metabolic and pathophysiologic consequences that mimic gram-negative sepsis. Animals resistant to the effects of endotoxin appear to be protected by a genetic inability to manufacture native TNF-α. TNF-α activates neutrophils for oxidant generation, phagocytosis, degranulation, and adherence. In addition, Walsh et al. (1992) showed attenuation of the haemodynamic derangement and pulmonary dysfunction in a porcine model of sepsis using a monoclonal antibody directed against the TNF-α molecule [39] . However, the early pulmonary hypertension and hypoxemia, recognized as cyclooxygenase effects were not attenuated. Since the discovery of TNF-α, numerous other cytokines have been described and the interactions between various cells via cytokines have led to the concept of cytokine network. The understanding of these cytokines has greatly enhanced our understanding of ALI. Cytokines are a diverse group of biologically active proteins that are instrumental in the evolution of acute lung injury. In addition, cytokines mediate their influence through autocrine, paracrine, and endocrine effects. Because of TNF-α and interleukin (IL)-1 ability to begin inflammatory responses and to be present early in the evolution of ALI, have been termed early response cytokines (Fig. 1). Although TNF-α and IL-1 are not chemoattractant, they can induce the production of IL-8, a potent neutrophil and lymphocyte chemoattractant, from many cells, including endothelial cells, fibroblasts, epithelial cells, alveolar macrophages, and neutrophils [38]. IL-8 production from these cells is stimulus specific. Endothelial cells produce IL-8 in response to endotoxin, TNF-α, or IL-1, whereas pulmonary fibroblasts and epithelial cells only respond to TNF-α or IL-1. In animal models of ALI, antibodies to IL-8 afford protection against injury [40, 41]. Many cells produce IL-8 during ALI, but early in ALI the alveolar macrophage appears to be an important source of this cytokine. As ALI progresses, recruitment and activation of other cells produce IL-8 and maintain high levels of IL-8 in the lung. Most of the studies investigating cytokines in ALI focused the inflammatory

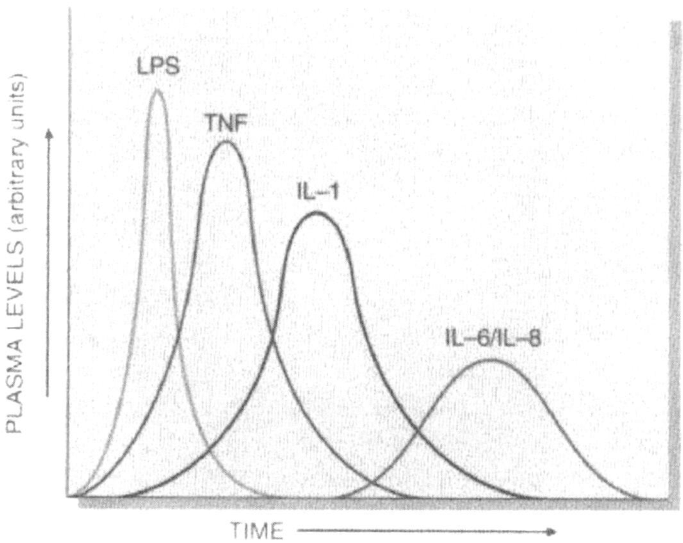

Fig. 1. Temporal evolution of cytokines in an experimental model of acute lung injury (ALI) induced by lipopolysaccharide (LPS).

function of cytokines. However, various cytokines also exhibit anti-inflammatory properties. Major anti-inflammatory cytokines include IL-1 receptor antagonist (ra), IL-4, IL-6, IL-10, IL-11, and IL-13. Specific cytokine receptor for IL-1, tumour necrosis factor-alpha, and IL-18 also function as pro-inflammatory cytokine inhibitors [42-46]. The main point is not only the production of pro-inflammatory cytokines but also the balance between pro-inflammatory and anti-inflammatory mediators. Several endogenous inhibitors of pro-inflammatory cytokines have been described, including IL-1ra, soluble tumour necrosis factor receptor, autoantibodies against IL-8, and anti-inflammatory cytokines such as IL-10 and IL-11 [47].

Experimental animals research suggest that parenchymal lung injury and an inflammatory response may be caused and perpetuated if mechanical ventilation results in alveolar overdistention and allows cyclic collapse and reinflation of alveolar units with tidal breathing [48, 49]. On the basis of these studies, pressure-limited, lung protective mechanical ventilatory strategies have been proposed for ARDS emphasising the need to open the lung and keep it open while avoiding alveolar overdistension [50]. Recently, different ventilation strategies (e.g., partial liquid ventilation, surfactant, prone position) have been studied in different animal models of ALI. Rotta and Steinhorn (1998) observed that partial liquid ventilation decreases pulmonary neutrophil accumulation in an experimental model of ALI induced by systemic endotoxemia [51]. The attenuation in pulmonary leukostasis in animals treated with partial liquid ventilation was equivalent to that obtained by a ventilation strategy that targets lung recruitment, such as high frequency oscillatory ventilation. Doctor et al. (2001) examine dose-response relationships regarding the efficiency of gas exchange and haemodynamic function during high frequency oscillation and partial liquid ventilation (HFO-PLV) of perfluorocarbon treated lung in a saline lavage-induced lung injury and suggest that this combination (HFO-PLV) is a novel strategy in the treatment of ALI [52] . Verbrugge et al. (1999) using an animal model of surfactant deficiency compared the effect of different ventilation strategies on oxygenation and inflammatory mediator release from the lung parenchyma [53]. Surfactant, partial liquid ventilation, and high PEEP improved oxygenation and reduced bronchoalveolar lavage fluid (BALF) protein levels. Broccard et al. (2000) observed in a model of lung injury initiated solely by mechanical ventilation a dependent predominance of tissue oedema and histological change in the supine position qualitatively similar to that developing in oleic acid-preinjured animals ventilated with the same peak transalveolar pressure and PEEP [54]. Prone position markedly attenuated these abnormalities. Van der Kloot et al. (2000) studied the effect of baseline ventilatory strategy and recruitment manoeuvres on end-expiratory lung volume and oxygenation in 18 dogs, using three models of acute lung injury: saline lavage, oleic acid injury and intratracheal instillation of *Escherichia coli* [55]. They concluded that responses to PEEP, tidal volume and recruitment manoeuvres differ among these models of ALI. The effectiveness of surfactant treatment in ALI in the adult is controversial. Waugh et al. (2000) [56] analyzed the effectiveness of early surfactant treatment in a phorbol-myristate acetate-induced ALI and observed that tracheal instillation of surfactant acutely elevate lung impedance in the first few hours after administration, and co-administration of PEEP appears to be critically important to counteracting these early effects of surfactant instillation on the lung. Brachenbury et al. (2001) showed that various surfactant treatment strategies were not effective in a model of HCl-induced ALI, but the lungs of these animals were recruitable with high frequency oscillation, as reflected by the acute and sustained oxygenation improvements [57]. These ventilation strategies are potential therapeutic options under investigation for the management of ALI.

How to develop an experimental model of acute lung injury?

How to develop an animal model of ALI?

The ideal animal model of ALI would first faithfully represent the aetiology and then reproduce, equally faithfully, the pathophysiologic phases that characterize the human syndrome, including exudative, proliferative, and fibrotic phases. Amongst them one could present:

Paraquat

Paraquat is an herbicide that accumulates predominantly in the lung and induces alveolar epithelial damage due to its action on type II pneumocytes (Fig. 2). This is an experimental model of diffuse alveolar damage, which by virtue of its low cost, rapid effect, and simplicity of administration has been used to study acute lung injury [58, 59]. In acute experiment the mortality rate is very high mainly in the presence of doses higher than 30 mg paraquat/kg. In order to develop a model of severe ALI 25 mg of paraquat/kg body weight is intraperitoneally injected. Recently, we observed the effects of different doses of paraquat on lung histology 24 hours after the injection of paraquat. Histological changes included interstitial oedema, intra-alveolar haemorrhage, inflammation with polymorphonuclear and mononuclear cells and hyaline membrane formation in rats, which received 25 and 30 mg paraquat/kg (severe ALI) (Fig. 3). Rats given 10 and 15 mg/kg present lungs with thickened alveolar membranes and increased

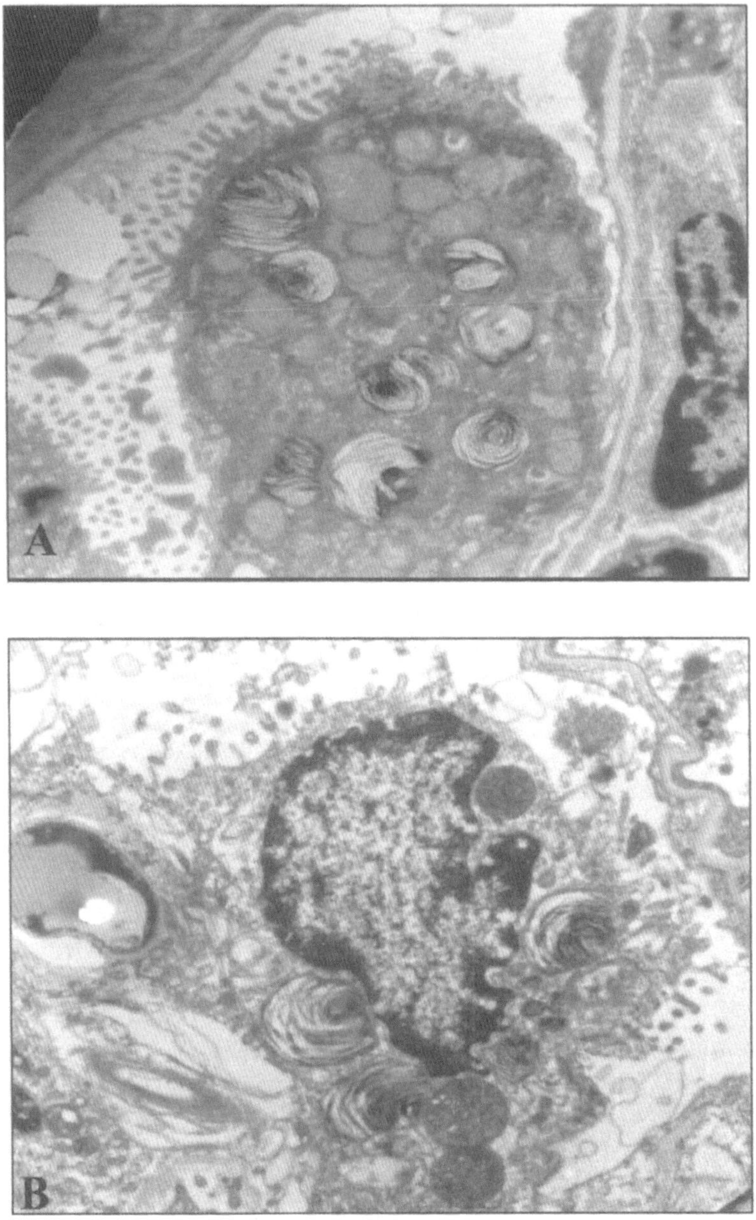

Fig. 2. Electron micrograph of lung from a rat 24 hours after intraperitoneal injection of saline (A) and paraquat (25 mg/kg) (B). Type II cells contains many lamellar bodies in paraquat-induced lung injury (B) (x5000).

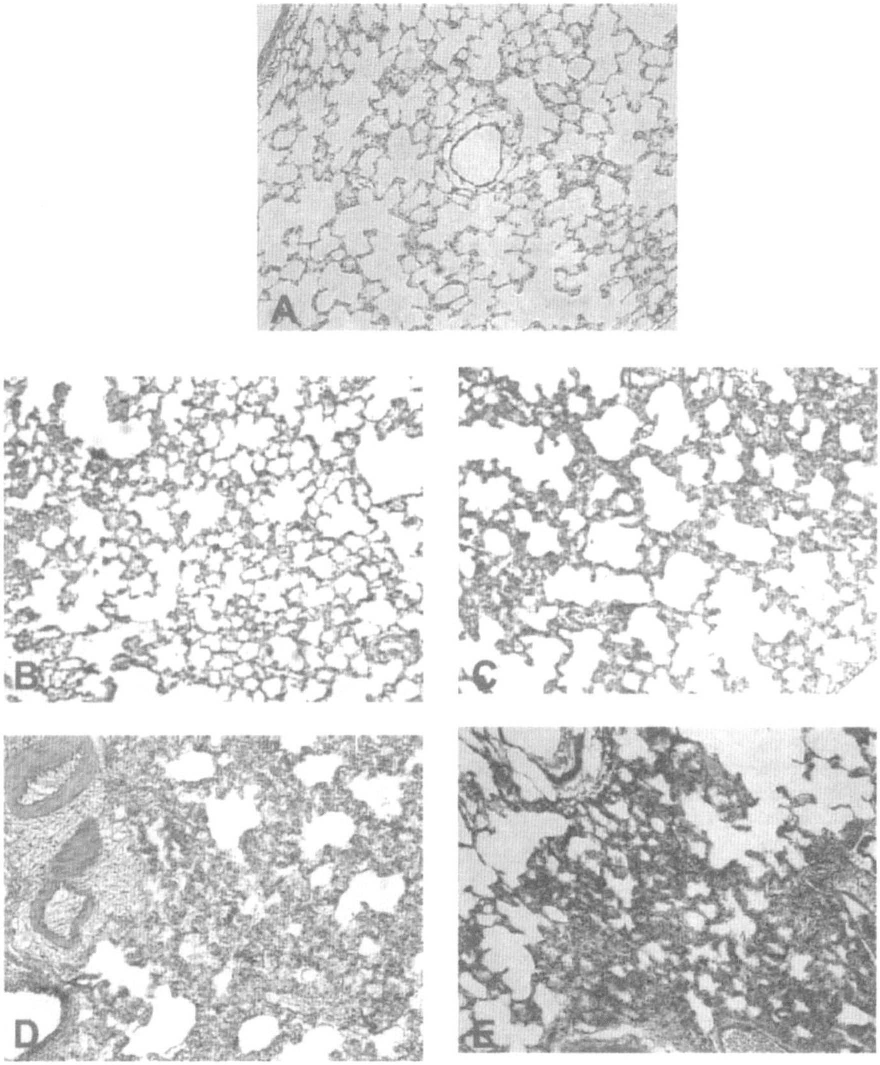

Fig. 3. Lung histology from the lungs of the control (A) and acute lung injury groups (10, 15, 25, and 30 mg/kg, B, C, D, and E, respectively). Photographs were taken at an original magnification of x100 from slides stained by HE.

cellularity, but did not demonstrate haemorrhage or hyaline membrane formation (mild ALI). The difference between the group that received 10 mg/kg and 15 mg/kg was demonstrated by the increment in cellularity and between 25 and 30 mg/kg was indicated by the augment in intra-alveolar haemorrhage [60].

Oleic acid

One of the most popular animal models of ALI is produced by injecting oleic acid (OA) directly into the pulmonary circulation. This 18-carbon unsaturated fatty acid with a single double bond is normally used in the synthesis of other fatty acids such as eicosatrienoic acid. The OA model is an unlikely paradigm for the aetiology of ALI (with the possible exception of ALI associated with fat embolization). However, in many other respects, it does resemble ALI, especially in its most acute aspects (Tables 3 and 4) [61]. No other model has been used as extensively to evaluate the risks and benefits of various treatment strategies before applying them to patients with ALI. Despite the use of different species, anaesthetic regimens, dosages of OA, and modes of support (mechanical ventilation, FIO_2), the pathologic sequence of findings is remarkably similar in most studies, and it is quite similar to that seen in ALI (Table 3). Because only 1 to 2 ml will reliably cause acute lung injury when administered to an animal weighing 25 kg, most investigators have injected pure OA as a single bolus directly into the pulmonary circulation {dog (45 and 90 mg/kg) [62], dog (90 mg/kg) [63], and baboon (35-125 mg/kg) [64]}. However, both smaller and larger doses have also been used [64]. At other times, the injection has been given in fractions, after sonication in saline, after dissolving the OA in ethanol, or as a continuous infusion over many minutes (0.1 ml/kg/h during 2 h (rabbit) [65]; 0.15 ml/kg during 30 min (piglets) [66]; 0.09 ml/kg during 60-90 min (dog) [55]. Each of these variations may alter the severity or extensiveness of the injury, resulting in different pathophysiological consequences.

Table 3. Pathologic similarities and differences between oleic acid (OA)-induced lung injury and acute lung injury (ALI) [61]

Phases	OA-induced injury	ALI
Exudative phase		
Proteinaceous Oedema	+++	+++
Intravascular Congestion	+++	++
Intravascular Coagulation	+	+
Endothelial cell necrosis	+++	++
Alveolar haemorrhage	++	++
Extravascular coagulation	++	++
Epithelial cell necrosis	+++	+++
Distribution	Focally diffuse, peripheral	Diffuse
Proliferative phase		
Type II cell proliferation	+++	+++
Mononuclear cell infiltrate	+++	+++
Resolution of oedema	+++	+++
Fibrotic phase		
Fibroblast proliferation	+	++
Fibrosis	+	++

Table 4. Comparison of nonpathologic features of oleic acid (OA)-induced acute lung injury with acute lung injury [61]

Feature	Comparison
Dependence of initial injury on inflammation	Comparable
Pulmonary sequestration of circulating cells	Comparable
Generation of reactive oxygen species	Comparable
Imbalance between procoagulant/fibrinolytic systems	Comparable
Prostaglandin production	Comparable
Leukotriene production	Different
Role of cytokines	Unknown
Severity of injury	
Protein leak	Comparable
Extravascular lung water accumulation	Comparable
Lung compliance	Comparable
Surfactant effects	Comparable
Nonbarrier endothelial function	Different
Multiorgan system failure	Unknown
Development of fibrosis	Uncertain
Development of pulmonary hypertension	Comparable
Mechanisms	Unknown

Saline lavage

Ashbaugh et al. suggested that loss of surfactant function might be responsible for the pattern of pulmonary pathophysiology in ALI [1] There are many experimental models that induce ALI by removing surfactant. Usually, with the animal in the supine position, one disconnects the tracheal tube from the ventilator and warmed sterile saline is instilled, using gravity, via a tracheal tube until a fluid meniscus level can be seen in the tracheal tube. After 1 min of apnoea, gravity drains the fluid and the recovered volume is measured. Ventilation resumes for 10 min after each lavage while PaO_2 determination continuously assesses lung injury. The repetition (up to eight times) of this procedure leads to the presence of an adequate injury (defined as PaO_2 less than 80 mmHg after 10 min of ventilation following lavage) [67].

Sepsis

Endotoxin was recognized as a potentially important mediator in the pathogenesis of ALI in 1974 when the infusion of *Pseudomonas* into sheep was shown to produce increased pulmonary permeability [15]. Thereafter, it was found that infusion of *E.coli* endotoxin in sheep produced a similar picture of non-cardiogenic pulmonary dysfunction [68]. Endotoxin is the LPS component of the cell walls of gram-negative bacteria. It is comprised of three major components: an oligosaccharide chain (O antigen), which is species specific; a core polysaccharide; and the lipid A region which anchors the complex to the cell. The lipid

A region accounts for the majority of the biologic activity of endotoxin. There are different methods of endotoxin induced ALI: intratracheal aerolization and instillation, intraperitoneal and intravenous injection [15, 51, 69-71]. The doses depend on the species and the means of administration. In addition, live *Pseudomonas aeruginosa* [39], *E. coli* or pneumococci could be used to induce ALI [55].

Summary

ALI is one of the most studied pathophysiologic processes occurring in the medical intensive care unit. Most of the current understanding about this severe clinical illness and the mediators associated with it has come from the study of relevant animal models. In the mid-1970s, the development of the sheep model of ARDS and, later, the porcine model led to the discovery of a wide variety of lipid mediators, amines, cytokine, proteases, etc. Parallel to the understanding of the pathogenesis of ARDS, a substantial number of new therapies began to emerge. However, because there are many mediators and the interaction of these agents is complex, true insight into the process has been slow in coming.

References

1. Ashbaugh DG, Bigelow DB, Petty TL et al (1967) Acute respiratory distress syndrome. Lancet 2: 319-323
2. Bernard GR, Artigas A, Bringham KL et al (1994). The American-European consensus conference on ARDS: definitions, mechanisms, relevant outcomes, and clinical trial coordination. Am J Respir Crit Care Med 149:818-824
3. Pepe PE, Potkin RT, Resus DR et al (1982) Clinical predictors of the adult respiratory distress syndrome. Am J Surg 144:124-130
4. Fein AM, Lippmann M, Hotzman H et al (1983) The risk factors, incidence, and prognosis of ARDS following septicemia. Chest 83:40-42
5. Bone RC, Grodzin CJ, Balk RA (1997) Sepsis: A new hypothesis for pathogenesis of the disease process. Chest 112: 235-243
6. Ryan SF (1990) Acute alveolar injury: experimental models. In: Gil J (ed) Models of lung disease. Marcel Dekker, New York, pp 641-733
7. Williwerth BM, Crawford FA, Young WG et al (1967) The role of functional demand on the development of pulmonary lesions during hemorrhagic shock. J Thorac Cardiovasc Surgery 54: 658-665
8. Pomerantz M, Eisman B (1968) Experimental shock lung model. J Trauma 8: 782-787
9. Sealy WC (1968) The lung in hemorrhagic shock. J Trauma 8: 774-781
10. Cook WA (1968) Experimental shock lung model. J Trauma 8: 793-796
11. Murray JF, and Staff of Division of Lung Diseases, National Heart, Lung and Blood Institute (1977). Conference Report-Workshop on mechanisms of acute respiratory failure. Am Rev Respir Dis 115: 1071-1078
12. Windsor ACJ, Mullen PG, Fowler AA (1993) Acute lung injury: What have we learned from animal models. Am J Med Sci 306:111-116

13. Flick MR (1986) Mechanisms of acute lung injury: What we have learned from experimental animal models. Crit Care Clin 2: 455-470
14. Staub NC (1971) Steady state transvascular water filtration in unanesthetized sheep Cir Res 28:135-139
15. Brigham KL, Woolverton WC, Blake LH et al (1974) Increased sheep lung vascular permeability caused by *Pseudomonas* bacteremia. J Clin Invest 54: 792-804
16. Craddock PR, Fehr J, Brigham KL et al (1977) Complement and leukocyte mediated pulmonary dysfunction in hemodialysis. N Engl J Med 296: 769-774
17. Hammerschmidt DE, Weaver LJ, Hudson LD et al (1980) Association of complement activation and elevated plasma C5a with adult respiratory distress syndrome. Lancet 1: 947-949
18. Till GO, Johnson KJ, Kunkel R (1982) Intravascular activation of complement and ALI: Dependency on neutrophils and toxic oxygen metabolites. J Clin Invest 60: 1126-1135
19. Henson PM, Larsen GL, Webster RO et al (1982) Pulmonary microvascular alterations and injury induced by complement fragments: Synergistic effect of complement activation, neutrophil sequestrations and prostaglandins. Ann NY Acad Sci 348: 287-300
20. Hosea S, Brown E, Hammer C et al (1980) Role of complement activation in a model of adult respiratory distress syndrome. J Clin Invest 66: 375-382
21. Stevens J, O'Hanley PT, Shapiro J et al (1986) Effects of anti-C5a antibodies on the adult respiratory distress syndrome in septic primates. J Clin Invest 77: 1812-1816
22. Rabinovici R, Yah C, Hillegass L et al (1992) Role of complement in endotoxin/platelet activity factor-induced lung injury. J Immunol 149: 1744-1750
23. Dehring DJ, Steinberg SM, Wismar BL et al (1987) Complement depletion in a porcine model of acute respiratory disease. J Trauma 27: 615-626
24. Flick MR, Horn JK, Hoellfel JM et al (1986) Reduction in total hemolytic complement activity with Naja haje cobra venom factor does not prevent endotoxin induced lung injury in sheep. Am Rev Respir Dis 133: 62-67
25. Brigham K, Meyrick B (1986) Endotoxin and lung injury. Am Rev Respir Dis 133: 913-927
26. Peterson MP, Huttemeier PC, Zapol WM et al (1982) Tromboxane mediates acute pulmonary hypertension in sheep extracorporeal perfusion. Am J Physiol 243: H471-H479
27. Gnidec AG, Sibbald WJ, Cheung H et al (1988) Ibuprofen reduces the progressive permeability edema in an animal model of hyperdynamic sepsis. J Appl Physiol 65: 1024-1032
28. Byrne K, Carey PD, Sielaff TD et al (1991) Ibuprofen prevents deterioration in static transpulmonary compliance and transalveolar protein flux in septic porcine acute lung injury. J Trauma 31: 155-166
29. Garcia JG, Noonan TC, Jubiz W et al (1987) Leukotrienes and the pulmonary microcirculation. Am Rev Respir Dis 136: 161-169.
30. Gadaleta D, Davis JM (1994) Pulmonary failure and the production of leukotrienes. J Am Coll Surg 178: 309-319
31. Rabinovici R, Bugelski PJ, Esser KM et al (1993) ARDS-like lung injury produced by endotoxin in platelet-activating factor-primed rats. J Appl Physiol 74: 1791-1802
32. Bachofen A, Weibel ER (1977) Alterations of the gas exchange apparatus in adult respiratory insufficiency associated with septicemia. Am Rev Respir Dis 116: 589-615
33. Meyrick B, Ryan US, Brigham KL (1990) Acute effects of *Escherichia coli* endotoxin on the pulmonary microcirculation of anesthetized sheep. Lab Invest 62: 355-362
34. Heflin AC, Brigham KL (1981) Prevention by granulocyte depletion of increased vascular permeability of sheep lung following endotoxemia. J Clin Invest 68:1253-1260
35. Shasby DM, Vanbenthugsen KM, Tate RM et al (1982) Granulocyte mediated acute edematous lung injury in rabbits and isolated rabbit lungs perfused with phorbol myristate acetate: role of oxygen radicals. Am Rev Respir Dis 125: 443-447
36. Brigham KL, Meyrick B, Berry JC et al (1987) Antioxidants protect cultured bovine lung endothelial cells from injury by endotoxin. J Appl Physiol 63:840-850
37. Hinson J, Hutchison A, Ogletree M et al (1983) Effect of granulocyte depletion on altered lung mechanics after endotoxemia in sheep. J Appl Physiol 55: 92-99

38. Kelley J (1990) Cytokines of the lung. Am Rev Respir Dis 141: 765-788
39. Walsh CJ, Sugerman HJ, Mullen PG et al (1992) Monoclonal antibody to tumor necrosis factor ??attenuates cardiopulmonary dysfunction in porcine gram negative sepsis. Arch Surg 127: 138-145
40. Mulligan MS, Jones ML, Bolanowski MA et al (1993) J Immunol 150: 5585-5595
41. Sekido N, Mukaida N, Harada A et al (1993) Prevention of lung reperfusion injury in rabbits by a monoclonal antibody against interleukin-8. Nature 365:654-657
42. Wakabayashi G, Gelfand JA, Burke J et al (1991) A specific receptor antagonist for interleukin 1 prevents *Escherichia coli* induced shock in rabbits. FASEB J 5: 338-343
43. Canonico AE, Brigham KL (1997) Biology of Acute Injury. In Crystal RG, West JB (eds) The Lung. Scientific Foundations. Lippincott-Raven Publishers, Philadelphia, pp 2475-2498
44. Opal SM, DePalo VA (2000) Impact of basic research on tomorrow's medicine anti-inflammatory cytokines. Chest 117: 1162-1172
45. Cassatella MA, Meda L, Bonora S, et al (1993) Interleukin 10 (IL-10) inhibits the release of pro-inflammatory cytokines from human polymorphonuclear leukocytes. Evidence for an autocrine role for tumor necrosis factor and IL-12 in mediating the production of IL-8 triggered by lipopolysaccharide. J Exp Med 178: 2207-2211
46. Parsons PE (2000) Mediators and mechanisms of acute lung injury. Clin Chest Med 3: 467-476
47. Pittet JF, MacKersie RC, Martin TR et al (1997) Biological markers of acute lung injury: prognostic and pathogenetic significance. Am J Respir Crit Care Med 155: 1187-1205
48. Dreyfuss D, Soler P, Basset G et al (1988) High inflation pressure pulmonary edema: respective effects of high airway pressure, high tidal volume, and positive end-expiratory pressure. Am Rev Respir Dis 137: 1159-1164
49. Bowton DL, Kong DL (1989) High tidal volume ventilation produces increased lung water in oleic acid injured rabbit lung. Crit Care Med 17: 908-911
50. Snyder JV, Froese A (1987) The open lung approach: concept and application. In: Snyder JV and Pinsky MR (eds) Oxygen Transport in the Critically Ill. Year Book Medical Publishers, Chicago, pp 374-395
51. Rotta AR, Steinhorn DM (1998) Partial liquid ventilation reduces pulmonary neutrophil accumulation in an experimental model of systemic endotoxemia and acute lung injury. Crit Care Med 10: 1707-1715
52. Doctor A, Price B, Bhargava N et al (2001) High frequency oscillatory ventilation of the perfluorocarbon-filled lung: dose response relationships in an animal model of acute lung injury. Crit Care Med 29: 847-854
53. Verbrugge SJC, Uhlig S, Neggers SJCMM et al (1999) Different ventilation strategies affect lung function but do not increase tumor necrosis factor-alpha and prostacyclin production in lavaged rat lungs in vivo. Anesthesiology 91: 1834-1843
54. Broccard A, Shapiro RS, Schmitz LL et al (2000) Prone positioning attenuates and redistributes ventilator-induced lung injury in dogs. Crit Care Med 28: 295-303
55. Van der Kloot TE, Blanch L, Youngblood M et al (2000) Recruitment maneuvers in three experimental models of acute lung injury. Effect on lung volume and gas exchange. Am J Respir Crit Care Med 161: 1485-1494
56. Waugh JB, Op't Holt TB, Olson LE et al (2000) Surfactant treatment impairs gas exchange in a canine model of acute lung injury. Crit Care Med 28: 2887-2892
57. Brackenbury AM, Puligandla OS, McCaig LA et al (2001) Evaluation of exogenous surfactant in HCl-induced lung injury. Am J Respir Crit Care Med 163: 1135-1142
58. Delaval PM, Gillespie DJ (1985) Pulmonary dysfunction during paraquat-induced lung injury: A model of acute alveolar injury. Crit Care Med 13:1056-1060
59. Smith P, Health D, Kay JM (1974) The pathogenesis and structure of paraquat-induced lung fibrosis in rats. J Pathol 114:57-67
60. Rocco PRM, Negri EM, Kurtz PM et al (2001) Lung tissue mechanics and extracellular matrix remodeling in acute lung injury. Am J Respir Crit Care Med (in press)

61. Schuster DP (1994) ARDS: Clinical lessons from the oleic acid model of acute lung injury. Am J Respir Crit Care Med 149:245-260
62. Derks CM and Jacobovitz-Derks D (1977) Embolic pneumopathy induced by oleic acid. Am J Pathol 87: 143-158
63. Schoene RB, Robertson HT, Thorning DR et al (1984) Pathophysiological patterns of resolution from acute oleic acid lung injury in the dog. J Appl Physiol 56: 472-481
64. Johanson WG Jr, Holcomb JR, Coalson J (1982) Experimental diffuse alveolar damage in baboons. Am Rev Respir Dis 126: 142-151
65. Furue S, Mikawa K, Nishina K et al (2001). Therapeutic time-window of a group IIA phospholipase A2 inhibitor in rabbit acute lung injury: correlation with lung surfactant protection. Crit Care Med 29: 719-727
66. Enrione MA, Papo MC, Leach CL, et al (1999) Regional pulmonary blood flow during partial liquid ventilation in normal and acute oleic acid-induced lung injured piglets. Crit Care Med 27: 2716-2723
67. Lachmann B, Robertson B, Vogel J (1980) In vivo lung lavage as an experimental model of the respiratory distress syndrome. Acta Anaesthesiol Scand 24: 231-236
68. Brigham K, Bowers R, Haynes J (1979) Increased sheep lung vascular permeability caused by *E. coli* endotoxin. Circulation 45: 292-297
69. Van Helden HP, Kuijpers WC, Steenvoorden D et al (1997) Intratracheal aerolization of endotoxin (LPS) in the rat: a comprehensive animal model to study adult (acute) respiratory distress syndrome. Exp Lung Res 23: 297-316
70. Rotta AT, Gunnarsson B, Hernan LJ et al (1999) Partial liquid ventilation influences pulmonary histopathology in an animal model of acute lung injury. J Crit Care 14: 84-92
71. Faffe DS, Seidl VR, Chagas PSC, Gonçalves de Moraes VL, Capelozzi VL, Rocco PRM, Zin WA (2000) Respiratory effects of lipopolysaccharide-induced inflammatory lung injury in mice. Eur Respir J 15: 85-91

Animal Models of Asthma

J. G. Martin, J.-P. Lavoie

Models are devised to allow the study of the components of the physiological system involved in a disease process. The ability to study the response of the system to perturbations, such as inciting stimuli or response modifying agents, for example drugs or neutralizing antibodies, permits conclusions to be drawn concerning cause and effect relationships in the putative cascade of events in the disease. A satisfactory model of human disease is one that not only reproduces one or more of the key elements of the disease but is reproducible and readily accessible to investigators. Models have been developed classically by driving physiological systems with various stimuli that may or may not be encountered in a physiological context, such as allergen or gaseous pollutants, or at least not in the concentrations used to elicit responses in the animal. One of the lessons that the successful development of such a model teaches is that exuberant responses of otherwise normal physiological systems are often at the root of diseases such as asthma. Furthermore, the characteristic that distinguishes the affected animal or human subject may not be clearly outside the range spanned by a normal population. The concordance of several alterations in function may be required to place the host on the susceptible end of a scale describing the risk of disease. Diseases of the above type are generally the result of the interaction of environmental factors and several risk-related genes. In some cases single gene alterations may have sufficiently profound consequences for function that disease results. In such cases modeling of the disease in animals requires another approach. One such approach is the design of a defective gene in an animal. The advent of transgenic and knock-out technologies has allowed investigators to delete or over-express gene products of interest while examining the consequences of these interventions on physiological functions. This intervention is confined to murine models to date. This paper will not address models based on genetic approaches.

An important consideration in the development of a model of disease is the choice of species and strain of animal. In some instances the choice of sub-strain may be important. The guinea pig is notoriously hyperresponsive to contractile agonists and so is often used for studies of airway responses. Large animals are often used when detailed physiological measurements, such as the partitioning of pulmonary responses into large or small airways/parenchymal contributions to increase in lung impedance. Mice have become the favored species for studies where an immunological mechanism is under consideration. Improvements in measurement techniques for lung function and provocation testing have made mice of interest also from the standpoint of airway hyperresponsiveness.

What has been modeled?

Asthma is a multifaceted disease that comprises various degrees of airway inflammation, airway hyperresponsiveness, and airway narrowing. One or more of these manifestations has been re-created through the use of quite a few animal models. Airway inflammation that is eosinophil rich and that also involves an increase in the number and in the activation state of other leukocytes has been successfully induced. Likewise, airway hyperresponsiveness to methacholine, histamine, or other contractile agonists, as well as airway narrowing, have been demonstrated. Two of the recognized triggers for asthma are allergen sensitization and exposure and the inhalation of increased volumes of dry air. Models employing these triggers have been touted to be appropriate models of allergen and exercise-induced asthma, respectively. The former has been much more extensively explored.

Allergic asthma

A predisposition to the development of sensitivity to common aeroallergens has long been recognized to be associated with asthma. The fact that the inhalation of allergen provokes bronchoconstriction has also been interpreted as indicating that aeroallergens are frequent causes of airway narrowing in asthmatic subjects. The recognition that allergen triggers a biphasic response in some, although not all, asthmatics was a key factor in prompting the exploration of the mechanisms of these responses [1]. The early response is IgE mediated and a consequence of mast cell degranulation. The alterations in lung function are caused by both airway smooth muscle contraction and a leak of fluid and protein from microvessels. The responsible mediators are histamine (serotonin in some rodents), prostaglandin D_2, and the cysteinyl-leukotrienes (cys-LTs). Other IgE receptor-bearing cells such as eosinophils, neutrophils, and macrophages may also participate in the response, but their contribution is as yet unclear. The late response occurring several hours after challenge and lasting for several hours is more complex and involves the activation of T cells [2,3] and a cascade of events leading to the synthesis of cys-LTs and other mediators [4-6]. The development of a late response and airway inflammation following allergen challenge is often accompanied by an increase in the responsiveness of the airways to provocation testing with methacholine and other contractile agonists.

The increase in airway responsiveness to contractile agonists, so-called non-specific hyperresponsiveness, is non-agonist specific and therefore is a post-receptor mediated phenomenon. The mechanism is thus far obscure. Airway hyperresponsiveness (AHR) is potentially caused by altered airway smooth muscle function, reductions in impedance to airway smooth muscle contraction by changes in the mechanics of the airways or parenchyma, or architectural changes increasing the degree of airway narrowing effected by a given degree of airway smooth muscle contraction. Altered airway smooth muscle function is most likely to be at the root of AHR, either through increase in mass or contractility.

Exercise induced asthma

Airway narrowing following exercise has been reproduced by hyperventilation to equivalent levels while maintaining conditions isocapnic [7]. This finding has led to the hypothesis that changes in airway function secondary to hyperventilation are responsible for exercise-induced asthma. Hyperpnea-induced bronchoconstriction has been used interchangeably with exercise-induced asthma in the exploration of the mechanisms of airway narrowing. Interestingly this trigger causes airway responses in quite a number of species [8-10], hence it may be not the sensitivity to the stimulus but rather the exuberant response in asthmatic subjects that is at fault. Not all the steps in the process have been dissected, but the thermal stress of conditioning the inspired air causes cooling and perhaps drying of the airway lining fluid.

Animal models

In the modeling of asthma, both large and small animal have been used. As the research strategies have changed there has also been a move away from large to small animal models, with various advantages and disadvantages. Large animals have in the past had the advantage that the measurements of lung function were of a quality comparable to those employed in the detailed characterization of lung mechanical function in human subjects. Now it is possible to obtain high-quality and reliable measurements even in the mouse, through the use of suitably designed small animal ventilators [11]. Despite this possibility many investigators have used so-called non-invasive lung function assessment for small animals, which is of uncertain validity in relationship to the precise site of the airway reaction (upper or lower airways).

Allergic asthma

Canine models

The dog has been used to develop a model of sustained AHR in association with sensitization and exposure to allergen. Dogs that are sensitized in the neonatal period to ragweed have been shown to develop AHR [12]. The mechanism of AHR has been attributed to altered airway smooth muscle (ASM) properties. The excised ASM from sensitized dogs can shorten more rapidly in response to a maximal stimulus than ASM from control animals [13]. This change is accompanied by a change in myosin light chain kinase activity [14,15]. This animal model is elegant but its potential is limited because of cost and the lack of reagents for the exploration of the underlying immunological mechanisms of the AHR.

Ovine models

The sheep has been extensively explored and has provided much useful information concerning the biochemical mediators of the late response. Indeed in only two animals, the sheep and the rat, has the late airway response been well characterized. Ascaris-sensitive sheep are used, which has the advantage that natural sensitization has taken place rather than the contrived protocols used for other species. Cys-LTs have been demonstrated to be important in mediating the late allergic response (LAR) [5], as well as kinins such as bradykinin and platelet-activating factor [16,17]. The model has also proven useful in the demonstration that the integrin VLA-4 is involved in the LAR and its antagonism is inhibitory to the response [18]. The sheep also serves as a model for the study of AHR that is induced by allergen challenge and can last for at least a week after challenge. An antagonist of VLA-4 administered after allergen challenge can reverse allergen-induced AHR [19]. LAR and AHR are also blocked by adhesion pathway inhibitors involving selectins [20].

Equine models

Heaves, also known as chronic obstructive pulmonary disease, is a form of recurrent airway obstruction and is a common condition of horses in Europe and North America, which is characterized by lower airway inflammation, reversible airflow obstruction, and bronchial hyper-responsiveness [21-23]. Similar to asthma, heaves is a spontaneously occurring condition that develops over a period of years. Initial signs may be limited to exercise intolerance; the frequency and severity of the coughing episodes increase as the disease progresses. In its most-severe form, an increased respiratory rate, flared nostrils, and double expiratory effort may be present, and a "heave line" caused by hypertrophy of the external abdominal oblique muscles may develop. The appearance and severity of the clinical signs tend to wax and wane and the duration of the attacks vary from days to weeks; horses may be asymptomatic between attacks. The airway obstruction is primarily due to bronchospasm and agonists reverse the obstruction within minutes. However, mucus hypersecretion and airway remodeling are also important contributing factors. An increase in pulmonary resistance and elastance is detected during disease exacerbation, whereas AHR is present both during clinical disease and remission.

Clinical signs of heaves can be induced in susceptible horses by the inhalation of dust from mouldy hay, and the airway obstruction is reversible in dust--free environments [21,22]. These observations led researchers to postulate that heaves is an allergic reaction to inhaled moulds and fungi present in hay. The positive passive cutaneous anaphylaxis test observed using sera from horses with heaves [23] and the elevated levels of IgE in bronchoalveolar lavage (BAL) [24] and serum [25] of affected horses are supportive of the involvement of a type I hypersensitivity reaction. Most horses have a positive skin reaction to common barn allergens, although horses with heaves tend to have a greater number of positive skin reactions [26]. Using in situ hybridization, we have recently shown that BAL cells from horses with heaves, similar to those of asthma patients, have increased expression of interleukin interferon (IL)-4 and IL-5 mRNA and decreased expression of interferon (IFN) which is consistent with a Th2 type cytokine response [27].

Heaves is characterized by a neutrophil recruitment into airway secretions following antigenic stimulation, and pulmonary eosinophilia is not a feature of the disease. After antigen challenge a delay of 5 h is expected before the initiation of neutrophil recruitment in lung tissues and the appearance of clinical signs of heaves [28]. This finding is reminiscent of the LAR in asthmatic subjects following allergen challenge. Histological lesions are more severe in the peripheral airways and resemble those of asthma, including epithelial detachment and regeneration, goblet cell hyperplasia, and hyperplasia of the bronchial smooth muscles [29,30]. Pulmonary radiographs are generally unremarkable even in severe cases, and the formerly held opinion that heaves shares a common etiopathogenesis with extrinsic allergic alveolitis (Farmers's lung) is incorrect.

Feline models

The cat is the second example of a spontaneous or natural asthma occurring in a species other than human. So-called feline asthma has been described to show clinical and histological features similar to those of human asthma. Respiratory distress, audible wheezing, and inflamed airways with eosinophilia was been reported to occur. It has also been used to show that allergen exposure causes airway remodeling with an increase in the airway glands, goblet cells, and the mass of airway smooth muscle [31], arguably the most-important change in airway structure induced by asthmatic inflammation. Airway secretions show Curschmann's spirals and Charcot-Leyden crystals. However, it appears that improved care of the animals with less parasitic infestation has made this condition uncommon.

Murine models

The mouse has been extensively used in recent times to evaluate various immunological and biochemical mechanisms of allergic airway responses. The principal advantage of this species is the extensive repertoire of reagents available to dissect the mechanisms of the various phenomena of interest. There are disadvantages, however, and some of these are substantive. Murine models are often sensitized by multiple exposures to allergen involving a priming dose and subsequent challenges through the airways or systemically. The varied protocols for sensitization are potentially crucial determinants of the degree of the AHR that is induced, as well as the pattern of airway inflammation. It is frequently difficult to compare the outcomes of different experiments because of the methodological differences. The lung of the mouse does not possess a bronchial circulation so that the airways are not supplied by systemic but by pulmonary vessels. The mechanisms of airway inflammation and the adhesion pathways involved in leukocyte migration may not pertain to larger animals and humans, in whom the systemic circulation provides much of the vascular supply to the airways.

An additional problem that investigators have faced in measuring lung function in mice is that of measuring airflow at the airway opening. There is no suitable pneumotachograph available for mice, because those commercially available have an excessive dead space and require animals to be either under-ventilated or ventilated adequately but with an excessive tidal volume. An alternative and satisfactory strategy is to use a body plethysmograph to measure volume changes of the chest wall and to derive flow, but this approach has not enjoyed much popularity. Many studies have been performed using non-invasive measurements of pulmonary function [32]. For this purpose animals are placed in a plethysmograph and measurements of pressure changes within the box are made. These pressure changes are a function of fluctuations in alveolar pressure caused by inspiratory and expiratory efforts. However, humidification and heating of the inspired gas also causes changes in box pressure. An index purporting to reflect airway constriction, termed Penh (enhanced pause), is used to measure pulmonary responses. This method is rather empirical and does not take into account the fact that the upper airways are reactive to most challenges, including allergen and methacholine. However, the changes in airway responsiveness using this method are associated with changes measured using more-conventional techniques [32]. The availability of a small animal ventilator specifically designed for the measurement of mouse lung mechanics has been a valuable tool for more-direct assessment of lung responses. The ventilator is attached via a small dead space to the animal and the excursion of the piston is used to obtain flow and volume signals [11]. With such a device detailed characterization of pulmonary mechanics is feasible.

Currently it has been shown that early responses to allergen challenge occur. These responses are usually IgE mediated, but it has been shown that typical allergic inflammation and AHR can occur in the absence of IgE [33]. Whether early airway responses occur in the absence of IgE does not seem to be have been addressed. No late responses have been demonstrated in the mouse, but airway inflammation that is rich in eosinophils follows allergen challenge. The eosinophilic airway inflammation that occurs in mice that are IgE deficient is dependent on CD4+ T cells [33,34]. AHR is also CD4+ T cell dependent [35,36]. In general, allergic inflammation, late airway responses, and AHR are associated with the expression of TH2 cytokines in the airway tissues and in cells in the BAL fluid. IL-4 and IL-5 have been particularly well evaluated and are certainly involved in certain aspects of the allergic response. IL-4 is important for immunoglobulin synthesis and is critical for switching to the IgE isotype. IL-5 is one of the most-important cytokines for the development of eosinophilia. IL-4 and IL–5 have been shown to be non-essential for the induction of AHR by allergen challenge in the mouse. IL-13, another TH2 cytokine, has emerged as a likely mediator of allergen-induced AHR [37, 38].

The mouse has also proven itself to be useful for the evaluation of the contribution of the CD8+ T cell to airway responses [39]. It appears that the CD8+ T cell can have both pro-inflammatory and anti-inflammatory roles depending on the experiment performed. In addition, T cells bearing the gamma-delta T cell receptor have been implicated in airway responses. These cells which are numerous in the airways and are frequently also CD8+ have been shown to be necessary for fully developed allergic inflammation and AHR.

Rodent models

The rat has been extensively explored as a model of allergic asthma. The development of a satisfactory model depends not only on the choice of species but also of strain or even substrain. The BN rat is perhaps the most-popular strain for study because it is a high IgE producer. This rat after active sensitization and allergen challenge has a high prevalence of early and late airway responses [40]. It develops an eosinophilic airway inflammation [41], but it is less spectacular than that found in the mouse. There is also evidence of T cell activation with a predominance of TH2 type cytokines expressed in the airways and BAL fluid [3]. By 24 h after allergen exposure, there is also AHR to inhaled contractile agonists such as acetylcholine, methacholine, and cys-LTs. The mechanisms of AHR are somewhat obscure, but are certainly T cell dependent [42]. AHR can be induced in allergen challenged animals that have been administered CD4+ T cells from sensitized donor rats. Late airway responses are somewhat better understood in that they are also CD4+ T cell dependent and are mediated by cys-LTs [4]. The cell sources of the cys-LTs are not established although macrophages and mast cells are likely candidates. Likewise the signals to these cells from the T cells have not been identified. Pre-treatment of T cells with anti-sense oligodeoxynucleotides for IL-4 has shown that the propagation of the signals within the airways following challenge is at least in part dependent on this cytokine [43].

Experiments using the technique of adoptive transfer have revealed that CD4 + T cells can induce allergen sensitivity in naïve recipient animals [44]. These animals display late responses and the typical pattern of inflammation after allergen challenge. However it has also been shown that CD8 + T cells can have a down-regulating action [45,46]. Indeed the BN rat has a relatively high CD4+ to CD8+ T cell ratio compared with other rat strains such as the Sprague-Dawley rat, suggesting that part of the responsiveness of the BN rat to allergen may relate to a deficiency of CD8+ T cells. Depletion of CD8+ cells in the Sprague-Dawley rat augments late airway responses in this animal [47], but does not cause the animal to have a degree of eosinophilia comparable to that of the BN rat. Clearly the atopic nature of the BN rat is determined by more than just the relative number of CD4 to CD8+ T cells. However, the CD8+ T cell is also a modulator of LAR in the BN rat because depletion of these cells also augments the airway response, including the degree of eosinophilia, as well TH2 cytokine and eotaxin expression [46]. The administration of CD8 + T cells from the lymph nodes of ovalbumin (OVA)-sensitized rats to sensitized recipients suppresses LAR and eosinophilia [45]. There is a reduction in TH2 cytokine expression and an increase in IFN-γ. However, the use of antisense oligonucleotides to inhibit IFN-γ expression by the transferred CD8+ cells did not restore the LAR but did affect eosinophilia, suggesting that the CD8+ cells inhibit the LAR by other mechanisms, whereas IFN-γ is an important regulator of eosinophilia (unpublished observations).

The CD8+ T cells are for the most part alpha-beta TCR-positive cells and are responsive to antigen presentation in conjunction with major histocompatibility class II molecules. Indeed the inhibitory effect of transferred CD8+ cells is only present when these cells are harvested from sensitized donors, implying a need for sensitization and clonal expansion of T cells that have the appropriate TCR. CD8+ gamma delta TCR-bearing cells are also a major source of IFN-γ and have been implicated in the mediation of tolerance in animals that are chronically exposed to OVA. These cells are also inhibitory of LAR when transferred to animals prior to sensitization to OVA, but not by IgE-dependent mechanisms. These cells inhibit the T cell response to OVA challenge, as evidenced by a reduction in T cell cytokines (unpublished observations).

Conclusions

Much useful information has been gleaned about the nature of asthma from modeling experiments using a variety of animal models. The choice of model has resided with the investigator and has not always been based on a careful consideration of the characteristics of the particular animal. Early models were based on the ability to take measurements of lung function, whereas more-recent models have been chosen based on the ability to dissect immunological and biochemical mechanisms of the responses. Allergen-induced models greatly exceed all other models of asthma and may have led to the misconception that no other triggers of asthma are of relevance. While a healthy skepticism concerning the pertinence of any model to human asthma is appropriate, the currently available models have been of enormous value in helping to unravel the pathogenesis of asthma.

References

1. Cockcroft DW, Ruffin RE, Dolovich J, et al (1977) Allergen-induced increase in non-allergic bronchial reactivity. J Clin Allergy 7:503-513
2. Bentley AM, Meng Q, Robinson DS, et al (1993) Increases in activated T lymphocytes, eosinophils, and cytokine mRNA expression for interleukin-5 and granulocyte/macrophage colony-stimulating factor in bronchial biopsies after allergen inhalation challenge in atopic asthmatics. Am J Respir Cell Mol Biol 8:35-42
3. Renzi PM, al Assaad AS, Yang J, et al (1996) Cytokine expression in the presence or absence of late airway responses after antigen challenge of sensitized rats. Am J Respir Cell Mol Biol 15:367-373
4. Martin JG, Xu L-J, Toh M-Y, et al (1993) Leukotrienes in bile during the early and the late airway responses after allergen challenge of sensitized rats. Am Rev Respir Dis 147:104-110
5. Wegner CD, Gundel RH, Abraham WM, et al (1993) The role of 5-lipoxygenase products in preclinical models of asthma. J Allergy Clin Immunol 91:917-929
6. Manning PJ, Rokach J, Malo JL, et al (1990) Urinary leukotriene E4 levels during early and late asthmatic responses. J Allergy Clin Immunol 86:211-220
7. Resnick AD, Deal EC, Jr., Ingram RH Jr, et al (1979) A critical assessment of the mechanism by which hyperoxia attenuates exercise-induced asthma. J Clin Invest 64:541-549
8. Omori C, Schofield BH, Mitzner W, et al (1995) Hyperpnea with dry air causes time-dependent alterations in mucosal morphology and bronchovascular permeability. J Appl Physiol 78:1043-1051
9. Yang XX, Powell WS, Martin JG (1997) Hyperpnea-induced bronchoconstriction is dependent on tachykinin-induced cysteinyl-leukotriene synthesis. J Appl Physiol 82:538-544
10. Parsons GH, Pare PD, White DA, et al (1989) Airway blood flow response to eucapnic dry air hyperventilation in sheep. J Appl Physiol 66:1443-1447
11. Gomes RF, Shen X, Ramchandani R et al (2000) Comparative respiratory system mechanics in rodents. J Appl Physiol 89:908-916
12. Becker AB, Hershkovich J, Simons FER, et al (1989) Development of chronic airway hyperresponsiveness in ragweed-sensitized dogs. J Appl Physiol 66:2691-2697
13. Antonissen LA, Mitchell RW, Kroeger EA, et al (1979) Mechanical alterations of airway smooth muscle in a canine asthmatic model. J Appl Physiol Respir Environ Exerc Physiol 46:681-687
14. Jiang H, Rao K, Halayko AJ, et al (1992) Ragweed sensitization-induced increase of myosin light chain kinase content in canine airway smooth muscle. Am J Respir Cell Mol Biol 7:567-573
15. Jiang H, Rao K, Liu X, et al (1995) Increased Ca2+ and myosin phosphorylation, but not calmodulin activity in sensitized airway smooth muscles. Am J Physiol 268:L739-746
16. Abraham WM, Burch RM, Farmer SG, et al (1991) A bradykinin antagonist modifies allergen-induced mediator release and late bronchial responses in sheep. Am Rev Respir Dis 143:787-796
17. Abraham WM, Stevenson JS, Garrido R (1989) A possible role for PAF in allergen-induced late responses: modifications by a selective antagonist. J Appl Physiol 66:2351-2357
18. Abraham WM, Sielczak MW, Ahmed A, et al (1994) Alpha 4-integrins mediate antigen-induced late bronchial responses and prolonged airway hyperresponsiveness in sheep. J Clin Invest 93:776-787
19. Abraham WM, Gill A, Ahmed A, et al (2000) A small-molecule, tight-binding inhibitor of the integrin alpha(4)beta(1) blocks antigen-induced airway responses and inflammation in experimental asthma in sheep. Am J Respir Crit Care Med 162:603-611
20. Abraham WM, Ahmed A, Sabater JR, et al (1999) Selectin blockade prevents antigen-induced late bronchial responses and airway hyperresponsiveness in allergic sheep. Am J Respir Crit Care Med 159:1205-1214
21. Lowell FC (1964) Observations on heaves: an asthma-like syndrome in the horse. J Allergy 35:322-330
22. Jean D, Vrins A, Lavoie JP (1999) Monthly, daily, and circadian variations of measurements of pulmonary mechanics in horses with chronic obstructive pulmonary disease. Am J Vet Res 60:1341-1346

23. Eyre P (1972) Equine pulmonary emphysema: a bronchopulmonary mould allergy. Vet Rec 91:134-140
24. Schmallenbach KH, Rahman I, Sasse HHL, et al (1998) Studies on pulmonary and systemic *Aspergillus fumigatus*-specific IgE and IgG antibodies in horses affected with chronic obstructive pulmonary disease (COPD). Vet Immunol Immunopathol 66:245-256
25. Eder C, Crameri R, Mayer C, et al (2000) Allergen-specific IgE levels against crude mould and storage mite extracts and recombinant mould allergens in sera from horses affected with chronic bronchitis. Vet Immunol Immunopathol 73:241-253
26. Evans AG, Paradis MR, O'Callaghan M (1992) Intradermal testing of horses with chronic obstructive pulmonary disease and recurrent urticaria. Am J Vet Res 53:203-208
27. Lavoie JP, Maghni K, Desnoyers M (2001) Neutrophilic airway inflammation in horses with heaves is characterized by a Th2-type cytokine profile. Am J Respir Crit Care Med (in press)
28. Fairbairn SM, Page CP, Lees P, et al (1993) Early neutrophil but not eosinophil or platelet recruitment to the lungs of allergic horses following antigen exposure. Clin Exp Allergy 23:821-828
29. Kaup FJ, Drommer W, Damsch S, et al (1990) Ultrastructural findings in horses with chronic obstructive pulmonary disease (COPD) 2: pathological changes of the terminal airways and the alveolar region. Equine Vet J 22:349-355
30. Robinson NE (2001) International Workshop on Equine Chronic Airway Disease. Michigan State University 16-18 June 2000. Equine Vet J 33:5-19
31. Padrid P, Snook S, Finucane T, et al (1995) Persistent airway hyperresponsiveness and histologic alterations after chronic antigen challenge in cats. Am J Respir Crit Care Med 51:184-193
32. Hamelmann E, Schwarze J, Takeda K, et al (1997) Noninvasive measurement of airway responsiveness in allergic mice using barometric plethysmography. Am J Respir Crit Care Med 56:766-775
33. Mehlhop PD, Rijn M van de, Goldberg AB, et al (1997) Allergen-induced bronchial hyperreactivity and eosinophilic inflammation occur in the absence of IgE in a mouse model of asthma. Proc Natl Acad Sci USA 94:1344-1349
34. Hogan SP, Mould A, Kikutani H (1997) Aeroallergen-induced eosinophilic inflammation, lung damage, and airways hyperreactivity in mice can occur independently of IL-4 and allergen-specific immunoglobulins. J Clin Invest 99:1329-1339
35. Gavett SH, Chen X, Finkelman F, et al (1994) Depletion of murine CD4+ T lymphocytes prevents antigen-induced airway hyperreactivity and pulmonary eosinophilia. Am J Respir Cell Mol Biol 10:587-593
36. Hogan SP, Koskinen A, Matthaei KI, et al (1998) Interleukin-5-producing CD4+ T cells play a pivotal role in aeroallergen-induced eosinophilia, bronchial hyperreactivity, and lung damage in mice. Am J Respir Crit Care Med 157:210-218
37. Wills-Karp M, Luyimbazi J, Xu X, et al (1998) Interleukin-13: a central mediator of allergic asthma. Science 282:2258-2261
38. Mattes J, Yang M, Siqueira A, et al (2001) IL-13 induces airways hyperreactivity independently of the IL-4r alpha chain in the allergic lung. J Immunol 167:1683-1692
39. Renz H, Lack G, Saloga J, et al (1994) Inhibition of IgE production and normalization of airways responsiveness by sensitized CD8 T cells in a mouse model of allergen-induced sensitization. J Immunol 152:351-360
40. Eidelman DH, Bellofiore S, Martin JG (1998) Late airway responses to antigen challenge in sensitized inbred rats. Am Rev Respir Dis 137:1033-1037
41. Elwood W, Barnes PJ, Fan Chung K (1992) Airway hyperresponsiveness is associated with inflammatory cell infiltration in Brown-Norway rats. Int Arch Allergy Immunol 99:91-97
42. Mishima H, Hojo M, Watanabe A, et al (1998) CD4+ T cells can induce airway hyperresponsiveness to allergen challenge in the Brown Norway rat. Am J Respir Crit Care Med 158:1863-1870
43. Molet S, Ramos-Barbon D, Martin JG, et al (1999) Adoptively transferred late allergic response is inhibited by IL-4, but not IL-5, antisense oligonucleotide. J Allergy Clin Immunol 104:205-214

44. Watanabe A, Mishima H, Renzi PM, et al (1995) Transfer of allergic airway responses with antigen-primed CD4+ but not CD8+ T cells in Brown Norway rats. J Clin Invest 96:1303-1310
45. Suzuki M, Taha R, Ihaku D, et al (1999) CD8+ T cells modulate late allergic airway responses in Brown Norway rats. J Immunol163:5574-5581
46. Allakhverdi Z, Lamkhioued B, Olivenstein R, et al (2000) CD8 depletion-induced late airway response is characterized by eosinophilia, increased eotaxin, and decreased IFN-gamma expression in rats. Am J Respir Crit Care Med 162:1123-1131
47. Olivenstein R, Renzi PM, Yang JP, et al (1993) Depletion of OX-8 lymphocytes from the blood and airways using monoclonal antibodies enhances the late airway response in rats. J Clin Invest 92:1477-1482

Optimization of Ventilation and Perfusion Matching

G. HEDENSTIERNA

In this chapter the distribution of pathology in acute respiratory failure (ARF) and acute respiratory distress syndrome (ARDS) will be discussed as well as the distributions of ventilation and lung blood flow (perfusion) and the consequences for ventilation-perfusion matching (V/Q). Finally, techniques to improve V/Q matching will be presented.

Distribution of pathology

ARF/ARDS is characterized by pulmonary infiltrates caused by extravasation of fluid, producing protein-rich pulmonary oedema that is later followed by fibrosis [1]. The infiltrates can be seen on the X-ray as densities. Computed tomography (CT) investigations have shown that most of the densities are in the dependent regions, indicating an influence of gravitational force [2-4]. The densities have an attenuation of around 0 Hounsfield units (HU) which means that they do not contain air. They are qualitatively similar to the densities (atelectasis) seen during anaesthesia, but quantitatively much larger. Thus, in ARDS patients the amount of densities may account for up to 70-80% of the lung area on the CT compared to 4-8% in the healthy lung, anaesthetized subjects. The apical regions are less compromised and the hilar and basal regions are more affected. The right and left lower lobes may be reduced in size and completely airless because of increased pressure in the abdominal cavity that pushes the diaphragm cranially [5].

Distribution of ventilation

In healthy, spontaneously breathing subjects, ventilation increases down the lung so that the dorsal region is better ventilated than the ventral region in the supine position. Anaesthesia and muscle paralysis alters the distribution, ventilation being preferentially directed towards ventral and mid regions, and the bottom-most areas are non-ventilated [6]. The morphological correlates to these changes are atelectasis in the bottom of the lung (no ventilation) and, most likely, airway closure in the regions above the collapsed lung tissue [7]. The latter reduces ventilation if closure is intermittent (i.e., airways close during expiration and reopen during inspiration). If closure is continuous, ventilation will be abolished and the non-ventilated parenchyma will eventually collapse and add to already existing atelectasis. The speed by which the collapse occurs depends on the oxygen fraction in the closed region [8]. If the subject has been breathing air prior to the closure of the airway, collapse will take hours. If breathing pure oxygen collapse appears within minutes [9]. In ARF/ARDS ventilation also goes to the upper lung regions, a finding that may not be too surprising in view of the collapsed or consolidated dependent lung regions that are thus non-ventilated [4]. The extent at which ventilation is affected differently in the isogravitational plane, compared to the healthy lung, has not been studied. It is reasonable to believe that there is a shift of ventilation away from basal regions towards the apex, in view of the larger amount of collapse and consolidation in the regions near the diaphragm [5].

Distribution of perfusion

There are few studies on pulmonary perfusion in ARDS patients. However, it is well known that, in healthy subjects, blood flow increases down the lung, in the gravitational plane [10]. In addition, there is an uneven distribution within an iso-gravitational level that may even exceed gravity [11]. The mechanisms are not fully established. Mechanical, positive pressure ventilation may impede venous return and flow through the lung so that cardiac output is reduced, and will also force blood flow down towards dependent lung regions, in particular if a positive end-expiratory pressure (PEEP) is applied [10]. This is hardly desirable since collapsed and consolidated lung tissue is mainly located in the dependent regions and thus is more perfused. On the other hand, PEEP may recruit lung tissue and reduce the visible "pathology". The net effect on perfusion of these non-ventilated regions (i.e. "shunt") is mostly beneficial but not always. In addition, the non-inflated tissue is relatively under-perfused as indicated by the discrepancy between the shunt fraction and the non-inflated tissue fraction (e.g., 30% of shunt with 60% of non-inflated tissue). This is caused by persisting hypoxic pulmonary vasoconstriction and, possibly, by mechanical compression of vessels in the consolidated region. This has been shown in experimental oleic acid oedema - dependent, consolidated lung regions being less perfused than during baseline, before oedema [12].

A frequent finding in ARDS is pulmonary hypertension [3]. When comparing pulmonary artery pressure and CT-scan data, a positive correlation between the mean pulmonary artery pressure and the lung weight has been shown [4]. What is the cause and effect is not clear. An increase in pulmonary artery pressure may induce an increase of lung oedema (i.e., an increase in lung weight). On the other hand, an oedematous lung may lead to an increase in pulmonary artery pressure by compression of pulmonary vessels. Whichever the independent variable may be, an average of 1 mmHg increase of pulmonary artery pressure was associated with a 14% increase of lung weight [4].

Ventilation/perfusion matching (VA/Q)

The gas exchange impairment is strongly related to the amount of disease (i.e., the non-inflated tissue mass). Thus, the impairment of arterial oxygenation and the venous admixture (shunt) correlate with the quantity of non-inflated lung tissue [4]. This suggests that the shunt fraction (i.e., perfusion of the non-inflated tissue) is the main cause of hypoxemia in patients with ARDS. The correlation between the amount of non-aerated lung tissue and hypoxemia and venous admixture might be anticipated. However, venous admixture does not separate true shunt (perfusion of non- ventilated, atelectatic or consolidated lung regions) from regions that are poorly ventilated in relation to their blood flow, causing low ventilation-perfusion ratios (low VA/Q). In studies on ARDS patients with the multiple inert gas elimination technique for assessing the distribution of VA/Q ratios, the major finding has been a large shunt, from around 20 to 70 % of cardiac output [13]. This fits with non-aerated tissue being the major or single cause of hypoxemia in ARDS, by producing shunt regions. Some patients may in addition show an increased perfusion of the low VA/Q regions but the majority has little of other disturbances. This is surprising, because one might have expected that the marked decrease in lung volume in ARDS promotes airway narrowing and airway closure therefore contributing to impeded ventilation and the creation of "low VA/Q" regions. There may be two explanations to this. One is that alveoli are less stable than normally, and collapse as soon as their dimensions are reduced (i.e., when their ventilation is diminished). Another is that the open lung regions retain their dimensions so those airways are not reduced in size.

Optimization of VA/Q

Different ventilatory modes have been tried for improving VA/Q and gas exchange in patients with ARF/ARDS as well as in experimental studies. Only a few of these modes will be discussed here in order to illustrate the effects on ventilation distribution, gas exchange and lung integrity.

Positive end-expiratory pressure, PEEP, is frequently used as a means of improving oxygenation of blood. It can be considered as an extension of positive pressure ventilation. PEEP increases lung volume and may open up collapsed lung regions. Such recruitment should improve oxygenation. However, the additional increase in intrathoracic pressure further impedes cardiac output and forces lung blood flow further down the lung [14]. This may result in an increased fractional perfusion of remaining atelectatic lung tissue, causing shunt to increase [15]!

PEEP may cause over-distension of alveoli and even damage the so called volo/barotrauma. It may mainly occur in upper lung regions because of their larger inflation. However, in ARDS, the damage seems to predominate in the lower lung region [16]. This has been proposed to be due to "shear stress failure" (i.e., the opening and closing of lung units with each tidal breath) [17]. Recently it has been shown in animal experiments that cyclic collapse and the reopening of dependent lung tissue occurs. Thus, in a porcine oleic acid oedema model, as high PEEP of 20-25 cm H_2O was needed to minimize the collapse and recruitment of each breath [18]. If cyclic collapse is the mechanism of volo/barotrauma, PEEP should be advocated to prevent intermittent collapse of the lung units. Such use may not be in conflict with the concept of protective ventilation which has been shown to improve outcome. However, much higher PEEP levels than normally used may be needed. On the other hand, a large tidal volume will not be as important to reopen collapsed tissue as if the PEEP level is low [18]. Thus, a small tidal volume that is part of the protective strategy, can more easily be used without promoting severe collapse.

Inverse ratio ventilation

The change in the inspiratory to expiratory (I:E) ratio from the conventional 1:2 to 2:1-4:1, the so called inverse ratio ventilation (IRV) was initially reported to improve oxygenation, sometimes dramatically [19]. IRV is normally performed in the pressure-controlled mode, which results in an early rapid increase in airway pressure and inspiratory flow. This rapid flow increase was thought to open up closed airways and the long inspiratory phase to promote alveolar recruitment. Although these may be possible mechanisms, the major effect is more likely executed by an interrupted expiration due to the short expiratory time. This creates an intrinsic PEEP that keeps alveoli recruited. Comparisons with conventional mechanical ventilation (CMV) with an extrinsic PEEP of the same magnitude as that produced intrinsically by IRV showed no advantage for the IRV technique [20]. It may be hypothesised that IRV could promote aeration of lung units with long time constants, due to the short expiratory time that is available, and would keep more collapsible units open to a higher degree than CMV. However, experimental data suggest the opposite. Thus, upper, already well aerated lung regions become even more aerated with IRV and lower, dependent regions are less expanded in comparison with CMV with essentially the same mean airway pressure and extrinsic/intrinsic PEEP (20 and 17 cm H_2O in CMV and IRV, respectively) [21]. Lung blood flow distribution, assessed by the injection of radioactive microspheres, showed no consistent difference between the two ventilatory modes, but shunt assessed by the multiple inert gas elimination technique, was much higher with IRV. This suggests that the major difference between the two modes is in the aeration and recruitment of alveoli and this was better with CMV.

Prone position

To rotate the patient from the supine to the left or right side is a common treatment of the intensive care patient in order to prevent bed sores and to facilitate the elimination of secretions. However, the positioning of the patient may also improve gas exchange. The prone position has been shown to increase oxygenation, sometimes dramatically in ARF/ARDS, but not all patients respond [22, 23]. The relative ease to prone the patient makes the treatment tempting and it seems reasonable to test. Whether the prone position improves outcome is less certain and a recent multicenter study by Gattinoni [24] showed no benefit in survival of the whole study group. However, the most severely affected patients seemed to do better with prone positioning.

The prone position is maintained for a few hours after which the patient is turned to the supine position for a similar time period. The pattern is then repeated for as long as necessary. Thus, one may argue that the rotation per se is the treatment, but the common finding is that oxygenation improves in the prone position and deteriorates when the patient is in the supine position [23].

The mechanism behind the improved gas exchange in the prone position is not fully understood. However, there are different observations that, taken together, provide a reasonable explanation. One piece of information is the pleural pressure difference between upper, non-dependent and lower, and dependent lung regions are smaller in the prone compared to the supine position in anaesthetized dogs [25]. Since airway minus pleural pressure (ΔP) is an important determinant of ventilation, it follows that if ΔP varies between upper and lower lung regions, ventilation distribution will be similarly uneven, and the smaller the difference the more even is the distribution. The reduced ΔP in the prone position may be related to the shape and regional compliance of the chest wall, the shape and weight of the lung and forces acting on the diaphragm. Moreover, in the supine position, the more compliant part of the chest wall is up (the anterior part of the rib cage) whereas in the prone position, the stiffer, dorsal part of the rib cage is up. This may possibly affect the ventilation distribution so that less goes to upper (dorsal) regions in the prone position. Support for this view was the finding of improved oxygenation in ARDS patients when the rib cage excursions were restricted in the supine position by the application of sand bags on the rib cage [26].

Another piece of information is that lung perfusion is more evenly distributed, in the gravitational plane, when prone, both in healthy humans [27] and in animal experiments [28]. Finally, the matching of ventilation and perfusion shows less variation in the prone position in anaesthetised, mechanically ventilated pigs [28].

Spontaneous breathing

Another aspect is whether to maintain some spontaneous ventilation in severe lung damage. Airway pressure release ventilation (APRV) allows an essentially unrestricted spontaneous breathing from a pre-set positive airway pressure, with the addition of short releases of the airway pressure to a pre-set lower airway pressure, mimicking an expiration and subsequent inspiration. Putensen and co-workers showed better oxygenation in experimental animals, and subsequently in human patients who where breathing spontaneously as little as 10% of their total ventilation in an APRV mode (also called BIPAP), compared to 100% mechanical ventilation [29, 30]. We found, in a porcine oleic acid model, a dose dependent improvement in oxygenation with increasing fraction of spontaneous ventilation [31]. Moreover, the animals that had been breathing spontaneously (between 50 and 100% of total ventilation) showed a reduction in the pulmonary artery pressure and an increase in PaO_2 6 hours after induction of lung damage compared to earlier phases of lung damage. On the other hand, pigs on continuous mechanical ventilation showed no recovery during the study period.

Pharmacological treatment

Another approach to improve V/Q matching is to use vasoactive drugs that dilate vessels in the ventilated parenchyma or constrict vessels in the non-ventilated lung. Since access to the non-ventilated lung is difficult, treatment focuses on vasodilation. Nitric oxide (NO) is a potent vasodilator produced in the endothelium and that diffuses to the vascular smooth muscle to exert its effect. Inhalation of NO produces dilation in the ventilated lung, and since inhaled NO does not reach the non-ventilated parenchyma, no dilation occurs. Blood flow is therefore diverted away from non-ventilated to ventilated tissue and the shunt is reduced [32]. This can not be achieved by intravenous administration of a NO donor, for an example nitroglycerin or nitroprusside. These drugs cause vasodilation throughout the vascular tree. The dilation in the non-ventilated lung may even be greater than in the ventilated tissue, because of the blunting of hypoxic vasoconstriction in the shunt region. The shunt may therefore go up when an intravenous vasodilator is given.

As many as 30-40% of intensive care patients do not respond to inhaled NO [33]. The causes are not fully understood, but observations have been made that show the consequences of inhaling NO are not as simple as one might have thought. The inhaled NO can be scavenged so that it can not exert its effect. The inhalation of NO stimulates the production of vasoconstrictors such as endothelin, that counter the vasodilation [34]. Finally, inhaled NO appears to cause vasoconstriction in non-ventilated lung parenchyma by the release of a blood-borne mediator [35]. The degree of redistribution of blood flow and the degree of pressure decrease in the pulmonary artery depends on the amount of ventilated and non-ventilated lung.

The use of vasoactive substances to optimize the V/Q matching can be further discussed. Suffice it to say that the nebulization of vasodilating agents into the airways may produce effects similar to those of inhaled NO [36]. However, since no systemic effect might be desired, nebulization may be less safe. Nebulization does not preclude a number of dangerous side effects which can be seen in NO therapy.

Conclusion

Acute respiratory failure is characterized by a pulmonary oedema and fibrosis with a gravitational orientation, that causes atelectasis and consolidation in dependent lung regions, but may spare upper, non-dependent regions. This affects the distribution of inspired air so no ventilation goes to the dependent regions whereas upper regions may be overinflated. Blood flow is only modestly reduced in the dense regions, creating a shunt. Other forms of ventilation-perfusion mismatch are mostly of minor importance. Different ventilatory modes may be used in an attempt to open up collapsed or consolidated regions and to direct ventilation and perfusion. Prone position appears to improve V/Q matching. Spontaneous breathing also seems to be advantageous in improving oxygenation. To switch from full mechanical ventilation to partial or full spontaneous breathing may be the road of the future. At least further testing is worthwhile.

References

1. Rinaldo JE, Rogers RM (1982) Adult respiratory-distress syndrome. Changing concepts of lung injury and repair. N Eng J Med; 306:900-909
2. Rommelsheim K, Lakner K, Westhofen P et al (1983) Das respiratorische Distress-Syndrome der Erwachsenen (ARDS) im Computer Tomogram. *Anaesth Intensivther Notfallmed*; 18:59-64
3. Maunder RJ, Schuman WP, McHugh JW et al (1986) Preservation of normal lung regions in the adult respiratory distress syndrome. Analysis by computed tomography. *JAMA*; 255:2463-2465
4. Gattinoni L, Pesenti A, Bombino M et al (1988) Relationships between lung computed tomographic density, gas exchange, and PEEP in acute respiratory failure. *Anesthesiology*; 69: 824-832
5. Puybasset L, Cluzel P, Gusman P et al (2000) Regional distribution of gas and tissue in acute respiratory distress syndrome. I. Consequences for lung morphology. *Intensive Care Med*; 26; 857-869
6. Tokics L, Hedenstierna G, Svensson L et al (1996) V/Q distribution and correlation to atelectasis in anesthetized paralyzed humans. *J. Appl. Physiol.*; 81: 1822-1833
7. Hedenstierna G (2000) Anesthesia and Gas Exchange. In: *Pulmonary and Peripheral Gas Exchange in Health and Disease.* Roca J, Rodriguez-Roisin R, Wagner PD, eds. Marcel Dekker Inc.: 177-198
8. Dantzker DR, Wagner PD, West JB (1975) Instability of lung units with low VA/Q ratios during O_2 breathing. *J Appl Physiol*; 38(5):886-895
9. Rothen HUB, Sporre G, Engberg G et al (1995) Prevention of atelectasis during general anaesthesia. *Lancet* 345: 1387-1391
10. West JB, Dollery CT, Naimark A (1964) Distribution of blood flow in isolated lung: relation to vascular and alveolar pressures. *J Appl Physiol*, 19:713-724
11. Glenny RW, Lamm WJ, Albert RK, Robertson HT (1991) Gravity is a minor determinant of pulmonary blood flow distribution. *J Appl Physiol*, 71:620-629
12. Schuster DP, Haller J (1990) Regional pulmonary blood flow during acute pulmonary edema: a PET study. *J Appl Physiol*; 69: 353-361
13. Mélot C (1994) Ventilation-perfusion relationships in acute respiratory failure. *Thorax*; 49: 1251-1258
16. Gattinoni L, Bombino M, Pelosi P et al (1994) Lung structure and function in different stages of severe adult respiratory distress syndrome. *JAMA*; 271: 1772-1779
17. Muscedere JG, Mullen JB, Gan K, Slutsky AS (1994) Tidal ventilation at low airway pressures can augment lung injury. *Am J Respir Crit Care Med*; 149: 1327-1334
18. Neumann P, Berglund JE, Mondejar EF et al (1998) Effect of different pressure levels on the

dynamics of lung collapse and recruitment in oleic acid-induced lung injury. *Am J Resp Crit Care Med*; 158: 1636-1643
19. Tharratt RS, Allen RF, Albertson TE (1988) Pressure controlled inverse ventilation in severe adult respiratory failure. *Chest*; 94: 755-762
20. Lessard MR, Guerot E, Lorino H et al (1994) Effects of pressure controlled ventilation with different I:E ratios versus volume controlled ventilation on respiratory mechanics, gas exchange and hemodynamics in patients with adult respiratory distress syndrome. *Anesthesiology*; 80:983-991
21. Neumann P, Berglund J, Andersson LG et al (2000) Effects of inverse ratio ventilation and positive end-expiratory pressure in oleic acid-induced lung injury. *Am J Respir Crit Care Med*; 161: 1537-1545
22. Douglas WW, Rehder K, Beynen FM et al (1977) Improved oxygenation in patients with acute respiratory failure. The prone position. *Am Rev Respir Dis*; 115: 559-566
23. Mure M, Martlin Cr, Lindahl S (1997) Dramatic effect on oxygenation in patients with severe acute lung insufficiency treated in the prone position. *Crit Care Med*; 25: 1539-1544
24: Gattinoni L (2001) Prone positioning in ALI: clinical application. Simposia Mostra Anestesia Ranimazione e Terapia Intensiva (SMART); Milano.
25. Wiener-Kronish P, Gropper MA, Lai-Fook SJ (1985) Pleural liquid pressure in dogs measured using a rib capsule. *J Appl Physiol*; 59: 597-602
26. Brazzi L, Ravagnan I, Pelosi P, Gattinoni L (1999) Prone position in anaesthesia and intensive care. *Care Crit Ill*; 15: 5-10
27. Nyrén S, Mure M, Jacobsson H, Larsson SA, Lindahl SGE (1999) Pulmonary perfusion is more uniform in prone than supine position: Scintigraphy in healthy humans. *J Appl Physiol*; 86: 1135-1141
28. Mure M, Domino KB, Lindahl SGE et al (2000) Regional ventilation-perfusion distribution is more uniform in the prone position. *J Appl Physiol*; 88: 1076-1083
29. Putensen C, Räsänen J, Lopez FA (1994) Ventilation-perfusion distributions during mechanical ventilation with superimposed spontaneous breathing in canine lung injury. *Am J Resp Crit Care Med*; 150: 101-108
30. Putensen C, Mutz NJ, Putensen-Himmer G, Zinserling J (1999) Spontaneous breathing during ventilatory support improves ventilation-perfusion distributions in patients with acute respiratory distress syndrome. *Am J Respir Crit Care Med* 159:1241-1248
31. Neumann P, Hedenstierna G (2001) Ventilatory support by continuous positive airway pressure breathing improves gas exchange as compared with partial ventilatory support with airway pressure release ventilation. *Anesth Analg*; 92: 950-958
32. Rossaint R, Falke KJ, Lopez F et al (1993) Inhaled nitric oxide for the adult respiratory distress syndrome. *N Engl J Med*; 328:399-405
33. Manktelow C, Bigatello LM, Hess D et al (1997) Physiologic determinants of the response to inhaled nitric oxide in patients with acute respiratory distress syndrome. *Anesthesiology*; 87:297-307
34. Chen L, He H, Mondejar EF et al (2001) Endothelin -1 and nitric oxide synthase in short rebound reaction to short exposure to inhaled nitric oxide. *Am J Physiol.*; 281: H124-131
35. Hambraeus Jonzon K, Chen L, Freden F et al (2001) Pulmonary vasoconstriction during regional NO inhalation. Evidence of a blood-borne regulator of NO synthase activity. *Anesthesiology.*
36. Walmrath D, Schermuly R, Pilch J et al (1997) Effects of inhaled versus intravenous vasodilators in experimental pulmonary hypertension. *Eur Respir J*; 10:1084-1092

Alveolar Recruitment

L.M. BIGATELLO, P. CAIRONI

Hypoxemia can be relieved in two basic ways: by increasing the concentration of inspired oxygen (FiO_2) and by inflating the hypoventilated lung. Other mechanisms, such as hyperventilation and administration of hyperbaric o-xygen, have limited efficacy (the former) or are impractical (the latter). Our study reviews the mechanisms and effects of promoting alveolar inflation and recruitment in patients with acute respiratory failure.

It is clear that applying positive pressure at the airway improves gas exchange in patients with acute respiratory failure. This may occur through expansion of poorly ventilated alveoli, recruitment of previously collapsed alveoli, and also through a decrease of shunted blood flow. Thus, the mechanism of improved gas exchange with positive pressure ventilation (PPV) is complex, and can be difficult to sort out in each individual patient.

Positive pressure ventilation may also improve respiratory mechanics. This occurs because recruitment increases the volume of the aerated lung. However, since the lesion of acute lung injury (ALI) is inhomogeneous, positive pressure will cause variable volume changes throughout the injured lung, and while it may recruit some areas, it may over inflate and damage others.

Hence, choosing the appropriate way of administering PPV in patients with acute respiratory failure is not simple, and remains controversial.

Mechanism of improved gas exchange

PPV improves gas exchange in patients with acute respiratory failure. This observation was reported in the first description of the acute respiratory distress syndrome (ARDS) [1] and confirmed in successive publications, [2, 3] which emphasized the benefit of using positive end expiratory pressure (PEEP) together with a large tidal volume (V_T) to reverse the severe hypoxemia characteristic of this syndrome. The striking effect of PPV on arterial oxygenation in some of these patients promoted the use of unusually high levels of PEEP ("superPEEP"), consisting of 40 cm H_2O or more [3].

Although it is somewhat obvious that positive pressure applied at the airway facilitates the opening of alveolar units and thus affects gas exchange, the detailed mechanisms of the beneficial effects of positive pressure are less straightforward. The complexity of this topic surrounds two main issues: 1) the haemodynamic effects of PPV; and 2) the complex dynamics of lung insufflation and recruitment, including the role of the V_T and other inspiratory manoeuvres versus the recruitment by PEEP.

Haemodynamic effects of PPV

The haemodynamic effects of PPV have been considered through the years mainly as a negative factor associated with the use of high positive pressure at the airway, both in the form of large V_T and of high levels of PEEP. The effect of PPV on cardiac performance is mediated by several factors:1)the magnitude of the pressure applied at the thorax; 2) the patient's volume status; and 3) the fraction of pressure that is transmitted to the vascular structures inside the thorax.

The first two factors, although quite complex, were summarized by McGregor [4]. Increasing the thoracic pressure has two main effects: to decrease the venous return to the heart and to increase the ejection fraction. In ideal conditions of volume status and with mild pressure changes, these two opposing forces tend to produce an equilibrium, and very little is seen (as in every healthy surgical patient appropriately anesthetized and ventilated with PPV). However, if the positive intrathoracic pressure is high and/or the volume status is low, the negative haemodynamic effects of PPV will prevail, because veins are collapsible, and venous return to the heart will cease [5]. Hence, cardiac output (CO) and blood pressure will fall. Twenty-five years ago Quist et al. demonstrated in animals that increasing levels of PEEP caused a progressive decrease of CO until the circulating volume was fully restored with blood transfusions [6]. Although heart-lung interplay is far more complex, including the effects of ventricular interaction and autonomic reflexes, the basic principles mentioned here are sufficiently correct and clinically helpful.

The third factor relates to the fraction of positive pressure that is actually transmitted to the thoracic cavity. Under normal circumstances, when the compliance of both the lung and the chest wall are equal, exactly half of the pressure applied at the airway is transmitted across the lung. When the compliance of the lung is greatly diminished, a much lower fraction of the pressure applied is transmitted. This principle led early investigators to support the use of exceptionally high pressures [3]. While this is no longer customary, it is a common observation that clinically adequate levels of PPV can be well tolerated haemodynamically by patients with ARDS in virtue of their decreased lung compliance.

Thus, PPV can cause a decrease of CO in patients with acute respiratory failure. In most instances, this is an undesirable phenomenon. Not only because many of these patients are already haemodynamically unstable, but also because a low CO worsens hypoxemia through an increase of peripheral O_2 extraction and a consequent desaturation of the mixed venous blood entering the lungs. However, decreasing CO may occasionally have a positive effect on oxygen exchange. In patients with a significant shunt fraction due to alveolar consolidation and collapse, such as patients with ARDS, a decrease of CO may decrease the fraction of shunted blood. This may ultimately result in a more favourable distribution of ventilation and perfusion and increase the PaO_2 [7].

Mechanisms of recruitment

Simply stated, recruitment should occur when the fraction of pressure applied at the airway reaches an alveolus and becomes higher than the pressure that is keeping it closed. However, this pressure may include two components. One is the pressure existing on the outside of the alveolus, essentially due to the weight of the surrounding lung tissue, determined mainly by gravitational forces and the density of the lung tissue (oedematous lung weighs more than normal lung). The second is the pressure that may be necessary to open a collapsed alveolus, determined by factors such as Laplace's law (a higher pressure is needed to "pop open" a collapsed alveolus, as when inflating a balloon) and the absence of an effective surfactant layer.

Therefore, PPV may further inflate open alveoli and open collapsed alveoli. The term *recruitment* is best described by the second component. Positive pressure can be provided throughout the administration of the V_T and between respiratory cycles of PEEP. The mechanism by which PEEP improves gas exchange has been studied for the past thirty years, following a description of its beneficial effect on the PaO_2 in ARDS patients. Clearly, the PEEP increases functional residual capacity (FRC), as was demonstrated by Katz et al., [8] who showed that the increase of lung volume induced by PEEP in patients with acute respiratory failure was often higher than predicted on the basis of the measure static compliance of the respiratory system. This indicated that more aerated lung tissue must have been present as a result of the PEEP. In a similar experiment, Ranieri et al. demonstrate the occurrence of alveolar recruitment on the respiratory system when applying different levels of PEEP [9].

One of the obstacles in this research is the difficulty to accurately measure the FRC in a clinical setting. The estimate of the "end expiratory lung volume" [9] and a simplified helium dilution technique [10] have been used as a bedside index of recruitment. However, the visual demonstration of recruitment by PEEP was made possible by the application of computed tomography (CT) in the field of pulmonary pathophysiology. Gattinoni et al. demonstrated PEEP-induced lung recruitment on *chest CT scan*, in a series of papers that profoundly affected our way of thinking about the respiratory mechanics of ARDS. [11-13] However, even this visual demonstration has its limitations because a) quantification of recruitment remains indirect, and b) obtaining serial CT images in these patients is not always practical. The advent of the helical CT, which allows rapid and complete imaging of the lungs, may cause this system to become clinically applicable [14].

Currently, these phenomena are studied mainly through the determination of the static V-P curve of the respiratory system. With this technique, one can observe that lung inflation occurs on the linear segment of a curve. When recruitment occurs, the V-P curve presents an inflection, above which the slope (i.e., the compliance of the respiratory system) increases due to inflation of newly opened units [15, 16]. The combination of these physiological measurements with CT scan imaging of the lung has identified two general types of lung collapse [13]. One is simply due to the weight of the surrounding oedematous tissue, which causes *compression atelectasis*, and the other to a more complex combination of gas reabsorption and lack of surfactant (*absorption atelectasis*), which may require higher levels of PEEP. The above considerations indicate that lung recruitment in patients with acute respiratory failure is a complex phenomenon. Thus, choosing the appropriate way of recruiting the lung and/or the correct level of PEEP is not a simple task. In the following section, we will summarize the current views on this topic.

Choosing the level of PEEP

Many different methods have been proposed throughout the years for appling the most appropriate level of PEEP to patients with acute respiratory failure. While earlier recommendations suggested the use of very high pressures ("super-PEEP") to optimize recruitment, [3] most clinicians today tend to set a level that improves gas exchange without affecting systemic blood pressure. This method was first formalized by Suter et al. [17], who suggested to increase the PEEP until the arterial O_2 delivery no longer increased, due to a decrease of the CO ("best PEEP"). In day-to day practice, this is accomplished with the *PEEP test*, which consists of applying increasing levels of PEEP in steps of 2-3 cm of H_2O at 10-20 minute intervals and observing its effects on PaO_2, arterial blood pressure and, when available, CO.

More recently, when performing simple respiratory mechanics at the bedside, choosing the appropriate level of PEEP can be based on the measured P-V curve of the respiratory system. As discussed above, patients with ARDS often show an identifiable change of the slope in the early part of the P-V curve [15, 16]. At this point in the curve, often called the "lower inflection point", a significant portion of alveolar recruitment must occur. Amato et al. [18] suggested that applying a level of PEEP just above the lower inflection point would assure recruitment. In a series of 53 patients with severe ARDS, they identified a PEEP level of approximately 16 cm H_2O as the most favourable level to *open the lung*, improve PaO_2 and avoid the trauma associated with opening and closing of alveoli at end expiration. By combining the use of these PEEP values with low end inspiratory pressures, which resulted in a V_T of approximately 5-6 ml/kg of body weight, these authors reported a significant decrease in mortality [19]. To optimize recruitment, they also performed occasional *recruitment manoeuvres*, consisting in a prolonged end inspiratory pressure plateau (*e.g.*, 40 cm H_2O for 20 seconds). Thus, over the past few years, the P-V curve of the respiratory system obtained at the bedside has been used both to describe the mechanical characteristics of the lung and to set the ventilatory parameters of patients with ARDS [20]. When a characteristic sigmoidal curve is observed, the lower inflection point is used to set the PEEP level. A second inflection point, occurring after the steeper portion of the curve and called "upper inflection point", indicates over distention of lung units, and is used to set the end inspiratory pressure. In this way, one could ventilate ARDS patients assuring recruitment and avoid damage of the lung at both ends of the tidal ventilation. Figure 1 shows an idealized P-V curve with the characteristics discussed.

However, this approach has recently been challenged, as methods of studying lung recruitment at the bedside are becoming more precise. First, there is little theoretical basis to use the lower inflection point as the point of maximum recruitment. PEEP is an expiratory manoeuvre: at the end of a full lung deflation, PEEP prevents the collapsing alveolar. Hence, PEEP prevents derecruitment rather than inducing recruitment and it would be best determined on the deflation, rather than inflation part of the P-V curve. This has been observed in patients [21] and recently confirmed in a mathematical model [22]. Second, the way a P-V curve is constructed may significantly affect its ultimate shape. Even using the same technique (such as the "supersyringe") the resulting

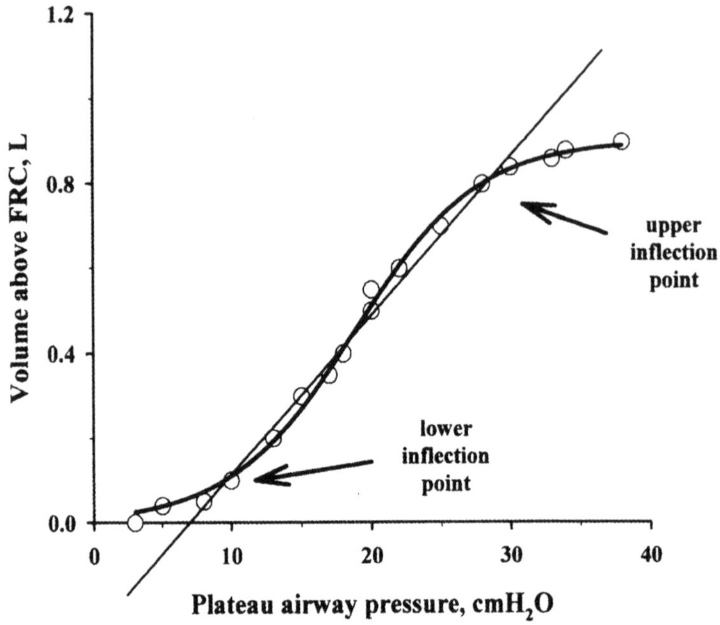

Fig. 1. Idealized P-V curve of the respiratory system in ARDS. It is suggested to set tidal ventilation between the two "inflection points". Modified from Ref. 20

P-V curve will vary depending upon the level of PEEP and the V_T used. Furthermore, the definition of the lower inflection point in literature and its visual interpretation by clinicians is not uniform [23]. Third, it seems unlikely that recruitment occurs at one discrete level of alveolar pressure, considering that in early acute respiratory failure lung injury is not homogeneous. Rather, recruitment and derecruitment are more likely to be dynamic events that occur around a range of alveolar pressures that vary among patients with respiratory failure of similar aetiology and within the same patient, as the injury evolves or as we change ventilatory settings.

These observations have their own physiological interest and important clinical implications. Jonson et al. studied the effect of varying the lung volume at which the P-V curve starts (the end expiratory lung volume) on the shape of the curve [24]. To no surprise, they found that curves starting from a clinically set PEEP value (average 11 cm H_2O) always occurred at a higher lung volumes than curves starting from a PEEP value of 0 cm H_2O and at a range of pressure well above the measured lower inflection point. More interestingly, they also observed that following a prolonged expiration of 0 cm H_2O, the ensuing P-V curve had a long linear segment with a high compliance, indicating ongoing recruitment throughout the insufflation.

Recent work in experimental animals [25] and in a limited number of patients [26] has expanded the above findings and provided further insight in the pathophysiology of lung recruitment and derecruitment. By combining classic respiratory mechanics and CT scan imaging of the lung, Pelosi et al. [25] confirmed, in dogs with oleic acid induced acute lung injury, that alveolar recruitment occurred throughout the entire V-P curve.

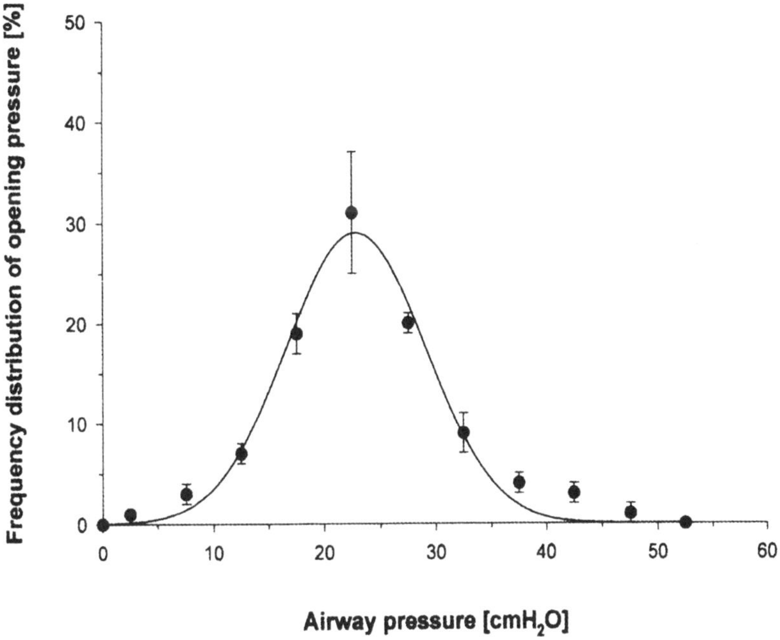

Fig. 2. Gaussian distribution of threshold opening pressures, with the highest frequency at 20-25 cm of H_2O. Modified from Ref. 25

These authors used a sigmoid function [27] to fit their datapoints on the P-V curve, confirming the validity of the mathematical model and its superiority over the visual inspection by a clinician [23]. Through the mathematical analysis of their P-V curve, they derived an *estimated threshold opening pressure*, the point on the curve at which a new increment in recruitment was observed. The striking finding of this experiment was that these opening pressures had a wide distribution fitting a Gaussian function, with the maximal frequency occurring at 20-25 cm H_2O (Fig. 2). Derecruitment, in a similar study on patients with early ARDS, [26] occurred over a lower range of pressures, between 0-15 cm H_2O. Figure 3 shows the effect of V_T in a dog with oleic acid induced acute lung injury: at both levels of PEEP (5 and 15 cm H_2O) increasing the V_T clearly recruited additional lung tissue.

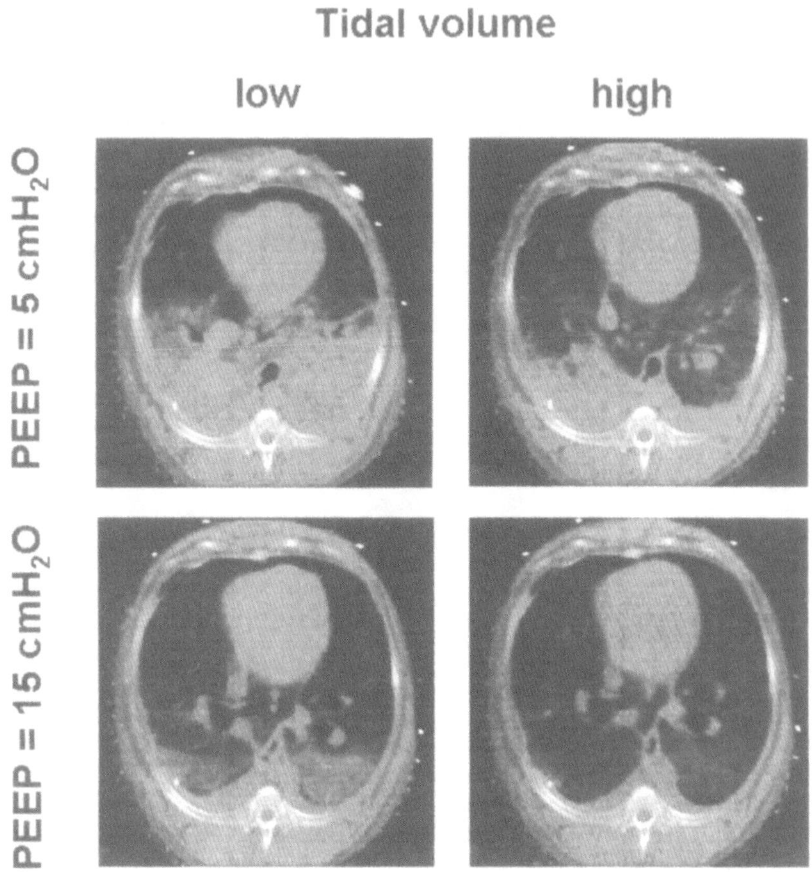

Fig. 3. End expiratory CT scan of a dog with ALI. At the same PEEP level (both 5 and 15 cm H_2O) increasing the V_T recruited a significant fraction of lung tissue. Modified from Ref. 25

Conclusions

Recruiting lung tissue improves gas exchange in patients with acute respiratory failure. Recruitment may also limit alveolar trauma at end expiration, cause alveolar trauma at end inspiration, and impair haemodynamics.

Hence, in order to provide the best degree of alveolar recruitment in patients one has to take in account complex and often opposing physiological phenomena. Recent data indicate that recruitment is a dynamic event that occurs throughout inflation of the lung, and that it can be maintained with moderate levels of PEEP. Our choices of ventilatory settings may no longer be dictated only by the desire to open more alveolar units, but by our general ventilatory philosophy. As evidence accumulates on the beneficial effects of low V_T ventilation, we have to find strategies that adequately permit the ventilation of the injured lung without inflicting further damage on it.

References

1. Ashbaugh D, Bigelow D, Petty T (1967) Acute respiratory distress in adults. Lancet 2:319-323
2. Pontoppidan H, Geffin B, Lowenstein E (1972) Acute respiratory failure in the adult. New Eng J Med 287:690-698
3. Kirby RR, Downs JB, Civetta JM, et al (1975) High level positive end-expiratory pressure in acute respiratory insufficiency. Chest 67:156-163
4. McGregor M, Sniderman A (1985) On pulmonary vascular resistance: the need for more precise definition. Am J Cardiol 55:217-221
5. Permutt S, Riley L (1963) Hemodynamics of collapsible vessels with tone: the vascular waterfall. J Appl Physiol 18:924-932
6. Qvist J, Pontoppidan H, Wilson R, Lever M (1975) Hemodynamc response to mechanical ventilation with PEEP. The effect of hypervolemia. Anesthesiology 42:45-55
7. Dantzker D, Lynch J, Weg J (1980) Depression of cardiac output is a mechanism of shunt reduction in the therapy of acute respiratory failure. Chest 77:636-642
8. Katz J, Ozanne G, Zinn S, Fairley H (1981) Time course and mechanism of lung volume increase with PEEP in acute pulmonary failure. Anesthesiology 54:9-16
9. Ranieri V, NT E, Corbeil C, Chasse' M et al (1991) Effect of positive end-expiratory pressure on alveolar recruitment and gas exchange in patients with the adult respiratory distress syndrome. Am Rev Respir Dis 144:544-551
10. Damia G, Mascheroni D, Croci M, Tarenzi L (1988) Perioperative changes in functional residual capacity in morbidly obese patients. Br J Anaesth 60:574-578
11. Gattinoni L, Pesenti A, Avalli L et al (1987) Pressure-volume curve of total respiratory system in acute respiratory failure. Computed tomographic scan study. Am Rev Respir Dis 136:730-736
12. Gattinoni L, Pesenti A, Bombino M et al (1988). Relationships between lung computed tomography density, gas exchange and PEEP in acute respiratory failure. Anesthesiology 69:824-832
13. Gattinoni L, D'Andrea L, Pelosi P et al (1993) Regional effects and mechanism of positive end-expiratory pressure in early adult respiratory distress syndrome. JAMA 269:2122-2127.
14. Malbuisson L, Muller J-C, Constantin J et al (2001). Computed tomography assessment of positive end-expiratory pressure- induced alveolar recruitment in patients with acute respiratory distress syndrome. Am J Respir Crit Care Med 163:1444-1450
15. Matamis D, Lamaire F, Harf A et al (1984) Total respiratory pressure-volume curves in the adult respiratory distress syndrome. Chest 86:58-66
16. Pesenti A, Marcolin R, Prato P et al (1985) Mean airway pressure vs. positive end-expiratory pressure during mechanical ventilation. Crit Care Med 13:34-37
17. Suter P, Fairley H, Isemberg M (1975) Optimum end expiratory pressure in patients with acute pulmonary failure. N Eng J Med 292:2984-2989
18. Amato M, Barbas C, Medeiros D et al (1995). Beneficial effects of the "open lung approach" with low distending pressures in acute respiratory distress syndrome: a prospective randomized study on mechanical ventilation. Am J Respir Crit Care Med 152:1835-1846
19. Amato M, Barbas C, Medeiros D et al (1998) Effect of a protective ventilation strategy on

mortality in the acute respiratory distress syndrome. New Eng J Med 338(6):347-354
20. Bigatello L, Hurford W, Pesenti A (1999) Ventilatory management of acute respiratory failure for Y2K. Anesthesiology 91:1567-1570
21. Holzapfel L, Robert D, Perrin F et al (1983) Static pressure-volume curves and the effect of positive end-expiratory pressure on gas exchange in adult respiratory distress syndrome. Crit Care Med 11:591-597
22. Hickling K (1998) The pressure-volume curve is greatly modified by recruitment. A mathematical model. Am J Crit Care Med 158:194-202
23. Harris R, Hess DR, Venegas J (2000) An objective analysis of the pressure-volume curve in the acute respiratory distress syndrome. Am J Crit Care Med 161:432-439
24. Jonson B, Richard J, Straus C et al (1999) Pressure-volume curve and compliance in acute lung injury. Am J Crit Care Med 159:1172-1178
25. Pelosi P, Goldner M, McKibben A et al (2001) Recruitment and derecruitment during acute respiratory failure. An experimental study. Am J Respir Crit Care 164:122-130
26. Crotti S, Mascheroni D, Caironi P et al (2001) Recruitment and derecruitment during acute respiratory failure. A clinical study. Am J Respir Crit Care Med 164:131-140
27. Venegas J, Harris R, Simon B (1998) A comprehensive for the pulmonary pressure-volume curve. J Appl Physiol 84:389-395.

How to Open an Atelectatic Lung

D.L.H. Poelma, B. Lachmann

Physiological background

The lung is composed of millions of alveoli, which can be seen separately. LaPlace was the first to draw attention to the pressure in a bubble, which depends on the surface tension at the air-liquid interface and the radius; this relation was later called after its discoverer: the Law of Laplace, $p = 2\gamma / r$ (where p = pressure, γ = surface tension, r = radius). In other words, at the same radius, the pressure necessary to avoid bubble collapse is higher as surface tension increases. As long as the surface tension is not zero, there still is a retractive force that normally could lead to bubble collapse. That this model is also valid for the lung was shown by von Neergaard, who eliminated the air-liquid interface by filling the lung with fluid, and discovered that the pressure required to fill a lung with fluid is only one-third to one quarter that to fill a lung with the same volume of air.

Based on this observation, von Neergaard concluded from his experiment that the pressure necessary to inflate a lung would be much higher if the surface tension of water or plasma acts at the air-liquid interface of the alveolus. He also concluded from these observations that there must be a substance acting at the air-liquid interface, which reduces the surface tension to a much lower figure than that of water or plasma. However, considering the law of LaPlace, stabilizing different-sized alveoli requires an additional mechanism, which changes the surface tension according to the surface area. All these perquisites are fulfilled by the pulmonary surfactant system.

Pulmonary surfactant system

Surfactant is a surface-active agent that forms a thin layer over the inner surface of the lung, controlling the surface tension in the lung. Of course, the primary function of controlling the surface tension is to regulate the exchanges between the air in the lung and the alveolar fluid. In this sense, surfactant provides valuable assistance for the passage of gases into the bloodstream, but it also inhibits the fluid from entering the air space and therefore keeps the lung dry.

Surfactant also stabilizes the relationship between surface tension and surface area. Without this adjustment, the effort required to expand the alveolus would be much greater, and during expiration the alveolus would collapse. In other words, surfactant minimizes the force required to expand an alveolus and prevents the alveoli from expiratory collapse.

The ability of surfactant to adjust surface tension means that alveoli of different sizes can respond to the same pressure independent of their size; in other words, smaller alveoli can expand by the same amount of pressure as larger alveoli. This is important because alveoli are connected to each other and if their expansion was not controlled, the point of attachment between two alveoli would be pulled further away by a large alveolus than a small alveolus can stretch, causing "shear forces" (Fig. 1).

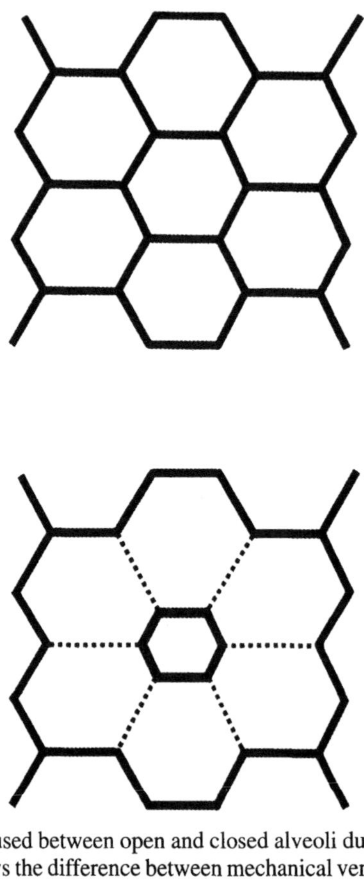

Fig. 1. Shear forces are caused between open and closed alveoli due to pulmonary interdependence of alveoli. This figure shows the difference between mechanical ventilation of normal alveoli (upper panel) and mechanical ventilation of the same alveolar unit after surfactant inactivation (lower panel)

This stretch is probably the major cause of structural damage and may be the basis, not only for formation of hyaline membranes, but also for the release of cytokines, thus triggering the pathophysiological mechanisms of acute respiratory failure. The alveoli maintaining their relative size to each other means that these shear forces are avoided, thus preventing damage to the alveolar wall.

Furthermore, repeated opening and collapse of alveoli leads to movement of surfactant into the smaller airways, as a result of compression of the surfactant film, when the surface of the alveolus becomes smaller than the surface occupied by the surfactant molecules [1, 2] (Fig. 2).

This loss of surfactant into the airways works together with the cilia to act as a direction control that ensures that mucus and inhaled particles move only in one direction (out of the lung) during the repeated compression and expansion of breathing. As long as there is a balance between synthesis, release of surfactant, and consumption of surfactant the lung will perform normally.

Using traditional artificial ventilation, the patient's lung collapses and reopens repeatedly. The alveoli decrease to a smaller size than usual, and more surfactant is lost into the airways, or forms non-surface active aggregates. This effect is emphasized by high tidal volumes and zero positive end expiratory pressure (PEEP), and finally results in surfactant deficiency at the air-liquid interface.

The immediate effects of the surfactant deficiency are an increase in pressures necessary to achieve the same volume changes. Less immediately obvious are the increased shear forces, due to the surfactant deficiency the alveoli are more prone to collapse, causing atelectasis, loss of surface tension regulation, alveolar shearing and shunt, resulting in both lower perfusion and pulmonary edema.

Whereas these results are undesirable in healthy patients, they can cause a serious life-threatening situation in diseased lungs. The obvious conclusion in order to maintain a sufficient gas exchange and preserve surfactant function and lung mechanics, is that the lung should be open throughout the respiratory cycle. This is exactly what the Open Lung Management achieves by opening the lung and keeping it open.

Open lung management

The implied rationale of Lachmann's editorial: "Open up the lung and keep the lung open"[3] leads to certain questions: What is an "open lung"? Why should we "open up the lung"? How should we "open up the lung" without risking barotrauma?

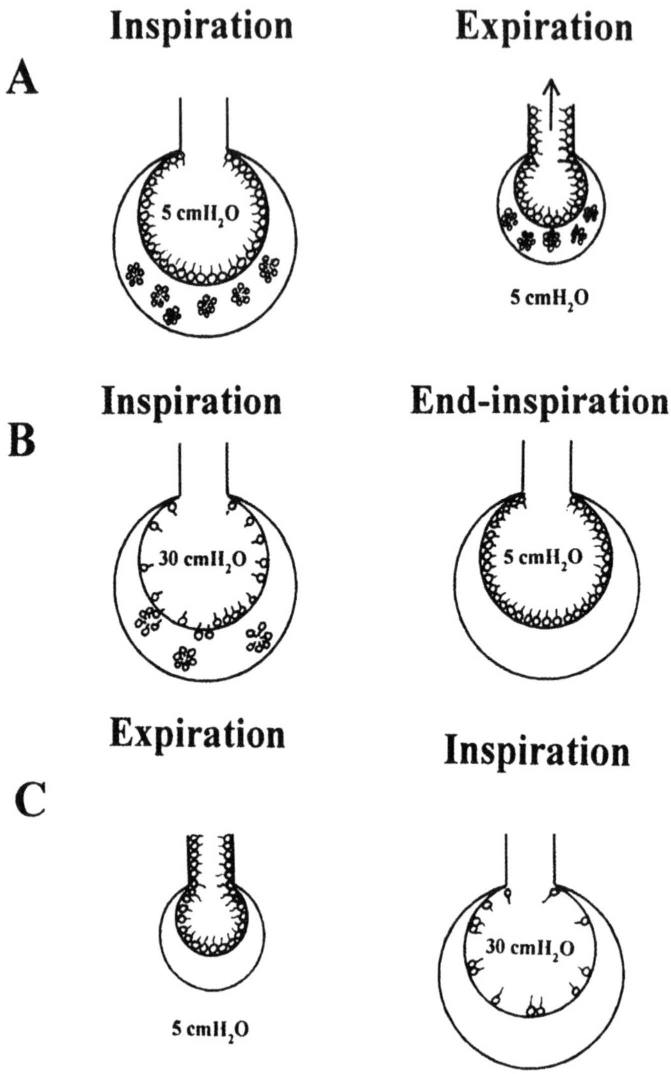

Fig.2. Diagram showing the balance between surfactant synthesis, release and consumption in the lung. A Balance between synthesis, release, and consumption of surfactant in the healthy lung. The pressure values given represent the intrapulmonary pressure needed to open up the alveolus. At the surface and the hypophase (micelles), there are sufficient molecules of surfactant. These micelles deliver the surfactant necessary to replace the molecules squeezed out during expiration.
B Imbalance between synthesis, release, and consumption of surfactant due to artificial ventilation. At the beginning of inspiration, there is an apparent deficiency of surfactant molecules but there is a respreading of molecules stored in the hypophase of the surfactant layer. At the end of expiration there is, in principle, enough surfactant on the surface.
C With the next expiration, surface active molecules are squeezed out and no surface active molecules are left in the hypophase for respreading, creating the situation where a serious surfactant deficiency follows

What is an "open lung"?

The "open lung" is characterized by an optimal gas exchange at the lowest possible mean airway pressure with tidal volumes less than 6 ml/kg body weight [3]. The intrapulmonary shunt is ideally less than 10%, which corresponds to a paO_2/FiO_2 ratio of more than 450. Due to the low mean airway pressure, hemodynamic deterioration is minimized [3, 4], and due to the low tidal volumes (equal to the driving pressures) the shear forces are diminished.

Why should we open up the lung?

The consequences of closed lung units have already been described extensively: arterial hypoxemia, intrapulmonary shunting, and atelectasis with high risk of infection, multiorgan dysfunction [5], and the development of ventilation-induced lung injury (VILI) [6, 7]. Ventilating a lung that is not homogenously open leads to situation where the artificial ventilation may cause lung damage, instead of being a therapy to overcome respiratory failure.

What does the open lung management mean?

Open Lung Management uses the characteristics of the healthy lung to keep the lung open throughout the respiratory cycle.

The process consists of three steps:

- Finding the opening pressure and the collapse pressure of the patient's lung
- Opening the lung
- Keeping the lung open

A short description of how this is done is given below and illustrated using patient data in Table 1; more information on the practical aspects of the Open Lung Management is available in the literature [3, 4, 8-11].

Practical considerations

The optimal equipment set-up consists of a time-cycled pressure-controlled ventilator and if possible a continuous blood gas monitor. Before looking for the opening and closing pressure, one has to make sure the patient is hemodynamically stable, if necessary administer fluids, and PEEP should be set between 15 and 20 cm H_2O, either as static or as auto PEEP, or as a combination of both. Fraction of inspired oxygen (FiO_2) is set to 100% (allowing detection of small atelectasis and preventing hypoxemia during the Open Lung procedure).

The following example demonstrates the Open Lung Management in a patient admitted to the intensive care unit due to thoracic trauma, with a body weight of 81 kg. The patient was ventilated in a volume-controlled mode, according to the NHI network trial (PEEP 11 cm H_2O, frequency 32, tidal volume 6 ml/kg body weight).

Under this condition the patient deteriorated overnight requiring a FiO_2 of 0.7, and this finally resulted in the blood gases as shown in Table 1.

Before the Open Lung Management was performed, the patient received 1 l of crystalloids and ventilator settings were switched to pressure-controlled ventilation with a PEEP of 20 cm H_2O, peak airway pressure (PAWP) of 26 H_2O an I:E ratio of 1:1, respiration rate 40, and FiO_2 of 100%.

To find the opening pressure, PAWP was increased for about 3 breaths (5 s) to 45 cm H2O, and then set back to 30 cm H2O. This resulted in a paO2 of 265 mmHg; from this paO2 it was concluded that the applied pressure of 45 cm H2O was too low to open up the lung. Therefore this procedure was repeated by increasing the recruitment pressure in 5-cm H2O steps up to 60 cm H2O, where paO2 did not further increase. The pressure causing the last increase in paO2 is called the opening pressure. In this patient the opening pressure was 55 cm H2O.

The next step was to find the minimal required upper pressure limit (MRUPL). After recruitment, peak pressure was lowered from 30 cmH_2O in 2- -cm steps, and during this procedure paO_2 was stable down to a peak pressure of 24 cmH_2O. Further reduction of PAWP was done in 1-cm steps. After reducing the PAWP to 23, a sudden decrease in paO_2 appeared. This means in this patient the minimal required upper pressure limit was 24 cm H_2O.

The next step was to find the minimal required lower pressure limit. Before lowering PEEP, the lung had to be recruited and PAWP was kept constant at 24 cm H_2O. paO_2 was unchanged down to a PEEP level of 17 cm H_2O. At a PEEP of 16 cm H_2O, paO_2 deteriorated. This means that in this patient the minimal required lower pressure limit was 17 cm H_2O

Another recruitment was required after this procedure, using the ventilator settings described above. The final ventilator settings resulted in a driving pressure amplitude of 7 cm H_2O, with accompanying tidal volume of 5.2 ml/kg body weight.

Despite these small tidal volumes, the patient was slightly hyperventilated ($paCO_2$ of 31 mmHg, equal to a CO_2 elimination of 480 ml/min in total). The increase of the frequency to 47 and the change of the I:E ratio to 60% of the inspiratory time led to a decrease of CO_2 elimination to 430 ml/min, resulting finally in a $paCO_2$ of 36 mmHg. The cause of the decreased CO_2 elimination was the increased total PEEP due to auto-PEEP and increased dead space ventilation.

After this FiO_2 was reduced to 0.3 and the patient was very stable for the next 2.5 h, with regard to hemodynamics and the gas exchange. After this time

Table 1. Representative data from a patient who responded as expected to the Open Lung Management

Increase RR to 47, I:E = 3:2	$PaCO_2$ = 36 mmHg VCO_2 = 435 ml/min TV = 395 ml = 4,9 ml/kg	Smaller pressure amplitude due to auto-PEEP and increased dead space ventilation

Action	**Data**	**Comments**
Patient at day 2: volume control ventilation with tidal volumes of 6 ml/kg	FiO_2 = 70% PEEP = 11 cm H_2O RR = 32, I:E = 1:2 TV = 6 ml/kg = 480ml PAWP = 26 cm H_2O SaO_2 = 92 % paO_2 = 72 mmHg $paCO_2$ = 48 mmHg	Slight hypoventilation
Switch to pressure controlled ventilation FiO_2 set to 100% I:E = 1:1, RR: 40 PAW 26 cm H_2O PEEP 20	SaO_2 = 100 % paO_2 = 140 mmHg $paCO_2$ = 39 mmHg	
Increase PAWP to 45 cm H_2O for 3 breaths (5 s), then back to 30	paO_2 = 265 mmHg	
1 min after stabilization increase PAW to 50 for 5 s, then back to 30	paO_2 = 350 mmHg	
1 min after stabilization increase PAWP to 55 for 5 s, then back to 30	paO_2 = 530 mmHg $paCO_2$ = 28 mmHg	
1 min after stabilization increase PAWP to 60 for 5 s, then back to 30	paO_2 = 531 mmHg $paCO_2$ = 28 mmHg	paO_2 does no further increase Opening pressure = 55 cm H_2O
Decrease PAWP to 28	No changes	
Decrease PAWP to 26	No changes	
Decrease PAWP to 24	No changes	
Decrease PAWP to 23	PaO_2 = 480 mmHg	The lung is collapsing Minimum required upper pressure limit = 24 cm H_2O
Recruit the lung (PAWP to 55, then 24		Reach opening pressure and set back just above minimum required upper pressure limit
PAWP 24, decrease PEEP to 18	No changes	
PEEP to 17	paO_2 = 541 mmHg	
PEEP to 16	paO_2 = 470 mmHg	Minimum required lower pressure limit = 17 cm H_2O
Set PEEP to 17 Increase PAWP to 55 for 5 sec (recruit) and back to 24	paO_2 = 544 mmHg $paCO_2$ = 31 mmHg VCO_2 = 480 ml/min	Optimal CO_2 removal requires VCO_2 of 430 ml/min
Decrease FiO_2 to 30%	paO_2 = 162 mmHg $paCO_2$ = 36 mmHg	Optimized patient ventilation at open lung

FiO_2 = Fraction inspired oxygen, PEEP = positive end expiratory pressure, RR = respiration rate, TV = tidal volume, PAWP = peak airway pressure, I:E = inspiration expiration ratio

the patient was accidentally disconnected from the ventilator, but the reconnection with the same ventilator settings resulted in a deteriorated gas exchange.

From this, one can see that the pressure required to open the lung is much higher, almost twice as high, as the pressure required to keep the lung open (Fig. 3).

Once again, if for any reason the patient is disconnected from the ventilator, i.e., suctioning, transport, bronchoscopy, one has to apply the previously found opening pressure to recruit the lung. The applied ventilator settings should be adjusted at least every 3-4 h to guarantee the minimal required pressures that keep the lung open.

Most important is that we have to understand that each patient's lung requires different opening pressures and different pressures to keep it open, and both of these are also continuously changing over time in the disease stage of each patient's lung.

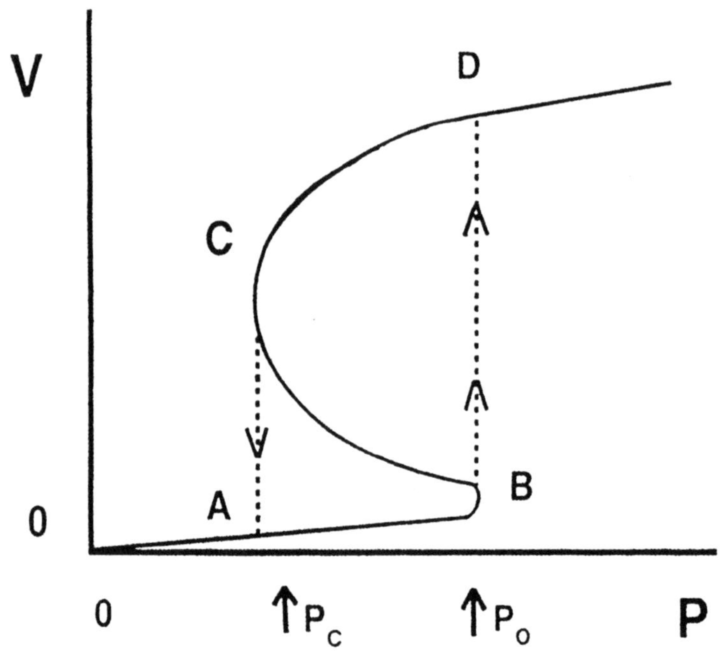

Fig. 3. Schematic drawing of a pressure-volume (P/V) curve showing the proposed mechanism of alveolar recruitment and collapse. With the increase of pressure during inspiration the corresponding change in volume is given by the P/V curve (solid line). At **A** the alveolus is still collapsed. It is not before point **B** that the critical opening pressure P_O is reached, the increase in alveolar volume is immediate (dashed line) and reaches **D**. The alveolus is recruited (note that the intra-alveolar pressure is the same at B and D). When the pressure is reduced to the closing pressure (P_C) at point **C** the change in volume follows the solid line and collapses again

References

1. Faridy EE (1976) Effect of ventilation on movement of surfactant in airways. Respir Physiol 27:323-334
2. Verbrugge SJ, Bohm SH, Gommers D, et al (1998) Surfactant impairment after mechanical ventilation with large alveolar surface area changes and effects of positive end-expiratory pressure. Br J Anaesth 80:360-364
3. Lachmann B (1992) Open up the lung and keep it open. Intensive Care Med 18:319-321
4. Lachmann B, Danzmann E, Haendly B et al (1982) Ventilator settings and gas exchange in respiratory distress syndrome. Nijhoff, The Hague
5. Ashbaugh DG, Bigelow DB, Petty TL, et al (1967) Acute respiratory distress in adults. Lancet II:319-323
6. Verbrugge S, Lachmann B (1998) Mechanisms of ventilation-induced lung injury and its prevention: role of surfactant. Appl Cardiopulm Pathophysiol 7:173-198
7. Dreyfuss D, Soler P, Basset G, et al (1988) High inflation pressure pulmonary edema. Respective effects of high airway pressure, high tidal volume, and positive end-expiratory pressure. Am Rev Respir Dis 137:1159-1164
8. Lachmann B, Jonson B, Lindroth M, et al (1982) Modes of artificial ventilation in severe respiratory distress syndrome. Lung function and morphology in rabbits after wash-out of alveolar surfactant. Crit Care Med 10:724-732
9. Böhm S, Vazquez de Anda G, Lachmann B (1998) The Open Lung Concept. In: Vincent J (ed) Yearbook of intensive care and emergency medicine. Springer, Heidelberg Berlin New York, pp 430-440
10. Hartog A, Vazquez de Anda GF, Gommers D, et al (2000) At surfactant deficiency, application of 'the open lung concept' prevents protein leakage and attenuates changes in lung mechanics. Crit Care Med 28:1450-1454
11. Vazquez de Anda GF, Hartog A, Verbrugge SJ, et al (1999) The open lung concept: pressure--controlled ventilation is as effective as high-frequency oscillatory ventilation in improving gas exchange and lung mechanics in surfactant-deficient animals. Intensive Care Med 25:990-996

Clinical Experience with Open Lung Management Experience in Trauma Patients

D. Schreiter, L. Scheibner, C. Josten

The pathomorphological substrate of lung contusion is a parenchymatous haemorrhage followed by an interstitial and alveolar oedema combined with a damage of the surfactant system [2] and resultant hypoventilation of these perfused but micro-atelectatic lung areas.

So the pathophysiological correlative is a dysregulation of the ventilation perfusion ratio, a right-to-left shunt [2, 7]. Typically the increase of FIO_2 cannot prevent the resultant severe hypoxia.

The consecutive disturbance of oxygenation represents the indication of the Open Lung Management.

This ventilation concept developed by Lachmann opens up atelectatic portions of the lung by means of a temporary high peak pressure and keeps the lung open by sufficiently high positive end expiratory pressure (PEEP) until the regeneration of the surfactant system [1, 3].

Patients

In a clinical trial from December 1997 to June 2001 we treated 38 patients after multiple trauma (ISS 43, PTS 32) including a severe chest contusion (AISR 5, PTST 14) and resultant disturbance of oxygenation (PaO_2/FIO_2-ratio 134 mm Hg) using the Open Lung Management.

Inclusion and exclusion criteria

There were included patients with a severe injury according to the definition of multiple trauma combined with serious chest contusion (AISR > 3, PTST > 7) and resultant disturbance of oxygenation (pO2/FIO2-ratio < 200).

Patients with left-sided heart failure had to be excluded. Patients younger than 14 years were also not included.

Patients with severe head injury and increased intracranial pressure were excluded as well. Even though 3 patients with severe head injury were treated according to the principles of the Open Lung Management taking the priority of the oxygenation disturbance into consideration.

In these 3 patients we measured the intracranial pressure and in addition to that we carried out a measurement of the blood flow in both Aa.cerebri mediae by means of Doppler ultrasonography [4].

Other contra indications were chronic obstructive pulmonary disease (COPD) and unstabilizable cardiovascular insufficiency.

Ventilator strategy and procedure of treatment

At the time of inclusion all patients were ventilated at a pressure controlled mode (IRV, bf 20/min, TV 6 ml/kg body weight, PEEP 10mbar). After connecting the patient to the monitoring system a subtle bronchoscopical airway cleaning was carried out.

The Open Up Manoeuvre itself was performed in deep sedation. Respirator settings were still pressure controlled (I:E ratio 2:1, PEEP 8-10 mbar). If not done before according to the patients need because of the poor oxygenation, the FIO_2 was set to 1 to make possible a better assessment of the ventilation-perfusion-ratio.

The breath frequency was increased to 80 per minute to create an intrinsic-PEEP, keeping the amplitude as low as possible during the application of the high peak pressures already. Based on these respirator settings the Open Up Manoeuver was carried out by increasing the peak pressure up to 50 mbar for 5 breaths. Subsequntly the peak interface pressure (PIP) was decreased back to 35 mbar watching circulation and oxygenation parameters. If no increase of the p_aO_2 up to 400 mbar could be achieved another Open Up Manoeuvre using a peak pressure of 65 mbar was carried out. In a few cases the oxygenation did not reach the level we expected, so a third Open Up Procedure was performed at a PIP of 80 mbar. After every manoeuvre the total PEEP had to be checked on making sure it was not lower than the calculated closing pressure of 20 mbar.

A global PEEP set at this level on the respirator could lead the patient into a critical cardiovascular situation. Therefore, we produced a regional dynamic PEEP by means of a pressure controlled inverse ratio ventilation at a high frequency. The expiration period is very short and so the affected injured lung areas are unable to empty completely. The remaining volume keeps the alveoli open. A set PEEP at a moderate level stabilizes the healthy unactive alveoli according to the above mechanism.

The levels of PIP and necessary minimal PEEP were based on experimental data [5, 6, 9, 10] and clinical experiences [8]. Using these calculated pressure levels the Open Up Procedure could be kept as short as possible. It took only some seconds because there was no need to detect the individual opening and closing pressures.

Looking for the best respirator setting we aimed at the lowest amplitude possible and a balance between deadspace and hyperventilation regulated by the breath frequency (60-100) leading to normocapnia and avoiding permissive hypercapnia.

After opening up the lung and keeping it open it was possible to reduce the FIO_2.

We avoided a disconnection of the system patient-respirator for 24 hours. If still necessary another Open Up Manoeuvre had to be carried out. After 24 hours we returned to the conventional pressure controlled mode and another bronchoscopy was performed. According to the patients actual oxygenation situation the Open Lung Management could be finished or had to be carried on.

Results

In most patients (n=19, 50%) the application of a PIP of 65 mbar was necessary to recruit successfully. In 8 patients 50 mbar were enough to open up the lung. The highest peak pressure required in 4 patients needed for successful recruitment was 80 mbar (Table 1).

Table 1.Demonstration of the required opening pressures of successful recruitment.*

Max. opening pressure		n	%
50	8	**21.1**	
55	2	5.3	
60	5	13.2	
65	19	50	**89.5**
70	0	0	
75	0	0	
	4	10.5	
80			**94.7***
	(2)*	(5.3)*	

*The aim of paO_2/FIO_2-ratio > 400 mmHg could not be reached in two cases

The median total PEEP level during the Open Up Manoeuvre was 39 mbar (37-42). During the Open Up Procedure tidal volumes of 490 ml (450-525)

were applied, representing a volume lower than the previous volumes (520 ml).

To keep the lung open a median total PEEP of 22mbar (21-24) was necessary. At a peak pressure of 33 mbar the resultant tidal volumes were 250 ml representing 3.5 ml/kg body weight.

A significant increase ($p = 0.001$) of the oxygenation ratio from 134 to 522 mmHg was achieved after the Open Up Manoeuvre and recruitment of the ventilation-disturbed pulmonary alveoli. The FIO_2 could be reduced to 0.6 after 1 hour, to 0.4 after 6 hours and to 0.3 after 24 hours.

In addition a clear-cut improvement in X-ray and CT could be shown. Impressive results were achieved in 6 patients when the procedure described above was performed under direct computed tomograph (CT) control (Fig.1 and Fig.2).

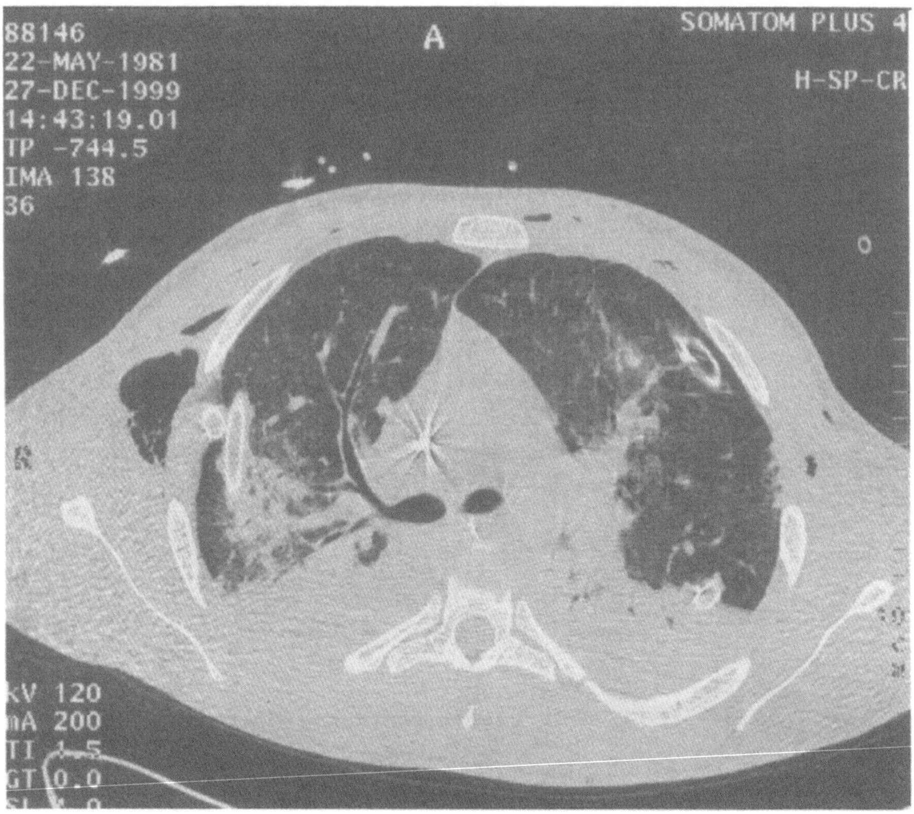

Fig. 1. CT-scan of a patient suffering from severe chest trauma before Open Up Manoeuvre

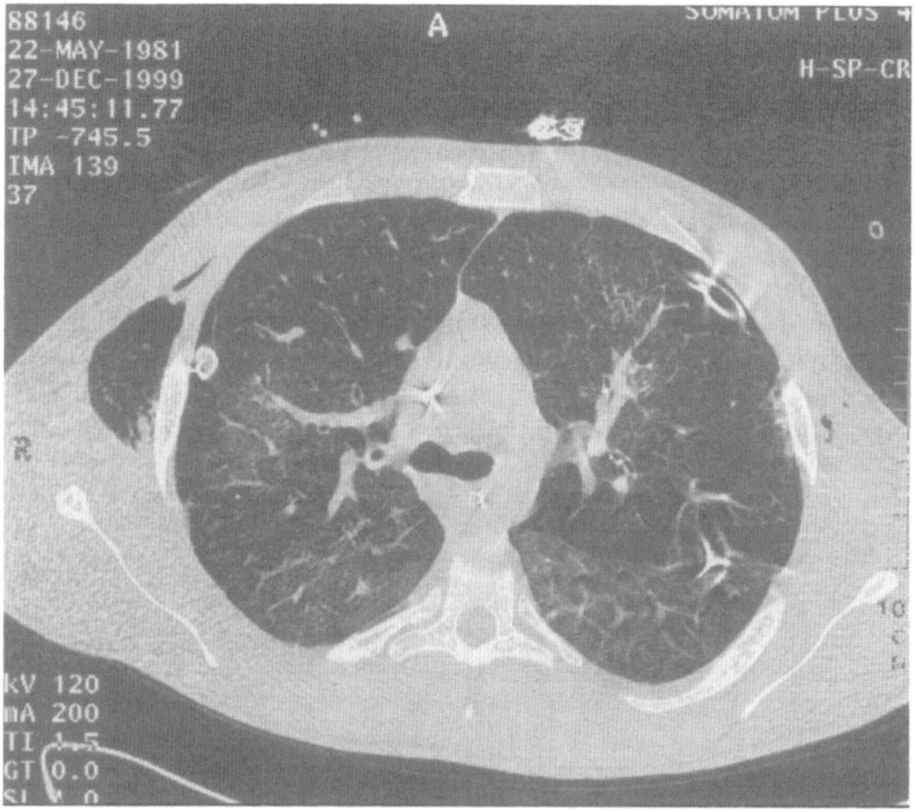

Fig. 2. Same patient 2 minutes after Open Up Manoeuvre

After approximately 34 hours the ventilation method could be changed back to a conventional one.

No patient developed a manifest acute respiratory distress syndrome (ARDS). Two patients died of extrapulmonary cause.

A significant decrease of the mean arterial pressure (MAP) was noticed during the Open Up Manoeuvre as well as a significant increase after reducing the peak pressure. There were no significant differences between MAP levels before and after Open Up.

According to the tendency of the MAP the intracranial blood flow showed a clear decrease during the application of the high opening pressure. But it returned to a flow level similar to the prevoius Open Up Procedure [4].

To make sure that there are no disturbances of perfusion of any system we carried out several laboratory analyses. There were no reported respirator changes.

Conclusions

The treatment of the ventilation perfusion disturbance after chest contusion using the Open Lung Management represents a causal therapeutic strategy. This ventilation method guarantees an impressive improvement of oxygenation and normocapnia. It eliminates atelectasis of the lung and prevents following complications. By ventilating the injured lung with low tidal volumes the Open Lung Management represents a lung protective strategy.

The Open Up Manoeuvre can be carried out using a PIP of 65 mbar guaranteeing a successful recruitment in most cases.

It is not a commonly used procedure. In our Intensive care unit it has been employed in cases of early stage of ARDS and especially in cases of severe chest trauma.

References

1. Böhm S, Lachmann B (1996) Pressure-control ventilation-Putting a mode into perspective. Int J Intensive Care. Spring.
2. Craven KD, Oppenheimer L, Wood LDH (1979) Effects of contusion and flail chest on pulmonary perfusion and oxygen exchange. J Appi Physiol: Resp Envir Exer Physiol 47: 729
3. Lachmann B (1992) Open up the lung and keep the lung open. Intensive Care Med 18: 319-321
4. Mende L, Katscher S, Engelmann L et al (2001) Hämodynamische Auswirkungen aktueller Beatmungsverfahren auf die zerebrale Perfusion. Intensivmed 38: 394-401
5. Sjöstrand UH, Lichtwarck-Aschoff M, Nielsen JB et al (1995). Different Ventilatory Approaches at Open lung. Intensive Care Med 21: 310-318
6. Wegenius GA, Sjöstrand UH, Svensson BA et al (1996). Radiological assessment of surfactant depletion lung injury. Applied Cardiopulmonary Pathophysiology 6: 119-129
7. Rutherford RB, Valenta J (1971) An experimental study of "traumatic wet lung". J Trauma 1 1: 146
8. Schreiter D, Abitzsch D, Scheibner L et al (1999) Das Open Lung Concept – Ein neues Beatmungsregime beim schweren Thoraxtrauma. Langenbecks Arch (Kongressband 1999): 909-912
9. Schreiter D, Scheibner L, Katscher S, Josten C (2000) Prevention of Acute Respiratory Failure by Optimal Ventilator Setting: The Open Lung Concept. Proceedings of 15th A.P.I.C.E. (Springer Verlag): 213-220
10. Steinert M, Schreiter D, Friedrich Th et al (1999) Thoracic surgery intensive care management of therapy in cases of serve injury of thorax with lesion of organs: thoracotomy after conditioning by the open-lung-concept (by Lachmann). J Thorac Cardiovasc Surg 47: 273

Semirecumbency Prevents Nosocomial Pneumonia in Mechanically Ventilated Patients

M.B. DRAKULOVIC, A. TORRES

Nosocomial pneumonia is the most common infection in the intensive care unit (ICU) [1]. Nosocomial pneumonia (NP) in mechanically ventilated (MV) or ventilator-associated pneumonia (VAP) typically refers to pneumonia developing after 48 hours following endotracheal intubation and MV [2]. Infections restricted to a series of MV patients within the ICU revealed that VAP accounts for approximately 90% of the infections in patients requiring assisted ventilation [3]. The European [4] and Spanish [5] multicenter studies have associated MV in ICU patients with almost 3-fold and 23-fold increased risk of NP, respectively, compared with non ventilated subjects. Furthermore, National Nosocomial Infections Surveillance (NNIS) system [6] reported approximately 9.3 times higher incidence density rates of VAP than nonventilator-associated pneumonia within the ICU, ranging from 2.6 times higher in the respiratory ICU to 19 times higher in the burn ICU. Nosocomial pneumonia is also a leading cause of death in ICUs [7], resulting in a significant 2 to 10-fold increase in the mortality rate [8-10] and the occurrence is shown to be an independent determinant of hospital mortality [11]. Recent inferences have been made, indicating that VAP markedly increases morbidity by affecting the ICU length of stay [12, 13] and the duration of MV [14, 15]. Two investigations reported that VAP caused a significant excess of the ICU length of stay in one clinical trial [12] and prolongation of the ICU hospitalization for 4 days in another clinical trial [13]. In addition, VAP increased almost 3-fold more than MV in a multicenter prospective study [14] or 9 days in a matched cohort investigation [15]. Finally, there is no doubt that VAP substantially increased the hospital costs for the survivors [16]. Papazian et al. estimated that each episode of VAP costs the hospital an additional $ 7 752 [15].

Pathogenesis of VAP includes two most commonly recognized pathogenic factors as bacterial colonization of gastric content and subsequent aspiration to the lower airways. The sequence of colonization from the stomach to the trachea in MV patients has been confirmed [17, 18] supporting the gastric role in NP development. Although some authors have failed to demonstrate the mechanism for gastric colonization [19, 20], there is supporting evidence that it is a significant risk factor for subsequent NP [21, 22]. It has been reported that the stomach, a sterile organ in healthy people (pH: 2) [21, 23], becomes colonized within 24 hours of ICU admission and in a series of traumatic, medical, surgical and neurological patients [24, 25] the initial colonization rates are almost 40%. Two investigations [21, 22] associated gastric bacterial overgrowth (103 -108/mL) with paralytic ileus and increasing pH, during the first 48 hours of MV. Most of the data emphasize gastric overgrowth with aerobic *Gram*-negative bacilli [21, 22], but high numbers of *Gram*-positive bacteria and fungi have been reported as well [24, 26]. Moreover, a retrograde colonization of the oropharynx from the stomach can be present when bacteria initially isolated in gastric fluid subsequently appear in pharyngeal [18] and tracheal secretions [17, 21, 22]. Finally this finding has been confirmed and extended by three other clinical trials [27-29] reporting that gastric bacterial overgrowth preceded two days to tracheal colonization in 27-45% MV patients during their ICU stay. Advanced age, underlying illness, malnutrition, administration of antacids and histamine H2-receptor antagonists [21-23, 29-32], delayed gastric emptying [33], coexistence of gastro-duodenal reflux [34, 35] and enteral feeding [36, 37] are factors predisposing gastric bacterial overgrowth. It is worth mentioning again that the gastric origin of oropharyngeal colonization (i.e., retrograde pharyngeal colonization) is a frequent event in intubated and MV patients with a nasogastric tube (NGT) in place [38]. Furthermore, the presence of a NGT through both the lower and upper esophageal sphincters renders them incompetent [39], facilitates regurgitation [i.e., gastroesophageal reflux (GER)] [38] and likelihood of subsequent aspiration of gastric content [40, 41] to lower airways.

The second important mechanism in the pathogenesis of VAP, aspiration of gastric contents colonized with bacteria corresponding with those isolated in the trachea aspirates [42], is a frequent event in MV patients [43], although cuffed endotracheal tubes are commonly used for prevention [44]. An incidence of aspiration of 40% and 70% have been reported in series of MV and tracheotomized patients, respectively [45, 46]. Factors that predispose patients to aspiration include host factors, such as impaired consciousness or recent thoracoabdominal surgery [21, 47-49] and external factors such as, tracheal and gastrointestinal tract instrumentation [50, 51]. It has recently been observed that both the supine position (i.e., lying flat in the bed) and the duration at which the patient is kept in that posture are the factors that increase the risk of aspiration of gastric contents to lower airways [40, 41].

In addition, relationship of aspiration with an enteral nutrition has been clearly confirmed [52]. Incident rates of enteral formula aspiration from 21 to 95% have been shown [53-55]. Also, the risk of aspiration in nutrition delivered through the duodenal or gastric tube has been demonstrated [56, 57]. One recent prospective cohort study [58] involving more than 1 000 patients in 16 ICUs has associated aspiration of gastric content in MV patients with an approximately 3-fold increase in the risk of VAP, compared with its absence in critically ill subjects. Furthermore, in two other clinical reports [43, 59] lung aspiration was determined as an independent predictor of NP in MV patients. Therefore, strategies aimed at preventing VAP will usually be focused on reducing the gastric colonization burden and decreasing the incidence of aspiration (i.e., on either of those two important risk factors for VAP).

Torres et al. hypothesized that semirecumbency (head of the bed elevated for 45 degrees angle from horizontal) could prevent aspiration as a risk factor for NP. In a randomized clinical design Torres et al. showed a significantly lower incidence of aspiration in patients nursed in the semirecumbent position compared to those in the supine position (4 154 counts per minute (cpm) versus 954 cpm: $p=0.036$, respectively). Furthermore, aspiration rates of time (expressed as difference in radioactivity count at 300 minutes and 30 minutes (initial)) from values of 2 294 ± 1 895 cpm in the supine position decreased to counts of 113 ± 77 cpm by applying an opposite nursing procedure (e.g., semirecumbency ($p=0.05$)). Moreover, microbiological analysis revealed far less incidence of retrograde pharyngeal and tracheal colonization within the semirecumbency compared to the supine position. Stated another way, bacterial agents isolated from pharyngeal, tracheal and gastric samples coincided in six of 19 (32%) patients in the semirecumbent position, and in 13 of 19 (68%) patients tested in the supine posture. The second randomized clinical trial of the same group [41] evaluated two body positions (supine and semirecumbency) on dynamics of GER in patients requiring MV and having NGT in place, and showed that the semirecumbent group clearly experienced significantly less aspiration of gastric content (expressed as radioactivity counting) to lower airways compared to the supine group (2.54 ± 0.49 cpm vs. 1.66 ± 0.45 cpm: $p < 0.01$, respectively). The authors concluded that semirecumbency reduces the incidence and risk of aspiration in MV patients and it might be a simple, prophylactic measure in preventing lung aspiration of gastric contents. Those findings have been further confirmed and extended by other investigators [60] showing a 3-fold risk of NP in patients lying in the supine position, during the first 24 hours of MV, which in turn resulted in a significant increase in the mortality rates compared to the alternate, semirecumbent position (30.2% versus 8.9%; $p< 0.001$, respectively). Therefore, only 5 patients needed to be treated in a semirecumbent position to prevent death from VAP. Furthermore, in two clinical trials [60, 61] the supine positioning within the first 24 hours of MV was also determined as an independent predictor of poor outcome.

Potts et al. [62] have shown significantly lower aspiration rates of enteral nutrition in NGT patients in the semirecumbent position compared to the patients to the supine position (98% *vs.* 21%; p<0.001, respectively).

In addition, powerful inferences have also been drawn about the effect of semirecumbency on GER [38, 63-65]. Two studies [63, 64] revealed that semirecumbency induced increasing esophageal clearance [66] and the disappearance of GER. This was further substantiated by Nagler and Spiro (1963) who demonstrated that, even in healthy subjects, the applied semirecumbent positioning induced disappearance of GER when lying in the supine position [65]. Ibanez et al. [38] showed scintigraphic evidence of GER in 67% of the patients in the semirecumbent position compared to 81% of the patients lying in the supine position.

In addition to those works, in the epidemiological study designed to identify risk factors predictive for nosocomial infections in ICU patients Fernandez-Crehuet et al. [67] confirmed that elevated head positioning (greater than a 30 degree angle) was protective against VAP. In a very recent clinical trial [68] designed to evaluate whether semirecumbency can reduce the incidence of VAP, 86 intubated and MV patients were randomly allocated to either the semirecumbent (39) or supine (47) positioning. The likelihood of clinically suspected and microbiologically confirmed pneumonia was assessed. The results have shown that clinically suspected pneumonia developed in significantly fewer patients nursed in semirecumbency compared to those maintained in the supine position [three of 39 (8%) *vs.* 16 pf 47 (34%); 95% CI for difference 10.0-42.0, p=0.003] and such difference was also true for microbiologically confirmed NP [semirecumbent: two of 39 (5%) *vs.* supine: 11 of 47 (23%); 95% CI 4.2-31.8, p=0.018]. These data suggest efficacy of the semirecumbent position, due to the number of patients that needed to be placed in that position to prevent an episode of VAP. Conceivably, authors tested modifiable risk factors as semirecumbency *vs.* supine positioning in a randomized clinical trial and confirmed that semirecumbency also lowers the incidence of VAP. Hence, maintaining the critically ill in the semirecumbent position represents an effective strategy for preventing VAP. Futhermore, the semirecumbency is a simple, non-cost and easy-to-apply measure to reduce NP in MV patients.

The benefit of the semirecumbent position has also been further reported [69]. In the patients with coma due to drug overdose, hospitalized in the toxicology ICU, Adnet et al. [69] found a significantly lower incidence of suspected aspiration pneumonia in cases who were discovered to be in semirecumbent, compared with subjects initially lying in the supine or in the lateral decubital posture. Semirecumbency is included amongst the seven most effective preventive strategies evaluated in randomized trials with respect to their potential influence to VAP [70].

Some professional practice guidelines [71, 72] and recommendations [73] suggest semirecumbency as a pneumonia prevention strategy. The 1994 Centers for Disease Control and Prevention (CDC) and Hospital Infection Control Advisory Committee (HICPAC), and the Guideline of prevention Nosocomial Pneumonia [71] classifies elevating the head of the bed at 30-45 degrees, if not contraindicated, as strongly recommended for all hospitals, and as considered effective by experts in the field, on the basis of strong rationale and suggestive but not definite evidence. Furthermore, the 1995 American Thoracic Society (ATS) Consensus Statement [72] states semirecumbency as a regimen with probable effectiveness, used widely in some clinical settings. Finally, in Kollef's recent recommendations for the prevention of VAP [73], semirecumbent positioning is rated as an effective preventive strategy for clinical use supported by at least one randomized, controlled investigation.

Two prospective studies [74, 75] have performed observational designs to determine the usual nursing position of the patients within their hospitalization in four ICUs [74] and in one respiratory ICU [75]. The results have shown that the most common nursing posture of subjects in ICUs was between 15-30 degrees elevation in the former study, and 23 degrees elevation angle in the latter investigation. Furthermore, only less than 25% of the patients were maintained in semirecumbency [74]. Consequently, although detailed clinical evidence, (i.e., three randomized trials) have shown that semirecumbency compared to supine positioning is associated with lower rates of aspiration [40, 41] and VAP [68], nevertheless MV patients have been rarely nursed in that position during their ICU hospitalization [74, 75]. This was further substantiated and extended by Cook et al. (2000) who conducted a Franco-Canadian cross sectional survey to determine the use, rationales against use and decisional responsibility for 7 of the most effective preventive strategies including semirecumbency [70]. They found that semirecumbent positioning was more often applied in the French than the Canadian ICUs (58.3% *vs.* 30.0%; $p=0.003$); the country as being a strong independent predictor of semirecumbency and nursing inconvenience was cited as a reason for the non-use of semirecumbent maintenance. Furthermore, semirecumbent positioning was significantly more often influenced by intensivists and bedside nurses in the Canadian compared to the French ICUs, whereas the general ICU policy determined semirecumbency to be more likely in France than in Canada (64.8% *vs.* 17.2%; $p < 0.001$). In another pilot study eighty-six percent of the studied patients were maintained in the supine positioning within their total respiratory ICU hospitalization [75].

These two studies in fact further portray the existing notion that detailed clinical evidence [40, 41, 68] and practice guidelines and recommendations [71-73] do not substantially have an impact on the use of semirecumbency as a VAP prevention strategy within critical care settings [70, 75].

In addition, a futher randomized clinical trial [68] on the incidence of VAP confirmed that patients in the supine body position compared to those in semirecumbency and cases with enteral nutrition *vs.* cases without enteral nutrition were almost 7 times and 6 times as likely to acquire VAP, respectively. Furthermore, the presence of both factors had an additive effect on the incidence of NP with the highest frequency (50%) seen in the subjects that were in the supine position being fed enterally. The incidence of VAP among the cases maintained supine without enteral nutrition was 10% and nearly close to the values (9%) found in the subjects fed enterally but nursed in the semirecumbent position. Conceivably, semirecumbency reduces the risk of VAP especially in patients fed enterally *via* NGT. Therefore, it is worth noting that in addition to 3 VAP prevention guidelines [71-73], the fourth, or the 1995 American Gastroenterological Association Guidelines for the use of enteral nutrition [76] also states raising the head of the patient's bed 30-45 degrees during feeding and one hour after, as a precaution which should be taken to limit complications of tube feeding. Existing evidence that the enteral route of nutritional support [77] is used in European [78] and Spanish [79] ICUs in 58% and 59.7%, respectively, that enteral feeding has a mean duration of approximately 10 days [80], that the often reported complications in MV enterally fed patients include a high incidence of GER [38], tracheal colonization [53, 81] and NP [36] further emphasize the need of maintaining semirecumbency in ICUs. However, although clinical practice guidelines represent the most efficient methods of identifying effective health care interventions [82-84], some preventive strategies are infrequently introduced in the ICUs [75], such as semirecumbency during enteral feeding [76].

In a recent Franco-Canadian survey VAP prevention guidelines were being implemented twice as much in the French than in the Canadian ICUs [70] and adherence for its two selected VAP preventive strategies in 179 hospitals participating CDC's NNIS system ranged from 93%-98% [85]. Recently confirmed, although guidelines represent an accessible source of detailed clinical evidence, they are not sufficient precursors of innovation for achieving evidence based health care [86]. Therefore, additional professional, educational and operational support for clinical innovations will probably accelerate the use of clinical evidence [86, 87]. The three present strategies are successfully embraced in a program aimed to prevent VAP, focusing its activity in the ICU [88-91].

A program to prevent VAP incorporates a continuous quality improvement concept [92] related to detailed clinical evidence, together with infection control procedures used for improvement and a multidisciplinary team approach [91]. Four prospective studies [88-91] designed to evaluate the impact of a program to prevent the incidence of VAP within ICUs have shown improved clinical outcomes [88-91] and reduced critical care costs [88, 89] due to program implementation. Kollef [93] described the components of PDSA (Plan-Do-Study-Act) model, that could simply be employed to develop a VAP prevention program incorporating research-based recommendations [71-73,76], which include semirecumbency as the most effective preventive strategy.

Finally, Hummel et al. [94] described a procedure for the continuous measurement of backrest elevation in critical care, using the pressure differential between two transducers attached to the bed frame. The transducer measurement procedure could be beneficial in the maintaining continuous quality improvement processes and research purposes on semirecumbency.

In conclusion, three final under stated comments are worth mentioning. First, semirecumbency reduces the incidence and risk of VAP, especially in patients fed enterally *via* NGT. Second, placing MV patients fed enterally *via* NGT in the semirecumbent position, if not contraindicated, is strongly recommended as effective, simple, inexpensive and is an easy-to-apply preventive strategy. Third, semirecumbency could be successfully introduced in critical care settings by programs for VAP prevention.

References

1. Vincent JL, Bihari DJ, Suter PM et al (1995) The prevalence of nosocomial infection in intensive care units in Europe: results of the European prevalence of infection in intensive care (EPIC) study. JAMA 274:639-644
2. Meduri GU, Johnson WG Jr (1992) International consensus conference: clinical investigation of ventilator-associated pneumonia. Introduction. Chest 102:551S-552S
3. Richards MJ, Edwards JR, Culver DH et al (1999) Nosocomial infections in medical intensive care units in the United States. Crit Care Med 27:887-892
4. Chevert S, Hemmer M, Carlet J et al (1993) Incidence and risk factors of pneumonia acquired in intensive care units: results from a multicenter prospective study on 996 patients. Intensive Care Med 19:256-264
5. Alvarez-Lerma F, Palomar M, Martinez-Pellus A et al (1997) Aethiology and diagnostic techniques in intensive care-acquired pneumonia: a Spanish multi-centre study. Clin Intensive Care 8:164-170
6. Keita-Perse O, Gaynes RP (2000) Surveillance and its impact. In: Jarvis WR (ed) Nosocomial pneumonia. Marcel Dekker, Inc., New York Basel, pp. 39-52
7. Leu HS, Kaiser DL, Mori M et al (1989) Hospital-acquired pneumonia: attributable mortality and morbidity. Am J Epidemiol 129:1258-1267
8. Fagon J-Y, Chastre AJ, Hance P et al (1993) Nosocomial pneumonia in ventilated patients: a

cohort study evaluating attributable mortality and hospital stay. Am J Med 94:281-288
9. Craig CP, Connelly S (1984) Effect of intensive care unit nosocomial pneumonia on duration of stay and mortality. Am J Infect Control 12:233-238
10. Cunnion KM, Weber DJ, Broadhead WE, et al (1996) Risk factors for nosocomial pneumonia: comparing adult critical care populations. Am J Respir Crit Care Med 153:358-362
11. Fagon J-Y, Chastre J, Vuagnat A et al (1996) Nosocomial pneumonia and mortality among patients in intensive care units. JAMA 275:866-869
12. Ibrahim EH, Ward S, Sherman G et al (2000) A comparative analysis of patients with early-onset vs. late-onset nosocomial pneumonia in the ICU settings. Chest 117:1434-1442
13. Heyland DK, Cook DJ, Griffith L et al (1999) The attributable mortality and morbidity of ventilator-associated pneumonia in critically ill patients. Am J Respir Crit Care Med 159:1249-1256
14. Markowicz P, Wolff M, Djediani K et al (2000) Multicenter prospective study of ventilator-associated pneumonia during acute respiratory distress syndrome. Incidence, prognosis and risk factors. ARDS study group. Am J Respir Crit Care Med 161:1942-1948
15. Papazian L, Bregeon F, Thirion X et al (1996) Effect of ventilator-associated pneumonia on mortality and morbidity. Am J Respir Crit Care Med 154:91-97
16. Wiblin RT (1997) Nosocomial pneumonia. In: Wenzel RP (ed) Prevention and control of nosocomial infections. Williams and Wilkins, Baltimore, pp. 807-819
17. Daschner F, Kappstein I, Engels J et al (1988) Stress ulcer prophylaxis and ventilation pneumonia: prevention by antibacterial cytoprotective agents. Infect Control Hosp Epidemiol 9:59-65
18. Goularte TA, Lichtenberg, Craven DE (1986) Gastric colonization in patients receiving antacids and mechanical ventilation: a mechanism for pharyngeal colonization. Am J Infect Control 14:88-92
19. Palmer LB, Donelen SV, Fox G et al (1995) Gastric flora in chronically mechanically ventilated patients: relationship to upper and lower airway colonization. Am J Respir Crit Care Med 151:1063-1067
20. Cade JF, Mc Cwat E, Singanporia R et al (1991) Uncertain relevance of gastric colonization in the seriously ill. Intensive Care Med 18:210-217
21. Atherton TS, White DJ (1978) Stomach as a source of bacteria colonizing respiratory tract during artificial ventilation. Lancet ii:968-969
22. Du Moulin GC, Hendley-White J et al (1982) Aspiration of gastric bacteria in antacid-treated patients: a frequent cause of postoperative colonization of the airway. Lancet ii:242-245
23. Reusser P, Zimmerli W, Scheidegger D et al (1989) Role of gastric colonization in nosocomial infections and endotoxemia: a prospective study in neurosurgical patients on mechanical ventilation. J Infect Dis 160:414-421
24. Ewig S, Torres A, El-Ebiary M et al (1999) Bacterial colonization patterns in mechanically ventilated patients with traumatic and medical head injury. Am J Respir Crit Care Med 159: 188-198
25. Bonten MJM, Gaillard CA, van Tiel FH et al (1994) The stomach is not a source for colonization of the upper respiratory tract and pneumonia in ICU patients. Chest 105:878-884
26. Drakulovic MB, Bauer TT, Torres A et al (2001) Initial bacterial colonization in patients admitted to a respiratory intensive care unit: bacteriological pattern and risk factors. Respiration 68:58-66
27. Kahn RJ, Brimioule R, Vincent JL (1982) Influence of antacid treatment on the tracheal flora in mechanically ventilated patients (Abstr). Crit Care Med 10:229
28. Hillman KM, Riodan T, O'Farrell SM et al (1982) Colonization of the gastric content in critically ill patients. Crit Care Med 10:444-447
29. Donowitz LG, Page MC, Mileur GL et al (1986) Alteration of nosocomial gastric flora in critical care patients receiving antacid and cimetidine therapy. Infect Control 7:23-26
30. Kappstein I, Schulgen G, Friedrich T et al (1991) Incidence of pneumonia in mechanically ventilated patients treated with sucralfate or cimetidine as prophylaxis for stress bleeding: bacterial colonization of the stomach. Am J Med 91:125S-131S

31. Apte MN, Konrad RD, Medheker PT et al (1992) Gastric colonization and pneumonia in intubated critically ill patients receiving stress ulcer prophylaxis: a randomized, controlled trial. Crit Care Med 20:590-593
32. Garvey MB, Mc Cambey AJ, Tuxen VD (1989) Effects of gastric alkalinization on bacterial colonization in critically ill patients. Crit Care Med 17:211-216
33. Heyland KD, Tougas G, King D et al (1996) Impaired gastric emptying in mechanically ventilated critically ill patients. Intensive Care Med 22:1339-1344
34. Inglis TJT, Spreat JL, Gibson JS et al (1993) Gastroduodenal dysfunction and bacterial colonization of the ventilated lung. Lancet 341:911-913
35. Wilmer A, Tuck J, Frans E et al (1999) Duodenoesophsgeal reflux and esophageal mucosal injury in mechanically ventilated patients. Gastroenterology 116:1293-1299
36. Jacobs SJ, Chang RW, Lee B et al (1990) Continuous enteral feeding: a major cause of pneumonia amongst ventilated intensive care unit patients. J Parent Ent Nutr 14:353-357
37. Spilker AC, Hinthorn RD, Pingelton SK (1996) Intermittent enteral feeding in mechanically ventilated patients: the effect of gastric pH and gastric cultures. Chest 110:243-248
38. Ibáñez J, Peñafiel A, Raurich JM et al (1992) Gastroesophageal reflux in intubated patients receiving enteral nutrition: effect of supine and semirecumbent positions. J Parent Ent Nutr 16:419-422
39. Mittal RK, Stewart WR, Schirmer BD (1992) Effect of a catheter in the pharynx on the frequency of transient lower esophageal sphincter relaxations. Gastroenterology 103:1236-1240
40. Torres A, Serra-Batlles J, Ros E et al (1992) Pulmonary aspiration of gastric contents in patients receiving mechanical ventilation: the effect of body position. Ann Intern Med 116:540-543
41. Orozco-Levi M, Torres A, Ferrer M et al (1995) Semirecumbent position protects from pulmonary aspiration but not completely from gastroesophageal reflux in mechanically ventilated patients. Am J Respir Crit Care Med 152:1387-1390
42. Torres A, El-Ebiary M, Gonzales J et al (1993) Gastric and pharyngeal flora in nosocomial pneumonia acquired during mechanical ventilation. Am Rev Respir Dis 148:352-357
43. Torres A, Aznar R, Gatell JM et al (1990) Incidence risk and prognostic factors of nosocomial pneumonia in mechanically ventilated patients Am Rev Respir Dis 142:523-528
44. Mc Crae W, Wallace V (1981) Aspiration around high volume, low pressure endotracheal cuff. BMJ 2:1220-1221
45. Cameron JL, Reynolds J, Zuideme DG (1973) Aspiration in patients with tracheostomies. Surg Gynecol Obstet 136:68-70
46. Spray BS, Zuideme DG, Cameron JL (1976) Aspiration pneumonia: incidence of aspiration with endotracheal tubes. Am J Surg 131:701-703
47. Huxley JE, Viroslav J, Gray RW et al (1978) Pharyngeal aspiration in normal adults and patients with depressed consciousness. Am J Med 64:564-568
48. Bishop RF, Anderson CM (1960) The bacterial flora of the stomach and small intestine in children with obstruction. Arch Dis Child 35:487-491
49. Oliveras L, Segovia A, Revuelta R (1974) Tube feeding and lethal aspiration in neurological patients: a review of 720 autopsy cases. Stroke 5:654-657
50. Cross AS, Roup B (1981) Role of respiratory assistance devices in endemic nosocomial pneumonia. Am J Med 70:681-685
51. Haley RW, Holton TM, Cutler DH et al (1981) Nosocomial infections in US hospitals, 1975-1976. Estimated frequency by selected characteristics of patients. Am J Med 70:947-959
52. Pingelton SK, Hinthorn DR, Lui C (1986) Enteral nutrition in patients receiving mechanical ventilation. Am J Med 80:827-832
53. Kingston GW, Phang PT, Leathley MJ (1991) Increased incidence of nosocomial pneumonia in mechanically ventilated patients with subclinical aspiration. Am J Surg 161:589-592
54. Winterbauer RH, Durning RB, Barron E et al (1981) Aspirated nasogastric feeding solution detected by glucose strips. Ann Intern Med 95:67-68
55. Schonhofer B, Barchfeld T, Haidl P et al (1999). Scintigraphy for evaluating early aspiration

after oral feeding in patients receiving prolonged ventilation via tracheostomy. Intensive Care Med 25:311-314
56. Benya R, Mobarhan S (1991) Enteral alimentation: administration and complications. J Am Coll Nutr 10:209-219
57. Strong RM, Condon SC, Solinger MR et al (1992) Equal aspiration rates from post pylorus and intragastric-placed small bore nasogastric-feeding tubes: a randomized prospective study. J Parent Ent Nutr 16:59-63
58. Cook DJ, Walter SD, Cook RJ et al (1998) Incidence of and risk factors for ventilator associated pneumonia in critically ill patients. Ann Intern Med 129:433-440
59. Celis R, Torres A, Gatell JM et al (1988) Nosocomial pneumonia, a multivariate analysis of risk and prognosis. Chest 93:318-324
60. Kollef MH (1993) Ventilator-associated pneumonia. A multivariate analysis. JAMA 270:1965-1970
61. Kollef MH (1995) The identification of intensive care unit-specific outcome predictors: a comparison of medical, surgical and cardiothoracic intensive care units from single institution. Heart-Lung 21:60-66
62. Potts GR, Zaroukian HM, Guierro AP et al (1993) Comparison of blue dye visualization and glucose oxidize test strip methods for detecting pulmonary aspiration of enteral feeding in intubated patients. Chest 103:117-121
63. Stanciu C, Bennet JR (1974) Oesophageal acid clearing: one factor in the production of reflux oesophagitis. Gut 15:852-857
64. Stanciu C, Bennet JR (1977) Effects of posture on gastro-oesophageal reflux. Digestion JR 15:104-109
65. Nagler R, Spiro MH (1963) Persistent gastroesophageal reflux induced during prolonged gastric intubation. N Engl J Med 269:495-550
66. Helm FJ, Dodds JW, Riedel RD et al (1983) Determinants of esophageal acid clearance in normal subjects. Gastroenterology 85:607-612
67. Fernandez-Crehuet R, Diaz Molina C, De Irala J et al (1997) Nosocomial infection in intensive care unit: identification of risk factors. Infect Control Hosp Epidemiol 18:825-830
68. Drakulovic MB, Torres A, Bauer TT et al (1999) Supine body position as a risk factor for nosocomial pneumonia in mechanically ventilated patients: a randomized trial. Lancet 354:1851-1858
69. Adnet F, Borron SW, Finot M-A et al (1999) Relation of body position at the time of discovery with suspected aspiration pneumonia in poisoned comatose patients. Crit Care Med 27:745-748.
70. Cook D, Ricard J-D, Reeve B, et al (2000) Ventilator circuit and secretion management strategies a Franco-Canadian survey. Crit Care Med 28:3547-3554
71. Tablan OC, Anderson LJ, Arden NH et al (1994) Guideline of prevention nosocomial pneumonia: Part I. Issues on prevention of nosocomial pneumonia, 1994. Infect Control Hosp Epidemiol 15:588-625
72. American Thoracic Society Ad Hoc Committee of the Scientific Assembly on Microbiology, Tuberculosis and Pulmonary Infections (1995) Hospital-acquired pneumonia in adults: diagnosis, assessment of severity, initial antimicrobial therapy and preventive strategies: a consensus statement. 153:1711-1725
73. Kollef MH (1999) The prevention of ventilator-associated pneumonia. N Engl J Med 340: 627-634
74. Reeve BK, Cook DJ (1999) Semirecumbency among mechanically ventilated patients: a multicenter observational study. Clin Intensive Care 10:241-244
75. Grap MJ, Cantley M, Munro CL et al (1999) Use of backrest elevation in critical care: a pilot study. Am J Crit Care 8:475-480
76. American Gastroenterological Association (1995) American Gastroenterological Association Medical Position Statement: Guidelines for the use of enteral nutrition. Gastroenterology 108:1280-1314

77. Cerra FB, Benitez RB, Blackburn GL et al (1997) Applied nutrition in ICU patients: a consensus statement of the American College of Chest Physicians. Chest 111:769-778
78. Preiser JC, Berre J, Carpentier Y (1999) Management of nutrition in European intensive care units: results of a questionnaire. Working Group of Metabolism and Nutrition of the European Society of Intensive Care Medicine. 25:95-101
79. Planas M (1995) Artificial nutritional support in intensive care units in Spain. The nutritional and Metabolic Working Group of the Spanish Society of Intensive Care Medicine and Coronary Units (SEMIUC). Intensive Care Med 21:842-846
80. Montejo JC (1999) Enteral nutrition-related gastrointestinal complications in critically ill patients: a multicenter study. The Nutritional and Metabolic Working Group of the Spanish Society of Intensive Care Medicine and Coronary Units. Crit Care Med 27:1447-1453
81. Pingelton SK (1989) Enteral nutrition as a risk factor for nosocomial pneumonia. Eur J Clin Microbiol Infect Dis 8:51-55
82. Grimshaw JR (1996) Towards effective professional practice. Therapie 51:233-236
83. Grimshaw JW, Hutchinson A (1995) Clinical practice guidelines- do they enhance value for money in health care? Br Med Bull 51:927-940
84. Woolf SH, Grol R, Hutchinson A et al (1999) Clinical practice guidelines: the potential benefits, limitations and harms recommending how to care for patients. BMJ 318:527-530
85. Manangan LP, Banerjee SN, Jarvis WR (2000) Association between implementation of CDC recommendations and ventilator-associated pneumonia at selected US hospitals. Am J Infect Control 28:222-227
86. Bero LA, Grilli R, Grimshaw JM et al (1998) Closing the gap between research and practice: an overview of systemic reviews of interventions to promote implementation of research findings. BMJ 317:465-468
87. Wyatt JC (2000) Practice guidelines and other support for clinical innovation. J R Soc Med 93:299-304
88. Kalleghan Si, Salemi C, Padilla S et al (1993) An effective continuous quality improvement approach to the prevention of ventilator-associated pneumonia. Am J Infect Control 21:322-330
89. Nicotra D, Ulrich C (1996) Process improvement plan for the reduction of nosocomial pneumonia in patients on ventilators. J Nurs Care Qual 10: 18-23
90. Jouner GA, Salisbury D, Bollin GE et al (1996) Utilizing quality assurance as a tool for reducing the risk of nosocomial ventilator-associated pneumonia. Am J Med Qual 11:100-103
91. Kaye J, Ashline V, Erickson D et al (2000) Clinical care bug team: a multidisciplinary team approach to reducing ventilator-associated pneumonia. Am J Infect Control 28:197-201
92. Berwick DM (1989) Continuous improvement as an ideal in health care. New Engl J Med 320:53-56
93. Kollef MH (1999) Epidemiology and risk factors for nosocomial pneumonia. Emphasis on prevention. Clin Chest Med 20:653-670
94. Hummel R, Grap MJ, Sessler CN et al (2000) Continous measurment of backrest elevation in critical-care: a research strategy. Crit Care Med 28:2621-2625

Acute Bronchial Asthma: Indications for Intensive Care

R. BRANDOLESE

Our understanding of the basic mechanisms and hence the treatment of bronchial asthma has greatly improved in recent years, such that most asthmatics are able to sustain a normal active life with simple and safe treatment [1, 2]. Nevertheless the incidence and the severity of asthma continue to increase despite advances in therapy [3], and a rise in fatal or near-fatal asthma has been reported in some Western countries [1, 4]. Although a number of explanations have been put forward, including the excessive use of bronchodilators [5, 6] and environmental factors, the reason for this unexpected increased rate is still unclear. Therefore, an acute attack is still hazardous in asthmatics, and occurs even when their monitoring and treatment have been optimized [7, 8].

In some patients acute asthma may be refractory even to aggressive therapy, so that mechanical ventilation is required [9, 10]. Based on our current understanding of ventilator-induced lung injury, ventilation of asthmatic patients has to avoid excessive lung inflation by limiting tidal volume administration and by prolonging expiratory time in order to facilitate lung emptying and to decrease dynamic pulmonary hyperinflation despite consequent hypercapnia [11]. Among more than 400 episodes of mechanical ventilation in acutely ill asthmatics patients reported in the literature for the years 1965-1984, the mortality rate was about 16%. In comparison, the mortality rate among mechanically ventilated patients with adult respiratory distress syndrome is still > 50% [12].

In all episodes of acute, severe asthma, signs of respiratory distress (tachypnea, paradoxical movement of thoracoabdominal compartment) were associated with rapid deterioration of airflow obstruction, shortly leading to severe gas exchange impairment [13, 14]. Near-fatal asthma is the consequence of asphyxia with hypercapnia and respiratory acidosis, rather than cardiac arrhythmia [15]. Arterial hyperlactatemia is frequently present during acute severe asthma and is a constant finding during treatment of a severe asthma attack. Lactate levels are as high as 7.72 mmol/l, but are of no prognostic value

[14]. Hypoxemia is a well-recognized characteristic of severe asthma. The mechanism of hypoxemia in patients with status asthmaticus requiring mechanical ventilation has been investigated by Rodriguez-Roisen et al. [16]. They demonstrated that mismatching in ventilation-perfusion ratio distribution is the major determinant of hypoxemia, whereas pulmonary shunt may be important only during 100% O_2 breathing [16]. In this connection it is noteworthy that hypoxemia may be worsened for a short interval by administration of bronchodilators, such that O_2-enriched gas flow should always be associated with medical therapy [17].

Ventilation-perfusion mismatching can also cause hypercapnia [17]. However, because of the sensitivity of the respiratory centers to changes in arterial carbon dioxide tension ($paCO_2$), any increase in $paCO_2$ will be immediately offset by an increase in alveolar and total ventilation, provided that the ventilatory pump can sustain the ventilatory mechanical load [18]. Whereas hypoxemia is due to a defect of the lung as a gas exchange organ, hypercapnia is a hallmark of failure of the ventilatory pump to sustain adequate alveolar ventilation [18].

Acute asthma is characterized by both hypoxemia and hypercapnia. Because anatomical shunt is minimal, arterial oxygen tension (paO_2) is generally improved by supplemental O_2 administration through a nasal catheter or facial mask. In contrast, worsening of $paCO_2$ can require institution of mechanical ventilation to sustain an adequate alveolar ventilation. During mechanical ventilation because of acute severe asthma, mixtures of helium/oxygen are used, and it has been observed that Heliox administration improves oxygenation, reducing the arterial-alveolar oxygen gradient $(A\text{-}a)O_2$.Therefore it is possible to reduce the inspiratory O_2 fraction in order to maximize the helium concentration and thus permit the full benefits of Heliox on lung mechanics in even the most severely ill asthmatics [18]. The institution of mechanical ventilation in patients with status asthmaticus (SA) can require muscle paralysis [19] in order to hinder baro- and/or volotrauma, to which this group of patients are particularly susceptible because of hyperinflation [20]. Severe life-threatening (SLTA) asthma needs to be identified in order to target hospital strategies to those patients presenting risk factors. In a case-control study of SLTA in adults, 70 patients with SLTA admitted to an intensive care unit were compared with 239 asthmatic subjects admitted for general medical treatment. The risk of developing SLTA increased with age and the asthmatics admitted to the intensive care unit (ICU) had experienced a hospital admission in the last year because of SLTA. No difference was noted between the two groups in sociodemographics, sex, or quality of life. In contrast, SLTA patients demonstrated deficiencies in the management of an acute attack [21]. Recent guidelines for diagnosis and treatment of severe asthma have indicated that the fundamental indication for admission of an acutely ill asthmatic patient into the ICU is a $paCO_2$ > 50 mmHg (6 7 KPa) and rapidly increasing, despite aggressive medical treatment [1, 20]. Although a rise in $paCO_2$ is such an important issue in severe asthma, the mechanism(s) of hypercapnia in asthma has not been adequately explored.

According to the classical proposal of Roussos and Lakynthinos [22], hypercapnia may be determined by three causes: (1) a depressed central drive; (2) important mechanical defects of the chest wall; (3) respiratory muscle fatigue. Although none of these conditions has been investigated directly in acute ill asthmatics patients, some results obtained during induced bronchoconstriction can provide an useful insight into possible mechanisms leading to hypercapnia in acutely ill asthmatics. Indeed it has been shown that the central drive measured by mouth occlusion pressure is increased during histamine--induced bronchospasm in both normal subjects and asthmatics, such that a depression of the respiratory centers seems unlikely in acute asthma.

Both the chest wall mechanics and the respiratory muscle contractility are normal in asthmatic patients with severe airflow obstruction [23]. However, the marked rise in lung volume determined by the massive increase in airway resistances during acute attack profoundly alters the chest wall mechanics, as well as the respiratory muscle pressure generating capability, causing respiratory muscle fatigue.

An increase in lung volume (dynamic pulmonary hyperinflation) is usually observed during a spontaneous acute attack or induced bronchoconstriction, partly because of changes in the position of the pressure-volume curve of the lung [23] and partly because of dynamic events such as: (1) the increase in airway resistance, which unduly slows the rate of lung emptying and prevents full decompression of the lung; (2) a decrease of the expiratory time related to increasing frequency of breathing (tachypnea); and (3) an increased post--inspiratory activity of inspiratory muscles (PIA) [23]. Breathing at high lung volumes enhances the elastic work of breathing. Because of the co-existing rise in airway resistance, the work of breathing can increase to a level that cannot be accomplished by the respiratory muscles, the pressure-generating capability of which is impaired by pulmonary hyperinflation, which causes changes in force-length operational range as well as in geometrical arrangement [24, 25]. The association of excessive ventilatory load and impaired ventilatory pump could lead to respiratory muscle fatigue and exhaustion, and hence to respiratory failure.

This hypothesis is suggested by some indirect evidence. Firstly, the morphological changes in the airways of asthmatics who died because of an acute attack. It has been shown that these airways are characterized by a narrow diameter, with diffuse mucus plugging in the lumen, massive inflammation of the bronchial wall, and bronchial smooth muscle hypertrophy [26]. These morphological changes account for the massive rise in flow resistance observed in spontaneous and induced bronchospasm, as well as in the few actual measurements performed in mechanically ventilated asthmatics, such as those reported in Table 1.

Table1. Respiratory mechanics in three young asthmatic patients during the 1st day of mechanical ventilation in the control mode

Variable	Patient 1	Patient 2	Patient 3
Sex	F	F	F
Age (years)	36	17	28
$\dot{V}E$ $l \cdot min^{-1}$	8.4	9.5	9.6
f $b \cdot min^{-1}$	12	13	12
VT l	0.70	0.73	0.80
TE s	3.1	2.9	3.7
PEEPi cmH_2O	12.9	13.9	8.0
ΔFRC l	0.81	0.30	0.48
Crs $l \times cmH_2O$-1	0.044	0.060	0.040
Rrs $cmH_2O \times l^{-1} \cdot s$	36.5	17.8	33.1

VE: Minute ventilation; f = ventilatory frequency; V_T = inflation volume; TE= expiratory time; PEEPi = intrinsic positive end-expiratory pressure; ΔFRC=difference between the static equilibrium volume of the respiratory system and the functional residual capcity during mechanical ventilation; Crs = static respiratory compliance; Rrs = respiratory resistance after subtraction of endotracheal tube and measuring equipment; Each measurement represents the average of 5-7 breaths. Patients were receiving therapy.

These data also show that the severe rise in resistance was associated with a predictable, remarkable degree of dynamic pulmonary hyperinflation, i.e., the end-expiratory lung volume was well above the relaxed functional residual capacity (FRC). This is further illustrated in Fig. 1 in which an intrinsic positive end-expiratory pressure (PEEPi) amounting to 20 cm H_2O is also shown. It has been recognized that PEEPi is systematically associated with dynamic pulmonary hyperinflation in mechanically ventilated patients with severe airway obstruction [27]. Figure 1 shows that both dynamic hyperinflation and PEEPi are significantly reduced by epinephrine administration (0.1 mg i.v.) because of the potent relaxant effect on bronchial smooth muscle.

Clearly these findings in mechanically ventilated asthmatics support the hypothesis of impending respiratory muscle fatigue because of heavy ventilatory load, i. e., the increased flow resistance plus the inspiratory threshold load due to PEEPi [28] has to be faced, while the respiratory muscle contractility is jeopardized by pulmonary hyperinflation. However, the paper of Wheatley et

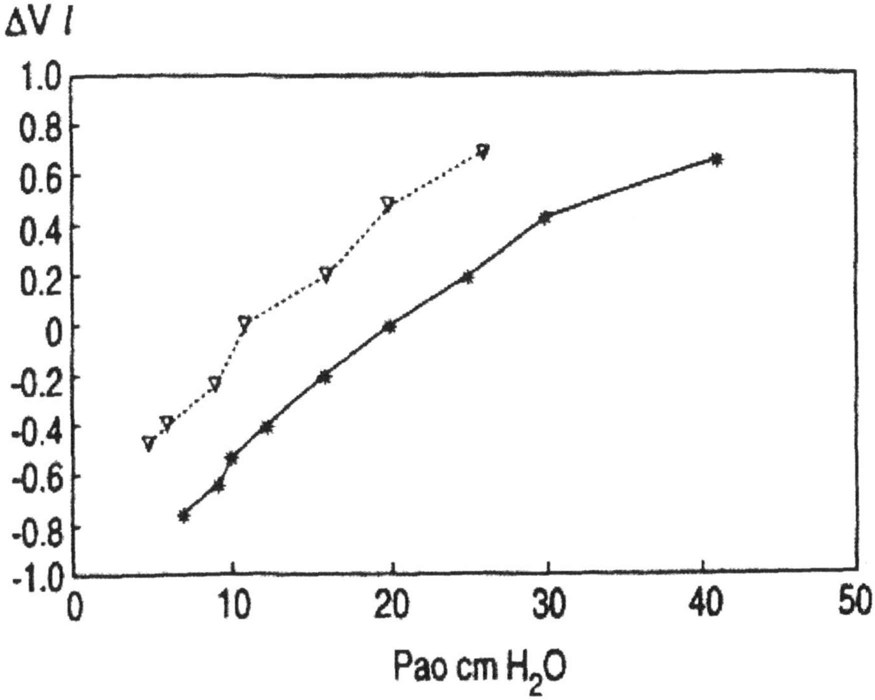

Fig. 1 Static relationship between volume (V) and pressure at the airway opening (Pao) in a critically ill asthmatic patient (female, 32 years) on the 1st day of (controlled) mechanical ventilation, before (*) and after (∇) 0.1 mg of adrenaline i.v. Experimental points have been obtained with the interrupter technique during relaxed expiration. ΔV=0 represents the end-expiratory lung volume during regular mechanical ventilation. The value of Pao at ΔV=0 provides the level of intrinsic positive end-expiratory pressure (PEEPi). Since the patient is dynamically hyperinflated, the relaxed expiration continues well below the end-expiratory lung volume during regular ventilation. However, although the expiratory time was about 30 s, the static equilibrium volume was not reached, because of the extremely high flow resistance. Adrenaline produced an important bronchodilatation as shown by the decrease of PEEPi from 20 to 10 cmH_2O, without changes in the slope of the ΔV=Pao relationship

al. [23] is noteworthy, raising the possibility that hyperinflation in asthmatics might be advantageous, not only by improving the airway patency and inspired gas distribution while decreasing the inspiratory flow resistive work, but also by minimizing the total respiratory muscle work and hence minimizing energy expenditure.

The results reported in Table 1 and Fig. 1 have important implications for mechanical ventilation in asthma. Firstly, the evidence of marked pulmonary hyperinflation support the conclusion of Darioli and Perret [29] that controlled hypoventilation might be indicated in acutely and severely ill asthmatics, in order to prevent pulmonary barotrauma due to excessively high volumes. Secondly, the ventilatory setting should be adjusted in order to minimize PEEPi and its adverse hemodynamic, cardiac, and mechanical effects. Thirdly, detection of PEEPi is important for two reasons: (1) application of external PEEP, if a patient is flow limited, lower than the pre-existing value of PEEPi might help to unload the respiratory muscles with the ventilatory modes requiring the patient's co-operation, e. g. assist ventilation, pressure support ventilation etc.; and (2) low level of external PEEP might be used with face mask ventilation during severe asthma attacks to prevent tracheal intubation [30, 31].

Severe hypoxemia, signs of respiratory distress, and rapidly deteriorating airflow obstruction are important indications to keep acutely ill, asthmatic patients under close observation and to use aggressive medical treatment. If, despite that therapy, $paCO_2$ reaches 50 mmHg and rises, mechanical ventilation support is required. It is fundamental to reduce the risk of life-threatening asthma and admission to ICU. In a study the impact of inhaled corticosteroids and beta agonists on the risk of life-threatening asthma was evaluated. Using multi-regression analysis it was demonstrated that a high level of inhaled beta-agonists was related to an increased risk of ICU admission, whereas a high level of inhaled corticosteroids was associated with a decreased a risk of ICU admission. [32]. The prognosis of asthma in adults is not as well described as that of chronic obstructive pulmonary disease. Longitudinal studies indicate that severe asthma has a poor prognosis, with the development of permanent lung function impairment and hospitalization and mortality. Asthmatic patients with previous admission to ICU are at high risk of severe asthma complications [33]. Therefore it is mandatory to identify those asthmatic patients who are at risk of developing SLTA in order to institute, promptly, an adequate treatment.

References

1. Guidelines for the diagnosis and management of asthma. National Institutes of Health (1991) National Institutes of Health, Bethesda, Md.
2. Higenbottam T, Hay I (1990) Has the treatment of asthma improved ? Chest: 98: 706-712
3. Hanael JL, Barber RG (1998) Critical management of the asthmatic patient. Curr Opin Pulm Med 4: 48-54
4. Buist AS, Vollmer WM (1990) Reflections on the rise in asthma morbidity and mortality: J Am Med Assoc 264: 1719-1720
5. Burrows B, Lebowitz MD (1992) The beta agonists dilemma. N Engl J Med 326:560-561
6. Spitzer WO, Suissa S, Ernest P et al (1992) The use of beta agonists and the risk of death and near death from asthma. N Engl J Med 326:503-506
7. Saetta M, Thiene G, Crescioli S, et al (1989) Asthma in a young patient with severe bronchial hyper responsiveness but stable peak flow records. Eur Respir J 2: 1008-1012
8. Pouw EM, Koeter GH, de Monchy JGR, et al (1990) Clinical assessment after a life-threatening attack of asthma: the role of bronchial hyperreactivity. Eur Respir J 3:861-866
9. Branthwhite MA (1990) An update on mechanical ventilation for severe acute asthma. Clin Intensive Care 1: 4-6

10. Armstrong RF, Bullen C, Cohen SL, et al (1990) Critical care algorithms of acute asthma. Clin Intensive Care 1: 46-47
11. Levy BD, Kitch B, Fanta CH (1998) Medical and ventilatory management of status asthmaticus. Intensive Care Med 24: 105-117
12. Gattinoni L, Brazzi L, Pesenti A (1991) Extracorporeal carbon dioxide removal in ARDS. In: Marini JJ Roussos C (eds) Update in intensive care and emergency medicine. Ventilatory Failure. Springer Verlag, Berlin Heidelberg New York, pp 308-317
13. Perret C (1989) Sudden asphyxia in asthma. In: Vincent JL (eds) Update in intensive care and emergency medicine. Springer Verlag, Berlin Heidelberg New York, pp 86-90
14. Rabbat A, Laaban JP, Boussairi A, Rochemaure J (1998) Hyperlactatemia during acute severe asthma. Intensive Care Med 24:304-312
15. Molfino NA, Nannini LJ, Martelliu AN, Slutsky AS (1991) Respiratory arrest in near fatal asthma. N Engl J Med 324: 285-288
16. Rodriguez-Roisen R, Ballester E, Roca J, et al (1989) Mechanism of hypoxaemia in patients with status asthmaticus requiring mechanical ventilation. Am Rev Respir Dis 139:732-739
17. West JB (1988) Respiratory physiology, ventilation, blood flow, and gas exchange. In: Murray J, Nadel J (eds) Textbook of respiratory medicine, vol.1. Saunders. Philadelphia, pp 47-84
18. Schaeffer EM, Pohlman A, Morgan S, Hall JB (1999) Oxygenation in status asthmaticus improves during ventilation with helium and oxygen. Crit Care Med 27: 2666-2670
19. Lemos JM de, Carr RR, Shalansky KF, et al (1999) Paralysis in critically ill: intermittent bolus pancuronium compared to continuous infusion. Crit Care Med: 2648-2655
20. Khadadah ME, Onadeko BO, Mustafa HT, Metwali KE (2000) Clinical feature and outcome of management of severe acute asthma in intensive care unit. Singapore Med J 41: 199-201
21. Kolbe J, Fergusson W, Vamos M, Garrett J (2000) Case control study of severe life threatening asthma (SLTA) in adults: demografic, health care and management of acute attack. Thorax Dec 55: 1007-1015
22. Roussos C, Lakynthinos S (1991) Ventilatory muscle fatigue and failure. In: Update into intensive care and emergency medicine. Springer Verlag, Berlin Heidelberg New York, pp 125-152
23. Wheatley JR, West S, Cala SJ, Engel LA (1990) The effect of hyperinflation on respiratory muscle work in acute induced asthma. Eur Respir J 3: 625-632
24. Cormier Y, Lecours R, Legis C (1990) Mechanism of hyperinflation in asthma. Eur Respir J 3: 619-624
25. Decramer M (1989) Effects of hyperinflation on the respiratory muscles. Eur Respir J 2: 299-302
26. Saetta M, Di Stefano A, Rosina C, et al (1991) Quantitative structural analysis of peripheral airways and arteries in sudden fatal asthma. Am Rev Respir Dis 143: 138-143
27. Broseghini C, Brandolese R, Poggi R, et al (1991) Respiratory mechanics during first day of mechanical ventilation in patients with pulmonary edema and chronic airway obstruction. Am Rev Respir Dis 143: 138-143
28. Gottfried SB, Rossi A, Milic-Emili J (1986) Dynamic hyperinflation, intrinsic PEEP, and mechanically ventilated patients. Intensive Care Dig 5: 30-33
29. Darioli R, Perret C (1984) Mechanical controlled hypoventilation in status asthmaticus. Am Rev Respir Dis 129: 385-387
30. Rossi A, Brandolese R, Milic-Emili J, Gottfried SB (1990) The role of PEEP in patients with chronic obstructive pulmonary disease during assisted ventilation. Eur Respir J 3: 818-822
31. Donner CF, Appendini L, Patessio A, et al (1992) Continuous positive airway pressure (CPAP) improves the efficiency of pressure support mask ventilation with acute respiratory failure. Am Rev Respir Dis 145: 526-530
32. Eisner MD, Lieu TA, Chi F et al (2001) Beta agonists, inhaled steroids and the risk of intensive care admission for asthma. Eur Respir J 17: 233-240
33. Lange P (1999) Prognosis of adult asthma. Monaldi Arch Chest Dis 54: 350-352

Esophageal Pressure in Anaesthetized Patients: Difficulties and Frequent Mistakes

J.O.C. AULER JR., C.R. FERNANDES

Indirect measurement of pleural pressure, with the use of a balloon inserted in the esophagus, had been initially proposed by Luciani in 1878, nevertheless, this procedure only became popular from the work of Buytendijk in 1949 [1]. Measurement of esophageal pressure (Pes) is an extremely useful method for the evaluation of respiratory mechanics (chest wall and lung). Several investigations allowed to estimate the values of elasticity and resistance of the lung and thoracic wall.

There are three methods for recording of esophageal pressure:

1. Through the introduction of a balloon-catheter in the stomach. A thin esophageal balloon, coupled to a catheter, is inflated with air and connected to a pressure transducer in its distal extremity;
2. Through a catheter filled up with liquid, adequately positioned in the esophagus and distally coupled to an appropriate pressure transducer; and
3. Through the use of small micro-transducers directly positioned in the interior of the stomach [2].

The widely employed technique for the measurement of esophageal pressure comprises the use of a balloon-catheter system compatible with standard dimensions. The perimeter of the balloon should ideally correspond to the perimeter of the esophagus (4 to 4.8 cm for adult humans). In practice, latex balloons, 0.1 mm thick and 5 to 10 cm long, with a perimeter of 3.2 to 4.8 cm are the most appropriate. In adult patients, 100 cm long polyethylene catheters with an inside diameter of 1.4 mm are conventionally used [1]. Adequate systems exist for children and infant patients.

Difficulties

Positioning of the esophageal balloon

One of the most difficult and important stages of the procedure is the appropriate positioning of the balloon into the esophagus of an anaesthetized patient in supine position, in order that the measurement of pleural pressure is obtained as accurately as possible. Errors previously committed in the right positioning of the patient resulted in errors in the indirect measure of the pleural pressure and distortions in the calculation of respiratory mechanics.

In their study, carried out in non-anaesthetized human patients in supine and prone positions, Knowles JH et al. [3] found contradictory values of esophageal pressure suggesting that in the supine position such a difference of values could be due to a compression of the stomach exerted by mediastinum contents, particularly the heart, and inferred that values of the esophageal pressure obtained from this position could not accurately reproduce the pleural pressure.

Baydur A et al. [4] confirmed the technique of an esophageal balloon, conventionally situated 10 cm far from the cardia, by means of an "occlusion test" performed in non-anaesthetized patients in different conditions of sitting and lateral and supine positions. The authors have concluded that the measures of esophageal pressure in certain individuals in the supine position, with the balloon conventionally positioned, did not reveal any changes in the pressure of the pleural surface [4]. Only with the re-positioning of the balloon at a different level location could be found where the "occlusion test", through simultaneous measurements of esophageal and mouth pressures, could approximate the unit. Exclusively in this location the estimate of pulmonary mechanics, based on esophageal pressure, would be presumably valid.

Considering the difficulty of introducing the balloon with the patient under anaesthesia and muscle relaxation, the precise definition of the correct positioning of the balloon-catheter in order that the pressure of the pleural surface is correctly transmitted, the majority of studies execute the positioning before the anaesthetic induction. In an awaken patient, the balloon is introduced as far as the stomach; progressively, the balloon is removed at the negative curve that signals the cardia localization. Approximating 10 centimeters more of the balloon is then withdrawn from this point, in order to make it lodged in the conventional position for an adequate measurement of the pleural pressure. In their attempt to validate the balloon technique in paralysed patients, Westbrook et al. [5] and Rehder et al. [6] carried out a manual compression of the thorax with occluded airways, having detected records that made them believe that esophageal pressure (ΔPes) and tracheal pressure (ΔPt) were rather similar, however, quantitative data was not tailored.

Higgs et al. [7] executed similar indirect measurements of pleural pressure with the introduction of an esophageal catheter in anaesthetized patients with halothane 1CAM, nitrous oxide 70% and oxygen. Patients were kept under spontaneous breathing and simultaneous measures of the tracheal and esophageal pressures were carried out with the use of the "occlusion test". With the balloon conventionally positioned 10 centimeters from the cardia, the authors were capable of finding an adequate correlation between ΔPes and ΔPt in the majority of individuals. However, in some individuals a re-positioning of the balloon was necessary. The authors have concluded that the balloon technique, used in anaesthetized patients in supine position, can reliably reproduce the measurement of changes occurred in the pleural pressure [7].

Other authors [8, 9] have used the "occlusion test" in the supine position before induction of anaesthesia for the purpose of validating the balloon technique while it was maintained and fixed in this position.

Pelosi et al. [10] studied two groups of normal and obese individuals: in both groups, with patients under anaesthesia and before muscular paralysis, confirmation of the measurement of esophageal pressure was verified in the supine position through the "occlusion test" during the occurrence of a few respiratory strains. In obese patients the correct position of the balloon was adjusted through thorax X-ray.

Ruiz et al. [11] fixed the catheter in the position where a maximal variation of esophageal pressure had been found during ventilation under positive pressure.

There are few studies which verify the positioning of the balloon in patients under anaesthesia and muscle relaxation. It is known that during the supine position mediastinum structures come down over the esophagus that is further increased with muscular relaxation. It is therefore questioned whether the values of the esophageal pressure accurately reveal the indirect measure of the pleural pressure with the same positioning of the balloon and before muscular relaxants are administered.

We have recently carried out a comparative study between pleural and esophageal pressures in 9 anaesthetized and paralysed patients submitted to coronary bypass grafting. All patients had their chest cavity drained due to mammary internal artery dissection. An esophageal balloon was conventionally maintained at a 10 cm distance from the cardia, as confirmed by thorax X-ray, and the volume of the balloon consisted of 1 ml of air. Measurement of esophageal pressure was carried out by means of a long and multi-perforated drain positioned into the left pleural inter-space at the level of the medium axillary line. Simultaneous measurements of pleural and esophageal pressures were carried out in different levels of the end expiratory positive pressure (PEEP) in the supine position and under different degrees of supine thorax elevation, i.e., 45 and 60 degrees with a PEEP of 5 cm of H_2O. It has been identified that the measurement of the esophageal pressure, with the balloon conventionally positioned 10 cm far from the cardia, exclusively corresponds to the pleural pressure in anaesthetized and paralysed patients in supine position when a medium PEEP of 5 to 10 cm of H_2O is applied, or when the patient is in a half-sitting position of 45 and 60 degrees. Measurement of the esophageal pressure in adult human patients, under anaesthesia and paralysed and in the supine position, ventilated with zero end expiratory pressure (ZEEP) or with high levels of PEEP (15 cm of H_2O), does not correspond to the measurement of pleural pressure [12].

Introduction of the catheter into the esophagus

In the majority of cases related in the literature, positioning of the balloon is usually performed before anaesthetic induction, due to the flexibility of the catheter, which requires indispensable co-operation of the patient in swallowing and adequate positioning. Another alternative, for the introduction of the catheter in anaesthetized individuals, is a rigid tube of latex that is driven throughout the stomach and positioned at a distance of 35 to 40 cm from the superior dental arcade. The eligible position of the balloon must be precisely confirmed through a thorax X-ray.

Manoeuvres of manual compression of the thorax in paralysed patients, associated with occluded airways carried out with the purpose of simultaneous recording of esophageal (ΔPes) and tracheal pressures (ΔPt), are in our observation inconsistent for an adequate positioning of the balloon in view that contingent on thorax morphology, weight and physical structure of individuals as well as on the existence of developed mammary glands. These values could be considerably controversial [12].

Measurement errors

Equipment

In order to avoid errors, the system for signal monitoring should be appropriate and installation procedures should be precise. This system comprises pressure transducers coupled to a signal conditioner that is, in turn, connected to an analogic digital converter, and very often to specific software, for carrying out estimates and recording. An accurate selection of transducers should be made considering that measures do not admit a significant margin of error. Therefore, high sensibility piezoelectric transducers would be the most adequate.

Equipment employed for protocol procedures should be properly adjusted and calibrated before it is used and set at regular intervals as well. Furthermore, the accuracy of the measurements and the margin of tolerance of errors should be thoroughly recognized. The equipment must be calibrated by certified equipment bearing valid connections with recognized domestic and international standards. There must be a definition for methods and procedures and calibration records should be carefully kept. Appropriate environmental conditions should be offered for calibration and measurement procedures during the execution of the protocol. Adequate conditions for the handling, preservation and storage of the equipment for the purpose of maintaining the precision and accuracy of the calibration is mandatory.

The most common errors, that cause inaccurate measures of pressure, are possibly related either to an incorrect choice of equipment and/or to its inadequate calibration. The narrow range of values does not admit tolerance; negligible measurement mistakes are significantly important in the achievement of final results.

Inflation of the balloon

The importance of the volume of air in the interior of the balloon is recognized by the fact that increased volumes are predisposed to high pressures and potential sources of measurement errors. A curve of compliance of the balloon should be achieved in order to eliminate this variable that eventually interferes with final results. With a calibrated syringe, a three-way stopcock and a calibrated transducer, a pressure-volume curve must be executed with the addition of 0.1 ml of air. In general, the curve becomes flat with volumes between 0.2 and 5 ml of air. Ideally, the administration of 0.5 ml of air would be preferable for the inflation of the balloon as well as adequate pressure measurements [1]. Before each inspection the volume of air in the interior of the balloon should be considered to discard whatever possibility of drainage.

Cardiac bruit

Heartbeat distorts the curves of esophageal pressure, particularly accentuated in the individuals in supine position, independent of the method that has been employed. Heartbeat bruit could be minimized with the use of wide balloons, smaller than 10 cm and with a perimeter of 4.8 cm, positioned in a specific location of the esophagus where cardiac artifacts are less noticeable [4]. The existence of signal conditioners would be fundamental for enabling the filtering of this noise without interfering with the absolute values of the pressure curves. Another alternative would be through the estimates carried out by specific software that considers the midrange of heartbeat signals and takes into the account the cardiac cycle period.

Mechanical ventilation

In anaesthetized and paralysed individuals, mechanically controlled and under ventilation, the absence of PEEP or the use of high PEEP values result in significant differences between esophageal and pleural pressures giving origin to errors in respiratory mechanics; therefore a PEEP between 5 to 10 cm of H_2O is used to approximate Pes and Ppl values.

Esophageal wave

During esophageal contraction not only is the baseline of the esophageal pressure increased but also the amplitude. These contractions are easily detected and data should not be considered unless Pes has returned to its baseline. These curves are different than those shown in the respiratory cycle and their presence can be, within a certain frequency, evidenced.

Conclusion

In our experience the esophageal balloon catheter method is a reliable tool to obtain pleural pressure measures in anaesthetized and paralysed patients. However, some points should be observed

1. The correct positioning of the balloon part of the catheter in the lower third of the esophagus should be checked.
2. In anaesthetized paralysed patients, together with respiratory manoeuvres, thoracic X-ray is useful to check the right positioning of esophageal catheter.
3. The compliance curve of the balloon should be used to fill the correct volume of air.
4. In mechanical ventilated patients the best correlation between pleural and esophageal pressure was observed with PEEP levels varying from 5 to 10 cm of water.
5. High sensitive transducers and reliable equipment should be employed to obtain the data from esophageal pressure.

References

1. Zin WA, Milic-Emili J (1998) Esophageal pressure measurement. In: Tobin MJ (Ed) Principles and Practice of Intensive Care Monitoring. McGraw-Hill, New York pp 545-552
2. Gilbert R, Peppi D, Auchinloss JH (1979) Measurement of transdiaphragmatic pressure with a single gastric-esophageal probe. J Appl Physiol 47:628-30.
3. Knowles JH, Hong SK, Rahn H (1958) Possible error using esophageal balloon in determination of pressure-volume characteristics of the lung and thoracic cage. J Appl Physiol 14:525-530
4. Baydur A, Behrakis PK, Zin WA et al (1982) Simple method for assessing the validity of the esophageal balloon technique. Am Rev Respir Dis 126:788-91
5. Westbrook PR, Stubbs SE, Sessler AD et al (1973) Effects of anesthesia and muscle paralysis on respiratory mechanics in normal man. J Appl Physiol 34:81-86.
6. Rehder K, Mallow JE, Fibuch EE et al (1974) Effects of isoflurane anesthesia and muscle paralysis on respiratory mechanics in normal man. Anesthesiol 41:477-485
7. Higgs BD, Behrakis PK, Bevan DR et al (1983) Measurement of pleural pressure with esophageal balloon in anesthetized humans 59:340-343
8. Baydur A, Sassoon CSH, Stiles CM (1987) Partitioning of respiratory mechanics in young adults: Effects of duration of anesthesia. Am Rev Respir Dis 135:165-172
9. D'Angelo E, Robatto FM, Calderini E et al (1991) Pulmonary and chest wall mechanics in anesthetized paralyzed humans. 70:2602-2610
10 Pelosi P, Crossi M, Ravagnan I et al (1996) Total respiratory system, lung, and chest wall mechanics in sedated-paralyzed postoperative morbidly obese patients. Chest 109:144-151
11. Ruiz Neto PP, Auler Jr JOC (1992) Respiratory mechanical properties during fentanyl and alfentanil anaesthesia. Can J Anaesth 39:458-65
12. Fernandes C, Auler Jr JOC (2001) Comparative study between esophageal and pleural pressure in anesthetized humans at different levels of PEEP. Abstract (accepted) ASA Meeting – New Orleans – October 2001. (Anesthesiology in press)

Haemodynamic and Metabolic Evaluations by Rebreathing Methods

M. GIRARDIS, C. LOMBARDINI, A. PASETTO

Cardiac output (CO) is a key parameter to assess the haemodynamic status, the cardiac performance and the therapeutic management in critical patients. In anaesthesia and intensive care practice, the methods most often used to measure CO are the classical thermodilution by a pulmonary artery catheter and the transpulmonary thermodilution by a femoral artery catheter [1, 2]. These methods are invasive and require a time period for catheter positioning. Therefore, they can not be used in low-risk patients and in emergency wards. Trans-esophageal echo-Doppler, even if less invasive, is expensive and requires high skilled personnel [2]. To solve the above limitations, new methods have been proposed to measure CO at the bedside. Rebreathing methods seem to be ideal in mechanically ventilated patients because they are non-invasive, continuous, not time consuming and inexpensive. The physiological basis, the different techniques and the clinical application of rebreathing methods will be discussed in the following paragraphs.

Rebreathing techniques

Rebreathing methods, regardless of the tracer gas and the technique used, involves the lungs as a tonometer that estimates the concentration of physiological (e.g., O_2 and CO_2) or chemically inert, soluble gases in arterial (Cax) and mixed venous blood (Cvx). In addition, the analysis of alveolar gases allows to measure the uptake or excretion (Vx) of the tracer gas [3]. Therefore, according to the Fick principle and under a steady state condition, the blood flow through the lungs (i.e., pulmonary capillary blood flow, PCBF) can be calculated as follows:

PCBF = Vx * (Cax-Cvx) [1]

Indeed, rebreathing methods are able to measure the pulmonary blood flow that effectively participates in gas exchange. Therefore, PCBF is the equal to right cardiac output (CO) minus right to left shunts (Qshunt):

PCBF = CO – Qshunt [2].

In normal subjects, anatomical and physiological shunts account for less than 6% of CO at rest and less than 3% during exercise, a value within the experimental error of the methods currently used for measuring CO [4]. Therefore, in normal subjects PCBF is assumed to be equivalent to CO. By contrast, in critical patients Qshunt is normally larger than 10% and varies with the pulmonary and cardiovascular conditions. Oxygen concentration (O2) in inspired mixture, end-expiratory positive pressure, ventilatory mode and posture further affect the entity of pulmonary shunt and venous admixture. Therefore, PCBF can be significantly different from total CO and a parallel method for estimating Qshunt is needed to calculate CO from alveolar gas analysis [3].

As regards to the parameters of equation 1, Vx is generally measured by monitoring the inspired and expired volumes of tracer gas over a finite period or on a breath by breath basis. Cax is estimated from the partial pressure of gases in alveoli, the alveolar to arterial pressure difference and the solubility constant (when inert gases are used), or by the dissociation curve (when dealing with O_2 and CO_2). The crucial step is the determination of Cvx. In most rebreathing techniques using inert gases, it can be assumed that Cvx is essentially zero. Due to the infrequent application in clinical practice, these methods will not be reviewed in the paper [3]. Similar to inert gases, partial CO_2 rebreathing technique eliminates the need for measuring $CvCO_2$ since it is assumed unchanged during the rebreathing manoeuvre [4] (see below). The different techniques for estimating Cvx both using O_2 and CO_2 will be described in the following paragraphs.

O_2 *techniques*

In the O2 rebreathing technique, the subject rebreathes from a bag with a volume equivalent to a functional residual capacity containing CO2 (8-10%) and N2 (90-92%) [5]. Six to eight seconds from the onset of rebreathing, alveolar PO2 (PAO2) achieves a plateau that is maintained up to additional 5-10 s. PAO2 values at the plateau is believed to reflect PO2 in mixed venous blood (PvO2). To convert PvO2 to O2 concentration (CvO2), the haemoglobin concentration and blood pH should be measured or assumed. CaO2 can be directly measured by gas analysis of arterial blood or derived by the assessment of the peripheral O2 blood saturation. VO2 is normally measured before the rebreathing manoeuvre in a steady state condition. Apart for the complexity of the procedure and the calculations, this technique has never been applied in critically ill patients because it can induce hypoxia, and pulmonary V/Q ratio inhomogeneities impair the achievement and the shape of the PAO2 plateau before recirculation.

CO_2 *techniques*

Compared to O_2, CO_2 as tracer gas presents several advantages: 1) CO_2 is absent in inspired gases; 2) CO_2 is an high-soluble gas, thereby PCO_2 in alveolar gas ($PACO_2$) is equivalent to PCO_2 in arterial blood ($PaCO_2$) and 3) the slope of CO_2 dissociation curve is linear in a large physiological range, thereby the $CxCO_2$ can be easily calculated as long as the pH and oxyhaemoglobin concentration are provided or unchanged during rebreathing. As mentioned above, the volume of CO_2 expired by unit of time (VCO_2) and the concentration of CO_2 in arterial blood can be easily estimated by the analysis of expired flow and CO_2 in expired gases. This is usually performed before the rebreathing manoeuvre in all but one of the techniques proposed by Farhi et al. [6]. To estimate PCO_2 in mixed venous blood three different manoeuvres are available: breath holding, single breath and total rebreathing. These three methods induce a transitory interruption of CO_2 elimination that leads to $PACO_2$ increasing toward $PvCO_2$, up to recirculation.

Breath Holding

PvCO2 is estimated by breath holding at different intervals or by varying CO2 in an inspired mixture and at breath-holding times. These manoeuvres provide the relationship between PACO2 and the gas-exchange ratio (R). The extrapolated point for $R = 0$ (i.e., the point at which gas exchange has stopped or at PCO2 equilibrium) is the value of oxygenated PvCO2. This method requires a high degree of subject co-operation and assumes that both VCO2 and CO remain constant over the period needed to construct the curve between PACO2 and R. Although this method has been proposed in ventilated patients, today it is not utilized [7].

Single Breath Expirate

This interesting method is based on the continuous analysis of PO2 and PCO2 during a single slow exhalation [8, 9]. The instantaneous R can be easily measured by dividing the instantaneous values of PCO2 by the corresponding values of PO2 and then plotting the corresponding values of PCO2. PvCO2 can be estimated by R is equal to 0.32, which is the equilibrium point between PaCO2 and PaO2 (Haldane effect). A few assumptions should be made for an accurate estimation of CO by this technique: a linear relationship between PACO2 and R, the lung tissue does not buffer CO2 and the later expiration gases have a longer contact with capillary blood. The latter assumption is valid in a normal resting subject, but is not valid in a patient with impaired V/Q distribution. Therefore, this method has never been used for clinical measurements.

Total Rebreathing

The subject rebreathes from a bag containing a mixture of CO_2 and O_2 (to avoid dangerous hypoxemia during the manoeuvre) at a specific rate and for approximately 20 seconds. A PCO_2 plateau value of CO_2 (i.e., the $PvCO_2$) is normally achieved within 6 seconds and indicates the equilibrium between capillary blood and alveolar gases. If a plateau is not obtained during the rebreathing manoeuvre, the measurement can be repeated by changing the volume of the bag or, alternatively, $PvCO_2$ can be estimated by extrapolation with an error lower than 2%. This method has been largely utilized in normal subjects both at rest and during exercise. This method is also in agreement with other literature. In a patient with cardiopulmonary dysfunction, total rebreathing showed a good precision only if $PaCO_2$ was measured directly [10-13]. In fact, the pulmonary V/Q mismatching may lead to a significant difference between end-tidal and arterial PCO_2, because of an increasing alveolar dead space fraction. It goes without saying that in critical patients the estimation of $PvCO_2$ is more reliable than the non-invasive estimation of $PaCO_2$.

One-step rebreathing method

The one-step rebreathing method has been developed to overcome the problems associated with other techniques and to measure all the variables needed for CO calculation in one step. The patient rebreathes (20-25 seconds) from a bag containing a known volume of CO_2 with a tidal volume and rate that leads to an initial drop of $PACO_2$. Thereafter, $PACO_2$ rises to a plateau and breath by breath analysis of expired CO_2 allows the calculation of VCO_2 and $PvCO_2$. To eliminate the bias of the change in lung CO_2 stores, $PACO_2$ ought to restore pre-rebreathing values within 10 seconds of rebreathing. If this is not the case, the rebreathing should be repeated with a different CO_2 volume in the bag [6]. So far, no data on the application of this method in critical patients has been published.

Partial rebreathing

To eliminate the need for a $PvCO_2$ estimation, a new CO_2 rebreathing technique was proposed [4-14]. By inserting a system consisting of a three-way valve and of a dead space between the mouth of the subject and the atmosphere, the patient rebreathes only a part of his exhaled gas. This leads to a reduction of CO_2 elimination and an increase of $PACO_2$. Therefore, CO is obtained by measuring the changes in VCO_2 and $PACO_2$ and by applying the differential form of the Fick equation. Since this technique causes an increase in blood CO_2 lower than that observed during total rebreathing, does not require an inspired special mixture and can be frequently repeated, it was recently automated in a CO monitor for clinical use ($NICO_2$). The validity of this technique relies on the assumption that $PvCO_2$ and dead space fraction (see above) did not change during the rebreathing, and that Qshunt can be estimated by inspired and arterial PO_2. Unfortunately, these assumptions are invalid in many circumstances, particularly in critically ill patients with pulmonary impairment. More insight for the application of partial rebreathing in the clinical field is needed.

The major disadvantages of using CO_2 as a tracer gas can be summarized as follows: 1) $PACO_2$ can be significantly different from $PaCO_2$ during exercise and in pulmonary diseases because of increasing of alveolar dead space; therefore, $PaCO_2$ must be measured directly by arterial blood; 2) the $PvCO_2$ estimation often requires a cumbersome calculation and 3) the arterial to mixed venous CO_2 difference and VCO_2 are very sensitive to changes in ventilation; hence, a slight deviation from a steady state condition can lead to a inaccurate CO determination.

In conclusion, rebreathing methods can not be considered an appropriate non-invasive alternative to CO monitoring in anaesthesia and intensive care practice because they only estimate the effective non-shunted PCBF. In a patient with cardiopulmonary diseases, PCBF is significantly lower than CO and non-invasive assessment of Qs is highly inaccurate. In spite of this, rebreathing methods may be useful non-invasive tool to optimize the ventilatory management (i.e., PEEP level) and for the metabolic monitoring (VO_2 and VCO_2) of critical patients.

References

1. Nilsson LB, Eldrup N, Berthelsen PG (2001) Lack of agreement between thermodiluition and carbon dioxide-rebreathing cardaic output. Acta Anaestesiol Scand 45(6): 680-685
2. BinderJC, Parkin WG (2001) Non-invasive cardiac output determination: comparison of a new partial-rebreathing technique with thermodilution Anesth Intensive Care 29(1): 19-23
3. Sackner MA (1968) Measurement of cardiac output by alveolar gas exchange. Hand of physiology-The respiratory system IV, chapter 13: 233-255
4. de Abreu MG, Quintel M, Ragaller M, Albrecht DM (1997) Partial carbon dioxide rebreathing: a reliable technique for noninvasive measurement of non shunted pulmonary capillary blood flow. Crit Care Med Apr 25(4): 675-683
5. Cerretelli E, Cruz JC, Farhi LE, Rahn H (1996) Determination of mixed venous O_2 and CO_2 tension and cardiac output by a rebreathing method. Resp Physiol 1: 258- 264

6. Farhi LE, Nesarajah MS, Olszowka AJ et al (1976) Cardiac output determination by simple one-step rebreathing technique. Respir Physiol 28:141-159
7. Knowles JE, Newman W, Fenn WO (1960) Determination of oxygenated mixed venous blood CO_2 tension by a breath holding method. J Appl Physiol 32: 782-787
8. Kim TS, Rahn H, Farhi LE (1966) Estimation of the true venous and arterial PCO_2 by gas analysis of a single breath. J Appl Physiol 21: 1338-1344
9. Arnold JH, Stenz RI, Thomson JH, Arnold LW (1996) Noninvasive determination of cardiac output using single breath CO_2 analysis. Crit Care Med 24: 1071-1705
10. Mahler DA, Matthay RA, Snyder PE et al (1985) Determination of cardiac output at rest and during exercise by carbon dioxide rebreathing method in obstructive airway disease. Am Rev Respir Dis 131: 73-78
11. Clausen JP, Larsen OA, Trap-Jensen J (1970) Cardiac output in middle-aged patients determined with CO_2 rebreathing method. J Appl Physiol 28: 337-342
12. Davis CC, Jones NL, Seales BJ (1978) Measurements of cardiac output in seriously ill patients using a CO_2 rebreathing method. Chest 73: 167-172
13. Binder JC, Parkin WG (2001) Non-invasive cardiac output determination: comparison of a new partial-rebreathing technique with thermodilution Anesth Intensive Care 29(1): 19-23
14. Gedeon A, Forstund L, Hedenstierna G et al (1980) A new method for non-invasive bedside determination of pulmonary blood flow. Med Biol Eng Comput 18: 411-418

Monitoring of Pulmonary Capillary Blood Flow and Alveolar Dead Space Using the Combined Methods of Volumetric Capnography and "Partial CO_2 Rebreathing" ($NiCO_2$)

B. ALLARIA

Data available in all operating theaters and intensive care units make it possible to obtain important information about the adequacy of the ventilation perfusion ratio (V/Q). This ratio, which is normally 0.8, decreases and increases in two specific conditions. It decreases in the case of poorly ventilated but perfused alveoli (increased shunt QS/QT) and it increases with well-ventilated but poorly perfused alveoli (increased alveolar dead space $V_{D\,ALV}$). In both of these cases, it is difficult for the pulmonary capillary to eliminate CO_2, in the first case due to inadequate ventilation and in the second because of inadequate perfusion. Thus, arterial CO_2 (p_aCO_2) increases and alveolar pCO_2 ($p_{et}\,CO_2$ of traditional capnography) decreases in both situations.

In every case in which the V/Q ratio is altered, $p_{ET}CO_2$ – which is normally equal to p_aCO_2 or shifts by no more than 5 mmHg – becomes significantly lower, and thus the $p_aCO_2 - p_{ET}CO_2$ gradient increases.

Therefore, the availability of two simple values (p_aCO_2 and $p_{ET}CO_2$) makes it possible to detect an alteration in the V/Q ratio.

$$\Delta\, CO2 = paCO_2 - p_{ET}CO_2 = 0 - 5 \text{ mmHg}$$

If $\Delta CO_2 > 5$ mg, we can suspect an alteration in the V/Q ratio.

However, ÄCO_2 increases both in the case of shunt increase (reduced V/Q) and in the case of reduced perfusion with increased $V_{D\,ALV}$ (increased V/Q).

In order to proceed with a diagnosis, we need two sets of information: (1) pulmonary capillary blood flow (PCBF) and (2) the volume of the alveolar dead space ($V_{D\,ALV}$).

Today, monitoring alveolar dead space is relatively simple using volumetric capnography. The instrument that performs this has been available for a number of years (CO_2SMOPlus), and it essentially uses a flow sensor and a capnograph to plot $P_{ET}CO_2$ against tidal volume (V_T), creating the curve illustrated in Fig. 1.

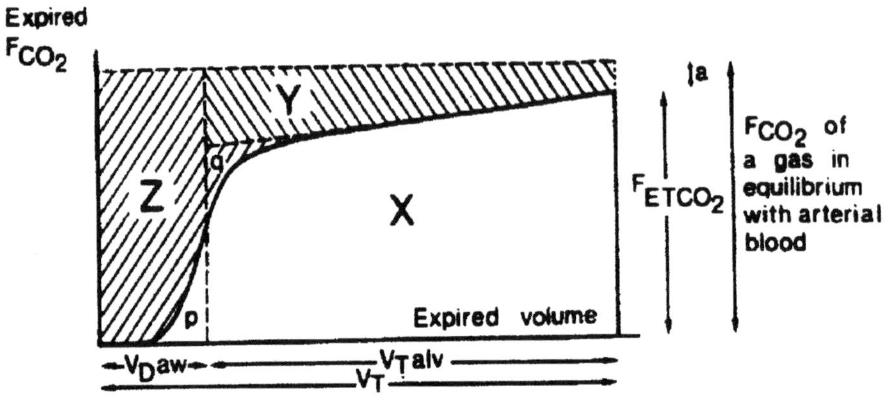

Fig. 1. Use of flow sensor and capnograph to plot $P_{ET}CO_2$ against tidal volume (V_T). x = Volume of expired CO_2, y = Vd alv, z = Vd aw, a = Δ CO_2

Consequently, by using this instrument we can obtain some information we need: the volume of the alveolar dead space ($V_{D\ ALV}$). Nevertheless, even with this information it is not always easy to detect whether an alteration in the V/Q ratio (and thus an increase in ÄCO_2 that, as we have indicated, is strictly correlated) is linked solely to an increase in dead space, or if there is a concomitant deficiency in alveolar ventilation. As shown in Fig. 1, volumetric capnography also makes it possible to monitor alveolar ventilation ($V_{T\ ALV}$), which is essentially the difference between V_T and $V_{D\ ALV}$: $V_{T\ ALV} = V_T - V_{D\ ALV}$.

For example, if we use increasing positive end-expiratory pressure (PEEP) values in acute respiratory distress syndrome (ARDS) to recruit alveoli, we may run the risk of disturbing alveolar perfusion, increasing the dead space, and diminishing effective alveolar ventilation. Here, what we mean by effective alveolar ventilation is not the type that simply recruits alveoli but the type that, in addition to recruiting them, also furnishes correct aeration.

As a result, when using volumetric capnography the PEEP that is best suited to the patient is the one that, at an equivalent V_t, will permit the best alveolar ventilation with the lowest $V_{D\ ALV}$.

However, it is widely known in both intensive care and in the operating theater that, in addition to information on aeration, it is also essential to have information on circulation. Here again, what interests us is not cardiac output in a broader sense but the quantity of blood per minute that has participated in aeration, thereby eliminating CO_2 and becoming rich in O_2. By using thermodilution, we can state that this blood quantity corresponds to cardiac output (COTD) less the amount that does not participate in aeration (venous admixture = VA).

The cardiac output that participates in aeration (or non-shunted pulmonary capillary blood flow = NS PCBF) is thus

$$\mathbf{NS\ PCBF = CO_{TD} - VA}$$

Since optimized artificial ventilation permits alveolar recruitment, it should reduce the shunted pulmonary capillary blood flow and thus improve NS PCBF. However, artificial ventilation, particularly with high PEEP levels, can diminish venous return and thus lead to an overall reduction in pulmonary capillary blood flow. As a result, it is always difficult to know if the ventilation technique that has been selected will make NS PCBF better or worse.

Therefore, it is important to have a monitoring technique that can keep NS PCBF under control. Moreover, NS PCBF monitoring would also make it possible to avoid the frequent calculation of DO_2 that, because it expresses not only cardiac output but also the O_2 content of the blood, is the general parameter that best allows us to monitor the possibility of oxygenating the body. A very incisive study published recently in *Critical Care Medicine* [1] has in fact demonstrated a strong correlation between NS PCBF and DO_2 in pigs with induced ARDS.

Since NS PCBF is the part of the cardiac output that participates in aeration, it is difficult to imagine that it would not be correlated with DO_2. To date, however, NS PCBF was difficult to gauge without using a Swan Ganz catheter and even when it was used, the formula

$$\mathbf{NS\ PCBF = CO_{TD} - VA}$$

was debatable because of the difficulty in obtaining an accurate measurement of the VA.

Volumetric capnography has contributed significantly to solving this problem, making it possible to measure VCO_2 (area x in Fig. 1), as we have seen above. This has allowed measurement of pulmonary capillary blood flow with the Fick method, using the variations in VCO_2 and $EtCO_2$ during rebreathing [2].

This method is based on the assumption that PCBF can be measured in ventilation without rebreathing and with rebreathing, according to the following formulae:

$$\mathbf{Q\ PCBF = \frac{VCO_2\ non\ rebr.}{CVCO_2\ non\ rebr. - C_aCO_2\ non\ rebr.}} \tag{1}$$

$$Q\ PCBF = \frac{VCO_2\ rebr.}{CVCO_2\ rebr. - C_aCO_2\ rebr.} \tag{2}$$

in which VCO_2 is the elimination of CO_2/min and $CVCO_2$ is the concentration of CO_2 in the arterial part of the alveolar capillary.

Assuming that PCBF remains constant during measurement, equations **(1)** and **(2)** can be combined as follows:

$$QPCBF = \frac{VCO_2\ non\ rebr. - VCO_2\ rebr.}{(CVCO_2\ non\ rebr. - C_aCO_2\ non\ rebr.) - (CVCO_2\ rebr. - C_aCO_2\ rebr.)} \tag{3}$$

The large quantity of CO_2 in the venous compartment allows us to assume that $CVCO_2$ remains constant with or without rebreathing over a short period of time.

We can thus eliminate the terms $CVCO_2$ - $CVCO_2$ and transform equation **(3)** as follows:

$$Q\ PCBF = \frac{VCO_2\ non\ rebr. - VCO_2\ rebr.}{(C_aCO_2\ rebr. - C_aCO_2\ non\ rebr.)} = \frac{\Delta VCO_2}{\Delta C_aCO_2} + \tag{4}$$

The technological development of the volumetric capnograph, which already permits the measurement of VCO_2 (CO_2SMOPlus), has led to a new instrument, the NICO_2. In addition to the potential offered by the previous device, this new instrument also makes it possible to plot $P_{ET}CO_2$ versus TV during rebreathing periods inserted automatically through a valve and a circuit, as shown in Fig. 2, thereby measuring ÄVCO_2 according to formula **(4)**.

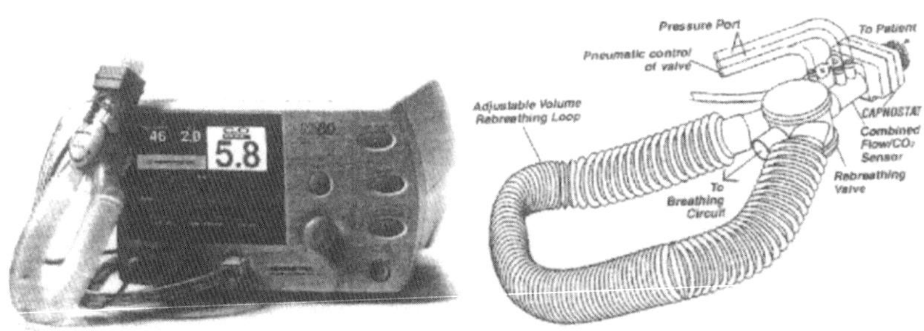

Fig.2. The NICO_2 device (non-invasive cardiac output) with the circuit for "partial rebreathing"

C_aCO_2 is calculated by measuring the $P_{ET}CO_2$, which is assumed as the equivalent of P_aCO_2, and the following formula is applied:

$$\mathbf{C_aCO_2 = [6.957\,(Hg) + 94.864] \times log.[1 + 0.1933\,P_aCO_2]} \quad \mathbf{(5)}$$

Given that, as we have stated repeatedly, $p_{ET}CO_2$ can also differ consistently from $p_{ET}CO_2$ in respiratory distress and hypovolemia, periodically it is useful to input the real p_aCO_2 value as assessed via hemogas analysis, in order to correct the unmeasured value.

The final formula is given below:

$$\mathbf{Q\ PCBF = \frac{\Delta VCO_2}{\Delta P_{ET}CO_2}}$$

The $NICO_2$ device thus measures the cardiac output component that participates in aeration, or in other words the parameter that we referred to above as

NS PCBF (non-shunted pulmonary capillary blood flow)

It is easy to see that when these data are available, it is then possible to arrive at the traditional value of cardiac output, adding the shunt value (QS/QT). In order to do this, this instrument uses a Nunn diagram that constructs the iso-shunt curves by plotting FiO_2 (x axis) versus P_aO_2 (y axis) replaced by SpO_2.

Based on our experience, the QS/QT value calculated using the Nunn diagram, is sufficiently correct if the shunt value is not high, but it is underestimated when it is important, as often occurs in severe cases of ARDS. It must be pointed out that if we use the $NICO_2$ device to evaluate cardiac output in routine situations (e.g., general anesthesia), the problem of high shunt values generally does not arise. On the other hand, if we use it to manage the artificial ventilation of the critical patient, the added value of this instrument lies mainly in the fact that it both measures NS PCBF and monitors $V_{D\ ALV}$, rather than in the opportunity it offers to measure cardiac output values non-invasively.

By allowing NS PCBF and $V_{D\ ALV}$ to be measured directly at the patient's bedside, the $NICO_2$ device offers us a new and noteworthy way of optimizing artificial ventilation in critical patients. While this is undoubtedly the most--interesting aspect of this new technique, the possibility it also offers for the non-invasive monitoring of cardiac output is equally welcome.

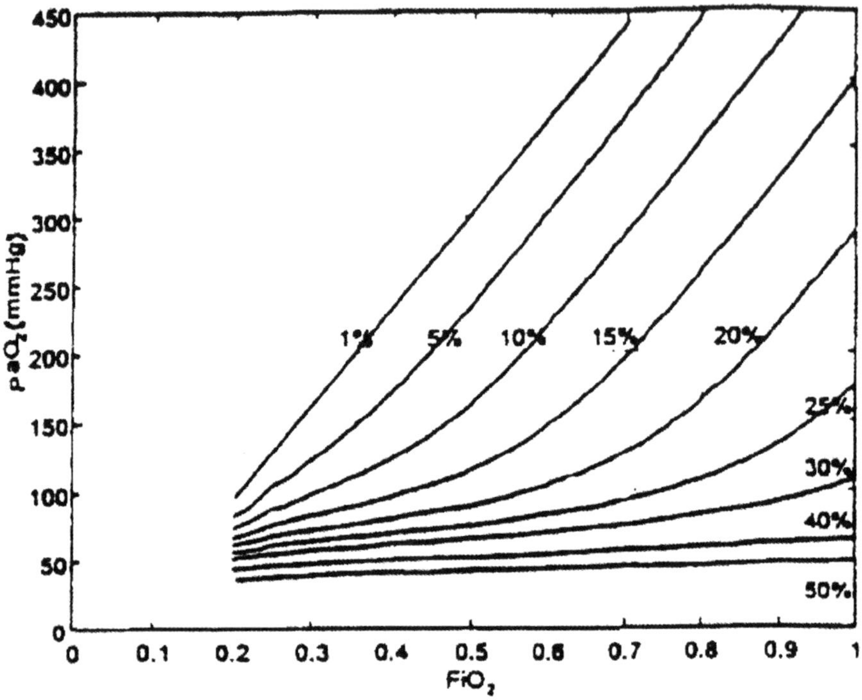

Fig. 3. Nunn diagram for evaluating the intrapulmonary shunt

References

1. Kanhai KJK, Strijdhorst H, et al (2000) Non invasive monitoring of non shunted pulmonary capillary blood flow in the acute respiratory distress syndrome. Crit Car Med 28: 1059
2. Jaffe MB (1999) Partial CO_2 rebreathing cardiac output. Operating principles of the NICO system. J Clin Monit Comp 15: 287
3. Nunn JF (1993) Applied respiratory physiology, 4th edn Butterworth, Oxford

Application of "Single Breath – Volumetric Capnography" Analysis in Open Lung Strategy
Description of a Monitoring Tool

T. TABOR

Open lung strategies – what they are, how to use them, and why they are important – have been discussed in great detail in recent years. These strategies propose we focus on sparing lung tissue from the damaging effects of positive pressure ventilation. In doing so we hope to reduce the time of ventilation and also the associated risks.

Open lung strategies in critical care (reanimation) focus on recruitment of alveolar spaces, in an effort to reduce shear forces between unequally ventilated lung fields. It is proposed that a well-recruited lung has the best defense against the damaging effects of these shear forces. There are many techniques to facilitate lung recruitment. One aspect of recruitment is detecting that the lung is either recruited, or more importantly, needs to be recruited. Herein lies the direction of this essay.

To detect when a lung is recruited or de-recruited, we need a monitoring tool that is simple to use clinically and will allow even inexperienced clinicians to recognize the associated events. One such potential tool could be the graph that is generated when exhaled CO_2 concentration (from mainstream capnography) and airway flow are instantaneously integrated to produce the volume of CO_2 (Fig. 1). This graph is referred to as the single breath CO_2 ($SBCO_2$) curve.

The $SBCO_2$ curve is a volume-based capnography waveform that begins at the onset of expiration and ends with the onset of the next inspiration. It is a reflection of CO_2 elimination by volume (Fig. 2), and presents the investigator with a precise view of certain components of pulmonary anatomy. It is similar in shape to the more commonly recognized time-based capnography; however, the information contained in this integration is quite different. The $SBCO_2$ curve provides visual details about airway deadspace, perfusion, and gas distribution that are unavailable when using the more-familiar time-based capnography tracing.

A description of the individual portions of the curve is helpful to understand

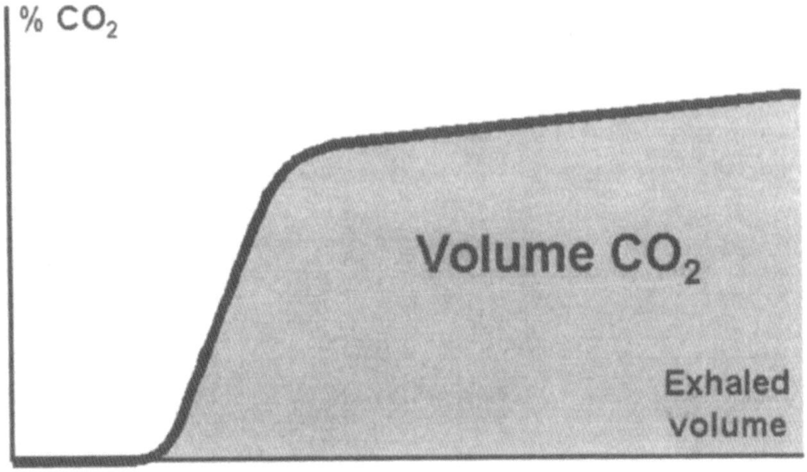

Fig. 1. Single breath CO_2 curve

the importance of this tool. The curve is generated by simultaneously measuring two signals. Airway flow and CO_2 concentration are collected from a sensor placed in the proximal airway. It is important to note that these signals must be collected exactly "in phase" with one another to avoid integration errors. In addition, the resolution of the data collection (sample rate) must be sufficient to adequately detail the evolving elimination of CO_2 volume. As a single sensor is placed in the proximal, it can only "see" a single-compartment lung (one airway, one alveolus, and one pulmonary capillary). The characteristics of the entire functional lung field are presented in a single curve.

The $SBCO_2$ curve is divided into regions. Each region describes a different portion of pulmonary anatomy, as well as the associated function (Fig. 2). Phase I represents gas eliminated from airway deadspace – pure airway deadspace. Phase II represents gas eliminated from fast or early emptying alveoli, and is considered transitional from pure airway gas to pure alveolar gas. Phase III represents pure alveolar gas. Phase III has a slightly positive slope in normal subjects. This is due to CO_2 being continuously excreted into alveolar gas as perfusion continues throughout exhalation.

Gas diffusion is a dynamic process, which occurs in two directions (O_2 into the capillary blood and CO_2 out) and continues throughout the respiratory cycle. It is imperative to visualize the constant evolution of ventilation, perfusion, and gas exchange as the $SBCO_2$ curve is produced in order to use the curve as a tool for monitoring events. While it is nearly impossible to graphically represent the

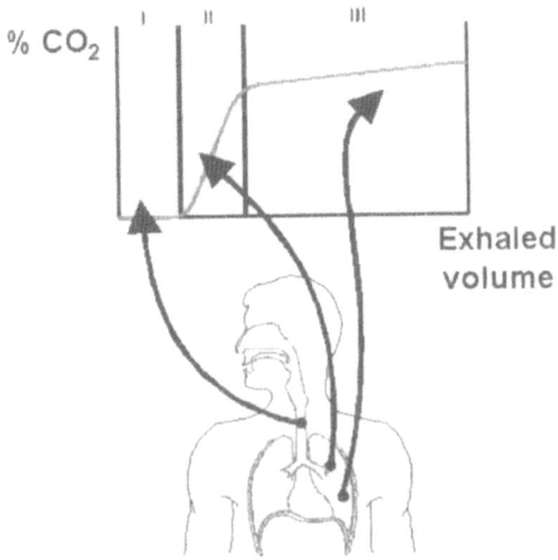

Fig. 2. Single-breath CO_2 curve divided into three phases reflecting pulmonary anatomy and associated function

delivery of O_2 to the pulmonary capillary bed, we can use CO_2 as trace gas to provide insight into O_2 delivery.

Phase II is considered transitional from pure airway gas to pure alveolar gas and contains volumes from both regions. To separate phase II and apply gas volumes to the appropriate category (either airway or alveolar), two lines are drawn in the graph (Fig. 3) . The first along the slope of phase III. The second

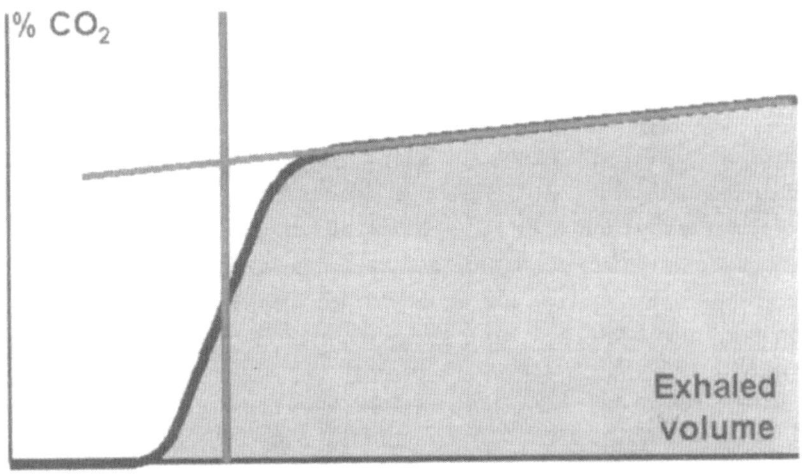

Fig. 3. Single-breath CO2 curve – separation of phase II and application of gas volumes to the appropriate category

line is drawn perpendicular to the x-axis and shifted left or right such that two equal triangles are formed. This exercise in geometry assumes that 50% of phase II gas is airway and the remaining 50% belongs to the alveolar regions. The results allow the division of the exhaled tidal volume to be sub-divided into airway deadspace volume and alveolar volume (Fig. 4).

The $SBCO_2$ curve can provide supplementary information about ventilation

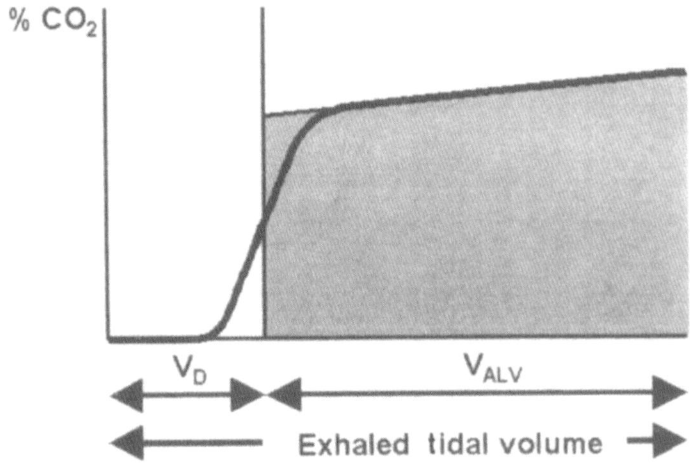

Fig. 4. Division of exhaled tidal volume into airway deadspace and alveolar volume

and perfusion if an additional line is added to the plot representing $paCO_2$ (Fig. 5). Placing the $paCO_2$ line on the plot defines additional areas. Area X represents the volume of CO_2 actually eliminated by the tidal volume. Area Z represents the amount of CO_2 that was not eliminated due to the presence of airway deadspace. Area Y represents the volume of CO_2 not eliminated due to the presence of alveolar deadspace. The entire rectangle represents the amount of CO_2 that potentially could be excreted in the breath if there were no airway deadspace or alveolar deadspace. This whole picture graphically represents the instantaneous relationship of physiological deadspace. Area X+Y+Z in combination presents the volume of potentially extractable CO_2, with area X representing the volume actually eliminated.

Physiological deadspace ratio is traditionally calculated as:

$$Vd/Vt = \frac{PaCO_2 - PeCO_2}{PaCO_2}$$

Using the areas created in Fig. 5 the same relationship can be explained:

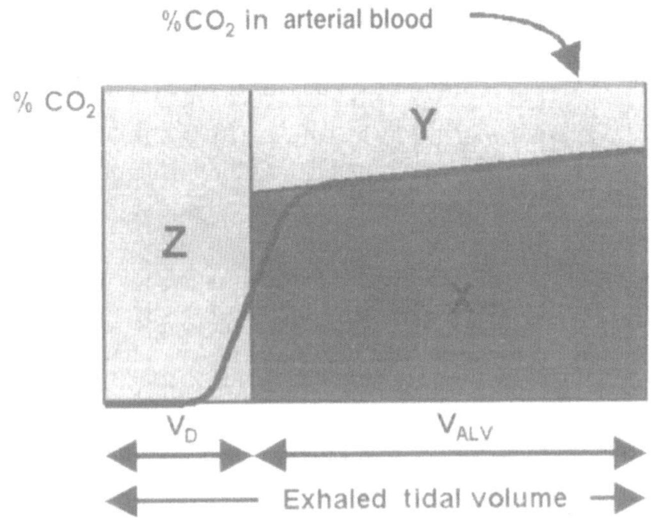

Fig. 5. $paCO_2$ addition to single-breath CO_2 curve

$$Vd/Vt = \frac{Y + Z}{X + Y + Z}$$

In graphic form, the relationship of eliminated to non-eliminated CO_2 volume is easier to comprehend and ultimately use in clinical practice. Changing physiological deadspace ratio is one goal of lung recruitment.

Thus far this essay has only described the generation of a curve produced by the integration of two signals. How can this be applied to the open lung strategies implied by the title? It is suggested that this curve is a graphic representation of a single-compartment lung with airway, alveoli, and capillary units being reduced to single components. How is this useful for managing open lung strategies? For the answers one must apply the monitoring tool to the subject being measured. If indeed we want to monitor recruitment and de-recruitment we have to imagine what this physiology looks like in a single-compartment lung model. How will the airway volume respond to a recruitment maneuver? How will the slope of phase III change? How does the slope of phase II respond to increased or decreased perfusion? What will these graphic representations tell us when applied to real patients?

The use of this tool, although in existence for many years, and its clinical significance has not been well documented. Experience in the intensive care unit is small when compared with the use of electrocardiography for example. It is the opinion of this author that $SBCO_2$ tells an interesting and important story about our patient's mechanism for eliminating CO_2. By using this unique view of CO_2 elimination, we gain insight into the delivery of O_2 and to the overall geometry of the lung anatomy. If we understand anatomy/physiology, realize the components of the monitoring tool and finally visualize what we are attempting to accomplish, then the utility of the $SBCO_2$ curve begins to become clear. Certainly more investigation is needed. Enough is currently known about $SBCO_2$ to make its contribution valuable to clinical decisions. Its final place in intensive care and other clinical areas depends on our daily evaluation of its responses in comparison with clinical observations. Only then will the total potential of this monitoring tool be realized. It is the intention of this discussion to indicate what is possible when the technique of measuring volumetric CO_2 is put to clinical use. It is hoped to encourage further investigation and application of this technique.

Suggested readings

1. Aitken RS, Clarke-Kennedy AE (1928) On the fluctuation in the composition of the alveolar air during the respiratory cycle in muscular exercise, J Physiol 65: 389-411
2. Arnold JH, Stenz RI, Thompson JE, et al (1996) Noninvasive determination of cardiac output using single breath CO_2 analysis, Crit Care Med 24:1701-1705
3. Brunner J, Thompson D (1993) Computerized ventilation monitoring, respiratory Care. J Adv Nurs 38:110-124
4. Fletcher R (1986) On-line expiratory CO_2 monitoring. Int J Clin Monit 3: 155-163
5. Fletcher R (1986) The single breath test for carbon dioxide, Berlins Arlöv, ISBN 91-7810-575-7
6. Fowler WS (1948) Lung function studies. II. The respiratory dead space. Am J Physiol 154: 405-416
7. Ream R, Schreiner MS (1993) Phase III slope of the CO_2 expirogram in patients with ARDS. Anesthesiology 79: A301
8. Ream RS, Schreiner MS, Neff JD, et al (1995) Volumetric capnography in children: influence of growth on the alveolar plateau slope, Anesthesiology 82: 64-73

How Permissive Should Hypercapnia Be?

G. Servillo, L. D'Amato, R. Tufano

The alteration of gas exchange is one of the main characteristics of acute respiratory distress syndrome (ARDS), and the first approaches aim to normalize blood gas values. Large tidal volumes and high peak inspiratory pressure were used, restricted only for the risk of pneumothorax and hemodynamic impairment. An evolving body of experimental studies, conducted over the last decades, have demonstrated ventilator-induced lung injury (VILI). They also demonstrated that mechanical ventilation with high peak inspiratory pressure induces a "dose"-dependent exudative pulmonary edema, correlated more to high tidal volume excursion than to high inspiratory pressure [1, 2].

A protective ventilatory strategy against acute lung injury, widely accepted nowadays, consists of the delivery of lower tidal volumes during ventilation that causes, in most cases, a reduction of current volume and hypercapnia. In the context of protective mechanical ventilation, hypercapnia is not inevitable: lungs with a severe ARDS may present some peculiarities that are compatible with traditional ventilation, supporting normocapnia without extreme risk. The static volume-pressure curve of respiratory system provides useful suggestions on this subject [3, 4]. However, the aim to support normocapnia during severe ARDS is not realistic. Both mechanical characteristics of the lung and increased $paCO_2$ lead to higher than average ventilation values. This ventilation is directed towards the relatively normal lung fractions that are exposed to a very elevated "specific ventilation" [5]. The proposal to accept the increased $paCO_2$ probably arose from the observation of some patients with chronic obstructive pulmonary disease, in which a slow and progressive $paCO_2$ increase is considered as an adaptation mechanism to eliminate CO_2 with reduced respiratory work [5, 6].

The progressive increase of hypercapnia allows patients with chronic respiratory failure to fairly well tolerate the severe respiratory acidosis. Chronically elevated $paCO_2$ in the range of 75 - 110 mmHg does not seem to cause symptoms in such patients, as long as significant arterial oxygen desaturation is avoided.

The main purpose of this paper is to evaluate a controversial issue, namely the degree of respiratory acidosis that can be tolerated. We start with a review of the physiological and pathophysiological effects of hypercapnia.

Local and systemic effects of hypercapnia

The most-important consequences of hypercapnia for the function of any organ result from a complex interplay between local effects of CO_2 on proton concentration and effects mediated by the activation of the sympathoadrenergic system [7, 8]; the latter are subject to important interspecies variation, and are heavily influenced by anesthesia. However, the bulk of investigation in this field has been done on isolated preparations and anesthetized animals, with relatively few studies performed in humans. Therefore, extrapolation of most experimental results to the clinical situation must be done with extreme caution.

Acute hypercapnia has a myriad of effects, concerning almost all physiological functions. In the following, we shall focus on effects of potential significance to the intensivist.

Because of the free diffusibility of CO_2 across cell membranes, a sudden increase in extracellular $paCO_2$ will decrease the intracellular pH (pHi). Due to the abundance of carbonic anhydrase in the cytosol, intracellular acidosis occurs rapidly [9]. The latter is responsible for most of the effects of hypercapnia. However, several immediate or late compensatory mechanisms are able to partly compensate for the variations in pHi in presence of a severe hypercapnia. In fact, a reduction of pHi (6.9 - 7.2) does not modify the cellular energy state. As a hypothesis, a severe acidosis may have a protective effect on the hypoxic cell. Finally, acidosis inhibits the activity of contractile elements and deregulates the electrical properties of the excitable cells.

Hypercapnia induces an acute deterioration of ventricular performance. The myocardial response to acute respiratory acidosis is mainly characterized by an impairment in contractility, which is entirely reversible [10]. The principal mechanism responsible for the fall in cardiac contractile force is explained by a rapid diffusion of CO_2 into cells, with consequent intracellular acidosis, which interferes with myofilament responsiveness to calcium, as recently reviewed [11].

CO_2 is a potent coronary vasodilator, and hypercapnia produces a substantial increase in coronary flow, together with a rise in coronary sinus paO_2 [12], independent of myocardial oxygen consumption [13]. Response to CO_2 is likely to be different in the presence of heart failure or diminished coronary reserve.

The hemodynamic response to hypercapnia is characterized by an increase in cardiac output, heart rate, and stroke volume, and a decrease in systemic vascular resistance [14, 15]. This response represents the balance between the depressant effects of CO_2 on mechanical performance and its indirect effects on peripheral chemoreceptors and vasomotor centers, which improve both sympathetic nervous activity and catecholamine secretion. On the other hand, hypercapnia may adversely affect right ventricular performance in patients with previously impaired right ventricular systolic function. Respiratory acidosis induces pulmonary arteriolar vasoconstriction, thus leading to pulmonary hypertension and an increase of both end-diastolic and end systolic right ventricular volumes [16].

The hypercapnia rise to arrhythmogenic effects, especially ventricular ones, requires further investigation.

Increased pCO_2 produces a rightward shift of the oxygen dissociation curve, promoting the release of O_2 to the tissues. This effect is related to two mechanisms: the increase in H^+, as CO_2 is hydrated in carbonic acid, and the formation of carbamino compounds from the reaction between CO_2 and N-terminal amino acids of the hemoglobin chains. The decreased affinity of hemoglobin for O_2 may compromise the O_2 loading in alveolar capillaries, an effect of minimal significance when paO_2 is in the normal range, but dramatic in the presence of pulmonary disease and hypoxemia [17].

Hypercapnia acts on the central nervous system by reducing intracellular and extracellular pH; the effects on the O_2 consumption of the brain are controversial, even though available studies suggest that the O_2 demand of the brain does not change or even decreases in hypercapnic conditions [18-20].

In normal subjects hypercapnia increases the cerebral blood flow [21, 22]; this effect is partly mediated by the concomitant arterial hypertension, which increases cerebral perfusion pressure, and in part by cerebral vasodilatation, which reduces cerebral vascular resistance.

Hypercapnia reversibly increases intracranial pressure because of the enlargement of cerebral blood volume secondary to the diminished vascular tone in the face of maintained or raised vascular pressure [23, 24].

Theoretically, CO_2 has anesthetic properties on the basis of its lipid solubility, but anesthesia by CO_2 alone requires a much higher partial pressure (> 200 mmHg) [25]; in addition to being an anesthetic, CO_2 also has stimulant properties on the central nervous system, the best-known being the stimulation of respiratory drive, which becomes maximal for $paCO_2$ in the range of 100 - 150 mmHg [7].

Acute hypercapnia reduces the contractility and the endurance of skeletal muscle, in particular that of diaphragm [26, 27]; it would be interesting to know how fast the respiratory muscles recover their strength and endurance upon return to normocapnia after hypercapnic exposure of a few hours or a few days. This would indicate whether weaning from the ventilator might be difficult.

Normoxemic hypercapnia increases the secretion of epinephrine, norepinephrine, adrenocorticotropic hormone, cortisol, aldosterone, and antidiuretic hormone [7, 8, 28, 29].

The inhalation of up to 10% CO_2 has no effect on airway resistance, but probably reduces the expiratory flow because it causes a laryngeal narrowing [30].

Hypercapnia has been shown experimentally to increase sodium and chloride absorption in the gut [31], but whether it increases the risk of acute gastrointestinal bleeding by stimulating gastric secretion of H^+ remains to be established.

The high level of CO_2 in the portal venous blood increases portal resistance and reduces portal flow, whereas slight changes in the opposite direction are noted in the hepatic arterial circulation, with an overall reduction of total hepatic blood flow [32].

Studies on dogs have shown that mild acute normoxic elevations of $paCO_2$ (70 mmHg) led to either a moderate fall [33] or a moderate increase of renal vascular resistance, with relatively little impact on renal blood flow and glomerular filtration rate. More-severe acute respiratory acidosis ($paCO_2$ >100 mmHg) results in more-pronounced renal vasoconstriction, with a concomitant fall of renal blood flow, glomerular filtration rate, and possibly urine output [33].

Protective role of increased $paCO_2$

The increased $paCO_2$ produced by permissive hypercapnia per se plays a protective role. Historically, CO_2 has been utilized for therapeutical aims as, for example, in carbon monoxide poisoning to accelerate carbon monoxide clearance, and in vascular surgery, especially during carotid endoarterectomy, to augment cerebral perfusion. An increasing body of literature suggests that respiratory acidosis can exert protective effects on tissue injury in several different organ systems, including the central nervous system, the myocardium and the lung. Many studies have demonstrated that hypercapnic acidosis (HCA) due to adoption of smaller tidal volumes protects against acute lung injury, independent of the ventilatory strategy employed. This led us to suppose that the beneficial effects of permissive hypercapnia in patients with ARDS may be due in part to the ventilatory strategy, with lower tidal volumes that per se may limit the risk of VILI due to the reduction of lung stretch, and in part to HCA.

Shibata et al. [34] demonstrated that HCA might possess a direct protective role in ischemia-reperfusion and free radical lung injury produced by purine and xanthine oxidase, and this role would exist independent of the ventilatory strategy employed. The authors demonstrated that HCA, generated by altering the inspired fraction of CO_2 in the isolated buffer-perfused rabbit lung, had no adverse microvascular effects and prevented the increase in capillary permeability following acute lung injury induced by ischemia-reperfusion or by free radicals. Finally, they demonstrated that HCA inhibited in vitro the activity of xanthine oxidase, a pivotal enzyme in ischemia-reperfusion injury.

Buffering HCA to normal pH with buffer solutions, such as $NaHCO_3$, Carbicarb, or THAM, greatly attenuated the protective effect of HCA. The exact mechanisms of the deleterious effects of buffering HCA are unclear. One possible explanation involves the suggestion that HCA, and then H^+, protects against ischemia-reperfusion lung injury via alterations of amiloride-sensitive Na-H exchange channels. Hence, buffering HCA might involve alterations in the functional opening status of microvascular ion channels, resulting in altered pulmonary fluid regulatory mechanisms [35]. Many beneficial effects of acidosis are due to the reduction of cellular respiration and of O_2 consumption, which may further benefit an imbalance between supply and demand, in addition to greater O_2 delivery. In the myocardium HCA is highly protective against ischemia-reperfusion injury, because acidosis may prevent intracellular calcium overload by preventing cellular influx of Ca^{2+}, increasing intracellular binding, and decreasing sarcoplasmatic release. This reduces contractility and O_2 demand, possibly explaining the protective effect of acidosis during myocardial ischemia [36].

For lung and myocardium, HCA is more protective than metabolic acidosis in terms of microvascular permeability. Probably this protective effect of HCA is at least partly dependent on "intracellular mechanisms", since extracellular acidosis induced by hypercapnia gives rise to a more-rapid increase in intracellular acidosis than acidosis due to a metabolic cause. This is due to the high solubility of CO_2 and its free diffusibility across cell membranes.

HCA also has an important protective role against hypoxic-ischemic brain damage. Vannucci et al. [37] demonstrated that elevated CO_2 has a neuroprotective effect, even when this is instituted for a period of only 2 h following ischemic-reperfusion brain injury, while hypocapnia is deleterious. During this study the authors also observed that cerebral blood flow was better preserved during hypercapnia and that the greater O_2 delivery promoted cerebral glucose utilization and oxidative metabolism. That is important for optimal maintenance of tissue high-energy phosphate reserves. Furthermore, the glutamate levels in cerebrospinal fluid were lower during hypercapnia, and this led us to suppose that the reduction of excitatory amino acid secretion might be involved in central nervous system protection.

HCA has also beneficial effects on inflammatory mechanisms, because it reduces neutrophil and macrophage activity, leukocyte superoxide formation, expression of cell adhesion molecules, phospholipase A_2 activity, and neuronal apoptosis [38, 39].

Controlled hypoventilation and permissive hypercapnia

Clinical studies on deliberate application of lower tidal volumes with permissive hypercapnia are few. The first study, in 1984, described the application of permissive hypercapnia in patients ventilated for asthmatic fit [40]. The encouraging results of this pioneering work showed a reduction of complications induced by mechanical ventilation and a decrease in mortality. Subsequently these results have been confirmed, and today the use of hypercapnic hypoventilation during asthma is accepted.

Some years later, Lee et al. [41], in a prospective randomized study, compared ventilation with low tidal volumes with traditional ventilation in two groups of patients without pulmonary pathology undergoing surgery. In the group treated with lower tidal volumes, a small reduction of oxygenation was observed, while normocapnia was preserved in every patient.

The idea of ventilation with low tidal volumes and low pressure for patients with ARDS came into clinical practice when Hickling et al. [42] showed that limiting peak pressure and consequently tidal volume, and accepting the presence of hypercapnia, the outcome of ARDS patients seemed to improve.

Recently, five randomized studies comparing the different ventilatory strategies utilized to reduce VILI have been published. Amato et al. [43] reported beneficial effects in 53 patients with severe ARDS by application of principles of recruitment and preservation of pulmonary volume. Patients were randomized into two groups: a control group treated with high tidal volumes, that affered normal paCO2 values, without limits for airway pressure, and a group treated with protective ventilation, in which therapeutic aims were the limitation of tidal volumes and inspiratory pressures and the reduction of minute volume, accepting the presence of hypercapnia and making use of sedation and paralysis. The patients treated with this protective approach were ventilated with high positive end-expiratory pressure (PEEP), set according to the morphology of the volume-pressure curve, 2 cm above the inferior inflection point. The authors noticed a decrease in mortality in the group treated with protective ventilation, Stewart et al. [44] studied 120 patients with a high risk of ARDS, but without typical manifestations of the syndrome. These were separated in two randomized groups. The authors reported no significant differences in mortality, barotrauma incidence, and multiorgan failure between the group treated with lower tidal volumes and the group treated with conventional ventilation.

Brochard et al. [45] studied 116 patients with ARDS, randomized into two groups. The first group (treatment group) was treated with current volumes of 10 ml/kg, preserving an inspiratory pressure of 25 cm H_2O and accepting the occurence of hypercapnia. The second group (control group) was treated with current volumes of 10 ml/kg and with an adequate respiratory rate to preserve normocapnia. The level of applied PEEP was similar in the two groups and was selected according to blood gas parameters. The authors did not observe any significant decrease in mortality at 60 days, or any modifications in the duration of mechanical ventilation, pneumothorax incidence, and multiorgan failure.

In a study by Brower et al. [46], 52 patients with ARDS were studied and randomized into two groups. The first group was treated with protective ventilation, the second group with conventional volumes, preserving a plateau pressure in the range of 45 - 55 cm H_2O. In all patients, respiratory rate was selected to preserve normocapnia. In both groups, PEEP was selected according to the oxygenation; mortality was not different in the two groups.

The results of the last three studies are substantially different from those of Amato et al. [43]. However, these experimental studies suggest that the main mechanism involved in VILI is the cyclic collapse and recruitment of alveoli rather than pulmonary overstretching. VILI might be reduced by applying high PEEP selected according to the oxygenation. In the studies conducted by Stewart et al. [44], Brochard et al.[45], and Brower et al. [46], the PEEP level was selected according to oxygenation and it was not different in the two groups. A second possible explanation of the difference between the results of different works might be the respiratory rate in the group treated with protective ventilation. In this group, as in the study of Brower et al. [46], respiratory rate was increased to preserve normocapnia. So the benefit of decreased pulmonary overstretching, obtained with low tidal volumes, might be opposed by the increase in respiratory rate. Finally, the efficacy of ventilation with lower tidal volumes might be reduced by deleterious effects of hypercapnia and acidosis that are able to give rise to organ dysfunction. Even with such limitations, these studies have supplied new and important indications for ventilatory treatment in patients with ARDS. Firstly, they demonstrated that ventilation with plateau pressure £ 35 cm H2O is useful to reduce the risk of VILI and mortality. Secondly, an intentional decrease of tidal volumes does not seem to offer any advantage when applied in patients with only a risk of ARDS. Thirdly, PEEP can represent an efficacious means of reducing VILI and mortality when combined with the use of low plateau pressure.

Practical approaches to ventilation with permissive hypercapnia

During ventilation with lower tidal volumes and permissive hypercapnia we have to consider the following factors.

Absolute and relative contraindications

These directly depend on the adverse effects, previously described. The absolute contraindication to this ventilation with permissive hypercapnia is related to the powerful vasodilatory effect of $paCO_2$ on cerebral vessels. This excessive vasodilatation causes an augmentation of cerebral blood flow that results in a great increase in intracranial pressure, which might aggravate prior cerebral disorders, such as cerebral trauma or hemorrhage, space-occupying intracranial lesions, severe cerebral hypertension, and other cerebrovascular diseases. However, some authors suggest that in these particular conditions ventilation with permissive hypercapnia is possible, providing intracranial pressure is monitored and effects due to the increased $paCO_2$ are examined[47].

The relative contraindications concern the presence of ischemic cardiopathy, right ventricular dysfunction with pulmonary hypertension, uncorrected hypovolemia and severe metabolic acidosis.

Gradual increase of CO_2

Hypercapnia should be implemented progressively to allow the compensatory mechanisms to buffer HCA to normal pH. It has been recommended that the CO_2 increase should be implemented in steps of 10 mmHg/h up to a maximum level of 80 mmHg. If, for any reason, it is necessary that hypercapnia exceed 80 mmHg, it is strongly recommended to proceed much more slowly [48].

Safety limits and pH reduction

According to general agreement, an intervention is not required as long as a $paCO_2$ level below 80 mmHg and an arterial pH below 7.15 is maintained. When these values exceed safety limits, some authors do not use buffer solutions with a pH above 7, while other authors prefer a careful alkalinization with a slow administration of $NaHCO_3$.

Deep sedation

The necessity of deep sedation, in order to reduce the augmented respiratory drive and so to prevent severe discomfort, is generally admitted for intensive care unit patients as opposed to the need for neuromuscular blocking agents. Hickling et al. [49] reported that some patients tolerate fairly well permissive hypercapnia with spontaneous breathing, even if this gives rise to a severe tachypnea, suggesting that an adaptation of respiratory drive to HCA is possible, but differs in degree from patient to patient.

Monitoring

Monitoring during ventilation with permissive hypercapnia does not differ from the monitoring usually applied in conventional mechanical ventilation. The measurement of arterial blood gases remains the best assessment of arterial oxygenation; the arterial O_2 saturation should always be calculated when hypercapnia is implemented. An invasive hemodynamic monitoring is indicated and recommended in patients with known or suspected right or left ventricular dysfunction, prior pulmonary hypertension, coronary disease, or severe hypoxemia. Ophthalmoscopy is recommended to search for signs of increased intracranial pressure.

Weaning

For weaning from permissive hypercapnia, it is suggested to increase alveolar ventilation progressively in order to prevent cardiovascular instability. When patients remain hypercapnic for a short period of 24 h, with $paCO_2$ values above 80 mmHg, we consider adequate a rate of decrease in the range of 10 - 20 mmHg/h. If hypercapnia is maintained for more days and acidosis was treated with buffer agents, a too rapid reduction of $paCO_2$ leads to a metabolic alkalosis, with concomitant convulsivant effects and depression of respiratory drive. For these reasons the discontinuation of permissive hypercapnia should be more progressive, extending over at least 2 or 3 days [48].

Conclusion

In recent years, the literature has indicated the benefit of a protective ventilation approach with low tidal volumes and higher PEEP in ARDS. The effects of hypercapnia with such a ventilatory approach are not fully known. However, in the light of recent evidence, a re-evaluation of traditional concepts of hypercapnia is needed.

References

1. Webb HH, Tierny DF (1974) Experimental pulmonary edema due to intermittent positive pressure ventilation with high inflation pressure: protection by positive end-expiratory pressure. Am Rev Respir Dis 110: 556-565
2. Dreyfuss DG, Soler P, Basset G, et al (1988) High inflation pressure pulmonary edema: respective effects of airway pressure, high tidal volume, and positive end-expiratory pressure. Am Rev Respir Dis 137: 1159-1164
3. Servillo G, Svantesson C, Beydon L, et al (1997) Pressure-volume curves in acute respiratory failure : automated low flow inflation versus occlusion. Am J Respir Crit Care Med 155: 1629-1636
4. Servillo G, De Robertis E, Coppola, et al (2000) Application of a computerised method to measure static pressure volume curve in acute respiratory distress syndrome. Intensive Care Med 26: 11-14
5. Pesenti A (1990) Target blood gases during ARDS ventilatory menagement. Intensive Care Med 16: 349-351
6. Gothgen IH, Berthelsen PG, Rasmussen JP, et al (1993) Ventilation in ARDS and asthma: the optimal blood gas values. Scand J Clin Lab Invest 53 [Suppl 214]: 67-73
7. Nunn JF (1987) The effects of changes in carbon dioxide tension. In: Applied respiratory physiology, 3rd edn Butterworth, London, pp 460-470
8. Brofman JD, Leff AR, Munoz NM, et al (1990) Sympathetic secretory response to hypercapnic acidosis in swine. J Appl Physiol 69: 710-717
9. Thomas RC (1984) Experimental displacement of intracellular pH and the mechanism of its subsequent recovery. J Physiol (Lond) 354: 3-22
10. Tang WC, Weil MH, Gazmuri RJ, et al (1991) Reversible impairment of myocardial contractility due to hypercarbic acidosis in the isolated perfused rat heart. Crit Care Med 19: 218-24
11. Orchard C, Kentish J (1990) Effects of changes of pH on the contractile function of cardiac muscle. Am J Physiol 258: 967-981
12. Case RB, Greenberg H, Moskowitz R (1975) Alterations in coronary sinus PO_2 and O_2 saturation resulting from PCO_2 changes. Cardiovasc Res 9: 167-177
13. Wexels JC, Myhre ES (1987) Hypocapnia and hypercapnia in the dog: effects on myocardial blood-flow and haemodynamics during beta- and combined alpha- and beta-adrenoceptor blockade. Clin Physiol 7: 21-33
14. Blackburn JP, Conway CM, Leigh JM, et al (1972) $PaCO_2$ and the pre-ejection period: the $PaCO_2$ /inotropy response curve. Anesthesiology 37: 268-276
15. Prys-Roberts C, Kelman GR, Greenbaum R, et al (1967) Circulatory influences of artificial ventilation during nitrous oxide anaesthesia in man. II. Results: the relative influence of mean intrathoracic pressure and arterial carbon dioxide tension. Br J Anaesth 39: 533-548
16. Viitanen A, Salmenperä M, Heinonen J (1990) Right ventricular response to hypercarbia after cardiac surgery. Anesthesiology 73: 393-400
17. McLellan TM (1991) The influence of a respiratory acidosis on the exercise blood lactate response. Eur J Appl Physiol 63: 6-11
18. Siesjö BK (1980) Cerebral metabolic rate in hypercarbia – a controversy. Anesthesiology 52: 461-465
19. Berntman L, Dahlgren N, Siesjö BK (1979) Cerebral blood flow and oxygen consumption in the rat brain during extreme hypercarbia. Anesthesiology 50: 299-305
20. Prough DS, Rogers AT, Stump DA, et al (1990) Hypercarbia depresses cerebral oxygen consumption during cardiopulmonary bypass. Stroke 21: 1162-1166
21. Edvinsson L, McKenzie ET, McCulloch J (1993) Changes in arterial gas tensions. In: Cerebral blood flow and metabolism. Raven Press, New York, pp 524-552
22. Miller JD (1987) Cerebral blood flow variations with perfusion pressure and metabolism. In: Wood JH (ed) Cerebral blood flow. Physiologic and clinical aspects. McGraw-Hill, New York, pp 119-130

23. Lanier WL, Weglinski MR (1991) Intracranial pressure. In: Cucchiara RF, Michenfelder JD (ed) Clinical neuroanesthesia. Churchill Livingstone, New York, pp 77-110
24. Miller JD, Sullivan HG (1979) Severe intracranial hypertension. In: Trubuhovich RV, (ed) Management of acute intracranial disaster. Little Brown, Boston, pp 19-35
25. Eisele JH, Eger EI, Muallem M (1967) Narcotic properties of carbon dioxide in the dog. Anesthesiology 28: 856-865
26. Juan G, Calverley P, Talamo C, et al (1984) Effect of carbon dioxide on diaphragmatic function in human beings. N Engl J Med 310: 874-879
27. Gomes Vianna L, Koulouris N, Lanigan C, et al (1990) Effect of acute hypercapnia on limb muscle contractility in humans. J Appl Physiol 69: 1486-1493
28. Chen HG, Wood CE (1993) The adrenocorticotropic hormone and arginine vaspressin responses to hypercapnia in fetal and maternal sheep. Am J Physiol 264: 324-330
29. Raff H, Roarty TP (1988) Renin, ACTH and aldosterone during acute hypercapnia and hypoxia in conscious rats. Am J Physiol 254: 431-435
30. Butler J, Caro CG, Alcala R, et al (1960) Physiological factors affecting airway resistance in normal subjects and in patients with obstructive respiratory disease. J Clin Invest 39: 584-591
31. Charney AN, Feldman GM (1984) Systemic acid-base disorders and intestinal electrolyte transport. Am J Physiol 247: 1-12
32. Gelman S, Ernst EA (1977) Role of pH, PCO_2, and O_2 content of portal blood in hepatic circulatory autoregulation. Am J Physiol 233: 255-262
33. Bersentes TJ, Simmons DH (1967) Effects of acute acidosis on renal hemodynamics. Am J Physiol 212: 633-640
34. Shibata K, Cregg N, Engelberts D, et al (1998). Hypercapnic acidosis may attenuate acute lung injury by inhibition of endogenous xanthine oxidase. Am J Respir Crit Care Med 158: 1578-1584
35. Laffey JG, Engelberts D, Kavanagh BP (2000) Buffering hypercapnic acidosis worsens acute lung injury. Am J Respir Crit Care Med 161: 141-146
36. Laffey JG, Kavanagh BP (1999) Carbon dioxide and critically ill – too little of a good thing ? Lancet 354: 1283-1286
37. Vannucci RC, Towfighi J, Heitjan D, et al (1995). Carbon dioxide protects the perinatal brain from hypoxic-ischemic damage: an experimental study in the immature rat. Pediatrics 95:868-874
38. Allen DB, Maguire JJ, Mahdavian M, et al (1997) Would hypoxia and acidosis limit neutrophil bacterial killing mechanisms. Arch Surg 132: 991-996
39. Xu L, Glassford AJ, Giaccia AJ, et al (1998) Acidosis reduces neuronal apoptosis. Neuroreport 9: 875-879
40. Darioli R, Perret C (1984) Mechanical controlled hypoventilation in status asthmaticus. Am Rev Respir Dis 129: 385-387
41. Lee PC, Helsmoortel CM, Cohn SM, et al (1990) Are low tidal volumes safe? Chest 97: 430-434
42. Hickling KG, Henderson SJ, Jackson R (1990) Low mortality associated with low volume pressure limited ventilation with permissive hypercapnia in severe adult respiratory distress syndrome. Intensive Care Med 16: 372-377
43. Amato MBP, Barbas CSV, Medeiros DM, et al (1998) Effect of a protective-ventilation strategy on mortality in the acute respiratory distress syndrome. N Engl J Med 338:347-354
44. Stewart TE, Meade MO, Cook DJ, et al (1998) Evaluation of a ventilation strategy to prevent barotrauma in patients at high risk for acute respiratory distress syndrome. N Eng J Med 338: 355-361
45. Brochard L, Roudot-Thoraval F, Roupie E, et al (1998) Tidal volume reduction for prevention of ventilator-induced lung injury in the acute respiratory distress syndrome.Am J Respir Crit Care Med 158: 1831-1838
46. Brower RG, Shanholtz CB, Fessler BE, et al (1999) Prospective, randomized, controlled clinical trial comparing traditional versus reduced tidal volume ventilation in acute respiratory distress syndrome patients. Crit Care Med 27: 1492-1498

47. Gentilello LM, Anardi D, Mock C, et al (1995) Permissive hypercapnia in trauma patients. J Trauma 39: 846-852
48. Feihl F, Perret C (1994) How permissive hypercapnia should be? Am Respir Crit Care Med 150: 1722-1737
49. Hickling KG, Walsh J, Henderson SJ, et al (1994) Low mortality rate in adult respiratory syndrome using low-volume, pressure-limited ventilation wiyh permissive hypercapnia: a prospective study. Crit Care Med 22: 1568-1578

Capnography and Cardiac Output Determination

G. Murias, A. Villagra, L. Blanch

Since gas transfer across the alveolar capillary wall does not depend on active transport, the lung may be used as an aerotonometer, allowing the alveolar gas to equilibrate with the mixed venous blood. The analysis of this alveolar gas provides an indirect method for measuring mixed venous carbon dioxide tension ($pvCO_2$). The equilibration method, using a bag containing a high concentration of carbon dioxide in oxygen, has been shown to accurately measure oxygenated $pvCO_2$ and application of this method has led to the development of the non-invasive determination of cardiac output (CO) by the CO_2 rebreathing. Several studies have demonstrated the validity of this indirect Fick method in healthy subjects, in patients with cardiac dysfunction, in patients with obstructive airway disease, and in patients receiving mechanical ventilation [1-5].

Since the introduction to critical care of the balloon-directed thermistor-tipped pulmonary artery catheter in the 1970s [6], thermodilution CO measurements (TDCO) have been available at the bedside. Although inaccuracies of the method are known, it became the clinical "gold standard". However, soon after the introduction of the catheterization of the pulmonary artery, concerns about catheter safety appeared [7, 8], and some physicians recommended a moratorium in Swan Catheter catheter use [9-11].

Different approaches to non-invasive critical care monitoring have been suggested. Analyses of exhaled CO_2 and rebreathing techniques have been tested in the past for CO determination in the critical care setting. A close correlation was found between the rebreathing technique using arterial pCO_2 and the TD method in a variety of critically ill patients [2-5]. Unfortunately, the rebreathing method for CO determination was technically difficult and time consuming, factors that limited the routine use in the critical care arena. In order to reduce the technical burden of this method, the partial rebreathing technique for CO measurement (PRCO) has been developed (Non-Invasive Cardiac Output, NICO, Novametrix). PRCO technique allows non-invasive CO determination using the indirect Fick principle. PRCO may be performed automatically by inducing a periodic cyclic and transient increase of the instrumental dead space [12, 13].

A recent study was designed to assess the accuracy of a new device (NICO, *Novametrix*) to measure CO by using the PRCO method in mechanically ventilated critically ill patients (see Appendix), and to assess the hemodynamic effect of the transient $paCO_2$ increase induced by the PRCO method during the CO measurement.

Villagra et al. [14] studied 29 mechanically ventilated patients with a TD catheter in place. They measured CO simultaneously with the PRCO and TD method (TDCO), by delivering two 10 ml iced DW5% bolus during the 50-s rebreathing period. Up to four sets of CO measurements were performed in each patient, allowing at least 2 h between measurements. Unstable CO_2 readings were excluded. We also performed three TDCO measurements 1 minute before and after the PRCO period. Hemodynamic parameters were obtained 1 min before, during, and 1 min after the PRCO period. Variables were compared by one-way ANOVA. The simultaneous TD and PRCO measurements were compared by a concordance analysis. Villagra et al. [14] performed 101 CO measurements; 22 were discarded due to unstable CO_2 elimination. The bias of 79 measurements eligible for analysis was –0.35 ± 1.62 l/min and the 95% limits of agreement ranged from –3.51 l/min to 2.82 l/min. Considering CO variations at high CO values clinically less relevant, these authors performed the analysis only for CO of less than 7 l/min, and the bias was –0.07± 0.93 l/min and the 95% limits of agreement ranged from –1.90 l/min to 1.75 l/min. No changes in CO, heart rate, systemic or pulmonary pressures were observed before, during, or after the PRCO measurement. Although NICO cannot replace the pulmonary artery catheter, it offers an instantaneous, reasonably accurate, and totally non-invasive estimate of CO. The transient increase in $paCO_2$ caused during the rebreathing period does not induce significant changes in CO or hemodynamics.

A strong limitation of research in this field is the lack of a true gold standard. Clinical use has confirmed TDCO at this place, but limitations of the method are well known [15-19]. However, as a "clinical gold standard" TDCO provides information to physicians for medical decision-making. When evaluating another method, the new one must provide similar information in similar situations. In this scenario, lack of agreement between both methods does not describe which is correct and which is false. A comparison of CO measured by rebreathing techniques and TD is shown in Table 1. Differences between rebreathing methods and TDCO could also be explained by how far is the real CO from the measured value using either technique.

Clinicians must be alert to potential problems with CO_2 rebreathing techni-

Table 1. Comparison of cardiac output (CO) measured by two methods

	CO reference method	CO CO_2 rebreath	R value	Bias	Agreement
Franciosa [1]	5.9 ±1.6	5.5 ± 1.7	0.95	-	-
Davis et al. [3]	3.7 ± 1.3	3.6 ± 1.2	0.93	-	-
Mahler					
ARRD 1985	4.3 ± 0.9	3.4 ± 0.8	0.70	-	-
Blanch et al. [4]	5.5 ± 1.5	5.6 ± 1.5	0.91	0.12	1.85/-1.65
Neviere et al. [2]	-	-	0.96	-0.06	0.55/0.55
van Heerden et al. [5]	5.4 ± 1.6	4.7 ± 1.5	0.70	0.8	4.9/-3.3

que for CO measurement. Selection of the initial CO_2 concentration for the rebreathing bag might be important. Since the difference between $pvCO_2$ and arterial pCO_2 is only 6 mmHg, the estimate of $pvCO_2$ obtained after rebreathing from a bag containing a known concentration of CO_2 should be accurate. PRCO by itself measures the non-shunted blood portion of the cardiac output and the non-invasive method of shunt estimation is an adaptation of Nunn's iso-shunt plots [12]. Because high intrapulmonary shunt is quite common in critically ill patients further studies are needed to assess the accuracy of the PRCO method in patients with acute lung injury receiving mechanical ventilation. During the rebreathing period, elevation in minute ventilation induced by the increment of instrumental dead space during NICO measurement could have added thermal noise and might affect TDCO reproducibility [20, 21]. Finally, the CO_2-hemoglobin dissociation curve is linear only at values of pCO_2 above 30 mmHg (Table 2).

In summary, the PRCO method offers an instantaneous, reasonably accurate, and totally non-invasive estimate of CO in critically ill patients. NICO may have a place in intensive care unit provided that patients are not breathing spontaneously and not needing the measurement of pulmonary artery pressures.

Table 2. Potential problems with CO_2 rebreathing technique for CO measurement

- Selection of the initial CO_2 concentration for the rebreathing bag
- $pvCO_2$ and $paCO_2$ difference is only 6 mmHg
- The estimate of arterial pCO_2 (end-tidal pCO_2)
- Intrapulmonary shunted blood is not measured.
- Rebreathing maneuver to obtain a plateau can alter CO
- CO_2-hemoglobin dissociation curve is linear only at values of pCO_2 above 30 mmHg

References

1. Franciosa JA (1977) Evaluation of the CO2 rebreathing cardiac output method in seriously ill patients. Circulation 55:449-455
2. Neviere R, Mathieu D, Riou Y, et al (1994) Carbon dioxide rebreathing method of cardiac output measurement during acute respiratory failure in patients with chronic obstructive pulmonary disease. Crit Care Med 22: 81-85
3. Davis CC, Jones NL, Sealy BJ (1978) Measurements of cardiac output in seriously ill patients using a CO2 rebreathing method. Chest 73:167-172
4. Blanch L, Fernandez R, Benito S, et al (1988) Accuracy of an indirect carbon dioxide Fick method in determination of the cardiac output in critically ill mechanically ventilated patients. Intensive Care Med 14: 131-135
5. van Heerden PV, Baker S, Lim SI, et al (2000) Clinical evaluation of the noninvasive cardiac output (NICO) monitor in the intensive care unit. Anaesth Intensive Care 28: 427-430
6. Ganz W, Donoso R, Marcus HS, et al (1971) A new technique for measurement of cardiac output by thermodilution in man. Am J Cardiol 27: 392-396
7. Gore JM, Goldberg RJ, Spodick DH, et al (1987) A community-wide assessment of the use of pulmonary artery catheters in patients with acute myocardial infarction. Chest 92:721-727
8. Connors AF, Speroff T, Dawson NV, et al (1996) The effectiveness of right heart catheterization in the initial care of critically ill patients. JAMA 276:889-897
9. Robin DE (1985) The cult of Swan-Ganz catheter: overuse and abuse of pulmonary flow catheters. Ann Intern Med 103:445
10. Robin DE (1987) Death by pulmonary artery flow-directed catheter. Chest 92:727
11. Dalen JE, Bone RC (1996) Is it time to pull the pulmonary artery catheter? JAMA 276:916-918
12. Jaffe MB (1999) Partial CO_2 rebreathing cardiac output - Operating principles of the NICO system. J Clin Monit 15: 387-401
13. Capek JM, Roy RJ (1988) Nonivasive measurement of cardiac output using partial CO2 rebreathing. IEEE TransBiomed Engin 35:653-661
14. Villagra A, Murias G, Vatua S, et al (2000) Evaluation of the non-invasive CO_2 partial rebreathing method for cardiac output measurement in critical care. Intensive Care Med 26:S317
15. Snyder JV, Powner DJ (1982) Effects of mechanical ventilation on the measurement of cardiac output by thermodilution. Crit Care Med 10: 677-682
16. Stevens JH, Raffin TA, Mihm FG, et al (1985) Thermodilution cardiac output measurement. Effects of the respiratory cycle on its reproducibility. JAMA 253: 2240-2242
17. Harris AP, Miller CF, Beattie C, et al (1985) The slowing of sinus rhythm during thermodilution cardiac output determinations and the effect of altering injectate temperature. Anesthesiology 63: 540-541
18. Elkayam U, Berkley R, Azen S, et al (1983) Cardiac output by thermodilution technique. Effect of injectate's volume and temperature on accuracy and reproducibility in the critically Ill patient. Chest 84: 418-422
19. Bazaral MG, Petre J, Novoa R (1992) Errors in thermodilution cardiac output measurements caused by rapid pulmonary artery temperature decreases after cardiopulmonary bypass. Anesthesiology 77: 31-37
20. Wessel HU, James GW, Paul MH (1966) Effects of respiration and circulation on central blood temperature of the dog. J Appl Physiol 211: 1403-1412
21. Chatburn RL (1995) Measurement theory: accuracy issues in monitoring. In: Levine RL, From RE (eds) Critical care monitoring: from pre hospital to the ICU. Mosby Yearbook, St Louis, pp 17-42.

Appendix (adapted from reference 12)

The original indirect Fick equation

$$CO = \frac{VCO_2}{CvCO_2 - CaCO_2}$$

is rearranged in a different mode

$$CO = \frac{VCO_{2N}}{CvCO_{2N} - CaCO_{2N}} = \frac{VCO_{2R}}{CvCO_{2R} - CaCO_{2R}}$$

or

$$CO = \frac{DVCO_{2N} - DVCO_{2R}}{(CvCO_{2N} - CaCO2N) - (CvCO_{2R} - CaCO_{2R})}$$

where "N" means non rebreathing and "R" means rebreathing period. It is assumed that there is no change in cardiac output between the partial rebreathing period and the non-rebreathing period. As mixed venous CO_2 content (CvCO2) does not change during rebreathing, the equation could be rewritten as:

$$CO = \frac{\Delta VCO_2}{\Delta CaCO_2} \qquad \frac{\Delta VCO_2}{Sx\Delta PETCO_2}$$

The last can be used to measure non-shunted pulmonary capillary blood flow. By adding shunted flow, CO can be calculated.

Improvements in Percutaneous Tracheostomy: the Single-Step Rotational Dilation

G. FROVA

Until recently conventional surgical tracheostomy had a high overall morbidity and mortality rate in the ICU which was prevalently related to the underlying pathology. The mortality rate associated with the tracheostomy itself is very low, but complications such as bleeding, cellulitis-infection of the stoma and bad cosmetic results associated with the open procedure are still existing and relatively frequent. Several authors have substantiated the reduced incidence of bleeding and stomal infections with percutaneous tracheostomy (PT) in contrast with the surgical procedure [1, 2].

The success of the PT technique is the main reason which explains the gradual abandoning of the surgical procedure in adult ICU patients. Exhaustive reviews have reported the complications of surgical tracheostomy and the various methods of percutaneous tracheostomy [3, 4]. However, not all of the PT methods have simplified the procedure or are equally safe, because a reduced incidence of many intraoperative complications are dependent upon the experience and technical skill of the operator [5, 6, 7].

Performing tracheostomy with a percutaneous nephrostomy set based on the Seldinger technique and the gradual dilation of the stoma was the first innovation and has been reported as a safe procedure in the past years [8]; subsequently, many new instruments and technological refinements of the original procedure were described, but the original technique continues to be the most used and known method of PT [9].

The improvement attempts are characterized by four limiting aspects of Ciaglia's procedure: variable difficulty of entering, frequent pushing necessity, discontinuous dilation, and loss of time. To reduce duration and to abolish multiple dilation, modified forceps were inserted over the wire into the trachea and completely spread [10]. In the practice, the advantages of gradual dilation were lost with this new patented device and replaced by an uncontrolled transverse spreading. However, the indisputable advantages of the short skin incision resulted in difficulty during the introduction of the dilators and the tube.

The pathological consequences of pushing against the tracheal wall [11] are not completely clarified particularly as regards their clinical and functional significance. This potential damage was the basis for improvements of Ciaglia's original procedure (modification of number, size and shape of dilators; hydrophilic coating, etc.) and of the translaryngeal tracheostomy technique (TLT) [12]. TLT is the first single-step continuous dilation, but it is purely hypothetical that the necessity of pulling the tube through the tracheostomy tract with excessive force shall be less dangerous for tracheal cartilage than the opposite manoeuvre.

More recently a transcervical dilation procedure was proposed, based on a curved soft conical device (Ciaglia Blue Rhino). This shows the same theoretical difficulties in entering the trachea as evidenced with the multiple dilators original procedure. It has the same necessity to push the instrument against the tracheal wall with force when the incision is too small, the skin is particularly anelastic and the subcutaneous fat excessive, and it has the same risk of damage [13, 14]. However its advantage is the possibility of performing a rapid tracheostomy [15] in a continuous safe progressive single-step dilation.

A new transcervical procedure was recently ideated by the Author and developed in co-operation with Rüsch International (Esslingen, DE) in order to overcome all the described difficulties. It is based on the gradual insertion of a device into the trachea with a controlled rotating movement completely indifferent to the variable characteristics in rigidity of the tracheal wall. The procedure allows a continuous single-step dilation without the necessity of pushing against the wall itself.

Technical development

The new procedure was initially thought to overcome the difficulty met in introducing the first and second dilator of the Ciaglia set (Cook Critical Care, Bloomington, USA) or of its modified version (PercuQuick Rüsch) if the rigidity of the wall was excessive or the interanular space was calcified. The use of a metal orthopaedic screw mounted over the j-wire and inserted into the trachea with a rotating movement was successful in all cases presenting initial difficulties. The use of the screw allowed an easy dilation up to 5 mm diameter for subsequent insertion of the 1st and 2nd dilator, but the procedure was still discontinuous.

The next step was based on the possibility of a controlled rotation until reaching the appropriate diameter, eliminating the use of multiple devices, reducing the bleeding into the trachea between removal and insertion of many dilators and transforming the habitual necessity of pushing against the wall into pulling the device during rotation.

The kit (at the present time not yet commercially available) includes a scalpel, a catheter-introducing needle 14 G (2.3 mm OD) x 52 mm, a j-wire guide (1.25 mm OD) x 60 cm, a 10 mL syringe and plastic screws size 7, 8 or 9 (PercuTwist®) (Fig. 1). Separately available is the tracheostomy tube with its dilator-introducer (respectively 6.5, 7.5, 8.5 mm outer diameter for the corresponding sizes 7, 8, 9 inner diameter tracheostomy tube). The size of the tracheostomy tube is usually decided by the operator at the moment of the procedure in connection with patient's sex, age, weight and pathology.

The innovative device is the single-step dilator. It is a plastic device with two parts: the screw and the handle. The screw has twelve self-tapping threads, with diameters that increase from 2 mm to 13.6 (size 9), 12.3 (size 8) or 10.0 mm (size 7). Eight of the screws are distributed in the conical part with four screws in the cylindrical part. The self-tapping threads are covered with a hydrophilic coating. The handle has two different diameters, 20 and 25 mm, a feature which

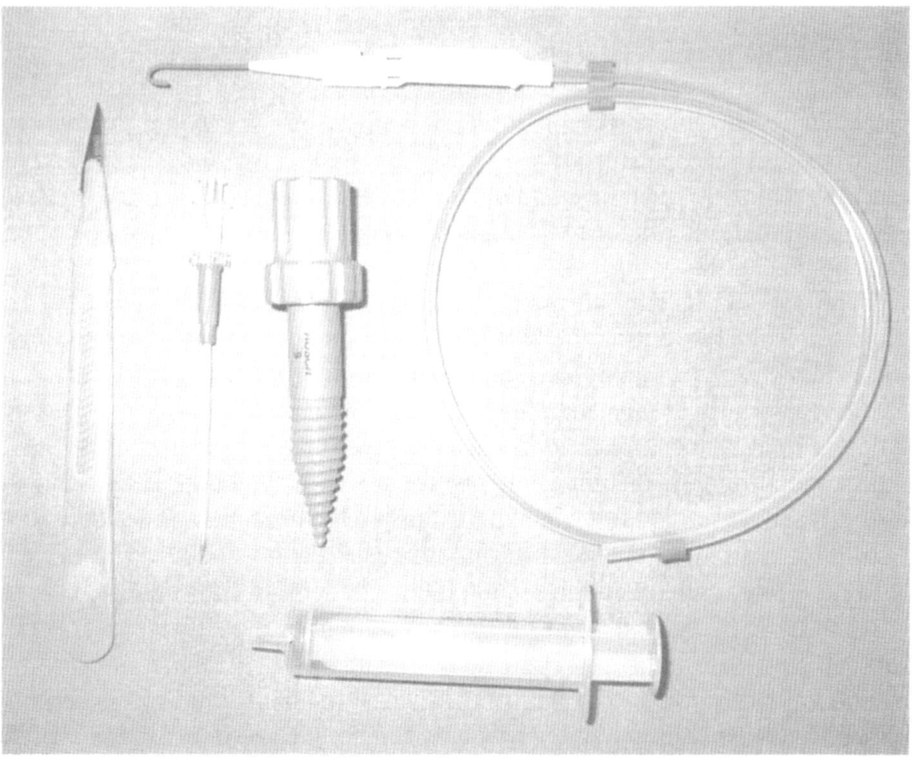

Fig. 1. The PercuTwist set

allows different rotary forces to be obtained. The kit can only be used once because the hydrophilic coating of the thread is destroyed when it is used.

Description of procedure

In addition to the tracheostomy set, two small basins (for antiseptic solution and water), sterile drapes and gauzes, water-based lubricant, suction catheters and an angulated adapter-connector for the tracheostomy tube (with a fiberscope port) are necessary. A sterile box with instruments for surgical tracheostomy and ligation of vessels should be at hand.

The instrumentation for continuous endoscopic guidance is absolutely necessary [16] and the use of a video-monitor is strongly recommended to visualize the endotracheal component of the procedure. The advantages are vessel identification with transillumination, the initial or final laryngoscopy, the confirmation of the midline puncture, the continuous control during the insertion of the screw and the final control of the distal part beyond the tracheostomy tube.

There is no need for a second surgical collaborator, because the procedure needs only one experienced operator plus a colleague performing the bronchoscopy, who oversees the administration of medications, the monitoring of vital functions and the adjustments of ventilatory settings. Moreover, a nurse is needed to help with materials and instrument procurement. It is more difficult to perform multiple dilator percutaneous tracheostomy without adequate surgical help [17].

The patients in ICU are monitored, nasally or orally intubated and on respiratory support; during the procedure, general anaesthesia with neuromuscular blockers is habitually used and the fraction of inspired oxygen is set at 1.0, independently of the patient's pathology. The patient's position is slightly different from the position used in open tracheostomy and the neck is maintained in an indifferent position as the one the patient will assume after tracheostomy. It is not useful to force in hyperextension the head and the neck because it is not necessary to evidence the inferior part of the trachea. The normal position is more safe for cervical spine trauma patients, it limits the increase in intracranial pressure and contributes to the creation of a shorter and more vertical tracheostomy tract. A roll under the shoulders is sometimes useful, while immobilization of the chin is always used by the Author; this is particularly advantageous in young over weight people with a very soft and mobile trachea.

Airway management can be performed by using different techniques. The procedure that is commonly used during percutaneous procedures is the partial withdrawal of the tracheal tube under endoscopic control until cricoid cartilage can be seen [17]. However, it is preferable to remove the tracheal tube and replace it by the insertion of a standard laryngeal mask [18]; this technique allows the evaluation of any potential damage induced by the tube on the laryngeal inlet, it eliminates the risk of loosing the airway, facilitates identification of the cricoid and the first ring, abolishes the possibility of puncturing the tube, its cuff or endoscopic instruments, and eliminates the risk of damaging the recurrent nerve branch when inflating the cuff between the cords and the cricoid [19].

After preparing and draping the patient, the bronchoscope is inserted into the laryngeal mask airway (LMA) adapter and the transillumination of the subglottic and tracheal region is obtained in order to look for the presence of vessels. The puncture of the skin is performed in the region between the cricoid and the 3rd ring after accurate palpation of anatomical landmarks. This has to be done exactly in the middle of the airway and accurately between the cartilages, preferably between the first and second ring. The endoscopic vision of the bulging mucosa into the tracheal lumen gives the signal for the correct position for the needle. Leaving the catheter in the trachea, the j-guidewire is pushed towards the carena and the catheter removed.

A 6-8 mm long vertical incision is made in the skin. The subcutaneous fat at the sides of the wire and the screw - after immersion for a few seconds in water - is then passed over the j-guidewire and then gently rotated clockwise without pushing it against the wall. A longer incision, commonly reported in the literature on percutaneous transcervical tracheostomy [8, 10, 17, 20], increases potential complications, such as stoma infection and scar evidence [21]. If the aim of the procedure is to obtain a very snug fit of the tracheostomy tube and a tighter tract, there is no reason to make a skin incision larger than the tip of the screw. If the primary dilational procedure is performed without a tissue dissection, the patient must be reintubated through the mouth in the event of accidental decannulation within the first 3 days of the procedure, while the tract is still immature [17]. Replacement of the tracheostomy tube in an emergent situation could be possible, but an experienced physician is needed as well as a Seldinger procedure with an introducer. Oherwise the results could be disastrous.

Depending on the variable depth of the trachea, the screw will appear into the airway after between 30 and 60 sec. When two or three threads are endoscopically visible, the controlled rotation can be continued by pulling the handle until the desired dilation is obtained. The device is removed by turning counter-clockwise. The tracheostomy tube mounted on the snug-fitting introducer, which has to be generously lubricated, is pushed over the j-wire guide until it is inserted into the trachea. The part of the introducer which is projected beyond the tip must be limited to 2 cm (Fig. 2).

The wire and the introducer are then removed, and the cuff is inflated. After tracheal suction, the patient is manually ventilated and then connected to the mechanical ventilator. Finally, endoscopic control is performed through the use of a tracheostomy tube to check its position and to evaluate the distal pre-carenal region for the presence of blood or clots in the main bronchi. A chest X-ray is routinely performed after the procedure.

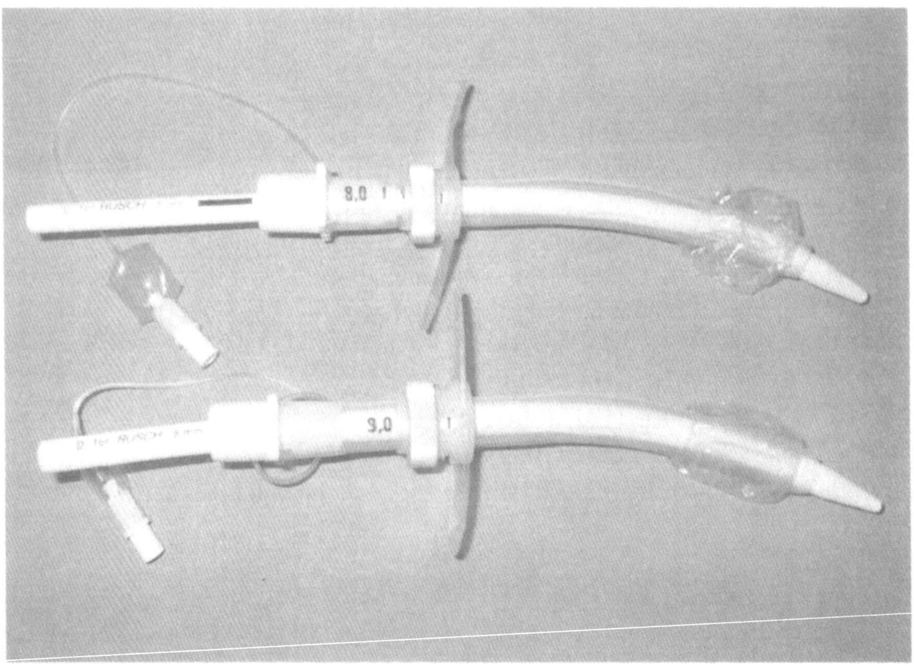

Fig.2. The size 8 and 9 introducers mounted on tracheostomy tubes

Indications and contraindications

Adult intubated ICU patients are the main indication for the procedure, not different from other percutaneous procedures; the absolute contraindications are the same too and include urgency and children. The relative contraindications are as follows: head trauma with instable intracranial pressure, midline neck mass, severe uncorrected coagulopathy, impossibility to identify anatomical landmarks, prolonged intubation with the suspicion of tracheomalacia, venous vessels larger than 5 mm on the midline (to be ligated before), and neck infections or thyroid cancer. Some of the above may be positively influenced by the properties of the new percutaneous tracheostomy procedure.

Preliminary results

Using the new procedure 37 patients were tracheostomized in our ICU from December 2000 till June 2001. The procedures were performed by the Author. The entrance in trachea was the space between the cricoid and the 1st ring in 18 cases, between the 1st and the 2nd ring in 16 cases and between the 2nd and the 3rd ring in 3 cases. The size of the screw was n. 8 in 30 cases and n. 7 in 7 cases.

The procedure was considered easy in 33 patients, not easy but completed in 3, difficult and abandoned in favour of the multiple dilators procedure in one patient at the beginning. No difficulty was encountered during the insertion of the tracheostomy tube. The internal and external bleeding during and after the procedure was evaluated after the incision, after the screw removal, at the end of the procedure and during the following 48 hours. While minimal bleeding was frequently seen after the skin puncture and incision, an incredibly low rate of visible bleeding was present after the removal of the screw [22]. A small amount of blood was suctioned at the end of the procedure in 4 patients, but no blood or clots occluding bronchi were detected by endoscopy. Postoperative oozing in the first 48 hours, not unusual with PT, was absent in 36/37 patients. The mean time for the procedure was 3.8 minutes from the introduction of the needle until the tube endoscopic observation.

No relevant complication (subcutaneous emphysema, pnx, false route, bronchial obstruction and desaturation, evident or massive bleeding, posterior wall damage, infection and cellulitis in the first week) was observed. In 5/37 patients minor intraoperative problems occurred (1 change of procedure, 3 ring fractures, 1 postoperative oozing). Other problems consisted of: 1 broken cuff, 6 bent j-wires, 1 procedure was performed in two steps. All problems had no clinical relevance.

Conclusions

Tracheostomy presents a large number of advantages compared to conventional prolonged endotracheal intubation (i.e., an improvement of patient's comfort and the avoidance of laryngeal, cricoidal and high-tracheal injury), conventional surgical tracheostomy is still associated with a remarkable number of complications in the ICU, which percutaneous tracheostomy techniques have partially eliminated. Lower complication rates and the better cosmetic results could be obtained if the operator gives particular attention to some key points: control of the airways, to routinely use the continuous endoscopic guidance, to limit the length of skin incision and abolish any tissue blunt dissection. The extremely low incidence of bleeding is probably related to the small incision, the stretching of tissues during the progressive rotational dilation and the tampon effect of a tightly fitting tracheostomy tube.

The new procedure achieves the same results as any other percutaneous tracheostomy procedure, but with an adjunctive advantage: the possibility to obtain the dilation in a continuous controlled manner probably without the potential damage to the tracheal wall and without the inconvenience of a discontinuous procedure. The technique is also very easy to learn and very quick to perform. Results of the rotational dilation are extremely favourable with an incidence of complications lower than that usually reported with other percutaneous procedures. Nonetheless, only an extensive controlled clinical trial is required to confirm these preliminary results.

References

1. Friedman Y, Fildes J, Mizock B et al (1996) Comparison of percutaneous and surgical tracheostomies. Chest 110:480-485
2. Freeman BD, Isabella K, Lin N et al (2000) A meta-analysis of prospective trials comparing percutaneous and surgical tracheostomy in critically ill patients. Chest 118:1412-1418
3. Moe KS, Schmid S, Stoeckli SJ et al (1999) Percutaneous tracheostomy: a comprehensive evaluation. Ann Otol Rhinol Laryngol 108:384-391
4. MacCallum PL, Parnes LS, Sharpe MD et al (2000) Comparison of open, percutaneous, and translaryngeal tracheostomies. Otolaryngol Head and Neck Surg 122: 686-690
5. Byhahn C, Wilke HJ, Lischke V et al (2001) Bedside percutaneous tracheostomy: clinical comparison of Griggs and Fantoni techniques. World J Surg 25: 296-301
6. Ravat F, Pommier C, Dorne R (2001) Tracheostomie percutanée. Ann Fr Anesth Réanim 20:260-281
7. Dulguerov P, Gysin C, Perneger TV et al (1999) Percutaneous or surgical tracheostomy: a meta-analysis. Crit Care Med 27: 1617-1625
8. Ciaglia P, Firshing R, Syniec (1985) Elective percutaneous dilational tracheostomy. A new simple bedside procedure: a preliminary report. Chest 87:715-719
9. Bause H, Prause A (1999) Ratings and complications with minimally invasive percutaneous tracheotomy. Anaesthesiol Intensivmed Notfallmed Schmerzther 34:659-664

10. Griggs WM, Worthley LIG, Gilligan JE et al (1990) A simple percutaneous tracheostomy technique. Surg Gynecol Obstet 170:543-545
11. Walz MK, Schmidt U (1999) Tracheal lesions caused by percutaneous dilatational tracheostomy – a clinico-pathological study. Intensive Care Medicine 25:102-105
12. Fantoni A, Ripamonti D (1997) Tracheostomia translaringea: metodo non chirurgico. Intensive Care Medicine 3:193-198
13. Byhahn C, Wilke HJ, Halbig S et al (2000) Percutaneous tracheostomy. Ciaglia Blue Rhino versus the basic Ciaglia technique of percutaneous dilational tracheostomy. Anesth Analg 91: 882-886
14. Edwards SM, Williams JC (2001) Tracheal cartilage fracture with the Blue Rhino Ciaglia percutaneous tracheostomy system. European Journal of Anaesthesiology 18:487
15. Johnson JL, Cheatham ML, Sagraves S et al (2001) Percutaneous dilational tracheostomy: a comparison of single versus multiple-dilator techniques. Crit Care Med; 29:1251-1254
16. Kost KM (2000) Percutaneous tracheostomy: comparison of Ciaglia and Griggs technique. Crit Care 4: 143-146
17. Kost KM (1998) Tracheostomy in the intensive care unit setting. In: Myers EN, Johnson JT, Murry T (eds) Tracheotomy. Singular Publishing Group Inc, San Diego, pp 75-96
18. Dexter TJ (1994) The laryngeal mask airway: a method to improve visualization of the trachea and larynx during fiberoptic assisted percutaneous tracheostomy. Anaesth Intens Care 22:35-39
19. Asai T, Latto IP, Vaughan RS (1993) The distance between the grille of the laryngeal mask airway and the vocal cords. Is conventional intubation through the laryngeal mask safe? Anaesthesia 48:667-669
20. Hazard PB, Garrett HE, Adams JW et al (1988) Bedside percutaneous tracheostomy: experience with 55 elective procedures. Ann Thor Surg 46:63-67
21. Frova G, Concoreggi C, Galbiati P et al (1997) Percutaneous dilatational tracheostomy with mixed technique in ICU. British Journal of Anaesthesia A360:110
22. Frova G, Quintel M (2001) A simple new method for percutaneous tracheostomy: the controlled rotating dilatation. Intensive Care Medicine (submitted)

TRAUMA

The Challenges of Delivering Acute Medical Services to Trauma Patients in Remote Locations

D.J. PENNEY, A. FLABOURIS, M.J.A. PARR

Trunkey in 1983 proposed the concept of the 'trimodal distribution of trauma deaths', with 50% of deaths occurring immediately following an accident, 30% of deaths in the first 4 h, and 20% of deaths beyond 4 h [1]. The concept of the 'Golden Hour' of trauma stresses the importance of early medical intervention within the 1st hour to prevent the organ damage that may result in later in-hospital deaths. The applicability and accuracy of these concepts has been questioned, but prompt resuscitation and delivery of the severely injured patient to definitive care is a crucial determinant of improved patient outcome.

It is well established that severely injured patients have an improved chance of survival if treated in trauma centers within regionalized trauma systems [2]. A trauma center can be defined as 'a hospital where the medical staff have a commitment to provide 24 hour in-house cover by surgeons, anaesthesiologists, and support staff to care for trauma patients' [1]. Regionalization ensures volume through fewer centers, a factor that is said to be associated with improved outcome [3], but may also increase the physical distance between such trauma centers and the injured in remote locations. Thus the challenges for the delivery of trauma care to remote locations include issues related to transport vehicles, equipment, personnel performance, and access.

Physical environments

Remote locations present differing challenges for the provision of trauma services compared with urban areas. The physical environment can be highly variable, even within the same regions. Such environments create many challenges for emergency medical services (EMS). These include notification of injury, location identification and access, patient extrication, delivery of medical staff, and equipment performance in extreme conditions.

Each region has its own physical characteristic in which an EMS will operate. The responding trauma system must anticipate these problems and be appropriately structured and resourced to counter such challenges. However, a system that works well in one region, may not be appropriate for another, and so rigid system requirements are inappropriate.

Epidemiology

Remote locations, in terms of medical service provision, can be defined as areas where a subgroup of a population is separated from access to higher standards of service by distance or other barrier [4]. This subgroup may differ in both demographics and health from an urban population. Regional population demographics may also vary due to temporary or seasonal population migration or seasonal physical environmental changes.

The human activities at different regions may be unique and predictable. Data gathering and analysis for each region is essential for risk assessment. For example, within the national park regions of California, the overall occurrence of nonfatal events was recorded to be 9.2 people per 100,000 visits. The majority of injuries, 70% of all nonfatal injuries, were related to musculoskeletal or soft tissue injury, 38% of which involved the lower limbs. Overall mortality rate was 0.26 deaths per 100,000 visits, of which males accounted for 78% of deaths, with heart disease, drowning, and falls being the most-common cause of death [5]. Similar data were recorded in another survey, with a mortality rate of 0.28 per 100,000 person-days of exposure, 80% of non-fatal injuries being soft tissue injuries [6]. In the latter study, 39% of all injuries and illnesses required evacuation (1.5 per 1,000 person-days of exposure).

When compared with urban statistics, similar mechanisms of injury in remote locations carry a higher mortality [7, 8]. Motor vehicle accidents in nonurban areas have a higher mortality, especially in children and adolescents [9].

Although injuries in such remote locations are infrequent, careful planning and individual selection prior to exposure to such environments can help limit their occurrence. Similarly injury prediction through prior regional risk assessment and use of regional databases of injury occurrences can aid with planning and prevention of future similar injuries. Preventative and planning processes may be of greater significance for remote locations, considering the challenges such environments place upon trauma systems.

EMS system

Effective trauma management requires a system of care designed to manage the patient from the injury scene all the way through to rehabilitation. Importance needs to be focused on developing the system as a whole, as weak components of the system will lead to an overall failure.

Access to EMS

An easy, single-point, rapid-access activation process is essential for all trauma systems. Education of the general public in bystander trauma care allows for the mobilization of community resources, which can act as the first-line response. As a concept this is very cheap to administer, and given the current reluctance and inability of the lay public to play a role, there is real potential for a positive impact.

Most such systems however rely on a single telephone number for activation. Advancing telecommunication technology has made this service increasingly more widely available to remote locations, which in the past could not access such a service. Although travel time for EMS to injured patients can be very short, time to discovery of the injured is the greater time delay factor [10]

Transport vehicles

Primary response options are determined by factors such as distance from and to the site of definitive care, as well as geographical and climatic features. Motor vehicle and rotary or fixed-wing air response are among the available options. Cost is clearly a major factor, especially in underdeveloped countries. There have been no studies to clearly demonstrate one system is preferable to another in an urban environment.

For remote locations, each with its own unique characteristics, comparative study of choice of vehicles is impractical. Air or ground vehicles each have their own utility and crew capabilities. An EMS system should have recourse to several transport options in a continuously reviewed and evolving structure. More importantly, the choice of vehicle should be made in conjunction with the choice of the transport crew, as it may be the latter rather than the vehicle itself that have the greater impact upon patient outcome [11-14].

Factors such as the transport of appropriate personnel and equipment to the patient in as short a time as possible need to be balanced with consideration of maximal EMS crew safety. The safety of a commercial EMS helicopter service was examined in a safety study in 1988 in the United States where patient transport helicopters experienced twice the accident rate of air taxis, usually night and weather related, with human error being most frequently attributed as the cause [15]. Safety recommendations usually address weather conditions, pilot staffing and workload, night operations, pilot training and experience, equipment installation and performance standards, personnel protective clothing and equipment, and organization and management [16].

Ground transport is also not without risks. With all transport modalities there are important stressors, such as noise, vibration, acceleration forces, fatigue, and motion sickness, and the potential therapeutic limitations imposed by the transport environment.

Ambient environmental factors, such as altitude and temperature, can impact upon allowable vehicle size and performance. In all such circumstances, prior risk assessment, with multidisciplinary input, is crucial to the success of any trauma task

Personnel

A short on-scene time with a 'scoop and run' approach may be contrasted to a longer prehospital phase with a 'stay and stabilize' philosophy, which better describes circumstances in remote locations, for which the "run" phase is greatly exaggerated. The latter approaches require highly trained and skilled personnel with appropriate equipment. There is much debate over the benefit of the levels of training and skills of prehospital personnel. A recent review article by Spaite et al. [17] questioned that the primary determinant of outcome for trauma patients is the time interval from injury to the operating room, concluding that studies supporting the relationship are flawed and retrospective. The authors also reviewed articles for and against advanced life support (ALS) at the scene. They examined methodologies, results, and conclusions, and concluded no one study exists to convincingly support one approach over another. There is a desperate need for prospective, randomized controlled trials that compare ALS with basic life support prehospital care in victims of major trauma.

On-scene interventions range from simple to the sophisticated. Airway compromise and hypoxia are common at the scene of injury and result in a range of injury from irreversible brain damage and death to lesser insults that may profoundly influence outcome, especially in head-injured patients [18, 19]. The need for intervention is clear, how much intervention and by whom is less clear. Currently, even within the urban environment, the benefit of prehospital fluid administration and advanced airway management remains controversial [20, 21].

Within remote environments, risks in the delivery of scene resuscitation is greater and the timely availability of higher level "backup" support is less likely to be available. Rural environments not only have fewer available EMS [10], but have fewer advanced trained EMS personnel, who have less trauma exposure [22].

In such circumstances a "get it right the first time" approach would necessitate the delivery of the highest allowable level of care. This may require the use of trained and experienced medical [11-14], as opposed to paramedical, personnel. The latter approach would result in a greater "overtriage" rate for the level of personnel and equipment delivered to a remote location. Ultimately the acceptability of such rates needs to be based upon each region's unique environmental and injury pattern characteristics.

Emergency departments

Issues related to the availability of highly skilled hospital staff and their exposure to a sufficient number of trauma patients apply equally to the emergency departments of smaller rural hospitals as to prehospital EMS. Training, a trauma verification system, and integration of smaller hospitals into a wider trauma system can have a positive impact on patient outcome, especially for patients with more-severe injuries [23, 24].

Coordination of trauma care

Areas that have established regional plans to provide trauma care from the scene to rehabilitation have achieved dramatic reduction in preventable death rates [25]. Regionalization of trauma services involves the establishment of an injury database, regional plans, the identification of barriers to change, and the administrative support necessary for the efficient functioning of such services. Reasons for failure include lack of funds, political will, lack of awareness by society, and an underestimation of the resources and effort required to coordinate and integrate the system.

Coordination of trauma care in remote locations is even more challenging. The isolation of such populations, the desire to not medically disadvantage them, the infrequency of injuries, and the challenges of delivery of an urban equivalent system of trauma care to such regions need to be addressed. With developing technology, some medical care, in terms of advice, clinical expertise, and remote triage, can be delivered via advanced telemedical communication. Ideally each region, based upon their unique prior risk assessment, frequency, or injury occurrence and catalogue of available resources, should prepare and plan its own regional specific trauma response. An ongoing evaluation of all facets of such a response is vital as short- and longer-term regional variations evolve.

Conclusion

Patients injured within a remote environment will continually provide a challenge to all levels of trauma care providers. Strategies based upon detailed risk analysis and subsequent resource allocation and provision are essential for optimal service delivery. Such strategies would require continual re-evaluation and refinement. Remote environments should be incorporated within, and supported by, regional trauma systems. With the advancement in current technology, such support can be increasingly provided from a distant location.

References

1. Trunkey DD (1983) Trauma. Sci Am 249:20-27
2. Guss DA, Meyer FT, Neumann TS, et al (1989) The impact of a regionalized trauma system on trauma care in San Diego County. Ann Emerg Med 18:1141-1145
3. Sampalis JS, Denis R, Lavoie A, et al (1999) Trauma care regionalization: a process-outcome evaluation. J Trauma 46:565-579
4. Shepherd L, Auger T, Wisborg T, Williams J (2001) Trauma in rural and remote areas. In: Soreide E, Grande C (eds) Prehospital trauma care. Dekker, New York, pp 703-717
5. Montalvo R, Wingard DL, Bracker M, Davidson TM (1998) Morbidity and mortality in the wilderness. West J Med 168:248-254
6. Gentile DA, Morris JA, Schimelpfenig T, et al (1992) Wilderness injuries and illnesses. Ann Emerg Med 21:853-861
7. Flowe KM, Cunningham PRG, Foil MB (1995) Rural trauma. Surg Ann 27:29-39
8. Baker SP, Whitfield RA, O'Neil B (1988) County mapping of injury mortality. J Trauma 28:741-745
9. Baker SB, O'Neil B (1987) Geographic variations in mortality from motor vehicle crashes. N Eng J Med 316:1384-1387
10. Grossman DC, Hart LG, Rivara FP, et al (1995) From roadside to bedside: the regionalisation of trauma care in a remote rural county. J Trauma 38:14-21
11. Baxt WG, Moody P (1987) The impact of a physician as part of the aeromedical team in patients with blunt trauma. JAMA 257:3246-3250
12. Moylan JA, Fitzpatrick KT, Beyer J, Georgiade GS (1988) Factors improving survival in multisystem trauma patients. Ann Surg 207:679-685
13. Bartolacci RA, Munford BJ (1998) Air medical response to blunt trauma: effect on early survival. Med J Aust 169:612-616
14. Garner A, Rashford S, Lee A, Bartolacci R (1999) Addition of physicians to paramedic helicopter services decreases blunt trauma mortality. Aust NZ J Surg 69:697-701
15. Safety study-Commercial Emergency Medical Service Helicopter Operations (1988) National Transportation Safety Board, Washington, DC, report no. NTSB/SS-88/01
16. Geis C, Madsen P (2001) Working in the prehospital environment: safety aspects and teamwork. In: Soreide E, Grande C (eds) Prehospital trauma care. Dekker, New York, pp 83-97
17. Spaite DW, Criss EA, Valenzuela TD, Meislin HW (1998) Prehospital advanced life support for major trauma: critical need for clinical trials. Ann Emerg Med 32:480-489
18. Stocchetti N, Furlan A, Volta F (1996) Hypoxaemia and arterial hypotension at the accident scene in head injury. J Trauma 40:764-767
19. Chesnut RM (1995) Secondary brain insults after head injury: clinical perspectives. New Horiz 3:366-375

20. Owens TM, Watson WC, Prough DS, et al (1995) Limiting initial resuscitation of uncontrolled hemorrhage reduces internal bleeding and subsequent volume requirements. J Trauma 39:200--207
21. Bickell WH, Wall MJ Jr, Pepe PE et al (1994) Immediate versus delayed fluid resuscitation for hypotensive patients with penetrating torso injuries. N Eng J Med 331:1105-1109
22. Messick WJ, Rutledge R, Meyer AA (1992) The association of advanced life support training and decreased per capita trauma death rates: an analysis of 12,417 trauma deaths. J. Trauma 33:850-855
23. Rogers FB, Osler TM, Shackford SR, et al (1999) Study of the outcome of patients transferred to a level 1 hospital after stabilisation at an outlying hospital in a rural setting. J Trauma 46:328-333
24. Esposito TJ, Sanddal ND, Hansen JD, Reynolds S (1995) Analysis of preventable trauma deaths and inappropriate trauma care in a rural state. J Trauma 39:955-962
25. Cales RH (1984) Traumatic mortality in Orange County: the effects of the implementation of a regional trauma system. Ann Emerg Med 13:1-10

Trauma – Stabilization, Assessment, and Transportation

G. GORDINI, M. MENARINI

In the complex management of patients with severe trauma (severe trauma as defined by ISS15), the pre-hospital phase plays a fundamental role. As is often the case, the patient spends great part of the "golden hour" outside the hospital setting and in many European facilities, hospitalization (the time gap between the trauma-inducing event and arrival in the emergency ward) exceeds 1 h, especially in the case of events taking place in rural areas.

In the present paper we describe the state-of-the-art in pre-hospital treatment of trauma patients, derived from review of relevant literature and publications. Different views have contributed to a lively debate for several years.

Our conclusion - after examining the published material - is that it is not possible to draw and establish scientific evidence from said material, mainly for lack of randomized perspective studies; many researchers have in fact matched patients' groups which were not always comparable, either for their pathology or the degree of severity of their injuries. Spaite et al. [1] state that "apples and oranges" are mixed together, thus undermining the grounding of conclusions; many articles simply report experts' opinions and review limited case records.

We believe that a valid and realistic evaluation of the effectiveness of the pre-hospital treatment would need different reviews than those (often of a retrospective nature) concerning mortality.

The effects of pre-hospital treatment on morbility and mortality reduction for trauma patients are quite difficult to distinguish from the impact on the patient of subsequent actions carried out in the emergency room and other hospital wards.

In any case, the fact that a high percentage of deaths are incurred in pre-hospital settings (on the scene and during transportation) cannot be overlooked, thus further stressing the understanding that investments should be made on field emergency services.

Does a trauma system reduce trauma deaths?

Mortality and injury derived disabling outcome are widely believed to be reduced by the type of response provided by a "trauma system". The awareness of trauma relevance as a health issue [2] has led to the development of diverse intervention models (variations due to local health resources and culture), all nonetheless aimed at outlining a structured, consistent, and co-ordinated response. The main feature of the system consists of setting up of a network of facilities with integrated functions and assuring the care of all trauma patients with respect to their needs, while fully exploiting available resources ("inclusive system")

In particular, data from the United States have stressed that the setting up of a trauma system aimed at providing a multidisciplinary response, from the event scene to the hospital, does entail advantages in terms of outcome improvement. The trauma center is at the core of said systems. Some authors stress that, despite the fact that available data seem to favorably back trauma systems, further research is necessary with focussed studies that may provide stronger evidence concerning this positive association.

The direct center referral to hospitals specialized as trauma centers is a priority for pre-hospital emergency services, which would imply the definition of specific criteria for direct admission, based on diverse (physiological, anatomical, mechanical, and anamnestic) elements.

The issue of the assessment of the trauma victim at the accident scene is fundamental for emergency teams, as on the one hand it would guide the treatment [within the framework of the appropriate strategy for the given emergency medical services (EMS) system], while on the other hand directing the subsequent and appropriate hospital admission.

The staging of trauma patients, with respect to the severity of their condition, in terms of impairment of life functions, is based on scores grouping different evaluation criteria. The selection of scores takes into account not only their validity in terms of sensitivity, specificity and predictive value, but also whether they are easy to apply. Two scores should be mentioned here, which are widely used in pre-hospital care: the Glasgow Coma Scale (GCS) and the Revised Trauma Score (RTS).

The GCS score is widely believed to be reliable, by assuming that it can be easily applied and that the involved operators are strongly in agreement. As a matter of fact, several problems do question the effective reliability of the score system [3].

The GCS score should be derived from the assessment of cardio-respiratory stabilization, namely when hypoxemia and hypotension are not present; however, this does not always take place in the immediate post-trauma phase, when the emergency team carry out the primary assessment and treatment is initiated. Pre-hospital administration of sedatives and muscle relaxants (in EMS systems the percentage of patients arriving in the emergency room already sedated and with intubation is constantly increasing) hampers GCS reappraisal. The conclusion is that quite often the first GCS score is deemed sufficient, although made in far-from-optimal situations. The administration of short half-life drugs may be of help in establishing a "pharmacological window", whenever suitable. The utilization of the sole motor response has been suggested, as it is a good correlate of the total GCS [4].

Studies on GCS reliability should be carried out in the different trauma systems, as the related score - beside representing a threshold value for specific actions (e.g., endotracheal intubation, if GCS ≤ 8) - is calculated in many other prognostic assessment scores. An unreliable score would compromise all subsequent tests (for example, the result of head injury outcome would be invalidated).

The RTS is the most widely used system; while providing for consistent advantages, its limitations should also be taken into due consideration. Table 1 may be of some help in clarifying the matter [5]:

Table 1. Estimate of RTS sensitivity, specificity, and predictive value

Definition	Sensitivity[a)]	Specificity[b)]	Predictive value of a negative test[c)]	Predictive value of a positive test[d)]
ISS ≥ 18	38%	94%	96%	27%
ISS ≥ 20	56%	94%	98%	25%
Major emergency therapy[e)]	76%	94%	99%	25%

[a)] Percentage of patients with major injuries diagnosed by reduced RTS
[b)] Percentage of patients with minor injuries only, with maximum RTS
[c)] Percentage of patients with minor injuries only, of those with maximum RTS
[d)] Percentage of patients with major injuries of those with reduced RTS
[e)] Thoracotomy, laparotomy, emergency neurosurgery; immediate intensive care unit admission and death within 48 h

Independently from the criterion applied for centralization, the triage would always present some limitations, either entailing overtriage or undertriage. This would in its turn lead to the search for an "acceptability" threshold for over- and undertriage in order to reduce the number of improper admissions (facility overloading) on the one hand, and the admission of patients in unsuitable facilities, on the other (trauma patients dying outside trauma centers).

Can pre-hospital care reduce mortality in trauma victims?

Today the answer is that there is no sound scientific evidence enabling us to establish a universally accepted rationale for organizational and operational efforts carried out and implemented by EMS systems in order to achieve a drop in trauma deaths.

The classical study by Trunkey [6] on trauma mortality reported a trimodal mortality distribution (with three peaks: in the 1st hour; from the 1st to the 4th hour; later, after several days). Other more-recent studies have instead focussed on a different bimodal distribution.

In his study, Marson and Thomson [7] concluded that in a town in Brazil the setting up of an EMS facility has brought about a drop in mortality during the 1st hour, with a more even distribution in the following hours, which does not allow for the detection of the second peak in Trunkey's curve. According to the author, the setting up of an EMS system has produced the decrease in mortality for patients injured in motor vehicle crashes. Actually, the study lacks many elements which might enable it to support said conclusion unquestionably. There are no data on patients' trauma severity, on the incidence of severe head injuries, for example; the procedures really carried out; on the organizational and operational adjustments made in the hospital phase, if any. Sauaia et al. [8] reported a similar distribution. The question that may arise here is whether said distribution is simply a mere life prolongation of patients with injuries incompatible with survival, as generated by pre-hospital care.

Meislin et al. [9] reported a bimodal distribution, suggesting that it may be linked to the high percentage of blunt traumas found locally. This would reduce mortality in the 1st hour, while increasing mortality during the first 24 – 48 h. In blunt injuries, unlike penetrating injuries (widely represented in Trunkey's study), clinical presentations are less easily defined and only rarely is immediate surgery required for hemostasis. This picture is quite close to the situation in Europe, where blunt traumas are substantially prevalent.

What essentially can be stated at the moment is that pre-hospital care may influence time-to-death trend. Further understanding is required in order to see whether the action implemented has an actual impact on mortality drop in general terms.

Finding an adequate answer will not be easy, but it may be presumed that some useful elements will be derived from specific research studies on avoidable deaths, via the review by experts' panels and autopsies performed on all deceased patients, which might shed some light on unclear aspects of a given patient's treatment, a sign of farther reaching deficiencies in the system.

What strategy of pre-hospital intervention for trauma patients?

In a review of the efficiency of pre-hospital care, Pepe and Eckstein [10] stated that the intention to make matters simpler has instead further complicated matters. While defining an approach methodology for trauma patients, with its related protocols, is essential in order to assure a systematic action backed by specific rationale, it should however be emphasized that with respect to the clinical picture (type of injury, physiopathological impact), patient's needs may vary: for example, blunt trauma with head injuries presents different problems than a penetrating firearm chest injury.

But not solely. There are other variables, such as the distance from the trauma center, proficiency and skills of emergency team, availability of means of transportation. all of which play a relevant role in the definition of intervention strategies.

Once the trauma-inducing event has taken place and the force impacting on the person has produced more or less severe injuries (primary damage), the overall goal of health care is to minimize as much as possible the consequences of trauma, prevention of secondary damage. To this end, instruments should be found in order to curtail and stop the sequence of negative events (hypoxemia, hypotension, hypovolemia, hypercapnia) producing the progressive deterioration of the patient's condition, essentially via a common final pathway, here represented by the insufficient transport of oxygen to the cells.

In this instance, by leaving the opposition between basic life support (BLS) and advanced life support (ALS), "scoop-and-run" and "stay-and-play" aside, the operative application seems to be the definition of different strategies mainly related to the patient's type.

In United States case reports the percentage of penetrating injuries is quite high. For these patients the rapid center referral for definitive surgical procedure seems to be the most-rational and effective approach.

In Europe, where blunt injuries prevail (for the most part due to road accidents), an approach of this kind seems less suitable. An advanced approach aimed at the stabilization of cardiorespiratory parameters already during pre-hospital care and transportation appears more suitable.

If the above statement is true, it is necessary to find evidence of treatment measures implemented in the pre-hospital phase. The separation between BLS and ALS is not always univocal, and therefore the comparison of results of different studies may be put at risk or impaired.

In our opinion, reference may be made to ALS only if the following are included: advanced assessment capacity, endotracheal intubation, pleural decompression, mechanical ventilation, fluid infusion (fluid therapy). However, the mere classification is not enough as, in order to effectively validate an intervention strategy, the real incidence of procedure implementation on critical patients should be known, alongside the real clinical impact on relevant physiological parameters.

Merely reporting that patients have been treated by ALS teams does not necessarily mean that the envisaged maneuvers have actually been performed. The main concern about the performance of pre-hospital ALS treatment is that said approach might result in the loss of precious time with delay in definitive treatment performance.

Several elements may be brought against the above view. Firstly, whenever blunt traumas prevail, the need for emergency surgery is decidedly lower than in the case of penetrating injuries. Really advanced treatment in the field enables initiation of an "intensive" support, way before the arrival at hospital (intensive care is a way to treat a patient and not a physical place).

In a recent study, Sanson et al. [11] underline the need for ALS in a high percentage of trauma victims trapped inside motor vehicles, where their extrication would require a long time. Stocchetti et al. [12] reported a high percentage of hypoxemia and hypotension in patients with severe head injuries and concluded by stating that advanced care by an ALS team from the medical helicopter service may reduce these effects.

In short, Spaite et al. [13] and Delooz [14] underline that the fear of unnecessary delay on the trauma scene would be well-grounded only if operators in the pre-hospital setting have not been properly trained or lack specific experience.

This is quite relevant as sound conclusions may be effectively drawn on the real benefit of measures carried out, only if a good level of properly performed procedures is reached.

In a recent review, Liberman et al. [15] reported interesting data (derived from a meta-analysis of 174 articles). The mean time of stay on the scene was 18.5±3.8 min (11,323 patients) for ALS teams against 13.5±2.4 min (4,784 patients) for BLS teams ($P = 0.005$), but the total pre-hospital time was similar, namely 38.2±6.3 min for ALS and 36.2±9.3 min for BLS ($P = 0{,}271$). Definite conclusions might not be easily drawn from the above review, but certainly stating that the ALS treatment would increase the pre-hospital time becomes increasingly difficult. However, many studies comprising the present meta-analysis lack data on the total pre-hospital time, as well as a reference to the distance from the admission center. Moreover, the performance of procedures in the pre-hospital setting would enable the immediate start of the diagnostic phase and the continuation of life support upon arrival in the emergency ward. Within the overall framework of the patient's definitive treatment, and particularly for the trauma patient with shock, delaying endotracheal intubation (if suitable) and intravenous line placement until the arrival to the hospital emergency area in order to save a few minutes does not seem to produce relevant time advantages in terms of early intervention (need for diagnostic assessment).

The review of several maneuvers and procedures classified as ALS may further expand on the above remarks.

Winchell and Hoyt [16] reported an improvement in the survival of patients with severe head injury with intubation in the field. However, intubation was performed on only 50%. Murray et al. [17] drew opposite conclusions for a group of similar patients, but with an even lower percentage of intubations performed.

An operative strategy based on endotracheal intubation without any recourse to sedation and/or curarization would nevertheless by restricted to the treatment of patients with GCS = 3 – 4, and therefore in an extremely critical condition and for whom the benefit of a qualified treatment is probably rather limited. A rather interesting scenario would be unveiled here concerning the training of health staff for the performance of said procedure, with respect to manual skills as well as to the pharmacological approach supporting the maneuver.

Another useful intervention for life support is the treatment of hypertensive pneumothorax. Pleural decompression and chest drain produce an effective solution to a relevant cause of early death from chest injuries.

A study by Schmidt et al. [18] showed the effectiveness and safety of chest drain in the pre-hospital setting. Positive results are achieved via a simple thoracostomy [19].

Intravenous line placement has been mentioned in the literature. In particular several authors reported the uselessness of said procedure, as the subsequent fluid infusion may even be harmful for patients with uncontrolled bleeding. The main objection concerns the fact that the required time for intravenous line placement would stretch pre-hospital time. A more-detailed analysis shows that instead the scene time is not lengthened by attempts to place the intravenous line by expert staff, and also the intravenous line is placed during the performance of other procedures (extrication, limb immobilization) [20].

Hypovolemia induces the collapse of vein vessels, thus making subsequent placement much more difficult (for example during procedures or transportation). Having a venous access available does not necessarily mean an automatic "aggressive" infusion of fluids. Moreover, in the study by Bickell et al. [21], in a group of patients with delayed fluid infusion, an early venous line placement was performed. Having a venous line available is a necessary requisite when medication must be administered to facilitate endotracheal intubation. The main differences refer to the start of an aggressive infusion therapy in non-hospital setting, in particular for patients with shock.

It should be, however, recalled that many remarks are based on analyses of different patients and most of all for patients whose truly infused volumes are quite different from the targets effectively taken into consideration. In the case of crystalloid fluids at least a 3 : 1 ratio with respect to the presumed loss; 1 : 1 for colloids. Data report volumes that are quite distant from the theoretical values; this is for an infusion approach not performed with squeeze-bag, as the admission time is reduced. Also, the stratification of participating patients does not examine the actual incidence of head injury [22].

The choice of an intervention strategy ought to necessarily include the careful monitoring of the patient, in order to have a picture of the patient's condition and in particular the changes in life parameters induced by treatment, which do represent a tool for the objective outcome assessment with respect to the defined targets.

Performing the patient's intubation and activating the pulmotor in order to oxygenate him/her and keep his/her $paCO_2$ within physiological limits would not be enough; likewise an intravenous line placement and fluid infusion would not be a sufficient reason to presume that an effective hemodynamic response has been obtained. The definition of true effectiveness of the pre-hospital treatment can only derive from the analysis of responses detected up to the time of arrival in the emergency ward.

The chances to monitor the trauma patient's condition in the pre-hospital phase are limited, even more so than the options really available. Pulse oximetry may be of help in assessing the reached oxygenation level and peripheral perfusion (the pulse oximeter not reading any value might mean a condition of hypoperfusion and therefore hypovolemia) and the non-invasive monitoring of arterial blood pressure may provide for useful hemodynamic indications, particularly on macrocirculation. With the ECG, relevant rhythm disturbances may be detected.

An advanced intervention level requires a more-refined monitoring. A relevant role may be played by capnometry for ventilation assessment, particularly in the case of head injuries. The most widely applied guidelines envisage that the ventilation of patients with severe head injuries should assure normocapnia (thus avoiding the onset of hypocapnia inducing brain ischemia and hypercapnia inducing brain hyperafflux). With all its known limitations (first of all the gap between $ETCO_2$ and $paCO_2$), useful indications may also be considered, at least concerning markedly out-of-range capnia values (< 20 and > 50). The ideal condition would be having portable hemataerometers available, especially since pre-hospital ventilation time from intubation to arrival in the emergency ward may often exceed 30 min.

Pulmotors used in pre-hospital setting, although increasingly reliable, do not always ensure the precise delivery of set values. Non-negligible percentages of multiple trauma patients also present chest injuries requiring high-quality performance from the pulmotor. Beside paying attention to the values reported by the device, having a $paCO_2$ quantification and also time-based trends would certainly be quite useful.

Another aspect of positive pressure ventilation is also non-negligible, although often overlooked. It enables improvement of gas exchange on the one hand, while on the other hand producing hemodynamic effects that might become particularly relevant in trauma patients with hypovolemia. In said situations the consequence to be most feared is hypotension, with particularly harmful effects on severe head injuries. Setting ventilation in such a way that respiratory needs are satisfied with minimum hemodynamic impact would require ventilation monitoring.

The hemataerometry assessment upon arrival in the emergency ward (unpublished data) for patients with severe head injury and pre-hospital intubation, and admitted to the Resuscitation Ward of Ospedale Maggiore showed that for about one-half of the cases the $paCO_2$ value was in the 35 – 45 mmHg range, while for the other half at least 35% of cases reported values exceeding 45 mmHg, and for the remaining ones the values were below 35 mmHg. In the great majority of cases (93%), no severe hypoxemia was detected (defined as paO_2 60 mmHg.).

Another important issue concerns hemodynamic recovery and the assessment of fluid infusion effectiveness. At the state of the art, the end-points of volemic replacement are pressure values, with obvious limitations, as they do not report on the condition of microcirculation and organ perfusion.

The fear of worsening uncontrolled bleeding has brought many to believe that pre-hospital infusion should not be particularly aggressive; however, there is evidence that hypotension is a highly negative factor in terms of secondary brain damage. Not only that, Stocchetti et al. [12] showed that, while hypoxemia may be easily compensated, the same is not possible for arterial hypotension in multiple injury patients with severe trauma.

Recently Kreimeier et al. [23] reviewed the issue of permissive hypotension in trauma patients, drawing the conclusion that:

a) permissive hypotension seems a valid option for penetrating injuries (immediate surgery is necessary)
b) permissive hypotension, as fluid restriction, is not suitable for blunt trauma patients
c) permissive hypotension is contraindicated is patients with blunt and penetrating head injury

d) in elderly patients, increasingly present in trauma case reports, impairment of cardiovascular compensation mechanisms does not indicate permissive hypotension

The above conclusions are not far from guideline indications adopted in Italy (PTC) [24] setting as infusion goals definite pressure targets: PAS = 70 mmHg for penetrating trauma; PAS = 90 mmHg for blunt trauma without head injury; PAS ≥ 110 mmHg (or PAM = 90 mmHg) for blunt trauma with severe head injury.

If this results in a series of useful elements for the setting up of pre-hospital volemic replacement, then an objective assessment of what has already been obtained would take on additional relevance.

The monitoring of pressure upon arrival in the emergency ward as related to the quantity of infused fluids is essential in order to assess on the one hand the effectiveness of the adopted strategy, in order to reach the set pressure target, and on the other hand to collect data on how having reached the set targets has effectively produced a decreasing incidence of negative consequences for the trauma patient.

The mere macrocirculatory recovery is not sufficient to consider the state of shock fully overcome; even when the arterial blood pressure is back to normal, there could still be a compensated shock (with organ hypoperfusion, a deficit in the oxygen transport, DO_2) [25-27].

Base deficit (BD) and lactacidemia assessment upon arrival in the emergency ward (ideally already in pre-hospital setting) provides for some indications on microcirculation, although the general usefulness of these parameters should be further studied [28-31].

A study by Davis et al. [32] reported that the BD on admission in the emergency ward correlates with the fluid volumes and transfusions needed for volemic replacement.

Riexen et al. [33] reported that BD and lactacidemia are indicators of oxygen debt and are correlated with the onset of early acute respiratory distress syndrome (ARDS). Patients with early ARDS had higher BD and lactic acid levels than patients without this complication. Understanding whether the pre-hospital treatment would improve organ perfusion in terms of hemodynamic recovery (pressure targets) on the one hand, while on the other subsequently reducing the onset of early trauma complications and late mortality, could be quite useful.

The studies now taking place on "small volume resuscitation" with hypertonic-hyperosmotic solutions, following experimental data, pursue two goals: volemic replacement with macrocirculatory recovery (without excessive pressure rise) and improvement in organ perfusion with DO_2 increase via a direct action on microcirculation.

Moreover, but here we move on unknown ground, by reducing the incidence of secondary damage, pre-hospital treatment might decrease complications and therefore the number of days in intensive care units with relevant financial savings.

Does transportation influence trauma patient's outcome?

The transportation phase for the trauma patient is a delicate one, as it may be a potential source of additional worsening of general conditions, especially when the cardio-respiratory parameters have not been stabilized.

Helicopters are becoming quite popular and are increasingly used for the transportation of trauma victims, both for primary (from the accident scene to the trauma center) and secondary transportation (from the first admission hospital to the trauma center).

It should be underlined that having a medical helicopter service available offers advantages not with relation to the transport services provided, but primarily for the possibility of reducing the therapy-free interval, with an ALS team rapidly arriving on the accident scene and initiating the patient's treatment [34].

Helicopters effectively ensure a rapid center referral, but it should be remembered that the real advantages time-wise (especially when the presence of trauma pathology with shock does require hospitalization in the shortest possible time) are produced only with a careful management of the aircraft and a comparison with ambulance mileage. In effect, data from studies on emergency helicopter services report that sometimes the distance from the landing area near the hospital is such that an additional time span is necessary for the transportation to the emergency ward, de facto eliminating the advantage produced by recourse to the aircraft.

And not only that: emergency helicopter services have to face several constraints in their utilization (e.g., adverse weather conditions, lack of visibility, night time); being aware of these shortcomings would mean that within the trauma system (and the EMS system) resources enabling the fastest admission possible of the trauma patient should be co-ordinated with a sufficient number of ambulances assuring acceptable transportation time. Undoubtedly the geographic layout of the territory and hospital distribution will determine specific choices tailored to the area under consideration.

To date no definite data are available indicating that emergency helicopter services would ensure a drop in trauma deaths. The analysis of the advantage provided by the emergency helicopter service should be probably carried out from a different perspective than the mere decrease in admission time in trauma centers and should also comprise the treatment level provided by airborne teams, to be compared, in our opinion, with what is otherwise performed by ambulance teams.

Each EMS system should be designed in such a way that the integration of the road emergency vehicles and the helicopter services provides the maximum benefit for the trauma patient, by combining performance quality with time reduction before arrival in the emergency ward.

An issue which has been neglected is worthy of further analysis: does the type of emergency transportation influence the behavior of the ALS team? In other words, does the helicopter used as a means of transportation require an increased aggressiveness on the scene? Our experience, although not backed by objective data, leads us to conclude that the need for transportation by helicopter would spur the emergency team to carry out more-aggressive procedures before take-off in view of possible complications. For example, endotracheal intubation is performed in restless patients with moderate head injuries (GCS 9 – 13), in order to be more in control during flight and to avoid having to perform the procedure under difficult conditions. Some studies report that some procedures are performed in the health care compartment inside the helicopter, but certainly the limited space does not allow the performance of safe procedures. The patient's stabilization before helicopter transportation (or in any case the preparation in order to avoid emergency landing for treatment reasons before arrival) is in our opinion an unavoidable objective for the medical emergency helicopter service.

The lack of definite data does not allow us to conclude that this specific transportation strategy would entail specific benefits (lower incidence of iatrogenic complications) or impairments (increase in hospital admission time).

Besides these remarks, a concept should be stressed, which is becoming more relevant in the light of what we have previously reported. The transportation phase, which may be of non negligible duration, especially in the case of rural and/or mountain areas, should not be considered as a “passive” phase within the framework of the patient's diagnostic-therapeutic pathway, an unavoidable time span; as it cannot be reduced over a given limit (independently from the transport means of choice), it should be turned into a resource for the patient's treatment. Reference may be made here to “scoop-and-treat”, which would mean on the one hand the rapid application of focussed treatment, but mostly the monitoring of performed procedures (patient's condition, response to treatment) during transportation.

Pre-interhospital link

The response rationale of a system resides in the extent to which a linear diagnostic-therapeutic pathway can be ensured for trauma patients, without any time losses and interruptions in the emergency care chain.

The shift from pre-hospital to interhospital emergency area is an essential link to be build and strengthened. All actions performed in the field (in terms of procedures and time saving) are meaningful in the light of the speed by which the patient who has arrived in the emergency ward is treated by the trauma team.

We won't deal here with the issue of hospital management, but rather we would like to stress an essential concept. Having ALS teams available and the actual application of procedures that are deemed necessary allow - apart from the treatment per se - a direct connection with the trauma team, via the adoption of a shared language and the knowledge of procedures, available resources, and the response that must be assured.

Moreover, the choice of centralization for patients with severe trauma would require not only a strategy of pre-hospital intervention, but also the need to define simple approaches, also shared in the pre-alert phase, so that on patients' arrival in the emergency ward everything that might be needed for an emergency treatment would be ready.

The strength of the pre-interhospital interface is further increased whenever joint training programs are run (and more so when operations are provided both in the field and in the emergency ward) enabling health personnel to share the problems of their specific professional areas, and therefore to work more effectively during emergency situations.

Specific studies should be carried out for this sector concerning alert criteria for the trauma team (sensitivity and specificity of adopted criteria), in order to understand the extent to which the setting up of specific resources would produce a true time saving for the definitive treatment, in particular emergency surgery.

Several studies carried out in different areas have underlined an aspect that should not be neglected. An effective EMS, at least with respect to reduced admission time, will determine the arrival of severe traumas in the emergency ward at a higher rate than is usually the case whenever EMS systems are either ineffective or non-existent. The organization of the first hospital response is essential in order to ensure the suitable therapeutic level tailored to each patient [35, 36].

Conclusions

Reviewing the pre-hospital phase separately does not mean overlooking the need to ensure a treatment continuum to the trauma patient, but simply understanding whether what has been designed according to clinical and physiopathological knowledge finds correspondence in terms of effectiveness, namely whether the condition of patients with major trauma on arrival in the emergency ward is closer to the normality range (or at least to the set targets), vis-à-vis patients transported by BLS teams (scoop-and-run).

The lack of scientific evidence does not allow - at least at the moment - to design effective and universally shared intervention strategies. The designing of specific and methodologically correct studies seems to be pressing, if a rationale is to be found for what is performed on a daily basis by EMS systems all over the world, with the understanding that a single response model cannot be put forward, both concerning diverse systems and different types of patients.

What is however clear is that pre-hospital emergency care does represent an essential element for any trauma system, as it would seem likewise unthinkable not to establish a dedicated training structure for the specific training of emergency personnel, independently from their professional qualifications and roles.

References

1. Spaite DW, Criss EA, Valenzuela TD, et al (1998) Prehospital advanced life support for major trauma: critical need for clinical trials. Ann Emerg Med 32: 480-489
2. National Committee of Trauma and National Committee of Shock (1966) Accidental death and disability – the neglected disease. National Academy of Sciences/National Research Council Washington, D.C.
3. Marion DW, Carlier PM (1994) Problems with the initial Glasgow Coma Scale assessment caused by prehospital treatment of patients with head injuries: result of a national survey. J Trauma 36: 89-95
4. Ross SE, Leipold C, Terregino C, et al (1998) Efficacy of the motor component of the Glasgow Coma Scale in trauma triage. J Trauma 45: 42-44
5. Roorda J, van Beek EF, Stapert JW, et al (1996) Evaluation performance of the Revised Trauma Score as a triage instrument in the prehospital setting. Injury 27: 163-167
6. Trunkey DD (1993) Trauma. Sci Am 249:28
7. Marson AC, Thomson JC (2001) The influence of prehospital trauma care on motor vehicle crash mortality. J Trauma 50: 917-920
8. Sauaia A. Moore FA, Moore EE (1995) Epidemiology of trauma deaths. J Trauma 38: 185-188
9. Meislin H, Criss EA, Judkins D, et al (1997) Fatal trauma: the modal distribution of time to death is function of patient demographics and regional resources. J Trauma 43: 433-440
10. Pepe PE, Eckstein M (1998) Reappraising the prehospital care of the patient with major trauma. Emerg Med Clin North Am 16: 1-15
11. Sanson G, Di Bartolomeo S, Nardi G, et al (1999) Road traffic accidents with vehicular entrapment: incidence of major injuries and need for advanced life support. Eur J Emerg Med 6: 285-291
12. Stocchetti N, Furlan A, Volta F (1996) Hypoxemia and arterial hypotension at the accident scene in head injury. J Trauma 40: 764 -767

13. Spaite DW, Tse DJ, Valenzuela TD (1991) The impact of injury severity and prehospital procedures on scene time in victims of major trauma. Ann Emerg Med 20: 1299-1305
14. Delooz H (1991) Organization and implementation of emergency services in the treatment of major trauma. J Neurotrauma 6 [Suppl 1]: S1-S6
15. Liberman M, Mulder D, Sampalis J (2000) Advanced vs basic life support for trauma: meta-analysis and critical review of the literature. J Trauma 49: 584-599
16. Winchell RJ, Hoyt DB (1997) Endotracheal intubation in the field improves survival in patients with severe head injury. Arch Surg 132: 592-597
17. Murray JA, Demetriades D, Berne TV, et al (2000) Prehospital intubation in patients with severe head injury. J Trauma 49: 1065-1070
18. Schmidt U, Stalp M, Gerich T (1998) Chest tube decompression of blunt chest injuries by physicians in the field: effectiveness and complications. J Trauma 44: 98-101
19. Deakin CD, Davies G, Wilson A (1995) Simple thoracostomy avoids chest drain insertion in prehospital trauma. J Trauma 39: 373-374
20. Spaite DW, Valenzuela TD, Criss EA (1994) A prospective in field comparison of intravenous line placement by urban and non urban emergency medical services personnel. Ann Emerg Med 24: 209-214
21. Bickell WH, Wall MJ, Pepe PE (1994) Immediate vs delayed fluid resuscitation for hypotensive patients with penetrating torso injuries. N Engl J Med 331: 1105-1109
22. Kaweski SM, Sise MJ, Virgilio RW (1990) The effect of prehospital fluids on survival in trauma patients. J Trauma 30: 1215-1219
23. Kreimeier U, Prückner S, Peter K (2001) Permissive hypotension during primary resuscitation for trauma and shock. In: Vincent JL (ed) Yearbook of intensive care and emergency medicine. Springer, Berlin Heidelberg New York
24. Italian Resuscitation Council (1997) Prehospital trauma care manual. Fotocompositori, Bologna
25. Porter JM, Ivatury RR (1998) In search of end points of resuscitation in trauma patients: a review. J Trauma 44: 908-914
26. Scalea TM, Maltz S, Yelon J (1994) Resuscitation of multiple trauma and head injury: role of crystalloid fluids and inotropes. Crit Care Med 22: 1610-1615
27. Abou-Khalil B, Scalea TM, Trooskin SZ, et al (1994) Hemodynamic responses to shock in young trauma patients: need for invasive monitoring. Crit Care Med 22: 633-639
28. Dunham CM, Siegel JH, Weireter L, et al (1991) Oxygen debt and metabolic acidemia as quantitative predictors of mortality and the severity of the ischemic insult in hemorrhagic shock. Crit Care Med 19: 231-243
29. Siegel JH, Rivkind AI, Dalai S (1991) Early physiologic predictors of injury severity and death in blunt multiple trauma. Arch Surg 125: 498-508
30. Davis JW, Shackford SR, Holbrook TL (1991) Base deficit as a sensitive indicator of compensated shock and tissue oxygen utilization". Surg Gynecol Obstet 173: 473-476
31. Rutherford EJ, Morris JA, Reed GW (1992) Base deficit stratifies mortality and determine therapy. J Trauma 33: 417-422
32. Davis JW, Parks SN, Kaups KL, et al (1996) Admission base deficit predicts transfusion requirements and risk of complications. J Trauma 41: 769-774
33. Riexen D, Siegel JH (2000) Metabolic correlates of oxygen debt predict posttrauma early acute respiratory distress syndrome and the related cytokine response. J Trauma 49: 392-403
34. Nardi G, Massarutti D, Muzzi A (1994) Impact of emergency medical helicopter service on mortality for trauma in North-East Italy. A regional prospective audit. Eur J Emerg Med 1: 69-77
35. Mock CN, Jurkovich GJ, Amon-Kotei D, et al (1998) Trauma mortality patterns in three nations at different economic levels: implications for global trauma system development. J Trauma 44: 804-814
36. Arreola-Risa C, Mock CN, Padilla D, et al (1995) Trauma care systems in urban Latin America: the priorities should be prehospital and emergency room management. J Trauma 39: 457-462

Trauma Intensive Care: Early and Late Challenges

G. Nardi, L. Riccioni, E. De Blasio

The development of a trauma program, with a clinical service, trauma protocols, and a well-organized trauma team could be expected to improve the process of care and thereby outcomes after injury. An integrated model of trauma care allows better continuity of care, minimizes communication errors, and establishes the overall responsibilities for the whole process through the identification of a trauma team leader. Evidence supports the assertion that a fully implemented trauma system reduces mortality rate for severely injured patients [1]. Continuous quality improvement and performance monitoring are cornerstones in achieving the principal targets of the trauma program: reduction of preventable death after injury.

"Structure", "process" and outcome are the focal points for quality evaluation [2]. The definition of "structure" includes the resources and the individuals assembled to provide the required level of care, as well as their credentials. "Process" includes selection of the diagnostic pathway and priorities in therapeutic interventions.

A trauma program management was developed at our emergency department (ED), with the introduction of consensus-developed clinical practice guidelines and protocols, along with a quality improvement program. Performances were concurrently audited through outcome measures, including mortality rates related to patients Injury Severity Score (ISS), intensive care unit (ICU) and hospital length of stay, and costs.

As a result of the quality improvement programs, significant pitfalls in our trauma system were identified and the need to undertake innovative strategies was underlined.

Among the identified "process" pitfalls there were: frequent delay in the activation of a full trauma team, even in the case of patients who needed aggressive resuscitation; lack of written guidelines; a low compliance with ATLS recommendation for ED "emergency" radiographs; incomplete cervical spine clearance in patients with major trauma; excessive delay in long bone fracture stabilization as a result of a lack of consensus among anesthesiologists, orthopedic and neurosurgeons.

Until the end of 1998, trauma patients admitted to the ED were first evaluated by a surgeon who could request the assistance of anesthesiologists and other trauma specialists in cases of need. In an attempt to improve the quality of trauma care, we revised our organization and adopted a two-tier "trauma team" strategy. According to the new strategy, trauma patients are triaged in the prehospital setting or on admission to the ED and the full trauma team (an anesthesiologist in the role of team leader, a surgeon, a radiologist, and three ED nurses) is immediately activated whenever clinical conditions or accident dynamics fit the "alert" criteria for severe trauma. In all other cases, the trauma team is limited to the surgeon and two ED nurses, and the anesthesiologist is called whenever required.

Better practice guidelines were identified by extensive literature review, and a multidisciplinary consensus was achieved. The guidelines were then incorporated into written protocols to facilitate better adherence by all the physicians involved in the patients' care.

As part of the educational program, all anesthesiologists and trauma surgeons involved in trauma care followed an ATLS Course. Anesthesiologists also took part in the Italian Resuscitation Council Pre-hospital Trauma Care Course. The compliance with ATLS guidelines and the accuracy of the radiological diagnostic pathway were evaluated through audit performed an regular basis.

The more-relevant problem we had to face was the definition of the ideal pathway to treat multiple trauma patients with long bone fractures, as data in the literature are inconclusive and there were conflicting priorities among the different specialists.

Therefore this paper will focus mainly on this topic, with the aim of analyzing data from the literature concerning optimal timing of long bone fracture stabilization and presenting our own experience.

Long bone and pelvic fracture: which is the "ideal" time for fixation?

The currently employed criteria for triage consider fractures of two or more long bones as high suspicion criteria for major trauma. Recent studies have demonstrated that the incidence of femoral fractures in motor vehicle collisions increases dramatically with increasing impact energy. The presence of a femoral fracture is directly related to the change in velocity and was found to be less than 4% for crash at a speed lower than 25 km/h and 20% at about 50 km/h. Crash victims with femoral fractures have a significantly higher incidence of hemopneumothorax and bowel injuries; hemorrhagic head injuries are also more frequent, but this trend does not achieve statistical significance [3].

Therefore both prehospital and hospital clinicians should have a higher index of suspicion for bowel and chest injuries in blunt trauma victims who present with femoral fractures. Adili et al. [4] recently reported that in severe trauma patients the presence of bilateral femoral fracture was associated with a slight increase in the average ISS (32.0 vs. 29.2), but a threefold higher mortality rate than in cases of unilateral fractures (33.0% vs. 10.7%). Moreover, patients with orthopedic fractures are expected to face greater challenges regarding functional recovery than patients with the same ISS but without orthopedic injuries, and require a longer hospital stay and have a worst functional outcome even 12 months after admission [5]. The severely injured patients with orthopedic injury require a focused project to assure them the ideal treatment to improve their final outcome after injury. This approach may initially require additional resources, but it may bring about a reduction in hospital stay, with minor expenditures and a lower morbidity.

The way multiple trauma patients with major orthopedic injuries are treated and the timing of long bone stabilization may affect their final outcome. More than 20 years ago a few reports began to draw attention to the advantages of early fixation of limb fractures in the reduction of fat embolism [6]. Some years later Seibel et al. [7] found an association between pulmonary failure and the number of days the patients were kept in traction. Moreover, the use of traction in patients with severe multiple trauma was identified as the major risk factor for the development of multiple system organ failure, secondary sepsis, and poor outcome. Limb traction was shown to increase fat embolisms, and the enforced supine position was associated with the development of atelectasis and subsequent pulmonary infection. Traction use also increases narcotic requirements to control pain caused by motion at the fracture site. These findings were confirmed by Bone et al. [8] in a prospective randomized study. In the delayed stabilization group, increased pulmonary complications, acute respiratory distress syndrome, fat embolisms, pneumonia) were observed to result in longer ICU and hospital stay and increased cost.

Patients with musculoskeletal injuries frequently sustain concomitant injuries to the neurological and respiratory systems. The optimal timing of operative fixation for limb fractures in the presence of intracranial injuries or severe lung contusions remains controversial, as some recent reports raised concerns that early operative stabilization of fractures may be detrimental to neurological recovery [9] or be associated with increased risk of impairment of pulmonary functions. Concerns with early fixation in patients with brain injuries include secondary brain damage as a result of hypotension due to surgical bleeding, and complexity of controlling intracranial hypertension during orthopedic surgery.

In a review of 171 patients with severe head trauma associated with pelvic or lower extremity fractures, Scalea et al. [10] found no evidence that early fracture fixation negatively influences central nervous system outcomes or mortality.

Other authors have criticized the concept that early intamedullary nail fixation (IMN) of long bone fractures may result in a reduction in pulmonary complications, as worsening pulmonary function has been observed in patients with lung injury submitted to IMN [11], especially when a reamed nail was employed.

The EAST Practice Management Guidelines Committee recently performed a metanalysis [12] to analyze the existing evidence for or against early stabilization for long bone fractures. Although an extensive revision of the literature was performed, no class I data and only 6 class II studies were identified. Therefore there is insufficient evidence to support a standard of care on this topic and there is a clear need for large randomized studies. With these limitations the following level II recommendations were reported: "*Polytrauma patients undergoing long-bone stabilisation within 48 hours of injury have no improvement in survival when compared with those receiving later stabilisation. However there may be some patients who will have fewer morbidity. There is no evidence that early stabilisation has any detrimental effect. It is preferable to perform long bone stabilisation in polytrauma patients*."

Although these conclusions seems to favor the early fixation strategy, even in cases of severe brain injury, in patients not adequately resuscitated or with intracranial lesions that may require neurosurgery, the definitive treatment of limb fractures may be delayed up to 72 h. Recently, external fixation (EF) was proposed as a "bridge" to achieve the benefits of early fracture stabilization during early resuscitation, and postpone the additional stresses related to IMN until the patient is stabilized. In a large retrospective study of 324 patients with femur fractures, Scalea et al. [13] reported a median operating room time of 35 min for EF compared with the 135 min required for IMN as an average. The estimated blood loss associated with the two procedures was 90 ml for EF and 400 ml for intramedullary nailing. They therefore suggested that in cases of severe head or chest trauma associated with long bone fractures, a "damage control" strategy should be applied: patients should be treated with EF soon after admission and submitted to more elective definitive fracture fixation as soon as possible. The mean time to definitive fracture fixation after EF in the series of Scalea et al. [13] was 4 days. To reduce the excessive delay in long bone fracture stabilization, the "damage control" strategy as proposed by Scalea was endorsed and introduced in the ED guidelines at S. Camillo Hospital. Patients with orthopedic fractures who are hemodynamically stable and not at risk of developing intracranial hematoma are treated with early IMN. Patients who require aggressive resuscitation or have a high intracranial pressure are treated with EF as a temporary bridge, and definitive IMN is performed as soon as possible. Such a strategy has allowed us to avoid limb traction, with a favorable impact on the quality of nursing. However, only a few patients require this approach, as the majority can be successfully submitted to IMN within 24-36 h of injury.

Severe pelvic fractures: an underscored cause of exsanguination

Unstable pelvic ring disruptions are often associated with significant mortality and morbidity, especially in patients with multiple injuries. Early pelvic fixation should contribute to diminish ongoing bleeding. However, many patients with unstable pelvic fractures cannot sustain prolonged interventions such as internal fixation. Temporary anterior external fixation has been proposed as a tool to improve pelvic ring stability and allow a more-effective resuscitation [14]. In most cases intravascular volume resuscitation and pelvic external fixation are adequate in stopping the pelvic hemorrhage. However, a small percentage of patients may continue bleeding despite early application of a pelvic external fixator. The uncontrolled hemorrhage in pelvic fractures is usually the result of vascular disruption caused either by laceration of a vessel by a bony fragment or of shearing of vessels at their point of origin as the result of sudden distortion. In these cases the attempt to ligate the vessels by a surgical approach is usually ineffective and may worsen the situation. In patients who continue to present hemodynamic instability, transcatheter arterial embolisation (TAE) is the treatment of choice to stop hemorrhage. Wong et al. [15] reported a 100% success rate of embolization in a group of 17 hypotensive patients with unstable pelvic fractures. However, the mortality rate was 17.6%. The risk of death was statistically correlated with the time lapse from arrival to angiography (6.0 h vs 2.3 h in the survivors) and with the amount of blood received before embolization. Controversy exists over the issue whether or not pelvic external fixation is necessary before TAE [16, 17]. The application of an external fixator can reduce pelvic volume and contribute to effectively tamponade the low-pressure venous hemorrhage. However, it will probably be inadequate in the case of major bleeding from arterial vessels, and may cause a delay in angiography and embolization. In our clinical practice all the patients with pelvic ring disruption or with a fracture of the pelvis associated with retroperitoneal hematoma, or who require aggressive volume resuscitation, are submitted to early angiography, according to the ED guidelines shown in Fig. 1. External fixation of the pelvis is seldom applied and as soon as hemodynamic and coagulation are effectively restored, patients are considered as candidates for early internal fixation of the unstable pelvis. During the last 12 months, ten patients with unstable pelvic fractures were submitted to TAE. In one case TAE had to be repeated after 6 h. The final success rate was 100% and all the patients survived.

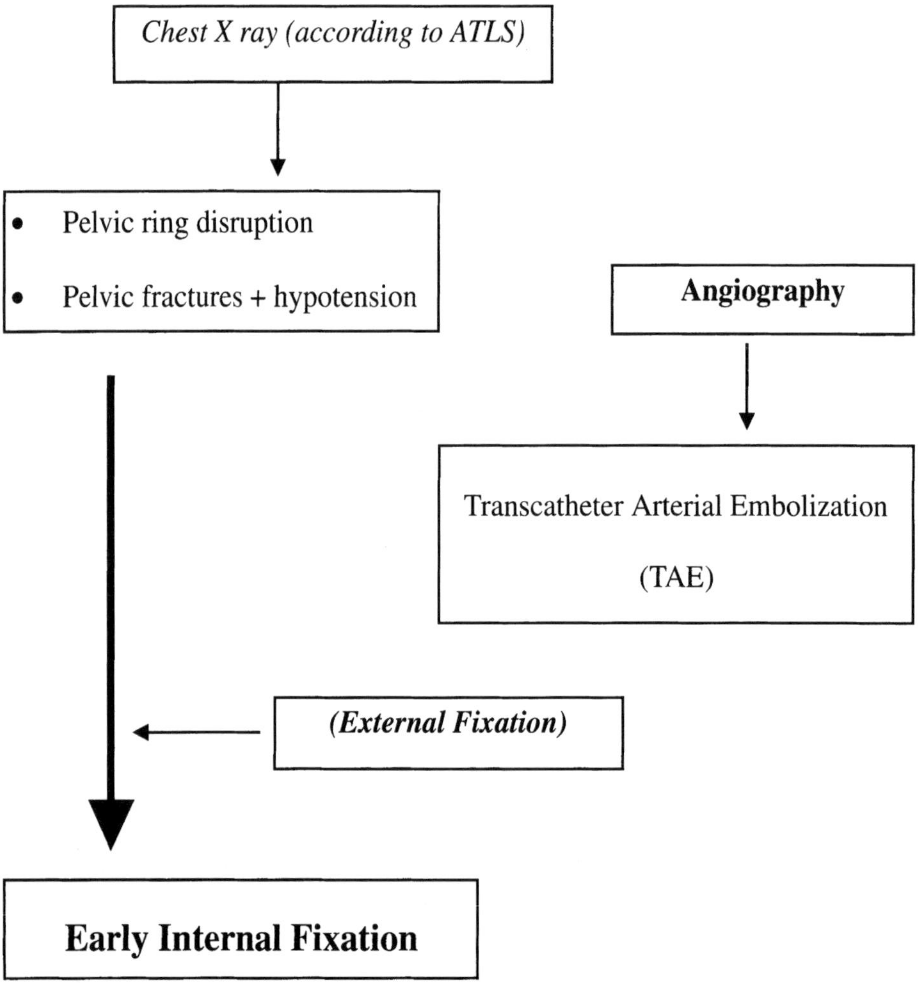

Fig.1. Recommended pathway for patients with pelvic fractures (S. Camillo's emergency department guidelines)

Results of the quality improvement program

As part of the quality improvement program, data of all major trauma (MT) victims (ISS ≥ 16) admitted to the ED during three comparable periods before (Jan-May 1998), during (Jan-May 1999), and after (Jan-May 2000) the implementation of the process, were retrospectively and prospectively collected and analyzed.

The number of MT patients admitted to the hospital increased from 39 during the first 5 months of 1998 to 106 in 2000. ISS was 30.2 ± 11.3 in 1998, 29.6 ± 13.7 in 1999, and 30.5 ± 12.9 in 2000 (Fig. 2). The percentage of patients submitted to chest, cervical spine, and pelvis X-rays on admission according to ATLS guidelines, rose from 20% to 96%. The mean time from hospital admission to surgical orthopedic stabilization (IMN or EF when required) for patients admitted to the ICU dropped from 12 days in 1998 to 4.6 in 1999 and 1.3 in 2000 (Fig. 4). In 2000, 86% of the patients with limb fractures who required surgery were treated within 36 h of admission versus 11% in 1998.

Jan-May	n	Males	Females	Age	ISS
1998	**39**	**27**	**12**	**41±19.6**	**30.2 ± 11.3**
1999	**86**	**60**	**26**	**42.2±17.3**	**29.6 ± 13.7**
2000	**106**	**77**	**29**	**41.8±21.2**	**30.5 ± 12.9**

Fig. 2. Demographics and severity scoring index

Hospital mortality, which was as high as 42% in 1998, was reduced to 20.8% 2 years later. ICU mortality dropped from 36% to 9%. ICU length of stay was reduced from 22 days to 12 as an average, and hospital length of stay for survivors from 45 to 38 days.

Conclusions

The implementation of a trauma program with clearly defined written guidelines and a multidisciplinary trauma team with a well-recognized leadership in a busy Level II ED has brought about tangible gains in performance within less than 2 years. The strict adherence to ATLS guidelines and the introduction of a policy of early fixation of fractures of femur, tibia, fibula, and pelvis appear to be key in improving clinical outcomes and reducing both the preventable death rate and hospital stay. The importance of a quality assurance approach must also be strongly emphasized.

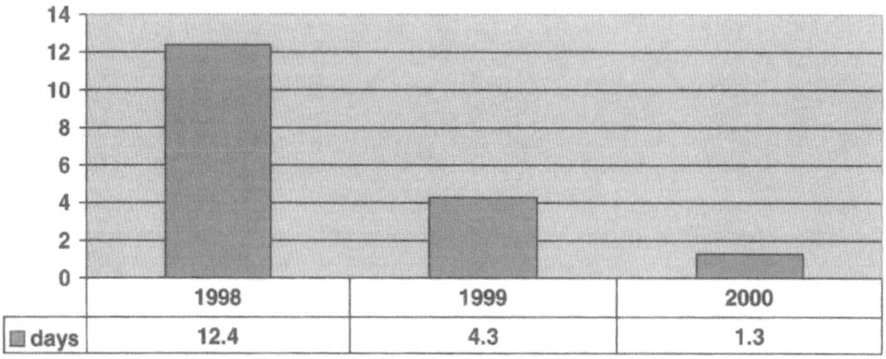

Fig. 3. Mean time from hospital admission to long bone fracture stabilization in patients with major trauma (Injury Severity Score 15)

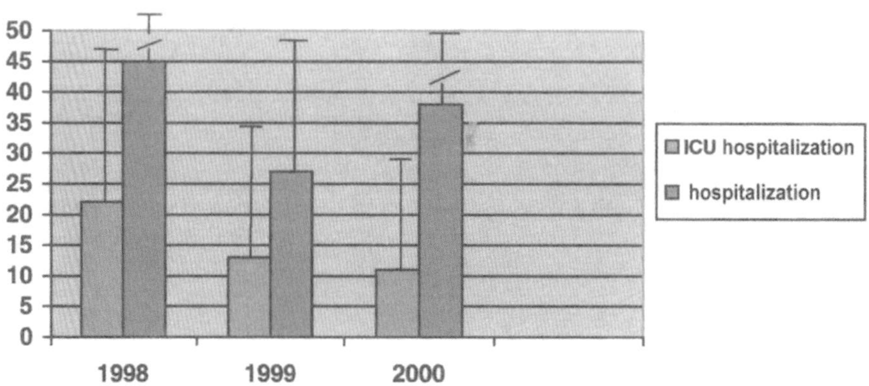

Fig. 4. Changes in intensive care unit (ICU) and hospital stay related to the different phases of the implementation of the program

References

1. Mullins RJ, Veum-Stone J, Helfand M, et al (1994) Outcome of hospitalized injured patients after institution of a trauma system in an urban area. JAMA 271: 1919-1924
2. Donabedian A (1988) The role of outcomes in quality assessment and assurance. JAMA 260: 1743-1748
3. Rastogi S, Wild BR, Duthie RB (1986) Biomechanical aspects of femoral fractures in automobile accidents. J Bone Joint Surg Br 68: 760-766
4. Adili A, Bhandari M, Lachowski RJ et al (1999) Organ injuries associated with femoral fractures: implication for severity of injury in motor vehicular collisions. J Trauma 46: 386-391
5. Michaels AJ, Madey SM, Krieg JC, Long W (2001) Traditional Injury Severity Scoring underestimates the relative consequences of orthopedic injury. J Trauma 50: 389-396
6. Riska E, Von Bonsdorf H, Hakkinen S, et al (1976) Fat embolisms in patients with multiple injuries. Injury 8: 110-116
7. Seibel R, La Duca J, Hasset JM, et al (1985) Blunt multiple trauma, femur traction and the pulmonary failure septic state. Ann Surg 202: 283-288
8. Bone LB, Johnson KD, Weigelt J, et al (1989) Early versus delayed stabilization of femural fractures: a prospective randomized study. J Bone Joint Surg Am 71: 336-340
9. Jaicks RR, Cohn SM, Moller BA (1997) Early fracture fixation may be deleterious after head injury. J Trauma 42: 1-6
10. Scalea TM, Scott J, Brumback RJ, et al (1999) Early fracture fixation may be "just fine " after head injury: no difference in central nervous system outcomes. J Trauma 46: 839-846
11. Pape HC, Auf'm'Kolk M, Paffrath T, et al (1993) Primary intramedullary femur fixation with associated lung contusion: a case of post-traumatic ARDS ? J Trauma 34: 540-548
12. Dunham CM, Bosse JM, Clancy VT, et al (2001) Practice management guidelines for the optimal timing of long-bone fracture stabilization in polytrauma patients: the EAST Practice Management Guidelines Work Group. J Trauma 50: 958-967
13. Scalea TM, Boswell SA, Scott JD, et al (2000) External fixation as a bridge to intramedullary nailing for patients with multiple injuries and with femur fractures: damage control orthopedics. J Trauma 48: 613-623
14. Tucker MC, Nork SE, Simonian PT, Chip Routt ML (2000) Simple anterior pelvic external fixation. J Trauma 49: 989-994
15. Wong Y, Wang L, Ng CJ, et al (2000) Mortality after successful transcatheter arterial embolization in patients with unstable pelvic fractures: rate of blood transfusion as predictive factor. J Trauma 49: 71-74
16. Agolini SF, Shah K, Jaffe J, et al (1997) Arterial embolization is a rapid and effective technique for controlling pelvic fracture hemorrhage. J Trauma 43: 395-399
17. Grimm MR, Vrahas MS, Thomas KA (1998) Pressure-volume characteristics of the intact and disrupted pelvic retroperitoneum. J Trauma 44: 454-459

Trauma Scoring Systems

F. DELLA CORTE, G.L. VIGNAZIA, M. CAVAGLIÀ

During the last 20 years many trauma-scoring indexes have been developed and their applicability seems to be important mainly because they could allow [1]:

- comparisons of the efficacy of different therapeutic interventions and outcome
- quick triage during the pre-hospital phases as well as priority treatments.

The traumatic event can be simplified as input (anatomical component and its related physiological consequence) and output (mortality and morbidity). The aim of a scoring system is to give a reliable output.

Since DeHaven's original work using injury scores [2], in 1952, several publications have been written regarding trauma gravity index. The weakness of these indexes is related to prediction of mortality. Its basis was developed as followed:

- Combination between anatomical and physiological parameters to obtain intermediate score; their sum determines the final score. As a consequence, an error can be amplified.
- Standardized combinations between different lesions as their effects on outcome were independent.
  Some lesions may have by themselves more lethal effects then those estimated by a simple adding model (i.e., extracranial lesions in a patients with traumatic brain injury have a more-devastating effect on outcome).

Furthermore, they did not consider both pre-existing chronic illnesses and age (recent scoring systems introduced these last data, i.e., the HARM score).

The ideal score system should finally include [3]:

1. a detailed anatomical description of the lesions and impact on outcome
2. a description of the traumatic agent and/or event dynamics, considering also the physiological parameters detected on the spot and on intensive care unit (ICU) admission.
3. the impact on outcome of pre-existing pathological conditions
4. forms easy to be filled in by any professional operator.

Evaluations and comparisons between different statistical analysis tools are described below.

Injury severity score

Injury severity score (ISS) is often preferred since it does not consider physiological parameters. ISS is based on the Abbreviated Injury Scale (AIS) developed in 1969 to select road accident patients according to their anatomical lesions. This scale considers 1,200 different kinds of lesion (subdivided into 6 different anatomical regions) and is graded from 1 (minor lesion) to 6 (lesion leading to death) (Table 1).

Table 1. Example of lesions evaluated by Abbreviated injury scale (AIS)

Lesions	Score
Shoulder pain (not specified)	0
Distortion of the wrist	1 (minor)
Tibial linear fracture	2 (moderate)
Head injury – coma on admission, lasting less than 1 h, without neurological sequelae	3 (serious)
Major hepatic fracture	4 (severe)
Incomplete laceration of thoracic aorta	5 (critical)
Brainstem laceration	6 (lethal)

Baker [4] used the AIS to calculate the ISS. Arbitrarily a score of "75" was attributed to lethal lesions (score of "6" on AIS), and the score of any other non-lethal lesion ranged from 1 to 75. To calculate the score of non-lethal lesions it is necessary to add the square values of the three highest scores obtained from AIS evaluation (Table 2).

Table 2. Injury severity score (ISS)

1. Evaluate for each anatomical region the most up-to-date AIS
2. Identify the highest AIS score on each anatomical region
    - Head - neck
    - Abdomen
    - Pelvic ring and limbs
    - Face
    - Thorax
    - Skin surface
3. Add the square values of the 3 highest scores

The variability among scores makes the ISS a non-linear scale. A score of

9 or 16 is common, 14 and 22 are less frequent, and 7 and 15 not obtainable. The final score should be calculated using the median of the values and not the mean. The most-important ISS limitation is the failure to include different lesions on the same region (since only the most-severe lesion is considered in obtaining the final score). Important lesions can be underestimated or even not counted.

New Injury Severity Score

Recently Osler [5], modifying the ISS, developed the New Iniury Severity Score (NISS). The upgraded ISS does not consider different anatomical regions. It is based on the score obtained from the three most-severe lesions. This simple modification made the score more reliable in predicting mortality, especially considering penetrating wounds. Balogh [6] published data on a study where 50% of patients enrolled showed a NISS higher than ISS. On this group, NISS also showed its reliability in predicting multiple organ failure. In an elegant study, Marsh [7] showed a higher predictability of NISS than of ISS when applied to a pediatric population. Both these studies did not demonstrate a higher accuracy of NISS when compared with ISS.

Trauma Revised Injury Score

The Trauma Revised Injury Score (TRISS) index (Table 3), developed in 1987, was based on Revised Trauma Score (RTS), ISS, and age [8]. Physiological parameters such as respiratory rate, blood pressure, and Glasgow Coma Scale are also considered. This score has been built on a statistical analysis of 25,000 patients enrolled on Major Trauma Outcome that identified independent variables related to outcome [9]. Each variable is multiplied by a database regression factor, and the score is obtained by adding three calculated values. This score is graded from 0 to 8, considering also decimal numbers (Table 3).

Table 3. Revised Trauma Score

Physiological parameters	Points	Ponderal factor
Respiratory rate (breaths/min)		
10–29	4	
>29	3	
6–9	2	0.2908
1–5	1	
0	0	

Table 3 Revised Trauma Score (continued)

Physiological parameters	Points	Ponderal factor
Systolic blood pressure (mmHg)		
>89	4	
76 – 89	3	
50 – 75	2	0.7326
1 – 49	1	
0	0	
Glasgow Coma Scale		
13 – 15	40	0.9368
9 –12	3	
6 – 8	2	
4 – 5	1	
3	0	

Death probability is calculated by the following equation:

$$Ps = 1/(1 + e^{-b})$$

e = natural log
b = $b_0 + b_1$(**RTS**) + b_2(**ISS**) + b_3(**A**)
RTS = Revised Trauma Score
ISS = Injury Severity Score
A = age. *A = 0* age < 55, *A = 1 age* > 55
b_0- b_3 = variable coefficient for closed and open trauma

The results express the injury survival probability. Conventionally, the TRISS values have to be obtained immediately at ICU admission. Values can be affected by resuscitation efforts that can alter physiological parameters.

TRISS applicability is simple and also enrols patients admitted to the ICU for more than 24 h. It is composed of an anatomical and physiological component and allows for trauma quantification.

This score is widely used to evaluate the therapeutic efficacy on traumatized patients.

TRISS represents a step further in the evaluation of traumatized patients.

The most-important limitations of TRISS are attributed to:

- Morbidity is not evaluated
- Difficulties in operator training, due to ISS
- Inter-observers variability [10], less evident for low and high Ps but relevant for Ps of 0.05 and 0.95. Patient data from different hospitals are sometimes not used.

Harbourview Assessment for Risk of Mortality

Proposed by West [11], this methodology is based on the fact that not only independent single injury but also some injury combinations can affect mortality. Furthermore, it considers previous pathologies and does not evaluate physiological parameters that are often inaccurate or lacking.

It comprehends 2,034 diagnostic codes regarding traumatic lesions and is derived from ICD-9-CM (International classification of disease – 9th revision). Codes are subdivided into 109 lesion categories, 51 of these constitute the final model (Table 4). Each category represents a group of similar anatomical lesions excluding burn injuries. Furthermore, 15 different mechanisms of lesion are considered as well as three interactions between category of lesion and 11 co-illnesses status.

Table 4 Some examples of variables included in the final model (OR = odds ratio

Independent variables	OR	Regression Coefficient
Constant β_0		- 4.709
Age related variables		
Age	0.81	- 0.216
age^2	1.01	0.011
Mechanism of injury		
Fall from a height	1.30	0.262
Collision with a motor-vehicle	3.15	1.148
Collision with a bike	0.5	- 0.698
Category of lesion		
Loss of consciousness > 24 h	95.17	4.556
Cranial fracture	1.84	0.612
Facial fracture	0.649	- 0.433
1 to 3 rib fracture	0.58	- 0.553
Fracture > 3 ribs	1.63	0.489
Haemothorax	2.16	0.771
Major splenic laceration	6.01	1.793
Co-morbidity		
Cirrhosis	19.2	2.954
Ischemic cardiopathy	2.68	0.984
Interactions		
Head injury and spinal trauma	2.12	0.750
Thoracic trauma and spinal trauma	5.01	1.611

The following formula gives the hospital mortality probability (Pm).

$$P_m = 1/(1+e^{-\beta})$$

e = natural logarithm

$\beta = \beta_0 + \beta_1(age) + \beta2(age^2) + \hat{a}_{80}$ (thoracic and spinal trauma)

β_0 = constant β1-80 = regression coefficients related to each independent variable. A category not present is given a value of 0. HARM allows for more--reliable mortality prediction than models based on AIS, also without evaluation of physiological data.

Lack of physiological data represents one of the limits of this model. In fact, if two patients of the same age, lesions, injury mechanism, and co-illnesses are considered, they would show the same mortality probability, independent of physiological parameters. It would be interesting to study changes in predictability of this model after adding physiological parameters.

Moreover, some diagnostic categories included in the final model represent a limit. It has been shown that psychosis present before trauma has a protective effect (OR = 0.16), but from a clinical point of view this is of little importance. Probably a bias exists in the final model due to the small number of patients enrolled in the study to create some model categories.

ICISS (International Classification of Disease-9 Based Injury Severity Score)

This model proposed by Osler [12] is based on ICD-9CM. Each category has been calculated using the Survival Risk Ratio (SRR). It includes categories from 800 to 959.9, with the exclusion of categories 958.0 = gaseous embolism, 958.4 = traumatic shock, and 958.5 = post-traumatic anuria. Using the database of North Carolina Discharge Registry, the SRR has been calculated by dividing the number of times that a lesion was present in surviving trauma patients by the number of times that the same lesion shows on NCHDR (on both survivors and dead patients). The value obtained represents the patient's survival probability with a considered lesion. Table 5 shows same examples of calculated SRR and the corresponding ICD categories.

$$\text{ICISS} = P_{\text{lesion survivor } 1} \times P_{\text{lesion survivors } 2} \times \ldots \times P_{\text{lesion survivor } n}$$

ICISS shows the probability of surviving any single lesion present after trauma. It is calculated as the product of SRR for each single lesion presented.

Table 5. 11 of the 99 most-lethal lesions considered in this model.

SRR	ICD-9	Description
0	852.35	Subdural hematoma with persistent state of coma
0.41	902.33	Portal vein lesion
0.65	901.41	Pulmonary artery lesion

Table 5. 11 of the 99 most lethal lesion considered in this model. (continued)

SRR	ICD-9	Description
0.72	808.9	Pelvic fracture
0.75	901.9	Thoracic aorta lesion
0.76	862.21	Bronchial lesion
0.76	902.10	Inferior caval vein lesion
0.79	863.9	Gastrointestinal lesion not specified
0.79	897.4	Limb amputation
0.79	806.04	C_1-C_4 fracture
0.79	902.42	Renal vein fracture

-severe lesions have a low SRR and low ICISS patients presenting more than one lesion tend to have a lower ICISS.

ICISS is more predictable than ISS, either alone or in combination with parameters like age, mechanism of lesion, and RTS in more-complex surviving models.

TTS (Trauma Thoracic Severity Score)

In clinical practice it is very difficult to have an early and accurate scale of trauma severity. In the United States, mortality related to thoracic trauma reaches 60%, pulmonary contusion combined with three or more rib fractures being the principle death cause. Recently, Pape [13] developed a predictive scoring system to evaluate the relationships between blunt thoracic trauma severity and patient outcome (in previous models thoracic trauma was defined by thoracic lesions according to AIS).

This score incorporates pulmonary contusions detected by three chest X rays timed on admission, 24 and 72 h later. Pulmonary laceration is defined as continuous air leakage following aspiration thoracic drainage or diagnosed during thoracotomy.

The criteria used to defined lesion severity take into consideration pulmonary contusion dimension, number of injured lobes and thoracic wall fractures (number of costal, sternal, and or clavicle fractures). Clinical criteria are used to define hemothorax, pneumothorax, and hypertensive pneumothorax. paO_2/FiO_2 ratio is calculated from the worst blood gas analysis during the first 24 h (Table 6).

Table 6. Thoracic Trauma Severity Score

Grade	PaO_2/FiO_2	Rib fracture	Pulmonary contusion	Pleural involvement	Age	Score
0	>400	0	none	none	<30	0
I	300-400	1-3	1 lobe unilat.	PT	30-41	1
II	200-300	3-6	1 lobe bilat. or 2 lobes unilat.	HT/HPT unilat.	42-54	2
III	150-200	>3 bilat.	< 2 lobes bilat.	HT/HPT bilat	55-70	3
IV	< 150	Flail chest	≥ 2 lobes bilat.	TPT	>70	5

PT = pneumothorax, HT = hemothorax, HPT = hemopneumothorax;
TPT = hypertensive pneumothorax

Score value varies between 0 and 25 and is obtained by adding the single category score. Parenchymal lesions show a different prevalence according to age. Young people (age range 21-40 years) show a higher incidence than old people (age range 51-70 years).

Pulmonary parenchymal lesions show a worse outcome than costal fracture (i.e., bilateral pulmonary contusion in association with hemopneumothorax or pulmonary laceration). Mortality is dramatically increased from bilateral involvement of thoracic wall injuries. Older persons (age > 70 years) are at higher risk for costal fractures than for pulmonary contusions. Furthermore, elderly people with severe thoracic trauma show almost 100% mortality.

TTS model seems to be the most-reliable score when compared with Thoracic ISS and AIS [14].

Comparison between different score models

Receiver Operating Characteristic Curve (ROC) (linear diagram developed in 1960 for electronic engineering) is the most commonly used statistical method in evaluating the efficacy of a predictive test.

It is obtained from the area under the curve of the following equation

Sensitivity * (1 – Specificity)

ROC = 1 is the ideal predicting value, while ROC = 0.5 is a causality predicting value. On a diagram where *x* represents 1 – Specificity and *y* represents Sensitivity, the most-reliable score models are those with ROC tangent to axis. Scores efficacy is also based on Hosmer-Lemeshov [15] calibration test, measuring differences between obtained and expected values. Since the best score has no difference between obtained and expected values, the best model shows a low calibration test value.

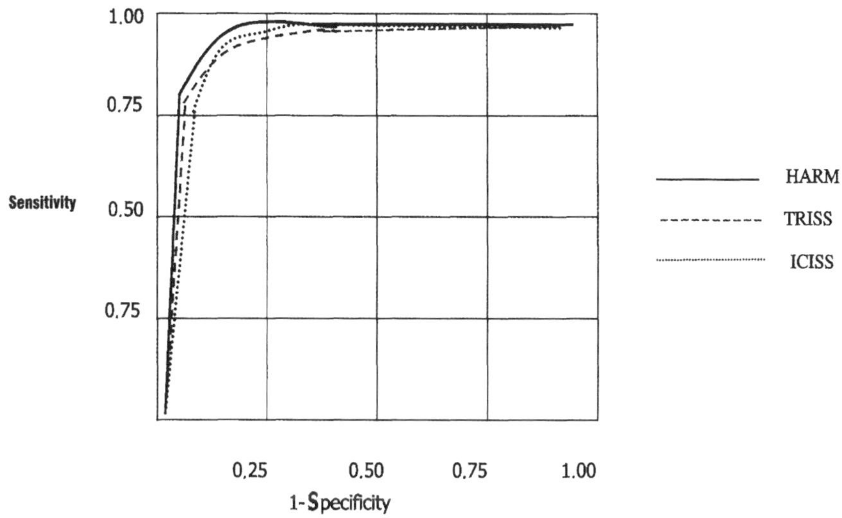

Fig. 1. ROC comparison of HARM, TRISS, and ICISS

Comparison of (Fig. 1) HARM, TRISS, and ICSS shows area under curve (AUC) values of 0.958, 0.946, and 0.940, respectively. According to West [11], HARM score has the highest AUC value relating to higher accuracy.

In comparison, Rutledge [16] reports conflicting results, showing that the ISS model is the less accurate and ICISS has better performances compared with TRISS.

It is clear that ICISS is more reliable when combined with physiological parameters (RTS and age). Figure 2 graphically shows comparisons between different models.

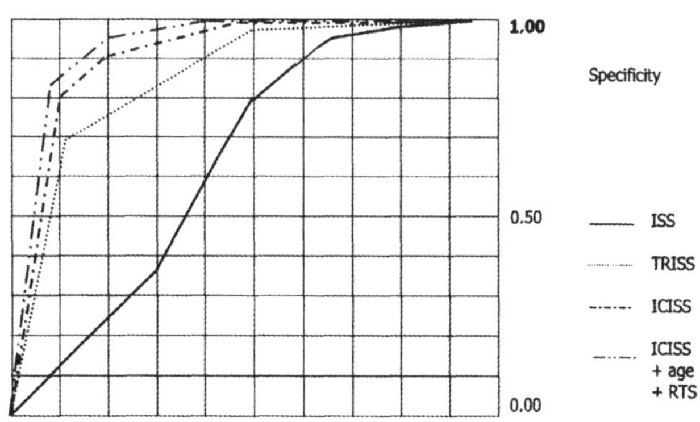

Fig. 2. ROC comparison of ISS, TRISS, ICISS and ICISS plus age plus RTS

Table 7 shows AUC corresponding to different severity score models.

Table 7. Severity score models and corresponding AUC

Models	AUC
ISS	0.0667
TRISS	0.877
ICISS	0.916
ICISS + age + RTS	0.950

Interesting are the conclusions of Pape [13] who showed the TTS superiority when compared with ISS or thoracic AIS. In Fig. 3 these data are presented graphically.

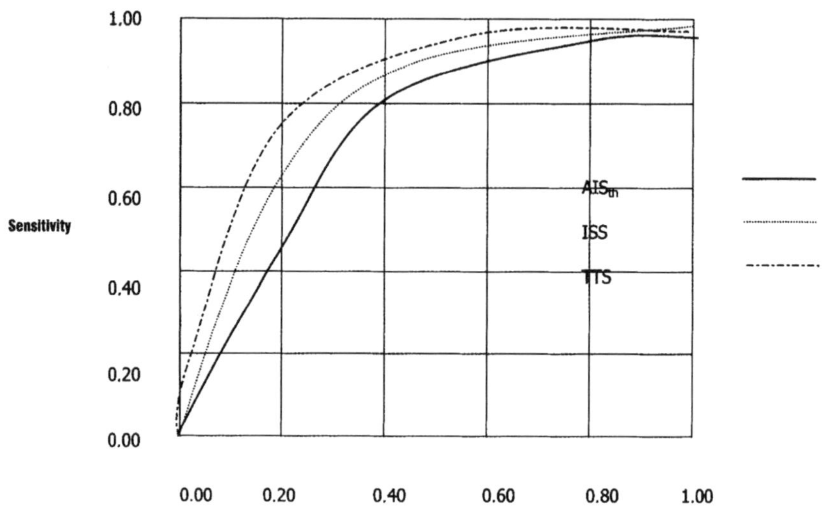

Fig. 3. ROC comparisons of thoracic AIS, ISS, and TTS

According to the gold standard of scoring system in trauma patients, none of the considered models completely satisfied the aims. The decision to adopt one model or another is based not only upon personal experience but also mainly upon the possibility of using reliable physiological parameters.

References

1. Brenneman FD (1998) Measuring injury severity: time for a change? J Trauma 44:580-583
2. DeHaven H (1952) The site, frequency and dangerousness of injury sustained by 800 survivors of light plane accidents. Crash injury research, Cornell University Medical College, New York
3. Dick WF, Baskett PJF (1999) Recommendations for uniform reporting of data following major trauma. The Utstein style. Resuscitation 42:81-100
4. Baker (1974) The Injury Severity Score: a method for describing patients with multiple injuries and evaluating emergency care. J Trauma 14:187-196
5. Osler T (1997) A modification of the Injury Severity Score that both improves accuracy and simplifies scoring. J Trauma 43:922-925
6. Balogh Z (2000) NISS predicts postinjury multiple organ failure better then ISS. J Trauma 48: 624-628
7. Marsh E (2001) The New Injury Severity Score and the evaluation of pediatric trauma. J Trauma 50:1106-1110
8. Boyd CR (1987) Evaluating trauma care: the TRISS method. J Trauma 27:370-377
9. Corbanese U (1996) Evaluation of trauma care: validation of the TRISS method in an Italian ICU. Intensive Care Med 22:941-946
10. Zoltie N (1993) The hit and miss of ISS and TRISS. BMJ 307:906-909
11. West T (2000) Harborview assessment for risk of mortality: an improved measure of injury severity on the basis of ICD-9-CM. J Trauma 49:530-541
12. Osler T (1996) ICISS: an international classification of disease-9 based Injury Severity Score. J Trauma 41:380-386
13. Pape HC (2000) Appraisal of early evaluation of blunt chest trauma: development of a standardized scoring system for initial clinical decision making. J Trauma 49:496-454
14. Wong DT (1996) A comparison of APACHEII score and TRISS for outcome assessment in intensive care unit trauma patients. Crit Care Med 24:1642-1647
15. Hosmer DW, Lemeshow S (1989) Applied logistic regression. Wiley, New York pp 142-143
16. Rutledge R (1998) The end of ISS and TRISS: ICISS, an international classification of disease, ninth edition-based prediction tool, outperforms both ISS and TRISS as predictors of trauma patients survival, hospital charges and hospital length of stay. J Trauma 44:41-49

Blast Injury

M. Muggia-Sullam

During the last 30 or 40 years, blast injury has become more and more common in certain countries. Most of these injuries are the result of terrorist activity or civilian conflicts. The leading countries are Great Britain, the former Yugoslavia, and Israel. Not only has the number of terrorist attempts grown, but also the magnitude and potency of blast munitions has increased over the years, thus augmenting the risk of severe injuries. Understanding the mechanism of explosions and the possible injuries inflicted by blast is crucial in an attempt to save wounded patients. Therefore, treatment of blast injuries should be part of the common knowledge of every surgeon and physician treating severely injured patients [1-4].

Blast injuries, as every terrorist attack, come at an unexpected time, aiming at killing and wounding as many people as possible. In addition, one of their purposes is to create chaos and confusion, in an attempt to paralyze daily activities. Hospitals treating these casualties should be prepared ahead of time, in order to get organized within the shortest possible time and admit an unknown number of patients with short notice [2, 4]. The amount of casualties admitted within this short period of time puts an enormous burden not only upon the hospitals, but also on the coroners who are trying to identify both the terrorist and the victims. Rapid identification of the perpetrators is crucial in the apprehension of accomplices and prevention of other attacks [5].

Blast injuries are usually classified into five types [6]:

1. Primary injury is caused by the primary blast wave and typically includes injuries to air-containing organs such as the tympanic membranes, lungs, and bowel, and may cause injuries to solid organs.
2. Secondary injury is caused by missiles propelled from within the explosive device or other debris. These cause penetrating injuries of various severity.
3. Tertiary injury is cause by displacement of the whole body against other objects or of extremities, causing amputations.
4. Flash burns that result from the extremely high temperatures caused by the explosion.

5. Crush injury caused by the collapse of buildings [2].

Only the first category is typical of blast, but often various types of injuries exist in the same patient. The treating physician should be aware of all the various possibilities, in order not to overlook hidden injuries. Once it was thought that most survivors of explosions suffered from secondary injuries. This is not true anymore, as several recent reports describe successful treatment of pure primary injuries. It has become clear that many factors influence the severity of primary injury.

A detailed description of the physical changes during an explosion is beyond the scope of this brief review, and can be found in other excellent articles [3, 6-9]. An explosion releases chemical energy by a process of detonation [6]. The force of the explosion depends on the velocity of detonation, which varies from 4000m/s to 8000m/s depending on the type of explosive. In recent years terrorists have used military explosives, which have a higher detonation velocity, therefore causing more damage. Following detonation, an expanding sphere of gas at high pressure and temperature is produced. The explosion creates a shock wave and a 'blast wind' that result from the expansion of gaseous products. The blast wave creates a pressure that reaches its maximum almost instantaneously. This high peak is followed by a negative pressure, which may contribute to the development of specific injuries, particularly eardrum perforations. The peak overpressure and its duration depend on the weight of the explosive used and the distance from the center of explosion. The blast wave propagates similar to a sound wave through and around objects. A large proportion of the shock wave is reflected off the ground and will reinforce the original wave. Similarly the shock wave is partly reflected by solid objects, and this effect too may reinforce the oncoming original shock wave. In closed spaces these effects may have a major influence on the creation of areas of overpressure much higher than expected by the size of the explosive. Therefore the severity of injuries and number of deaths is much higher in confined spaces. This has been shown by Katz et al. [10] who examined the results of an explosion inside a bus in Jerusalem. Some of the deaths occurred at a distance that only minor injuries would have been expected in an open place. On the other hand, passengers at a short distance from the explosion were only slightly injured, probably being protected by the seats of the bus. Recently these effects were stressed again by comparing casualties from explosions within busses in Jerusalem with victims of explosions in open space [11].

The blast wave creates in the body stress waves and shear waves [3, 6]. Stress waves have their maximal effects at air-fluid or air-tissue interfaces, therefore causing damage in the lungs, bowel, and auditory system. Shear waves cause most of the damage to solid or fluid-containing organs along their mesenteric attachments. Recent studies from Yugoslavia have found significant elevations in blood thromboxane A_2, prostacyclin and sulfidopeptide leukotrienes in blast casualties compared with nonblast patients. These changes suggest that blast injury causes a major physiological stress [1, 12].

Eardrum perforations were considered for a long time the hallmark of blast injury [7]. However various kinds of damage can be inflicted - an explosion may cause tinnitus, pain and dizziness, or deafness. These perforations depend not only on the distance from the explosion, but also on the position of the head at the time of the event, and on the presence of other objects that may have a protective effect [3]. Therefore, some patients with severe injuries may have intact eardrums. On the other hand, isolated eardrum perforation in survivors of explosions is not a marker of concealed blast injury. This finding may have a major impact on the decision to admit patients with eardrum perforations for observation for fear of development of pulmonary symptoms [13]. It seems safe to discharge these patients following a brief observation with no need for hospitalization. Every casualty should undergo an otoscopic examination, while further evaluation may be postponed, in most cases to ambulatory visits.

The most-common severe injuries seen in survivors are in the chest. Stress areas of great magnitude my result in disruption of the lung parenchyma that is particularly marked near the mediastinum, diaphragms and ribcage. These result in hemorrhage and leakage of interstitial fluid in the alveoli. Lung injury may vary from minor hemorrhages to full blown ‘blast lung’; often these injuries are accompanied by pneumothoraces. In addition some survivors are occasionally found in profound shock and hypoxia, without obvious hemorrhage. Recent laboratory investigations have found an immediate myocardial depression without a compensatory vasoconstriction. This effect may be a vagally mediated reflex that was prevented by bilateral cervical vagotomy in an experimental model [14, 15]. Some patients present with immediate pulmonary insufficiency with severe hypoxia. The typical chest radiograph shows the “butterfly lung” or ‘snowstorm’; namely white, opaque areas around the mediastinum. All the severely injured patients need immediate ventilatory support, which may employ innovative techniques [16, 17]. Often ‘loculated’ pneumothoraces are missed, as the spongy lung parenchyma is pushed towards the ribcage, and several thoracic drains may be needed in order to drain them properly. Ventilation may aggravate the patient’s cardiovascular condition and advanced hemodynamic monitoring techniques may be needed. The use of arterial waveform analysis, which is relatively noninvasive, may provide an accurate estimate of preload and may direct treatment [16, 18]. Contrary to common practice in trauma patients, the judicious use of sympathomimetic drugs may be helpful in treating shock caused by myocardial depression. Severe blast injury may be accompanied by pneumoperitoneum; this may worsen the hypoxia, hypercarbia, and shock. Rapid surgical decompression may have a dramatic effect, and should be considered whenever the patient's condition deteriorates [19].

Abdominal injuries as pure primary blast injuries are uncommon. As mentioned earlier, the bowel may be injured as it contains air and liquid or it may be torn at its mesenteric attachments. Primary blast injury to the bowel has been usually described following underwater explosions, and was considered almost nonexistent in survivors of air explosions. During the last few years several publications have described injuries to the jejunum and ileum following explosions in buses or in open air [10, 20]. Some of these injuries had an immediate presentation, while in others the diagnosis was delayed. It was postulated that there might be a mechanism of evolving damage to the bowel wall and delayed perforation. Therefore it has been suggested that patients exposed to a significant blast should be watched for at least 48 h [20]. (This in contrast to the previous statement that patients with isolated eardrum perforation may be discharged following a brief period of observation!)

Additional injuries were found to the spleen, without any additional damage. These peculiar injuries may have been caused by the sudden down movement of the diaphragm following the blast. A second possible mechanism may be that of tertiary injury, but as no other intra-abdominal injury was found in these patients, that would be unlikely [16].

Special environmental conditions may have major influences on the severity of injuries and their complications. The impact of blast inside a close space has already been stressed. Following two explosions in open spaces in Jerusalem, one at a marketplace, the other in an open mall, an outbreak of candidemia has been noticed. Air sampling revealed exclusive detection of *Candida* species and increased mold concentration in the market in comparison with the mall environment. Theses finding suggest a role for an exogenous, environmental source in the development of candidemia in these patients [21].

Patients who survive primary blast injuries may have long-term effects of their injury. Unexpectedly, despite extremely severe injuries, most patients who survived lung blast injury had normal lung function tests within a year of their injury [22]. Cernak et al. [12] found a variety of effects on the central nervous system; long-term alterations were shown in 30% of patients from blast injury in contrast to only 4% in other casualties. Obviously damage to the auditory system may have long-lasting sequelae.

Several studies have tried to classify blast injuries, as it became clear that common scoring systems are not optimal for these injuries. Mellor [3] divided blast casualties into four groups according to blast loading. Studying 216 servicemen killed in Northern Ireland he found that patients exposed to lower blast loading died primarily of head injuries, namely secondary injury [3]. Pizov et al. [16] proposed a blast lung injury severity scoring system, which is based on simple parameters of hypoxemia, chest radiographic abnormalities and barotrauma. The lung damage may be accurately estimated in the early hours after injury, and it may be helpful in determining patient management and prediction of final outcome [16]. Cernak et al. [1] studied 1,303 blast casualties and evaluated a quantitative assessment of subjective symptoms and measured changes in plasma cytokines, amino acids, and eicosanoids. They found that some grading systems failed to grade blast injury severity precisely, and that the addition of the subjective or functional impairments are important for scoring blast injury severity [1].

To summarize, blast injuries became common during the last decades. Knowledge of the pathophysiology and the possible inflicted injuries are essential in the successful management. Rapid organization and correct triage have paramount importance. Future studies should determine the specific neuroendocrine and humoral responses to blast injuries.

References

1. Cernak I, Savic J, Zunic G, et al (1999) Recognizing, scoring, and predicting blast injuries. World J Surg;23:44-53
2. Mallonee S, Shariat S, Stennies G, et al (1996) Physical injuries and fatalities resulting from the Oklahoma City bombing. JAMA 276:382-387
3. Mellor SG (1992) The relationship of blast loading to death and injury from explosion. World J Surg 16:893-898
4. Stein M, Hirshberg A (1999) Medical consequences of terrorism. The conventional weapon threat. Surg Clin North Am 79:1537-1552
5. Hiss J, Kahana T (2000) Trauma and identification of victims of suicidal terrorism in Israel. Mil Med 165:889-893
6. Mellor SG, Dodd KT, Harmon JW, Cooper GJ (1997) Ballistic and other implications of blast. In: Ryan JM, Rich NM, Dale RF, Morgans BT, Cooper GJ (eds) Ballistic trauma: clinical relevance in peace and war. Arnold, London pp 47-59
7. Cripps NPJ, Glover MA, Guy RJ (1999) The pathophysiology of primary blast injury and its implications for treatment. II The auditory structures and abdomen. J Roy Nav Med Serv 85:13-24
8. Guy RJ, Glover MA, Cripps NPJ (1998) The pathophysiology of primary blast injury and its implications for treatment. Part I: The thorax. J Roy Nav Med Serv;84:79-86
9. Guy RJ, Glover MA, Cripps NPJ (2000) The pathophysiology of primary blast injury and its implications for treatment. Part III: Injury to the central nervous system and the limbs. J R Nav Med Serv 86:27-31
10. Katz E, Ofek B, Adler J, et al (1989) Primary blast injury after a bomb explosion in a civilian bus. Ann Surg 209:484-488
11. Leibovici D, Gofrit ON, Stein M, et al (1996) Blast injuries: bus versus open-air bombings – a comparative study of injuries in survivors of open-air versus confined-space explosions. J Trauma 41:1030-1035

12. Cernak I, Savic J, Ignjatovic D, Jevtic M (1999) Blast injury from explosive munitions. J Trauma 47:96-104
13. Leibovici D, Gofrit ON, Shapira SC (1999) Eardrum perforation in explosion survivors: is it a marker of blast injury? Ann Intern Med 34:168-172
14. Irwin RJ, Lerner MR, Bealer JF, et al (1997) Cardiopulmonary physiology of primary blast injury. J Trauma 43:650-655
15. Irwin RJ, Lerner MR, Bealer JF, et al (1999) Shock after blast wave injury is caused by a vagally mediated reflex. J Trauma 47:105-110
16. Pizov R, Oppenheim-Eden A, Matot I, et al (1999) Blast injury from an explosion on a civilian bus. Chest 115:165-172
17. Sorkin P, Szold O, Kluger Y, et al (1998) Permissive hypercapnia ventilation in patients with severe pulmonary blast injury. J Trauma 45:35-38
18. Weiss YG, Oppenheim-Eden A, Gilon D, et al (1999) Systolic pressure variation in hemodynamic monitoring after severe blast injury. J Clin Anesth 11:132-135
19. Oppenheim A, Pizov R, Pikarsky A, et al (1998) Tension pneumoperitoneum after blast injury: Dramatic improvement in ventilatory and hemodynamic parameters after surgical decompression. J Trauma 44:915-917
20. Paran H, Neufeld D, Shwartz I, et al (1996) Perforation of the terminal ileum induced by blast injury: delayed diagnosis or delayed perforation? J Trauma 40:472-475
21. Wolf DG, Polacheck I, Block C, et al (2000) High rate of candidemia in patients sustaining injuries in a bomb blast at a marketplace: a possible environmental source. Clin Infect Dis 31:712-716
22. Hirshberg B, Oppenheim-Eden A, Pizov R, et al (1999) Recovery from blast injury. One-year follow-up. Chest 116:1683-1688

Prognosis in Cerebral Dysfunction in Patients with Head Trauma

N. LATRONICO, R. STEFINI, A. CANDIANI

In the case of acute diseases it is not easy at all to predict death or recovery
(Hyppocrates 400 B.C.).

Prevalence estimates for head trauma in the United States range from 2.5 million to 6.5 million individuals living with the consequences of traumatic brain injury (TBI) [1]. These estimates suffer from ascertainment bias, since they are based exclusively on information about hospitalized patients and those who die before hospitalization, while rates of hospitalization for TBI are declining, and care of persons with less-severe TBI is shifting from hospital admission to outpatient services [2]. Situation appears even more catastrophic when considering that road crashes account for most of the injuries, and that car use is rapidly increasing in many countries. It is estimated that by 2020 road crashes will have moved from ninth to third in the world ranking of disease burden [3].

Identifying effective treatments for head injury is thus of global health importance, and the reader could ask why the focus of this chapter is on outcome rather than on actually available and future treatments. The scope is to provide objective reasons why the outcome research may provide relevant and useful results for daily practice. The methodological basis for outcome research, as well as an overview on predictive variables and methods used to measure the outcome(s) of patients suffering from severe head trauma, are also presented.

Outcome and prognosis

The term outcome refers to what patients experience as a result of a disease and its treatment [4]. Prognosis refers to prediction of the possible outcomes of a disease and the frequency with which they can be expected to occur (e.g., complete recovery, disability, or death in head trauma). Patient characteristics, either demographic (e.g., age or sex), disease-related (e.g., level of coma), or co-morbid (e.g., chronic renal failure), may be used to more accurately or parsimoniously predict the outcome. These characteristics are called "prognostic factors" [5]. They are associated with the development of outcomes strongly enough to predict them, but do not (necessarily) cause them. Prognostic factors should be distinguished from "risk factors", which are the patient characteristics associated with the development of the disease: cigarette smoking is a well-known risk factor for lung cancer, however prognosis depends on histological type, tumor size and location, regional node involvement, and presence of metastases. Quiting smoking at that stage is irrelevant for prognosis [6]. Some examples pertaining to head trauma are given in Table 1.

Table 1. Examples of risk and factors in severe and mild brain trauma. GCS = Glasgow Coma Scale

Disease process: severe brain trauma		
Risk factors	**Prognostic factors**	**Outcome**
(those associated with the development of the disease)	(those associated with the development of outcomes)	(what patients may experience as a consequence of a disease and its treatment)
Driving a car being drunk	Fixed, dilated pupils GCS score of 8 Intracranial hypertension Compressed or absent basal cisterns on brain CT scan	Bad outcome[a] Good outcome[a] Brain ischemia Intracranial hypertension
Disease process: mild brain trauma		
Risk factors	**Prognostic factors**	**Outcome**
Many daily activities	Two or more episodes of vomiting[b]	Intracranial hematoma

[a] as defined in the Glasgow Outcome Scale (see Measuring the Outcome)
[b] from reference 13

Who is interested in outcome studies? And why?

Clinicians and researchers usually looking for different types of outcomes, not just death or survival, which may give clues to the disease process and stimulate specific research, are interested in outcome studies.

For example, age is an independent predictor of mortality, and mortality is higher in older than younger patients. However, this is not explained by an increased frequency of intracranial hematomas (a hypothesis based on presumed vascular fragility), which has led to the hypothesis that mechanisms of repair are degraded in the ageing brain. Prognostic variables also permit a more--accurate patient selection for treatment (those who may benefit from those who may not), improve the design and analysis of randomized clinical trials by permitting risk stratification (if age 50 years is a prognostic variable for survival, then the two study arms must have a comparable number of such patients), as well as adjustment for case mix in non-randomized studies [7].

As effective treatments are expected to improve the outcome, *health care organizations* are also interested in outcome studies for resources to be allocated efficiently. This aspect is particularly relevant in the highly technologically dependent specialty of Intensive Care Medicine, in which the role of several sophisticated monitoring devices is uncertain [8, 9].

Patients and their families are more interested in prognosis than in any other medical aspects of their disease process. Some physicians seem to ignore this simple principle, when indulging in detailed description of pathophysiology and diagnosis, while providing only vague, ambiguous information regarding prognosis. An even worse behavior is to predict a very bad outcome, no matter the real clinical condition, and to change it if the condition improves. In a recent Italian Consensus Conference on rehabilitation in head trauma [10], one of the authors (NL) personally witnessed how angrily patients and families' representatives emphasized the difficulty in obtaining trustworthy prognostic information from intensive care physicians and neurosurgeons. The following is a mother's comment. "Standing up in a crowded corridor I was told by a busy physician that my son' condition was extremely severe, and that the risk of death was almost 100%. Two days later the situation had changed dramatically. *Your son has responded well to treatments and has awakened, however the risk of permanent neurological damage is still high*, said a second physician. Three days later my son was discharged from the intensive care unit (ICU). After rehabilitation, he has recovered almost uneventfully. How can one believe in such physicians?".

Little clinical experience, medico-legal concern in case "the promise is not kept", absence of adequate premises and sufficient time, and perception of outcome prediction as a minor medical duty are some explanations. Reading the pertinent "statistics" literature is not an easy task for physicians, and represents a further impediment for the outcome research to be widely appreciated.

Evidence- or experience-based outcome prediction?

The science of outcome prediction has greatly evolved in recent years. In the United States it evolved from studies showing substantial geographic variations in the practice of medicine and surgery without any evident difference in patient outcomes. With escalating health care costs, there has been a growing interest in measuring the outcomes of medical intervention to determine the quality and appropriateness of medical care [4]. Improvement in the methodology of research, as well as refinement of statistical approaches, are playing a key role by providing better reference models for well-designed and clearly reported cohort studies [7]. This despite, the accuracy of individual outcome prediction models in head trauma, is far from optimal, and models can actually only supplement, not substitute, the clinical judgement and experience.

The ideal study for prognosis

As described above, variables predicting which patients do better or worse are called prognostic variables. It is usually impossible or unethical to randomize patients to different prognostic factors. Therefore, observational cohort studies, not experimental designs, are the best way to evaluate the increased risk associated with a prognostic factor. Good-quality prognostic studies are prospective in nature, and the initial set of variables potentially predicting the outcome is defined based on literature evidence and/or expert opinion. The prognostic study will (or will not) then confirm the variables as prognostic, and the initial patient group in which these variables are identified is called training or derivation set. For example, 34 variables were included in the initial Acute Physiology and Chronic Health Evaluation (APACHE) score after expert consultation. Subsequently, researchers found that only 12 of them actually affected survival [11]. Quality criteria for assessing prognostic studies are presented in Table 2 [5-7]. A final guide to decide whether a claim that a variable or, more likely, a set of independent variables is prognostic is to look for a second, independent sample of patients – the test set or validation set – in which variables are confirmed as predictive of the outcome. Table 2 also includes treatments, despite the fact that they are not, strictly speaking, prognostic factors. However they can modify the outcome and therefore, patients should have had the same treatment or equally effective treatments (in this case why use different treatments?) before an unbiased assessment of the prognostic ability of the study is delivered [7].

Table 2. Criteria for assessing the quality of papers dealing with prognosis[a]

Variables should be evaluated in a *representative sample* of patients assembled at a common point in the course of their illness, possibly at an early stage, perhaps at diagnosis
Follow-up should be sufficiently long and complete
Outcome should be objective, unbiased (examined by investigators blind to patients' clinical characteristics and prognostic factors), fully defined, appropriate
Prognostic variable should be clearly and objectively defined, including methods of measurement
Adjustment for important prognostic factors should have been done; validation in an independent group of 'test-set' or 'validation set' patients is desirable
Treatment subsequent to inclusion in cohort should be fully described

[a] Based on references 5-7.

Clinical prediction rules

In complex situation, like head trauma, several predictive variable are usually identified. Although the role of each variable can be individually examined, it is more useful to examine the impact of all of them together, and to determine how the variables interact with one another. Several types of multivariate statistical analyses are used to assess the relative contribution of variables (if any). If the predictive power of the variable(s) remains after considering other variables, it is called an independent prognostic variable. For example, both age and neurological severity (usually measured with the Glasgow Coma Scale, GCS) are independent prognostic variables, meaning that two patients with comparable GCS scores but different age are likely to have different outcomes (the older the age the worse the outcome), as well as two patients with comparable age and different GCS scores (the lower the GCS score the worse the outcome).

Variables found to be predictors can be converted into clinical prediction rules [12]. A pertinent example is the Canadian CT head rule for patients with minor head injury, in which five high-risk factors (failure to reach GCS of 15 within 2 h, suspected open skull fracture, any sign of basal skull fracture, vomiting $\geq$ 2 episodes, or age $\geq$ 65 years) and two additional medium-risk factors (amnesia before impact >30 min and dangerous mechanism of injury) were identified to allow doctors in emergency departments to order CT for their patients based upon strong evidence [13].

Prognostic studies in head trauma patients

In a recent paper Teasdale and Graham [14] commented: "The essential enigma regarding head injury is the uncertainty of its consequences, in particular, the variability in the outcomes for different patients after apparently similar initial injuries". It is the uniqueness of the person that makes the individual outcome difficult to predict, and emphasizes that a large number of patient characteristics (the prognostic variables) is needed to achieve the goal.

A second, more-basic problem is raised by Hill [15]: "If the brain is seen as the basis of the personality and is altered by the trauma, then, philosophically, it is difficult to argue that the person is the same as before". This problem is even more dramatic with children, whose brain is developing and no baseline is available. The critical point here is which outcome we can measure reliably.

Prognostic variables

A systematic review of published prognostic studies is out of the scope of this chapter. Furthermore, systematic reviews and meta-analysis are in their infancy in this field and criteria for judging quality are likely to change over the next few years [7]. The Brain Trauma Foundation has recently updated the guidelines for the management of severe head trauma, and a comprehensive evaluation of the published literature on the subject of prognostic factors in TBI has been included [16]. Age, GCS score, pupillary diameter and light reflex, hypotension, and brain CT features were identified as major prognostic variables. The reader is referred to this publication for details (*www.braintrauma.org*), however, conclusions should be taken cautiously since the criteria used to include studies in the analysis may be subjected to changes. Duration of anterograde or post-traumatic amnesia (PTA) is also a powerful predictor of outcome. This topic has recently been reviewed [17].

Despite the fact that many studies have used clinical information to derive predictive models, it was not until recently that high-quality studies with modern statistical modelling techniques were published providing reliable and easy-to-use prognostic models. Signorini et al. [18] demonstrated that five simple clinical variables can be identified that accurately predict the outcome: age > 50 years, GCS score, Injury Severity Score (ISS) (a summary measure of trauma to single or multiple body regions), a visible (or not) hematoma on brain CT, and pupil reaction to light [18]. After the initial training set of 372 patients, external validation was carried out on a new group of 520 patients (the test set or validation set, see Table 2) which corroborated the initial findings. The authors were then able to produce a "paper-and-pencil" *nomogram*, which can be used at the bedside to calculate the probability of survival of an individual patient. However, since the model is too pessimistic at low survival probabilities, its use is only recommended for proper stratification in therapeutic trials rather than for daily clinical decision-making, in which case withdrawing of treatments could be instigated inappropriately [19]. In a second study, the authors evaluated whether prognosis could be improved by adding to the five-variable baseline model the predictive value for survival of recording secondary insults (intracranial hypertension, hypo- and hypertension, low cerebral perfusion pressure, hypoxia, pyrexia, tachy- and bradycardia) [20]. Results showed that intracranial hypertension, defined as the total time that intracranial pressure (ICP) was above 20 mmHg up to 72 h after admission, adds substantial predictive value to the baseline model and is an independent predictor of bad functional outcome.

Taken together, these two studies [18, 20] represent the best-available evidence on outcome prediction in head trauma. They tell us that five simple variables already known when the patient is first admitted to the ICU combined with ICP derangement from this point on provide a useful set for accurately predicting outcome.

It must be emphasized, as the authors did, that the fact that the episodes of intracranial hypertension are predictive of death does not imply that a more--aggressive treatment to reduce or prevent them will improve survival. Likewise, the absence of any predictive power of hypoxia or hypotension does not mean that derangements in these physiological variables should be left uncorrected. As discussed above, prognostic variables are associated with the development of outcomes, but do not (necessarily) cause them, and treatment efficacy can only be addressed in a randomized controlled trial of adequate size. No such studies have been identified in a recent systematic review on ICP monitoring [21]. .

The prognostic role of genotype, gender, and associated injuries

Is the destiny written in the DNA?

In 1997 Teasdale et al. [22] demonstrated, by studying the apolipoprotein E (*APOE*) genotype on blood samples of head trauma patients, that variability in outcome can be, at least in part, genetically determined. In human beings there are three common alleles of APOE gene – epsilon2, epsilon3, epsilon4 – encoding three isoforms of the protein, E2, E3, E4. The protein has an active role in promoting repair processes after trauma by enhancing lipid transport to cell membranes, however the apoE E4 is the less active isoform. Furthermore, apoE E4 promotes rapid aggregation of amyloid beta-protein into amyloid fibrils with formation in the cerebral cortex of plaque-like deposits similar to those observed in Alzheimer disease. The hypothesis that patients with *APOE* epsilon4 could have a negative impact on prognosis was confirmed in a series of 93 patients, 63 with and 30 without *APOE* epsilon4;. 46% of patients with the allele died, were in a vegetative state or severely disabled at 6 months after trauma compared with 25% of patients without the allele. The data have been confirmed in other series [23, 24], including chronic TBI in boxers [25].

Clinical implications of these studies, if confirmed in larger series, could be relevant for determining prognosis, but also for advising patients with head trauma about the increased risk from further injury. Furthermore, a combination of previous head trauma and *APOE* epsilon4 genotype seems to act synergistically as risk factor for Alzheimer disease in later life.

Do females fare worse?

Head trauma is more than twice as likely to occur in men as in women. Recent data however suggest that females fare worse than males, and that gender is an independent prognostic factor. Kraus et al. [26], in a prospective cohort of 795 moderate and severe brain-injured patients, showed four independent factors predicting all-time mortality: gender, age, type of head trauma (penetrating or blunt) and GCS score [26]. Overall, the adjusted odds ratio for female gender was 1.75 (95% CI 1.09-2.82) indicating a 1.75-fold increase in risk of death. The greatest difference in mortality was demonstrated in patients over age 50 years (51.1% females, 28.4% males). Females were 1.57 times more likely to have a poor outcome (as measured by the GOS) than males (95% CI 0.80 -3.08), although this difference did not reach statistical significance. Results were not replicated in 1998 by Groswasser et al. [27], who actually showed a better outcome for women than men. However, only patients with severe head trauma were included, stratification was performed by the duration of unconsciousness (coma plus PTA) and outcome was estimated (not measured) by rehabilitation doctors as return-to-work status, which make the two studies difficult to compare [27]. In the study of Signorini et al. [18], female gender (as well as low alcohol consumption) was a predicting factor for bad prognosis only in the univariate analysis, but not in the multivariate logistic model. More recently, a meta-analysis has been published, which seems to confirm a worse outcome for female gender [28]. However, search strategy for detecting potentially useful papers was very limited (only Medline and English-language literature) and was actually based on eight papers. Quality analysis of selected papers was not reported, and patients with all-grade head trauma severity were analyzed. Finally, experts are reluctant, at the actual state of knowledge, in supporting formal meta-analyses on prognostic studies [7]. At present, no firm conclusion can be made as to whether or not gender is an independent prognostic factor in head trauma patients.

Do extra-cranial injuries matter?

The largest-ever published series that examined the influence of extracranial injuries on mortality rates in head-injured patients is that by Gennarelli et al. [29], which was based on data collected from 1982 to 1986 as part of the Major Trauma Outcome Study [29]; 49,143 patients were prospectively enrolled, of whom 16,524 were head trauma patients. Mortality was influenced by the presence of life-threatening to maximum extracranial injury (Abbreviated Injury Severity, AIS, 4 - 6) (*AIS* is a 6-grade classification of anatomical injury of body regions; grades are 1, minimal; 2, moderate; 3, severe; 4, life-threatening; 5 critical, survival uncertain; 6, maximum, virtually unsurvivable; *ISS* is a single-number measure derived by the AIS as the sum of squares of the three highest AIS grades; patients with an AIS of 6 are automatically assigned an ISS of 75) [30, 31] for all AIS grades of head injury, except grade 6 (maximum injury, including crush fracture, brainstem crush/laceration, decapitation, and spinal cord crush/laceration or transection). So, despite the authors commenting that mortality was little influenced by the presence of extracranial injury, actually more than a quarter of patients (25.6%) died because of an interaction between cranial and extracranial damage. More recently, Chesnut et al. [32] studied a prospective cohort of 717 severe head injury (GCS ≤ 8) patients to evaluate the role of extracranial insults in determining the outcome. Stratification was evaluated for age (0-39, ≥ 40 years), severe multiple trauma (AIS score ≥ 3: yes/no), hypotension (systolic blood pressure ≤ 90 mmHg: yes/no), and hypoxia ($paO_2 \leq 60$ mmHg: yes/no). Only hypotension and hypoxia were found to be strong predictors of bad outcome. Unfortunately important variables (GCS, pupillary reactivity, brain CT scan) were not considered for analysis, while others were categorized (age), when in fact less-arbitrary ways exist for exploring non-linear relationship with continuous variables [33]. AIS>3 was used as dichotomous variable, however AIS is calculated for several body regions, while ISS is a single-number summary measure linearly related to outcome [18]. Other studies have addressed the potential predictive value of associated extracranial injuries in head-injured patients [34], however small sample size, inadequate definition of prognostic variables, flawed statistical approach, and absence of validation set were common problems.

Available data indicate that extracranial injuries, as measured by ISS, have a role in determining the prognosis of patients suffering TBI. This role is independent of age, neurological severity, pupillary light reaction and evidence of hematoma on brain CT scan [18]. A single, high-quality, externally validated study yielded these results. Replication in other centers is awaited.

Measuring the outcome

The GOS is the most widely used method to assess the outcome after head injury, mainly because it is strongly related to severity, is easy to administer, can be applied to all cases, and has clinically relevant categories. These latter comprise death, persistent (permanent after 1 year) vegetative state, severe disability (dependent on daily support), moderate disability (able to use transport independently and to work in a protected environment), and good recovery (resumption of normal life despite minor neurological and psychological defects) [35]. An extended version (GOSE) has recently been proposed, in which each of the last three categories is further divided into two to increase sensitivity for those patients with ratings in the upper end of the scale [36].

Final considerations

Outcome in head trauma – what patients experience as a result of brain injury and its treatment – has almost infinite variations, which makes its prediction, the *prognosis*, a difficult task. However, outcome prediction is becoming a rigorous science based on probabilities, not prophecies, whose tools are *cohort studies*, not cards. Within this methodological frame, careful clinical observation and experienced judgement are essential for identifying the *prognostic variables*. Experience and evidence are intimately mingled, and neither can be renounced.

References

1. Centers for Disease Control and Prevention. National Center for Injury Prevention and Control. Epidemiology of traumatic brain injury in the United States (2000) Atlanta, Ga, USA www.cdc.gov/ncipc/dacrrdp/tbi.htm
2. Thurman D, Guerrero J (1999) Trends in hospitalization associated with traumatic brain injury. JAMA 282:954-957
3. Murray CJL, Lopez AD (1997) Alternative projections of mortality and disability by cause 1990-2020: Global Burden of Disease Study. Lancet 349:1436-1432
4. Gerszten PC (1998) Outcomes research: a review. Neurosurgery 43:1146–1156

5. Laupacis A, Wells G, Richardson SW, Tugwell P for the Evidence-Based Medicine working Group (1994) Users'guides to the medical literature. V. How to use an article about prognosis. JAMA 272:234-237
6. Sackett DL, Richardson SW, Rosenberg W, Haynes BR (eds) (1998) Evidence-based medicine. How to practice and teach EBM. Churchill Livingstone, Edinburgh
7. Altman DG (2001) Systematic reviews in health care. Systematic reviews of evaluations of prognostic variables. BMJ 323:224–228
8. Latronico N, Beindorf AE, Rasulo FA, et al (2000) Limits of intermittent jugular bulb oxygen saturation monitoring in the management of severe head trauma patients. Neurosurgery 46:1131–1139
9. Hall JB (2000) Use of the pulmonary artery catheter in critically ill patients: was invention the mother of necessity? JAMA 283:2577–2578
10. Allasia F, Cannoni I, Cattelani R, et al (2001) A report of the families' work group. G Ital Med Riabil 15:73-78
11. Knaus WA, Draper EA, Wagner DP, et al (1984) APACHE II: a severity of disease classification system. Crit Care Med 13:591-597
12. Wasson JH, Sox HC, Neff RK, Goldman L (1985) Clinical prediction rules: application and methodological standards. N Engl J Med 313: 793–799
13. Stiell IG, Wells GA, Vandemheen K, et al for the CCC Study Group (2001) The Canadian CT head rule for patients with minor head injury. Lancet 357: 1391–1396
14. Teasdale GM, Graham DI (1998) Craniocerebral trauma: protection and retrieval of the neuronal population after injury. Fundamental problems. Neurosurgery 43: 723–738
15. Hill H (1999) Traumatic brain injury: a view from the inside. Brain Inj 13: 839-844
16. Anonymous (2000) Guidelines for the management of severe head injury. A joint initiative of the Brain Trauma Foundation, the American Association of Neurological Surgeons, the Joint Section on Neurotrauma and Critical Care. Brain Injury Association,Washington, DC
17. Ahmed S, Bierley R, Sheikh JI, Date ES (2000) Post-traumatic amnesia after closed head injury: a review of the literature and some suggestions for further research. Brain Inj 14: 765-780
18. Signorini DF, Andrews PJD, Jones PA, et al (1999) Predicting survival using simple clinical variables: a case study in traumatic brain injury. J Neurol Neurosurg Psychiatry 66: 20-25
19. Murray LS, Teasdale GM, Murray GD, et al (1993) Does prediction of outcome alter patient management? Lancet 341: 1487-1491
20. Signorini DF, Andrews PJD, Jones PA, et al (1999) Adding insult to injury: the prognostic value of early secondary insults for survival after traumatic brain injury. J Neurol Neurosurg Psychiatry 66:26-31
21. Forsyth R, Baxter P, Elliott T (2001) Routine intracranial pressure monitoring in acute coma (Cochrane Review). In: The Cochrane Library, 3, 2001. Oxford: Update Software
22. Teasdale GM, Nicoll JAR, Murray G, Fiddes (1997) Association of apolipoprotein E polymorphism with outcome after head injury. Lancet 350:1069-1071
23. Friedman G, Froom, Sazbon L et al, (1999) Apolipoprotein E- 4 genotype predicts a poor outcome in survivors of traumatic brain injury. Neurology 52:244-248
24. Lichtman SW, Seliger G, Tycko B, Marder K (2000) Apolipoprotein E and functional recovery from brain injury following postacute rehabilitation. Neurology 55:1536-1539
25. Jordan BD, Relkin NR, Ravdin LD, et al (1997) Apolipoprotein E epsilon4 associated with chronic traumatic brain injury in boxing. JAMA 278:136-140
26. Kraus JF, Corinne Peek-Asa C, McArthur D (2000) The independent effect of gender on outcomes following traumatic brain injury: a preliminary investigation. Neurosurg Focus 8: 5
27. Groswasser Z, Cohen M, Keren O (1998) Female TBI patients recover better than males. Brain Inj 12:805-808
28. Farace E, Alves WM (2000) Do women fare worse: a metaanalysis of gender differences in traumatic brain injury outcome. J Neurosurg 93:539–545
29. Gennarelli TA, Champion HR, Sacco WJ et al (1989) Mortality of patients with head injury and extracranial injury treated in trauma centers. J Trauma 29:1193-1202

30. Civil ID, Schwab WC (1988) The Abbreviated Injury Scale, 1985 revision: a condensed chart for clinical use. J Trauma 28: 87-90
31. Copes WS, Champion HR, Sacco WJ, et al (1988) The Injury Severity Score revisited. J Trauma 28: 69-77
32. Chesnut RM, Marshall LF, Klauber MR, et al (1993) The role of secondary brain injury in determining outcome from severe head injury. J Trauma 34:216-222
33. Hastie TJ, Tibshirani RJ (1990) Generalised additive models. Chapman and Hall, London
34. Sarrafzadeh AS, Peltonen EE, Kaisers U, et al (2001) Secondary insults in severe head injury – do multiply injured patients do worse? Crit Care Med 29:1116-1123
35. Jennet B, Bond M (1975) Assessment of outcome after severe brain damage: a practical scale. Lancet I: 480-484
36. Wilson JTL, Pettigrew LEI, Teasdale GM (1998) Emotional and cognitive consequences of head injury in relation to the Glasgow Outcome Scale. J Neurotrauma 15:573-585

Respiratory Failure in Brain Injured Patients

P. PELOSI, G. COLOMBO, C. GAMBERONI

It is known that in brain injured patients the principal morbidity and mortality is frequently caused by cerebral nervous system injury and its neurologic consequences [1, 2]. Nevertheless, extracerebral organ dysfunctions are common in brain injured patients which increases morbidity and mortality [3, 4]. Among them, the most frequent complication is respiratory dysfunction including pulmonary oedema and pneumonia. It is now clear that there is an entire spectrum of pulmonary abnormalities caused either directly or indirectly by acute brain injury. Although respiratory problems seems to play a relevant role in the clinical management of brain injured patients, very few studies have investigated respiratory function abnormalities in this category of patients [5]. The aim of this review is to discuss: a) functional abnormalities; b) clinical treatment; c) possible prevention of respiratory function abnormalities in brain injured patients.

Definition of brain injury

Brain injury includes several clinical conditions, with markedly different pathophysiological mechanisms [6, 7]. For simplicity, in this review, we have defined as "brain injured patients" those who suffered from:

1) traumatic brain injury;
2) spontaneous haemorrhagic (subarachnoid or parenchymal or both) brain injury;
3) surgical brain injury (after trauma, haemorrhage, malignancies, etc).

It is possible, however, that pulmonary related problems and consequent prevention and treatment may be different between different categories of brain injured patients.

The role of extracerebral organ dysfunctions in brain injured patients

Recently, it has been emphasized that the outcome in brain injured patients is more frequently the result of a progressive dysfunction of organ systems remote from the site of the primary disease process (i.e., multiple organ dysfunction process) [8]. Table 1 summarizes the average prevalence of extracerebral complications (partitioned into overall and severe) in brain injured patients. Several reports indicate that medical complications after brain injury may significantly contribute to the overall mortality rate [3, 9, 10]. They found that pulmonary alterations accounted up to 50% of the deaths after brain injury. The mortality was significantly higher in patients with brain injury associated with at least one organ failure compared to patients with brain injury alone (65% vs. 17%, respectively). The occurrence of pulmonary failure was associated with an increase in the intensive care unit (ICU) and the duration of the hospital stay [11].

In summary, extracerebral organ dysfunctions and in particular pulmonary failure are important causes of morbidity and mortality in brain injured patients.

Table1. Prevalence of extracerebral organ dysfunctions in brain injured patients

		Total	Severe
Pulmonary	Pneumonia	40 %	25 %
	Embolism	1 %	100 %
Gut		40 %	5 %
Cardiac	Arrhythmia	30 %	5 %
	Cardiac failure	5 %	1 %
Metabolic	Electrolytes disorders	30 %	2 %
	Diabetes insipidus	7 %	7 %
Hepatic		25 %	4%
Haematologic		20 %	6 %
Renal		10 %	15 %

Why pulmonary complications occur in brain injured patients?

We can identify three major causes of pulmonary complications in brain injured patients: 1) neurogenic pulmonary oedema (NPE); 2) abnormalities in ventilation perfusion mismatch; 3) structural parenchymal abnormalities.

Neurogenic pulmonary oedema (NPE)

The most reported dramatic pulmonary complication in brain injured patients is NPE. In the 1960's Simmons et al. [12] reported that 85% of their series of combat casualties from Vietnam who died with a severe isolated head injury demonstrated a significant pulmonary pathology, including alveolar oedema, haemorrhage and congestion that was not the result of direct lung injury as chest trauma, so called NPE. However, NPE is very rare in civilians with brain injury, except in young patients with massive and usually rapidly fatal brain damage [13].

Ventilation perfusion mismatch

Several authors observed that the majority of brain injured patients with moderate to severe hypoxemia did not show evident radiographic abnormalities [14, 15]. Thus, it has been postulated that respiratory failure could occur without the presence of interstitial or alveolar oedema, due to ventilation perfusion mismatch [16, 17].

Three main mechanisms have been advocated:

1) redistribution in regional perfusion: a redistribution of ventilation and perfusion has been described in animals and men using the multiple inert gas technique [14, 18, 19]. There is some experimental evidence that ventilation perfusion matching is partially mediated by central nervous system (CNS), particularly in the hypothalamus [20];
2) pulmonary microembolisms could lead to increased dead space ventilation and ventilation perfusion mismatch [21, 22];
3) lung surfactant depletion: few experimental studies suggested that excessive sympathetic stimulation [15] and excessive hyperventilation [23], often present after brain injury, can reduce the production of lung surfactant which could lead to lung microatelectasis and ventilation perfusion mismatch.

We believe that the main reasons explaining respiratory insufficiency in brain injured patients are structural parenchymal abnormalities.

Structural parenchymal abnormalities in brain injured patients

We have identified five main causes of structural parenchymal alterations in brain injured patients: 1) abnormal breathing pattern; 2) release of inflammatory mediators; 3) release of catecholamines ("sympathetic storm"); 4) infectious processes; 5) "direct" trauma consequences as presence of lung contusion, pneumothoraces, pain-induced hypoventilation from rib fractures, etc.

Abnormal breathing pattern

Abnormal breathing patterns are commonly seen after brain injury. In particular, both hyperventilation and hypoventilation have been described. Hyperventilation is usually associated with periods of hypoventilation which can induce, together with a reduction in cough reflexes and impaired airway patency from inspissated secretions, alveolar atelectasis and consolidations [24].

Release of inflammatory mediators

Brain injury causes a marked release in the brain and in the systemic circulation of pro and con inflammatory agents which can lead to peripheral organ dysfunction, prevalently of the lung and to a moderate-severe immunodepression [25-27].

Thus, the release of these inflammatory mediators can lead to multiple organ failure where the lung parenchyma appears to be a preferential and more susceptible target. However, other possible mechanisms for brain injury-related symptoms of systemic inflammation include the high incidence of aspiration pneumonia in poor-grade patients, which can provide a nidus for systemic inflammation. Impaired pulmonary gas-exchange could further contribute to systemic inflammation, as invasive strategies of mechanical ventilation can cause volutrauma and barotrauma which in turn can trigger pulmonary cytokines release [28].

Release of catecholamines

Brain injury is followed by prolonged sympathetic hyperactivity, which may lead to hypertension and/or tachycardia. This circulatory hyperactivity induces an increase in cerebral blood volume and/or cerebral blood flow; hence, intracranial [29-31]. Moreover, the outcome after brain injury appears to be related to the intensity of the plasma catecholamines [32]. Catecholamines, and mainly norepinephrine, have been shown to produce two prevalent effects on the lung such as: 1) an increase of the alveolar capillary barrier permeability; and 2) an increase of the pulmonary lymph flow. In fact, several studies showed that increased permeability may be mediated by sympathetic activity [33, 34].

Infectious processes

Brain injured patients are characterized by an increased risk in developing ventilator associated pneumonia (VAP) [35, 36]. Its incidence is estimated in a range between 30-50% of the brain injured patients, being extremely severe in only 20-25% of the cases. Table 2 shows the independent risk factors for VAP

Table 2. The independent risk factors for ventilator associated pneumonia (VAP) in brain injured patients

Risk factors	**Risk**
Risk factors related to brain injury	
Altered conscience	6.6
Risk factors associated to the treatment of brain injury	
Aspiration	7.0
Emergency intubation	6.4
Mechanical ventilation > 3 deaths	2.3
Risk factors associated to the treatment of a general population of critically ill patients	
Reintubation	5.4
Age > 60 years	5.3
Supine position	4.8
Previous disease	3.6
Prior antibiotics	2.9

in brain injured patients. It is evident that altered conscience has been found to be an important independent risk factor for VAP in a majority of the studies which included these patients in their research. VAP can be arbitrarily divided in "early" pneumonia, if it occurs within the first 4 days after admission in ICU, and "late" pneumonia, if it occurs later than 4 days. "Early" pneumonia accounts for about 50% of the overall VAP during the intensive care unit stay [37].

Micro-organisms can be classified into potentially pathogenic micro-organisms (PPMs) and non-PPMs. PPMs are recognized by causing respiratory infections: Gram positive cocci such as *Streptococcus pneumoniae* and *Staphylococcus aureus*, Gram negative cocci such as *Moraxella catarrhalis*, and Gram negative rods such as *Haemophilus influenzae*, *Enterobacteriaceae*, *Acinetobacter* spp. and *Pseudomonas aeruginosa*. Non-PPMs are the microorganisms usually not involved in respiratory infections in the non immunodepressed host (*Streptococcus* viridans group, coagulase-negative *Staphylococci*, *Neisseria* spp., *Corynebacterium* spp., and *Candida* spp.) [38-40].

The most frequent etiologic agents of the "early" VAP include *Staphylococcus aureus* and the less frequent include *Streptococcus pneumoniae* and *Haemophilus influenzae*. On the contrary, the most frequent etiologic agents of "late" VAP were *Enterobacteriaceae*, *Acinetobacter* spp. and *Pseudomonas aeruginosa*.

Although the predominant pathogens of early onset pneumonia in patients with brain injury have been well established in several epidemiological studies, the precise relation of prior upper airway, tracheobronchial and gastric colonisation patterns with the development of pneumonia and microbial patterns has not been well investigated. In conclusion, patients with brain injury are characterized by a high incidence of VAP. Patterns of colonization and pneumonia suggest that these patients can suffer from an alteration of airway immune defence very early during their illness. The upper airways represent the most important reservoir of subsequent tracheobronchial colonization with early onset pathogens, which in turn is associated with early onset pneumonia (within 4 days). Both the upper airways and the stomach may be independent reservoirs for tracheobronchial colonization with late onset pathogens and late onset pneumonia. Preventive measures to reduce the incidence of early onset pneumonia in this population of patients may likely aim to an eradication of both upper and lower airway colonizers.

Lung morphological pattern in brain injured patients

The morphological pattern of the lung parenchyma in brain injured patients who developed respiratory insufficiency has not been fully investigated. The computed tomography (CT) has been used to better characterize the lung abnormalities of the patients with the acute respiratory distress syndrome (ARDS) [41]. Lung densities can be classified as : 1) normal lung; 2) ground-glass opacifications (i.e., mild increased attenuation with visible vessels); and 3) consolidation (i.e., markedly increased attenuation with no visible vessels). Recently, Goodman et al.[42] reported that the majority of patients with ARDS due to "direct" lung injury (i.e., pneumonia) shows areas of consolidations and areas of ground glass opacification that are presumably due to either less direct lung injury, atelectasis, or oedema from systemic effects of the lung injury. On the contrary, patients with ARDS due to "indirect" lung injury (i.e., extrapulmonary origin, because of abdominal surgical problems) are mainly characterized by multiple areas of ground-glass opacification and less consolidation areas. In other words, pneumonia is characterized by prevalent consolidation, while ARDS of extrapulmonary origin is characterized by prevalent atelectasis. We have recently investigated lung morphology of a group of patients with brain injury and severe respiratory failure (PaO_2/FiO_2 lower than 200 mmHg) due to VAP. An etiologic infectious agent was cultured by invasive techniques (bronchoalveolar lavage-BAL- or Brush) in all the patients with respiratory failure. Fig. 1 shows the representative chest X-ray and CT scan of the lung of a brain injured patient with respiratory failure. Although the gas-exchange was extremely compromised, the chest X-rays appeared relatively normal. However, the lung CT scans were characterized by important lung consolidations in the dependent regions. On the contrary, the non dependent regions appeared relatively healthy and well aerated, without any presence of ground-glass opacifica-

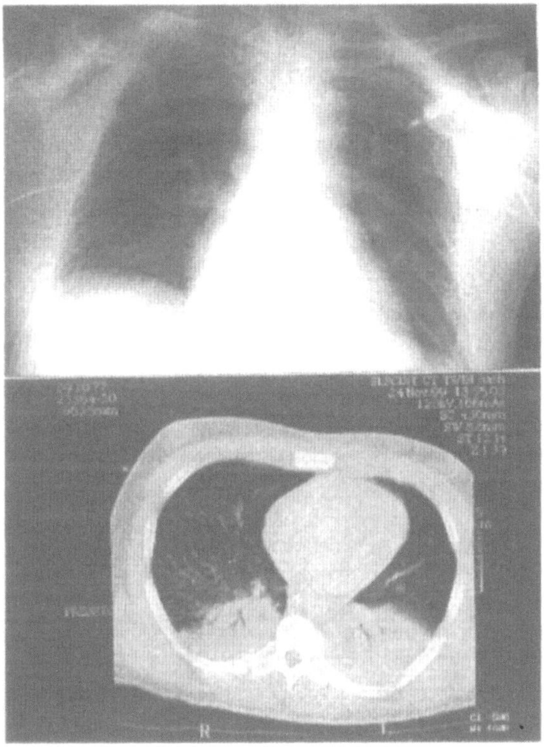

Fig. 1. Representative chest X-ray and (CT) scan image of a brain injured patient with respiratory failure. Note the absence of radiologic alterations in the chest X-ray, and the presence of the consolidations in the dependent lobes of the CT scan

tions. The presence of a normally aerated lung in the non dependent lung regions, and the posterior location of the densities can explain the imprecision of the chest X-ray to detect pulmonary alterations in these patients.

Respiratory mechanics in brain injured patients at 0 cmH_2O PEEP

Data relative to respiratory mechanics in brain injured patients are scanty [43]. We have recently investigated the modifications of respiratory mechanics in brain injured patients with and without severe respiratory failure and compared them to normal subjects under anaesthesia and paralysis [44]. We found that brain injured patients were characterized by: 1) increased intra-abdominal pressure and chest wall elastance; 2) increased airway resistance; and 3) altered pressure-volume curves of respiratory system and chest wall.

Increased intra-abdominal pressure and chest wall elastance

The intra-abdominal pressure (IAP) was increased in brain injured patients without respiratory failure compared to normal (13.1±3.2 vs. 8.5±2.8, $p<0.05$); in brain injured patients with respiratory failure IAP was further increased compared to patients without respiratory failure (16.2±3.3 vs.13.1±3.2, $p<0.05$). The IAP appeared to be correlated to the elastance of the chest wall ($r=0.69$, $p<0.001$). Similar correlation has been observed both in animal models and in normal subjects IAP was artificially altered, in obese subjects and in ARDS patients [45-48]. Moreover, increased IAP can lead to a reduction in lung volume favouring the occurrence of atelectasis, consolidation and infection. In our patients the elevated values can be explained by primary alterations of the gut physiology or oedema of the gastrointestinal tract. One of the organ systems manifesting signs of early dysfunction in isolated head injury is the gastrointestinal tract [49]. The apparent signs are gastroparesis, ileus, increased intestinal mucosal permeability and gastrointestinal bleeding associated with stress ulceration and coagulopathy [50]. There is a relationship between the severity of head injury and the incidence of gastroparesis. Although a number of factors have been postulated to contribute to the above phenomena, such as the use of opioids and sedatives, phenytoin, raised intracranial pressure, and elevated cytokines, increased sympathetic activity, the final common pathway of altered gastrointestinal function has not been well defined.

Increased airway resistance

Respiratory resistance can be partitioned into the "airway" and "viscoelastic" components.

We found that "airway" resistance was increased the in brain injured patients both with and without respiratory failure [44]. The increase in total resistance of the respiratory system (Rmax, rs) was mainly caused by an increase in total resistance of the lung (Rmax, L), while the contribution of total resistance of the chest wall (Rmax, cw) to Rmax, rs was rather small. The increase in Rmax, L was due to an increase in airway resistance in brain injured patients alone without severe respiratory failure, while the brain injured patients with airway resistance and viscoelastic resistance of the lung (DR, L) showed severe respiratory failure. It has been hypothesised that airway resistance increases after trauma and aspiration, but has never been proven [5]. Tantucci et al. [43] found an increase in airway resistance in a group of brain injured patients, but hypothesized that the increase was due to the concomitant hypocapnia.

It is well known that hypocapnia increases airway resistance in normal subjects. However, in our study, we controlled $PaCO_2$ within a physiological range, thus the increase in airway resistance was likely due to: 1) intrinsic alterations of the control of airway caliber; 2) increased thickness of the airway mucosa; and 3) reduction in lung volume.

The control of the airway caliber is regulated by the following: 1) the parasympathetic constrictor innervation of the lower airways; 2) the sympathetic innervation of the lower airways; 3) the vagal non adrenergic inhibitory system (NAIS); and 4) afferent fibers and axon reflexes [51]. It is possible that the alterations in the brain can influence the regulation of the neurologic control of the airway caliber, leading to airway constriction. On the other hand, an increase of the airway mucosa thickness is possible due to mucosal oedema caused by the systemic release of inflammatory agents. To explain the increase in airway resistance the reduction of lung volume alone is unlikely because we found an increase in airway resistance in brain injured patients without respiratory failure having a lung volume comparable to normal subjects. We believe that the altered control of the airway caliber is the most likely explanation, since a reduction in airway resistance after inhalation of an anticholinergic bronchodilator (e.g., ossitropium bromide) (Pelosi P., unpublished observation) was also observed. The role of other bronchodilators (β_2 agonists) and their optimal route of administration remains to be defined.

In conclusion, total lung and airway resistance are increased in brain injured patients with and without severe respiratory failure.

Pressure-volume curve of the total respiratory system, lung and chest wall

At positive end-expiratory pressure (PEEP) 0 cmH_2O the pressure-volume curve (P-V curve) of the respiratory system and of the chest wall were more curvilinear in brain injured patients with and without respiratory failure when compared to normal patients. The inflection point of the P-V curve of the respiratory system was mainly due to the chest wall component, being the P-V-curve of the lung substantially linear. This observation reinforces the hypothesis that alterations of the chest wall mechanics play a relevant role in the mechanical properties of the respiratory system in patients with brain injury.

Positive end-expiratory pressure in brain injured patients

PEEP is commonly used in patients with respiratory failure to improve oxygenation and respiratory mechanics [52]. However, the application of PEEP in brain injured patients is much more controversial.

PEEP can improve gas-exchange and respiratory mechanics when prevalent atelectasis is present [41]. More recently, relatively high levels of PEEP have been suggested not only to improve respiratory function but also to prevent or reduce ventilator associated lung injury in severely hypoxiemic patients [53, 54]. On the other hand, PEEP can increase the intracranial pressure by several mechanisms such as: 1) increased intrathoracic pressure which impairs venous return from the brain; and 2) the engorgement of epidural veins, resulting from transmitted positive intrathoracic pressure, which can compress the subarachnoid space and translocate cerebrospinal fluid to the intracranial vault. However, although the application of PEEP warrants caution for the above mentioned reasons, it has been suggested that moderate degrees of PEEP (lower or equal to 15 cmH_2O) [55] or very high levels of PEEP [56] can be safely used in the management of brain injured patients, particularly when pulmonary compliance is poor.

Elastance of the total respiratory system, lung and chest wall

We found that in brain injured patients with severe respiratory failure, PEEP markedly increased the elastance of the total respiratory system (Est, rs) and of the lung (Est, L), while decreased the elastance of the chest wall (Est, cw). The increase in Est, rs and Est, L suggests the prevalence of a stretching phenomena, while the decrease in Est, cw is likely due to the overall increase in lung volume with PEEP, which may place the thoracic cage in a more favourable part on the pressure-volume curve.

Resistance of the total respiratory system, lung and chest wall

PEEP significantly reduced airway resistance while markedly increasing DR, L (with no relevant influence on Rmax, cw) in both brain injured patients with and without severe respiratory failure. Thus, the resulting effect was a reduction in Rmax,rs and Rmax,L with PEEP. The results of the present study suggest that the decrease of Rmax, rs and the increase in DR, rs with PEEP can be ascribed mainly to the lung rather than to the chest wall. A reduction in airway resistance with PEEP has been previously reported in patients with respiratory failure and attributed to the increase in lung volume. However, DR, L markedly increased with PEEP, these data are in line with previous findings in pulmonary acute respiratory failure, indicating that stretching phenomena were prevalent. Although the physiologic meaning of DR,L is still unclear, these data suggest that stretching may affect the viscoelastic resistance of the lung tissue.

Gas-exchange and recruitment

PEEP can improve gas-exchange and respiratory mechanics when atelectasis is present. Raising the PEEP up to 15 cmH_2O did not significantly affect oxygenation in brain injured patients with VAP and severe respiratory failure; however, increased $PaCO_2$ in patients with brain injury and severe respiratory failure. The lack of response in oxygenation was paralleled by small alveolar recruitment induced by PEEP. Fig. 2 shows a representative CT scan of the lung at 0 and at 15 cmH_2O PEEP of a brain injured patient with severe respiratory failure. It is evident that PEEP only increased air bronchograms and did not modify alveolar consolidations. This finding is in line with recent observations that show prevalent consolidations and less recruitment with PEEP in patients

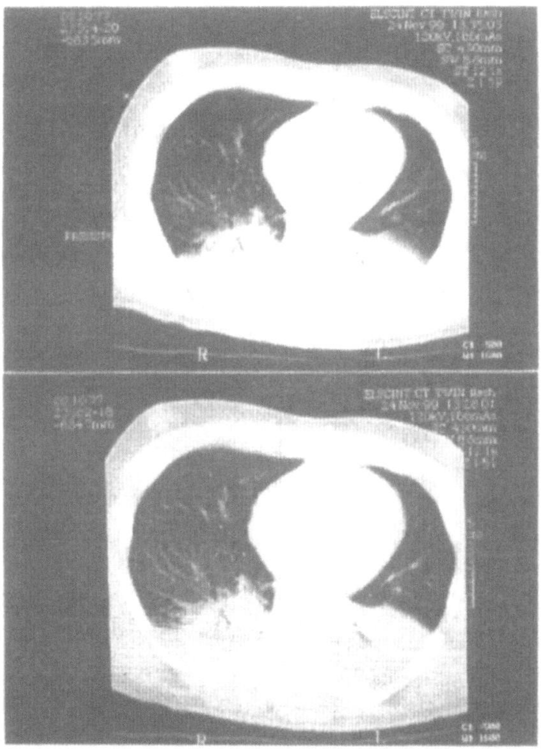

Fig. 2. Representative CT scan images of the lung at 0 and at 15 cmH_2O PEEP of a brain injured patient with severe respiratory failure. Note that PEEP does not modify alveolar consolidations, and only increases the air bronchograms.

with respiratory insufficiency due to pulmonary disease compared with those with respiratory failure due to extrapulmonary disease. The confirmation of poor lung recruitment by PEEP application in patients with VAP was obtained through an analysis of the changes of the P-V curves.

In normal subjects and in brain injured patients without respiratory failure the P-V curves of the total respiratory system and the lung thoroughly follow the same pattern, at different PEEP levels. On the contrary, in brain injured patients with respiratory failure, the P-V curves of the total respiratory system and the lung show a concavity towards the pressure axis, without any shift on the left, indicating alveolar stretching and poor alveolar recruitment.

Prevention of respiratory function abnormalities in brain injured patients

Since respiratory dysfunction plays a relevant role in the outcome of brain injured patients, it is extremely important to prevent it. Unfortunately, very few studies have investigated the efficacy of specific protocols to prevent respiratory dysfunction in these patients.

We believe that the main goals should be: 1) to prevent lung collapse and/or consolidation; 2) to prevent lung infections; and 3) to accelerate weaning from mechanical ventilation.

Prevention of lung collapse and/or consolidation

1) Mechanical ventilation could be useful in avoiding progressive collapsing and consolidation of the lung. However, many aspects in the ventilatory management are not clear:

- the superiority of controlled or assisted ventilation;
- the use of preventive recruitment manoeuvres and PEEP (applied before lobar consolidation occurrence);
- the routine use of prone position or kinetic therapy.

2) The use of fibroscopy to clear secretions could be used advantageously to reduce the formation of micro-macro atelectasis, consolidations and lobar infections. However, the excessive use of this technique can have negative effects on cerebral homeostasis [57].

3) Fluid balance: it is not clear if brain injured patients should be maintained more hypervolemic or hypovolemic. It is possible that excessive overfluid treatment can increase interstitial lung oedema and favour lung collapse. On the other hand, hypervolemia has been advocated for the treatment of these patients [58, 59].

4) Specific drugs

- low dose of corticosteroids could be useful to reduce the local and systemic inflammatory response. Up to now the routine use of corticosteroids is discouraged in brain injured patients [60]. However, all these studies were performed using high doses of corticosteroids. Recently, it has been shown that low dose corticosteroids can be useful in the treatment of ARDS and sepsis [61]. Thus the role of corticosteroids should be re-evaluated in the future studies.
- anti-sympathetic drugs (clonidine) and selective β_1 antagonist could be useful to reduce the negative systemic effects of the sympathetic storm [62, 63].
- bronchodilators (anticholinergic bronchodilators) could be useful to reduce airway resistance; thus, reducing the risk of micro-macro atelectasis and alterations in the ventilation perfusion mismatch (Pelosi P., unpublished observations).

Prevention of lung infection

1) Antibiotic prophylaxis with a cephalosporin of the second generation (cefuroxime or cefoxitin) can be useful to prevent "early" pneumonia. However, some studies reported an increased rate in "late" pneumonia if antibiotic prophylaxis is used for more than 24 hours [64].
2) Selective digestive decontamination (SDD) has been proposed to reduce the microbiological load in the oropharynx and in the stomach. Recently, a large metaanalysis, reported that SDD can be effective to reduce ICU stay and mortality when associated with i.v. prophylaxis [65].
3) Upright position: A recent randomized trial showed that upright position can be useful to reduce the VAP and the ICU stay in a general population of critically ill patients [66].
4) Continuous oropharyngeal aspiration has been found to reduce the oropharyngeal contamination and the occurrence of VAP [67].
5) Correct use of antiacid drugs: the routine use of antiacid drugs seems to be reasonable, because brain injured patients have an increased risk for gastric haemorrhage [68]. Recent randomized trials suggest that the use of H_2 antagonist reduce the incidence of clinically important gastric bleeding, with no increase in VAP [69].
6) Specific drugs

- Several drugs can reduce gut motility and favour uncoordinated peristalsis such as opioids [70], propofol [71] and low dose dopamine. The use of these drugs should be carefully monitored and limited in relation to the clinical situation.

- Prokinetic drugs, such as metoclopramide, cisapride [72] and erythromycin [73] could be useful to improve gut motility, likely reducing the unfavourable effects of IAP on the respiratory system [74] and the microbiological gastric colonization.

7) Nutrition is important for brain injured patients, but the respective role of enteral and parenteral nutrition is not clear [75, 76].

8) Personnel hygiene: protocols to regulate hygiene of the physicians and nurses are warranted. In particular, a careful handwashing policy seems to reduce the incidence of infections and improve the patients outcome [77].

9) ICU and hospital antibiotic policy: protocols to regulate the ICU and hospital antibiotics policy are warranted to reduce the risk of developing resistant micro-organisms and reduce costs [78].

Accelerate weaning from the ICU

1) Early tracheostomy: in brain injured patients, the technique and the optimal time for the procedure has not been yet defined. However, with the development of percutaneous techniques, the manoeuvre appears to be easier, safer and is associated with less complications. Tracheostomy appears to: 1) be better tolerated by the patients; 2) allow a better cleaning of the oropharynx; 3) reduce the incidence of sinusitis; 4) reduce anatomical alterations of the vocal cordae; 5) reduce the work of breathing. Thus, we believe that early tracheostomy may play a relevant role in the weaning and better clinical management of these patients [79].

2) Weaning trials (but not in head injured patients)

Two large randomized trials were performed in critically ill patients to investigate the optimal weaning procedure. T-tube tests and pressure supports were found equally effective in weaning the patients [80, 81]. However, in both studies brain injured patients were excluded. Thus, future trials are warranted when defining protocol weaning procedures in brain injured patients.

Conclusion

In conclusion, brain injured patients are at an increased risk for extracerebral organ dysfunctions, and in particular ventilator associated pneumonia. The occurrence of ventilator associated pneumonia increases the ICU and hospital stay, costs and the risk of death. The respiratory dysfunction is characterized by moderate to severe hypoxemia mainly caused by the presence of consolidation of the lower lobes. The chest X-ray may be misleading in interpreting lung morphology in these patients, thus a CT scan should be considered when the nature of hypoxemia is not completely understood. Respiratory mechanics are deeply affected by an increased intra-abdominal pressure, chest wall elastance and airway resistance. PEEP does not seem to be effective in improving respiratory function when VAP is the main cause of respiratory failure. Finally, strategies aimed to reduce the incidence of respiratory dysfunction and ventilator associated pneumonia have to be early applied after admission in the ICU. Further studies are warranted to better elucidate the pathophysiology and clinical management of respiratory dysfunction in brain injured patients.

Acknowledgements

We are particularly indebted to the medical and nursing staff of the Intensive Care Unit (Servizio Anestesia e Rianimazione B) of the Ospedale di Circolo-Varese, for their precious contribution and effort.

References

1. Kassell NF, Torner JC, Haley EC et al (1990) The international cooperative study on the timing of aneurysm surgery. Part 1: overall management results. J Neurosurg 73: 18-36
2. Kassell NF, Torner JC, Jane JA et al (1990) The international cooperative study on the timing of aneurysm surgery. Part 2: Surgical results. J Neurosurg 73: 37-47
3. Solenski N, Haley C, Kassell NF et al (1995) Medical complications of aneurysmal subarachnoid hemorrhage: a report of the multicenter, cooperative aneurysm study. Crit Care Med 23: 1007-1017
4. Clifton GC, Miller ER, Choi SC et al (2000) Lack of effect of induction of hypothermia after acute brain injury. NEJM 344: 556-563
5. Demling R, Riessen R (1990) Pulmonary dysfunction after cerebral injury. Crit Care Med 18: 768-774
6. Acheson RM (1964) The epidemiology of stroke. Lancet 1: 494-495
7. Cruz J, Minoja G, Mattioli C et al (1998) Severe acute brain trauma. In: Cruz J (ed) Neurologic and Neurosurgical Emergencies. WB Saunders Company, Philadelphia, pp 405-436
8. Knaus WA, Draper EA, Wagner DP et al (1985) Prognosis in acute organ-system failure. Ann Surg 202: 685-693
9. Le Roux PD, Elliott JP, Downey L et al (1996) Improved outcome after rupture of anterior circulation aneurysms: a retrospective 10-year review of 224 good grade patients. J Neurosurg 85: 39-49
10. Hernesniemi J, Vapalathi M, Niskanen M et al (1993) One-year outcome in early aneurysm surgery: a 14 year experience. Acta Neurochirurgica 122: 1-10
11. Gruber A, Reinprecht A, Illievich UM et al (1999) Extracerebral organ dysfunction and neurologic outcome after aneurysmal subarachnoid hemorrhage. Crit Care Med 27: 505-514
12. Simmons RL, Martin AM, Heisterkamp CA et al (1969) Respiratory insufficiency in combat casualties. Pulmonary edema following head injury. Ann Surgery 170: 39-44
13. Katsurada K, Yamada R, Sugimoto T (1973) Respiratory insufficiency in patients with severe head injury. Surgery 73: 191-199

14. Schumaker P, Rhodes G, Newell J et al (1979) Ventilation perfusion imbalance after head injury. Am Rev Respir Dis 119: 33-43
15. Beckman D, Bean J, Baslock P (1974) Neurogenic influence on pulmonary complications. J Trauma; 14: 111-115
16. Hoff JT, Nishimura M, Garcia-Uria J et al (1981) Experimental neurogenic pulmonary edema. Part 1: the role of systemic hypertension. J Neurosurg 54: 627-631
17. Garcia-Uria J, Hoff JT, Miranda S et al (1981) Experimental neurogenic pulmonary edema. Part 2: the role of cardiopulmonary pressure change. J Neurosurg 54: 632-636
18. Downing SE, Lee JC (1980) Nervous control of the pulmonary circulation. Annu Rev Physiol 42: 199-210
19. Fishman AP (1980) Vasomotor regulation of the pulmonary circulation Annu Rev Physiol 42: 211-220
20. Epstain F, Cooper K, Ward J (1988) Profound pulmonary shunting without edema following stereotaxic biopsy of hypothalamic germinoma. J Neurosurg 68: 303-307
21. Kaufman H, Moake J, Olson J et al (1980)Delayed and recurrent hematomas related to disseminated intravascular clotting and fibrinolysis in head injury. Neurosurgery 7: 445- 449
22. Hirashima Y, Nakamura S, Endo S et al (1997) Elevation of platelet activating factor, inflammatory cytokines, and coagulation factors in the internal jugular vein of patients with subarachnoid hemorrhage. Neurochem Res 10: 1249-1255
23. Forrest JB (1972) The effect of hyperventilation on pulmonary surface activity. Brit J Anaesth 44: 313-319
24. North J, Jennett S (1974) Abnormal breathing patterns associated with acute brain damage. Arch Neurol 31: 338-344
25. Nieto-Sampedro M, Berman MA (1987) Interleukin-1 like activity in rat brain: sources, targets, and effect of injury. J Neuro Res 17: 214-219
26. Holmin S, Schalling M, Hojeberg B et al (1997) Delayed cytokines expression in rat brain following experimental contusion. J Neurosurg 86: 493-504
27. Mathiesen T, Anderson B, Loftenius A et al (1993) Increased interleukin-6 levels in cerebrospinal fluid following subarachnoid hemorrhage. J Neurosurg 78: 562-567
28. Tremblay L, Valenza F, Ribeiro SP et al (1997) Injurious ventilatory strategies increase cytokines and c-FOS mRNA expression in an isolated rat lung model. J Clin Invest 99: 944-952
29. Rosner MJ, Nesome HH, Becker DP et al (1984) Mechanical brain injury: the sympathoadrenal response. J Neurosurg 61: 76-86
30. Neil-Dwyer G, Cruickshank JM, Doshi R (1990) The stress response in subarachnoid hemorrhage and head injury. Acta Neurochirurgica Supplementum 47(Suppl): 102-110
31. Dilraj A, Botha JH, Rambiritch V (1992) Levels of catecholamines in plasma and cerebrospinal fluid in aneurysmal subarachnoid hemorrhage. Neurosurgery 31: 42-51
32. Woolf PD, Hamill RW, Lee LA et al (1987) The predictive value of catecholamines in assessing outcome in traumatic brain injury. J Neurosurg 66: 875-882
33. Hurley JV (1978) Current views on the mechanisms of pulmonary edema. J Pathol 125: 59-80
34. Moss G, Staunton C, Stein A (1973) The centrineurogenic etiology of the acute respiratory distress syndrome. Am J Surg 126: 37-41
35. Langer M, Cigada M, Mandelli M et al (1987) Early onset pneumonia: a multicenter study in intensive care units. Intensive Care Med 13:342-346
36. Hsieh AH, Bishop MJ, Kubilis PS et al (1992) Pneumonia following closed head injury. Am Rev Respir Dis 146: 290-294
37. Langer M, Mosconi P, Cigada M et al (1989) Long-term respiratory support and risk of pneumonia in critically ill patients. Am Rev Respir Dis 140: 302-305
38. Torres A, Aznar R, Gatell JM et al (1990) Incidence, risk, and prognosis factors of nosocomial pneumonia in mechanically ventilated patients. Am Rev Respir Dis 142: 523-528
39. Kollef MH (1993) Ventilator-associated pneumonia. A multivariate analysis. JAMA 270: 1965-1970

40. Akca O, Koltka K, Uzel S et al (2000) Risk factors for early onset, ventilator associated pneumonia in critical care patients: selected multiresistant versus non resistant bacteria. Anesthesiology 93: 638-645
41. Gattinoni L, Pesenti A, Bombino M et al (1988) Relationship between lung computed tomographic density, gas exchange, and PEEP in acute respiratory failure. Anesthesiology 69:824-832
42. Goodman LR, Fumagalli R, Tagliabue P et al (1999) Adult respiratory distress syndrome due to pulmonary and extrapulmonary causes: CT, clinical and functional correlations. Radiology 213: 545-552
43. Tantucci C, Corbeil C, Chasse M et al (1993) Resistance in mechanically ventilated patients with severe neurological injury. J Crit Care 8: 133-139
44. Pelosi P, Colombo G, Gamberoni C et al (2000) Effects of positive end-expiratory pressure on respiratory function in head injured patients. Intensive Care Med 26: A450
45. Motoh T, Wayne J, Lamm WJE et al (1992) Volume infusion produces abdominal distension, lung compression and chest wall stiffening in pigs. J Appl Physiol 72: 575-582
46. Pelosi P, Foti G, Cereda M et al (1996) Effects of carbon dioxide insufflation for laparoscopic cholecystectomy on the respiratory system. Anesthesia 51: 744-749
47. Pelosi P, Ravagnan I, Giurati G et al (1999) Positive end-expiratory pressure improves respiratory function in obese but not in normal subjects during anesthesia and paralysis. Anesthesiology 91:1221-1231
48. Gattinoni L, Pelosi P, Suter PM et al (1998) Acute respiratory distress syndrome caused by pulmonary and extrapulmonary disease: different syndromes? Am J Respir Crit Care Med 158: 3-11
49. Power I, Easton JC, Todd JG et al (1988) Gastric emptying after head injury. Anesthesia 44: 563-566
50. McArthur CJ, Gin T, McLaren IM et al (1995) Gastric emptying following brain injury: effects of choice of sedation and intracranial pressure. Intensive Care Med 21: 573-576
51. Widdicombe J (1985) Control of airway caliber. Am Rev Respir Dis 131: S33-S35
52. Suter PM, Fairley HB, Isenberg MD (1975) Optimum end-expiratory airway pressure in patients with acute pulmonary failure. NEJM 292:284-289
53. Amato MB, Barbas CS, Medeiros DM et al (1998) Effects of a protective-ventilation strategy on mortality in the acute respiratory distress syndrome. NEJM 338:347-354
54. Ranieri VM, Suter PM, Tortorella C et al (1999) Effect of mechanical ventilation on inflammatory mediators in patients with acute respiratory distress syndrome: a randomized controlled trial. JAMA 282:54-61
55. Cooper KR, Boswell PA, Choi SC (1985) Safe use of PEEP in patients with severe head injury. J Neurosurg 63: 552-555
56. Miller RS, Nelson LD, Di Russo SM et al (1992) High level positive end-expiratory pressure management in trauma-associated Adult Respiratory Distress Syndrome. J Trauma 33: 284-290
57. Froman C (1988) Alterations of respiratory function in patients with severe head injuries. Brit J Anaesth 40:354-360
58. Ramming S, Shackford SR, Zhuang J et al (1994) The relationship of fluid balance and sodium administration to cerebral edema formation and intracranial pressure in a porcine model of brain injury. J Trauma 37: 705-713
59. York J, Arrillaga A, Graham R et al (2000) Fluid resuscitation of patients with multiple injuries and severe closed head injury: experience with an aggressive fluid resuscitation strategy. J Trauma 48: 376-380
60. Anderson P, Roberts I (1997) Corticosteroids in acute traumatic brain injury: systematic review if randomized controlled trials. BMJ 314: 1855-1862
61. Meduri GU, Headley AS, Golden E et al (1998) Effects of prolonged methylprednisolone therapy in unresolving acute respiratory distress syndrome: a randomized controlled trial. JAMA 280:159-165
62. Kariya N, Shindoh M, Nishi S et al (1999) Oral clonidine to control hypertension after head injury. Eur J Emerg Med 6: 77-79

63. Asgeirsson B, Grande PO, Nordstrom CH et al (1995) Effects of hypotensive treatment with α_2 agonist and β_1 antagonist on cerebral hemodynamic in severely injured patients. Acta Anaesthesiol Scand 39: 347-351
64. Sirvent JM, Torres A, El-Ebiabry M et al (1997) Protective effect of intravenously administered cefuroxime again nosocomial pneumonia in patients with structural coma. Am J Respir Crit Care Med 155:1729-1734
65. D'Amico R, Pifferi S, Leonetti C et al (1998) Effectiveness of antibiotic prophylaxis in critically ill adult patients: systematic review of randomized controlled trials. BMJ 316: 1275-1285
66. Drakulovic MB, Torres A, Bauer TT et al (1999) Supine body position as a risk factor for nosocomial pneumonia in mechanically ventilated patients: a randomized trial. Lancet 354: 1851-1858
67. Shorr AF, O'Malley PG (2001) Continuous subglottic suctioning for the prevention of ventilator associated pneumonia: potential economic implications. Chest 119: 228-235
68. Kamada T, Fusamoto H, Kawano S et al (1977) Gastrointestinal bleeding following head injury: a clinical study of 433 cases. J Trauma 17: 44-47
69. Marlowicz P, Wolff M, Djedaini K et al (2000) Multicenter prospective study of ventilator associated pneumonia during acute respiratory distress syndrome. Incidence, prognosis, and risk factors. Am J Respir Crit Care Med 161: 1942-1948
70. Wilder-Smith CH, Hill L, Wilkins J et al (1999) Effects of morphine and tramadol on somatic and visceral sensory function and gastrointestinal motility after abdominal surgery. Anesthesiology: 639-637
71. Freye E, Sundermann S, Wilder-Smith OHG (1998) No inhibition of gastrointestinal propulsion after propofol or propofol/ketamine-N_2O_2/O_2 anesthesia. Acta Anaesthesiol Scand 42: 664-669
72. McLaren R, Kuhl DA, Gervasio JM et al (2000) Sequential single doses of cisapride, erythromycin, and metoclopramide in critically ill patients intolerant to enteral nutrition: a randomized, placebo controlled, cross over study. Crit Care Med 28:438-444
73. Dive A, Miesse C, Galanti L et al (1995) Effect of erythromycin on gastric motility in mechanically ventilated critically ill patients: a double blind, randomized, placebo controlled study. Crit Care Med 23: 1356-1362
74. Wang XD, Soltesz V, Andersson R (1996) Cisapride prevents enteric bacterial overgrowth and translocation by improvements of intestinal motility in rats with acute liver failure. Eur Surg Res 28: 402-412
75. Taylor SJ, Fettes SB, Jewkes C et al (1999) Prospective, randomized, controlled trial to determine the effect of early enhanced enteral nutrition clinical outcome in mechanically ventilated patients suffering head injury. Crit Care Med 27: 2525-2531
76. Rapp RP, Young B, Twyman D et al (1983) The favourable effect of early parenteral feeding on survival in head injured patients. J Neurosurg 58: 906-912
77. Bischoff WE, Reynolds TM, Sessler CN, et al (2000) Handwashing compliance by health care workers: the impact of introducing an accessible, alcohol-based hand antiseptic. Arch Intern Med 160: 1017-1021
78. Scott G (2000) Prevention and control of infections in intensive care. Intens Care Med 26: 522-525
79. Diehl JL, El Atrous S, Touchard D et al (1999) Changes in the work of breathing induced by tracheotomy in ventilator-dependent patients. AJRCCM 159:383-388
80. Brochard L, Rauss A, Benito S et al (1994) Comparison of three methods of gradual withdrawal from ventilatory support during mechanical ventilation. Am J Resp Crit Care Med 150(4): 896-903
81. Esteban A, Frutos F, Tobin MJ et al (1995) A comparison of four methods of weaning patients from mechanical ventilation. Spanish Failure Collaborative Group. NEJM 332(6): 345-350

Blunt Chest Trauma

M. MUGGIA-SULLAM

Blunt chest injury is among the most-common types of injuries seen in modern civilization - most are caused by traffic crashes. They account for a large number of fatalities; many of them could be prevented by proper treatment. It is not the scope of this review to discuss in detail all the aspects of blunt chest trauma, but rather to concentrate on some topics. Some of them are common problems with simple solutions, others are more complex and controversial. Most of this review is based on excellent modern textbooks and on published guidelines. A short manual on management of trauma is the *ABC of Trauma* which is easily available [1]. Interested readers are referred to the outstanding book of Besson and Saegesser, which may be a bit outdated but is comprehensive and represents the personal experience of the authors [2].

Initial resuscitation

During the initial phase of resuscitation, respiratory distress should be detected and treated as soon as possible, as it carries a high mortality rate. Early endotracheal intubation is mandatory in any severely injured patient with any airway or ventilatory problem. However cardiac arrests in the emergency department (ED) frequently occur during or immediately following endotracheal intubation. There are several possible causes for cardiac arrest at that time. The most-common ones are failure to pre-oxygenate, esophageal intubation, intubation of the right main bronchus, and tension pneumothorax. Although tension pneumothorax may be rapidly lethal - one should check the proper position of the endotracheal tube before treating a presumptive tension pneumothorax. However, the diagnosis of a tension pneumothorax must be a clinical one, and waiting for a chest radiograph to confirm this diagnosis is a severe and often deadly pitfall. The next step, of paramount importance, is diagnosing and treating shock. Failure to correct hypotension greatly increases mortality rate. This is despite recent studies that indicated a possible benefit in penetrating trauma in maintaining a relatively low blood pressure until the time of surgical intervention. A massive hemothorax can interfere with ventilation and venous return; therefore it should be rapidly evacuated. However a massive hemothorax or a continuous massive bleeding is an indication for en emergency thoracotomy. Failure to recognize this condition may precipitate the patient's condition into irreversible shock, disseminated intravascular coagulation, and death [3-5].

ED thoracotomy

ED thoracotomy has gained popularity following several reports on its success in saving patients who would have otherwise died. But it should be remembered that most of these successful resuscitations followed penetrating injuries. The highest success rates have been reported for stab wounds to the chest. On the other hand success rates are extremely low, or almost non-existent, for blunt injuries. Therefore this procedure should be kept only for selected patients with blunt chest trauma. It is critical to distinguish between "no vital signs" and "no signs of life". The patient with "no vital signs" may be still alive, but has no measurable signs, like blood pressure or pulse, but demonstrates pupillary reactivity or respiratory effort. The patient with "no signs of life" has no vital signs, no movement or reflexes, no pupil reactivity, no corneal reflexes, no respiratory efforts, and no heart sounds or cardiac electrical activity. Patient outcome is dismal if an ED thoracotomy is done either in patients with blunt trauma or in patients arriving with no signs of life. ED thoracotomy permits the salvage of 30-57% of adult patients presenting with signs of life following an isolated cardiac injury and 13% without signs of life. In contrast, only 1-2% of patients with blunt trauma who require ED thotacotomy are salvaged, regardless of their physiological status at presentation. Similar results were obtained in children; when the cause of injury was blunt trauma, no child survived ED thoracotomy when vital signs were absent. Currently, patients arriving in extremis following blunt injury should undergo ED thoracotomy only if they show electrical cardiac activity. Most likely, no blunt trauma patient in arrest should undergo ED thoracotomy if vital signs are absent in the field or if there is evidence of an obvious head injury [3, 5, 6].

Injury to the chest wall

The commonest injury to the chest is a simple bruise followed by fracture to a single rib or several ribs. Often these injuries are missed, the patient discharged from the ED, only to be readmitted a couple of days later suffering from pneumonia secondary to atelectasis due to self-splinting of the chest-wall due to severe pain. Frequently the diagnosis can be made on clinical grounds or at least it should be suspected in any patient with local tenderness over the ribcage. The simplest cure is adequate treatment with painkillers. Some patients may require local infiltration with a local anesthetic; it should be remembered that several intercostal nerves must be blocked. An alternative method, for more--serious injuries is epidural analgesia, or epipleural analgesia. This will not only decrease pain and prevent the development of pneumonia, but may prevent deterioration of pulmonary failure, and may obviate the need for ventilatory support [5, 7].

Any massive hemo-pneumothorax must be properly drained. Up to 85% of chest injuries that need an intervention can be managed with a closed tube thoracostomy. Any physician treating wounded patients should be familiar with recommended techniques. The safest would be the open one, in order to prevent iatrogenic injuries. Often the chest drain is not placed correctly, either it is not inserted into the pleural space or it causes additional injury by penetrating the lung or going through the diaphragm into the spleen or liver. It has been suggested that laparoscopic trocars may be helpful in preventing these complications; but they have not met with widespread enthusiasm [5, 8, 9].

Antibiotics and chest tubes

A major morbidity associated with tube thoracostomy is development of empyema. The role of prophylactic antibiotics following the insertion of tube thoracostomy is controversial. It should decrease the incidence of this complication and it may reduce secondary pneumonia. Multiple factors contribute to the development of post-traumatic empyema that complicate the issue of proper recommendations. Among them are the circumstances of injury, associated injuries, and location and time of tube insertion, the technique used, and the expertise of the treating person. There is only level 3 recommendation for the use of prophylactic antibiotics, meaning that this recommendation is supported by available data but adequate scientific evidence is lacking. The current recommendation is to use a first-generation cephalosporin as prophylactic antibiotics and it should be used for no longer than 24 h. The available data suggest a reduction in the incidence of pneumonia, but not empyema, in patients with isolated chest trauma who need a chest tube [10].

Blunt cardiac injury

Much confusion exists about the true incidence of blunt cardiac injury (BCI), standard diagnostic modalities, and the appropriate monitoring and treatment that should be employed. The diagnosis of BCI depends directly on the aggressiveness of the treating physicians in seeking this diagnosis. No single test or combination of tests has proven consistently reliable in diagnosing BCI. This diagnosis should be suspected in any patient with an appropriate mechanism of injury [11-13]. At present the EAST recommendations are as follows [12].

Level I

An admission electrocardiogram (ECG) should be performed on all patients in whom there is suspected BCI.

Level II

1. If the admission ECG is abnormal (arrhythmia, unexplained ST changes, ischemia, heart block), the patient should be admitted for continuous ECG monitoring for 24 to 48 h. Conversely, if the admission ECG is normal, the risk of having a BCI that requires treatment is insignificant, and the pursuit of diagnosis should be terminated.
2. If the patient is hemodynamically unstable, an imaging study (echocardiogram) should be obtained. If an optimal transthoracic echocardiogram cannot be performed, then the patient should have a transesophageal echocardiogram (TEE).
3. Nuclear medicine studies add little when compared with echocardiography and, thus, are not useful if an echocardiogram has been performed.

Level III

1. Elderly patients with known cardiac disease, unstable patients, and those with an abnormal admission ECG can be safely operated on provided they are appropriately monitored. Consideration should be given to placement of a pulmonary artery catheter in such cases.
2. The presence of a sternal fracture does not predict the presence of BCI and, thus, does not necessarily indicate that monitoring should be performed.
3. Neither creatinine phosphokinase with isoenzyme analysis nor measurement of circulating cardiac troponin T are useful in predicting which patients have or will have complications related to BCI.

Most, if not all, of these recommendations may be applied at any ED treating trauma patients. Probably only patients who need further evaluation by means that are not available, such as TEE, should be transferred to another facility.

Blunt aortic trauma

Blunt injury to the thoracic aorta contributes to a large proportion of immediate deaths at the scene of car crashes. Other causes of this type of injury are collisions with pedestrians, falls from height, and crushing injuries. Debate exists about the best diagnostic modalities and the preferred operative procedure. Complicating issues are the facts that most of these patients suffer from additional injuries, some of them may be life threatening; in addition most diagnostic procedures are available only at larger and modern trauma centers. Only a few centers have the capability to repair a ruptured aorta and have enough experience to complete this procedure successfully [14-16]. According to the new EAST guidelines, currently there are no level I recommendations to support a standard of care [15].

Blunt aortic injury (BAI) should be suspected in any injured patient with a deceleration or acceleration mechanism. The most-common signs, but unusual, may be pseudocoarctation and intrascapular murmur. Absence of these signs does not rule out BAI. The first screening diagnostic tool may be the chest X–ray; but it should be remembered that a normal X-ray does not rule out severe trauma. The most-important chest X-ray findings include a widened mediastinum, obscured aortic knob, deviation of the left mainstem bronchus or nasogasrtic tube, and opacification of the aorto-pulmonary window, widened paratracheal and paraspinpous stripes, and apical capping. Contrary to previous thoughts, there is no correlation with hemo-pneumothorax or fractures of the thoracic skeleton.

Any patient with suspicion of BAI should undergo further evaluation. Aortic angiography remains the "gold standard" diagnostic modality; all other tests are compared with it. It is highly accurate with only a small percentage of false-positive findings due to anatomical abnormalities. Computed tomography of the chest (CTC) seems to be a rapid, readily available, and accurate diagnostic screening tool. The problem is that most authors recommend its use as a screening tool only to proceed to angiography in any patient with suspicious findings on CTC. The newer-generation helical or spiral CTC are much faster, more sensitive and probably have 100% negative predictive value. Once again, not every hospital has a modern CT, and its interpretation depends on available experts.

An additional diagnostic tool is TEE, which has gained popularity over the last few years. This too relies on specific training, and even in some large centers, TEE is not available on a 24 h basis. Its advantage is that it may be performed in the operating room during another procedure and it may detect and help in following small intimal tears. One of its disadvantages is that it does not visualize the ascending aorta and may miss injuries to the major aortic branches.

Most authors agree that prompt surgical repair gives the best chance to these patients, although delayed repairs have been described with success. This may represent natural selection, as the ones who were transferred to other centers and undergo surgery later may have lesser injuries. In some patients additional injuries or comorbid conditions may dictate medical therapy and delay in the surgical procedure until these problems are controlled. If surgery is delayed, blood pressure should be controlled by medical means. The most-devastating complications following surgery are paraplegia and renal failure that result from distal ischemia. Most likely some sort of distal perfusion is recommended, although highly experienced surgeons may prefer the clamp and sew technique. Recent developments have been reported with the use of endoluminal aortic stenting. This may prove in the future to be the best treatment for these patients.

In conclusion, every patient with suspected BAI should be screened. Probably this is best performed in a well-equipped center, saving precious time and possibly lives. To summarize, BCI is one the most-common types of injury. Most of these injuries may be easily diagnosed and treated following relatively simple procedures. More complicated injuries, especially BAI, should be diagnosed and treated in specialized centers. Future developments will probably find less- -invasive diagnostic and treatment modalities.

References

1. Driscoll P, Skinner D, Earlam R (eds) (2000) ABC of major trauma. BMJ Books, London
2. Besson A, Saegesser F (1989) A colour atlas of chest trauma and associated injuries. Wolfe Medical Publications, London
3. O'Neil BJ, Wilson RF (1996) Cardiopulmonary resuscitaion after trauma. In: Wilson RF, Walt AJ (eds) Management of trauma: pitfalls and practice. Williams and Wilkins, Baltimore, pp 28-50
4. Wall Jr MJ, Storey JH, Mattox KL (2000) Indications for thoracotomy. In Mattox KL, Feliciano DV, Moore EE (eds) Trauma. McGraw-Hill, New York, pp 473-482
5. Wilson RF, Steiger Z (1996) Thoracic trauma: chest wall and lung. In: Wilson RF, Walt AJ (eds) Management of Trauma: pitfalls and practice. William and Wilkins, Baltimore, pp 315-342
6. Biffl WL, Moore EE, Harken AH (2000) Emergency department thoracotomy. In: Mattox KL, Feliciano DV, Moore EE (eds) Trauma. McGraw-Hill, New York, pp 245-259
7. Cogbill TH, Landercasper J (2000) Injury to the chest wall. In: Mattox KL, Feliciano DV, Moore EE (eds) Trauma. McGraw-Hill, New York, pp 483-505

8. Lyass S, Simha M, Muggia-Sullam M (1995) Use of a laparoscopic trocar for tube thoracostomy - a rapid and safe method for chest tube placement. Eur J Emerg Med 2:96
9. Richardson JD, Spain DA (2000) Injury to the lung and pleura. In: Mattox KL, Feliciano DV, Moore EE (eds) Trauma. McGraw-Hill, New York, pp 523-543
10. Luchette FA, Barie PS, Oswanski MF, et al (2001) Practice management guidelines for prophylactic antibiotic use in tube thoracostomy for traumatic hemopneumothorax: EAST practice management guidelines work group. *http://www.east.org/tpg/chesttube.pdf*
11. Ivatury RR (2000) The injured heart. In: Mattox KL, Feliciano DV, Moore EE (eds) Trauma. McGraw-Hill, New York, pp 545-558
12. Pasquale MD, Nagy K, Clarke J (1999) Practice management guidelines for screening of blunt cardiac injury. EAST practice parameter workgroup for screening of blunt cardiac injury. *http://www.east.org/tpg/chapt2.pdf*
13. Wilson RF, Stephenson LW (1996) Thoracic trauma: heart. In: Wilson RF,Walt AJ (eds) Management of Trauma: Pitfalls and Practice. Baltimore, William & Wilkins, pp 343-360
14. Mattox KL, Wall Jr JW, LeMaire SA (2000) Injury to the thoracic great vessels. In: Mattox KL, Feliciano DV, Moore EE (eds) Trauma. McGraw-Hill, New York, pp 559-582
15. Nagy K, Fabian T, Rodman G, et al (2000) Guidelines for the diagnosis and management of blunt aortic injury. An EAST practice management guidelines workgroup. *http://www.east.org/tpg/chapt8.pdf*
16. Wilson RF, Stephenson LW (1996) Trauma to intrathoracic great vessels. in: Wilson RF, Walt AJ (eds) Management of trauma: pitfalls and practice. William and Wilkins, Baltimore, pp 361-387

Chest Trauma: Invasive Thoracic Procedures and Vascular Cannulation

G. Nardi, S. Minucci, G.P. Pino

Chest injuries cause one in every four trauma deaths in North America [1]. Among motor vehicle accidents (MVA) fatalities, about half the victims suffer chest trauma, and for 25% this is the primary cause of death [2]. Aortic injuries and blunt cardiac trauma (BCT) are leading causes of death in chest trauma patients, and yet diagnostic and therapeutic options for these clinical conditions are constantly under debate due to new technological advances.

Blunt cardiac trauma

The incidence and clinical relevance of heart lesions in blunt trauma are still to be precisely defined, due to confusion with regards to definitions and lack of recognized standards. While since 1992 it has been recommended that the term "myocardial contusion" should be avoided and "blunt cardiac trauma" used only in the case of severe arrhythmia or pump failure, many studies still use these definitions, making data in the literature potentially misleading.

Myocardial lesions can be caused either by the compression of the heart between the sternum and the spine, or by direct transfer of energy to the myocardium during the impact to the thorax, or because of rapid deceleration of the heart.

Myocardial dysfunction is frequently associated with blunt chest injury, with or without direct cardiac contusion, and the resulting impaired ventricular performance can complicate patient management and even be the cause of death.

In the case of direct injury to the heart, the definition of BCT can be employed. BCT refers to a huge spectrum of injuries, although it becomes important only when associated with significant symptoms, such as arrhythmia or hypotension, or when there are associated structural cardiac abnormalities, such as myocardial hemorrhage, or septal or free wall rupture, cases in which the right ventricle is more frequently involved. Other cardiac lesions may occur during blunt trauma, but this, however, is rare. Valvar lesions occur in about 1% of cases, and are predominantly of the aortic and mitral valves. Laceration, dissection, and thrombosis of the coronary arteries may lead to myocardial infarction and require prompt identification and surgery. These lesions have been found in 2% of cases in autopsy series [3].

Patients at risk of BCT should be recognized as such soon after injury and aggressively monitored. However, the diagnosis of BCT is not based on universally accepted criteria, and is often difficult to confirm, as the sensitivity and specificity of the different diagnostic tests is low. Electrocardiography (ECG) alone is unreliable in identifying BCT, as this type of injury is not characterized by any specific ECG abnormalities. Patients with blunt thoracic trauma frequently show transitory abnormal ECG associated with purely electrical phenomena unrelated to cardiac injury that can be caused by hemopneumothorax, subcutaneous emphysema, or tissue edema. The positive predictive value of ECG abnormalities is very low [4], although the negative predictive value is as high as 95%, and it has been documented that patients with normal ECGs are unlikely to develop cardiac complications after BCT [5]. ECG may be used to detect cardiac motion and structural abnormalities [6], but artificial ventilation and thoracic cage fractures or subcutaneous emphysema decrease the resolution of transthoracic ECG. According to a study of Salim et al. [7], transthoracic echocardiography correctly identified less than 50% of the patients who suffered BCT. Although more accurate, transoesophageal echocardiography (TEE) can rarely be used as an emergent diagnostic tool for trauma patients, as the technology is not always readily available and requires much experience. TEE would be best employed for patients at high risk for BCT, as determined by less invasive tests.

Recently, experimental studies have shown that troponin T and I are released after myocardial contusion, and that the amount of troponin released correlates with the total energy of the trauma [8]. Cardiac troponin serum levels have been used as an easy way to perform and repeat diagnostic tests to rule out BCT. However, troponin release can also occur as a result of global myocardial hypoperfusion, as in the case of severe hemorrhage and traumatic shock. Therefore, increases in troponin levels may mark a diffuse myocardial injury, even one not directly related to myocardial contusion [9]. Although the negative predictive value of cardiac troponin I (cTnI) is very high, the positive predictive value is much lower [7]. In their study, Salim et al. adopted as protocol the combined use of ECG and cTnI as a screening test for BCT in all patients admitted with evidence of significant thoracic trauma. A 12-lead ECG and cTnI serum level were ordered on admission and repeated 4 and 8 h later. The authors observed that in the case of abnormal findings in both tests the risk of developing myocardial dysfunction was 62%, while no cases of BCT were recorded when both initial ECG and cTnI were normal. They therefore recommend that patients with abnormal findings be closely monitored, while patients who on admission were found to have normal ECG and cTnI may be safely discharged in the absence of other injuries. Thorough heart examination is key to the correct diagnosis of BCT. In the absence of a prompt identification and without correct treatment, patients with undiscovered BCT are at high risk for perioperative complications [10].

Serious pulmonary contusions are often associated with myocardial dysfunction, even in the absence of direct trauma to the heart. Experimental studies suggest that two factors determine impaired myocardial performance: a reduction in right ventricular contractility and a significant increase of right ventricular afterload [11]. Preliminary data support the hypothesis that the depressed myocardial performance after isolated pulmonary contusion may be mediated by circulating neurohumoral factors, and that platelet-derived thromboxane may also be involved. Moreover, the increased afterload caused by a sharp rise in pulmonary resistance and pulmonary blood pressure may contribute independently to myocardial dysfunction. Patients with severe chest contusions should be monitored with a pulmonary artery catheter as soon as possible. However, due to the increase in pulmonary pressure, pulmonary capillary wedge pressure does not accurately estimate left ventricular end diastolic pressure, and hemodynamic data should be interpreted taking these limitations into account. Myocardial lesions without a direct trauma to the heart have also been reported in patients with severe head injuries. Myocardial damage develops most likely as the consequence of an abnormal release of norepinephrine, leading to coronary and pulmonary vasoconstriction, with the consequence of an increased right ventricular afterload and myocardial ischemia [12].

Recently a number of cases of blunt thoracic impact during sporting activities, which caused sudden collapse and death, have been reported. The majority of the documented cases were related to baseball impacts. At autopsies all the victims were found to be free from cardiac structural abnormalities. Interestingly, although a high percentage of the patients were given cardiopulmonary resuscitation within 3 min of the accident, cardiac rhythm could not be restored [13]. These episodes of sudden cardiac arrest after blunt thoracic impact are known as *commotio cordis* [14] and are related to cardiac arrhythmias [mainly ventricular fibrillation (VF)] without evidence of structural damage to the underlying chest organs. This condition has been reproduced in animal studies, and the risk of cardiac arrest has been correlated to the velocity of chest deformation and the amount of compression [15]. Although chest impacts can initiate VF during any phase of the cardiac cycle, there is nearly a fourfold increase in VF risk for impact during the T wave. Impact during QRS complex may lead to complete heart block [14]. A few episodes of commotio cordis occurred in victims wearing chest protectors designed to absorb or dissipate energy and reduce the force of impact [16]. These observations may help to explain some of the cases of unexpected prehospital death in trauma victims with no evidence of major injuries to any other body area.

Aortic injuries

Aortic injuries are the second most-common cause of death after blunt trauma. A recent review of 295 MVA fatalities has shown that as many as 12% of trauma victims had thoracic aortic tears [17] and an even higher percentage was reported in the past; 80% - 85% of the victims die at the scene or during prehospital transport, and only a small minority are admitted to hospital alive. However, if blunt aortic injuries (BAI) are not promptly diagnosed and treated, the majority of these patients will die within the first few days of hospitalization. A large multicenter study involving 274 patients with acute thoracic aortic injuries who reached the hospital alive, reported a mortality rate of 31%, with the majority of deaths attributable to traumatic aortic disruptions [18].

The most-common causes of BAI is motor vehicle collision with frontal or lateral impacts occurring with the same frequency [19]. Other causes of BAI include falls and pedestrian/vehicular collisions. The incidence of thoracic aortic injury is 12.7% in pedestrian fatalities, which is comparable to the incidence observed in motor vehicle collisions, as reported by Brundage et al. [20].

Patients who arrive at the hospital alive may present with a wide range of clinical symptoms, among which the most commonly reported are pseudo-coarction and intrascapular murmur. A transient hypotension at the scene with or without neurological impairment may also be related to aortic dissection. However, many patients may have a normal physical examination, and despite the enormous transfer of energy, less than half of patients with BAI have visible signs of chest wall injury [21].

Among the radiological signs, a widened mediastinum is the most frequently cited finding that triggers a suspicion of BAI. The widened mediastinum is usually defined as measuring more than 8 cm in width or as a mediastinal/chest width ratio of 0.38 or more [22]. Depression of the left main bronchus, tracheal shift to the patient's right, deviation of the nasogastric tube, indistinct aortic knob, or left apical cap are also considered strongly suggestive of BAI. However, BAI may occur despite a normal chest X-ray, and therefore a high level of suspicion should be always maintained in patients injured by significant deceleration mechanisms.

Angiography has been used as the gold standard diagnostic test for BAI. In recent years computed tomography of the chest (CTC) is taking on a greater role as the new generation of scanners, such as helicoidal or spiral CT, are very sensitive and have a negative predictive value very near to 100% [23, 24]. When helical or spiral CTC is used, angiography may be reserved for those patients with equivocal or indeterminate scans. TEE is also a very sensitive screening test, but requires specific training and expertise. In a recent study, Vignon et al. [25] compared TEE with contrast-enhanced helical CT in the diagnosis of BAI. TEE and CT were equally accurate in identifying all vascular injuries requiring surgery. However, TEE was more sensitive in detecting injuries involving the intimal or medial layers, which were conservatively treated.

TEE has serious advantages for use on unstable patients who cannot move to angiography or CT. However, TEE may miss injuries to the ascending aorta or the aortic branches.

Therapeutic management of BAI has changed recently. There is increasing evidence that limited aortic lesions (intramural hematoma, limited intimal flap) can benefit only from medical treatment alone, and that some patients with subadventitial rupture can benefit from delayed surgery [26]. In the extended or progressive lesions prompt surgical repair is considered the best approach by most of the authors. However, surgery may not be possible for all patients as BAI is often associated with multiple injuries, with severe head trauma bringing them beyond the upper limit of tolerance for thoracotomy. Moreover, in patients with intracranial hemorrhage or severe brain contusion, extracorporeal circulation must be avoided. In these patients a different approach is required. Pharmacological control of blood pressure with beta-blockers and/or nitroprusside is a cornerstone of the treatment when delayed or non-operative management is required. Nevertheless in patients with brain injuries hypotensive circulatory management is associated with a high risk of secondary cerebral ischemia, as normal cerebral perfusion pressure is required to assure brain perfusion.

The recent development of stent-graft technology has led to less-invasive strategies for the treatment of thoracic aortic injuries. The use of endovascular stent grafting to treat abdominal aortic aneurysms was first proposed in the early 1990s [27]; since then the applications of these techniques have gradually widened, and a few cases of endovascular stent-grafting to treat thoracic aortic injuries have been reported [28]. Fujikawa et al. [29] recently reported the first series of patients (6) with a rupture of the descending thoracic aorta, treated with endovascular stent-grafting. In this study the diagnosis of BAI was performed with CT scan, and angiography was subsequently performed to evaluate the exact site of the injury. Endovascular stent-grafting (ESG) was considered to be indicated only in cases of rupture below the left subclavian artery. Five of the six patients were treated within 8 h of injury. One patient died on day 6 due to a ruptured ascending aorta, and all others were discharged from the hospital. A follow-up CT scan revealed that in all these cases periaortic hematoma disappeared within 2 weeks.

We recently used ESG to treat a multiple trauma patient involved in a vehicular crash who presented with subarachnoid hemorrhage, unstable fracture of the pelvis, bilateral rib fractures with lung contusions, and fracture of the right femur. The patient was referred to our emergency department because of a progressively increasing dissection of the descending thoracic aorta. After ESG and internal fixation of the femur and the pelvic ring, the patient was discharged fully conscious and in good clinical condition.

Conclusions

Patients with BCT due to a major accident or those who present with arrhythmia or hemodynamic instability should be carefully examined to rule out BCT and aortic injuries. A normal ECG together with normal serial determination of troponin I can reasonably exclude the risk of BCT. Patients with abnormal findings should be submitted to further investigations, including TEE, and be closely monitored. TEE may be as sensitive as helical CT for diagnosing aortic injuries, but high technical skills and experience are required. The new ESG technology may increase the possibility of successfully treating patients with blunt thoracic aortic injury.

References

1. Advanced trauma life support program for doctors, 6th edn, American College of Surgeons
2. Kshettry V, Bolman R (1994) Chest trauma: assessment, diagnosis, and management. Clin Chest Med 15:137-146
3. Orliaguet G, Ferjani M, Riou B (2001) The heart in blunt trauma Anesthesiology 95: 544-548
4. Karalis DG, Victor MF, Davis GA, et al (1994) The role of echocardiography in blunt chest trauma: a thoracic and transesophageal echocardiographic study. J Trauma 36: 53-58
5. Christensen MA, Sutton KR (1993) Myocardial contusion: new concepts in diagnosis and management. Am J Crit Care 2: 28-34
6. Feghali NT, Prisant LM (1995) Blunt myocardial injury. Chest 108: 1673-1677
7. Salim A, Velmahos GC, Jindal A, et al (2001) Clinically significant blunt cardiac trauma: role of serum troponin levels combined with electrocardiographic findings. J Trauma 50: 237-243

8. Okubo N, Hombrouck C, Fornes P, et al (2000) Cardiac troponin I and myocardial contusion in the rabbit. Anesthesiology 93: 811-817
9. Edouard AR, Benoist JF, Cosson C, et al (1998) Circulating cardiac troponin I in trauma patients without cardiac contusion. Intensive Care Med 24: 569-573
10. Baum VC (2000) The patient with cardiac trauma. J Cardiothorac Vasc Anesth 48: 924-931
11. Moomey CB, Fabian TC, Croce MA, et al (1998) Determinants of myocardial performance after blunt chest trauma. J Trauma 45: 988-995
12. De Monte A, Petrei D, Nardi G, et al (1994) Fulminant neurogenic pulmonary oedema and transient myocardial depression do not contraindicate heart donation. Intensive Care Med 20 [Suppl 2]: 150
13. Maron BJ, Poliac LC, Kaplan JA, et al (1995) Blunt impact to the chest leading to sudden death from cardiac arrest during sports activities. N Engl J Med 333: 337-342
14. Link MS, Wang PJ, Pandian NG et al (1998) An experimental model of sudden death due to low-energy chest-wall impact (commotio cordis) N Engl J Med 338: 1805-1811
15. Bir CA, Viano DC (1999) Biomechanical predictor of commotio cordis. J Trauma 47: 468-473
16. Viano D, Bir CA, Cheney AK, Janda D (2000) Prevention of commotio cordis in baseball: an evaluation of chest protectors. J Trauma 49: 1023-1028
17. Horton TG, Cohn SM, Heid M, et al (2000) Identification of trauma patients at risk of thoracic aortic tear by mechanism of injury J Trauma 48: 1008-1014
18. Fabian TC, Richardson JD, Croce MA, et al (1997) Prospective study of blunt aortic injury: multicenter trial of the American Association for the surgery of trauma. J Trauma 42: 374-383
19. Katyal D, Mc Lellan BA, Brenneman FD, et al (1997) Lateral impact motor vehicle collisions: significant cause of blunt traumatic rupture of the thoracic aorta. J Trauma 42: 769-772
20. Brundage S, Harruff R, Jurkovich GJ Maier R (1998) The epidemiology of thoracic aortic injuries in pedestrians. J Trauma 45: 1010-1014
21. Lee J, Appel PL, Wohlmuth DA, Shoemaker WC (1997) Noncorrelation between thoracic skeletal injuries and acute traumatic aortic tear. J Trauma 43: 400-404
22. Nagy k, Fabian T, Rodman G, et al (2000) Guidelines for the diagnosis and management of blunt aortic injury: an EAST practice management guidelines work group. J Trauma 48: 1128-1141
23. Fabian TC, Davis KA, Gavant ML, et al (1998) Prospective study of blunt aortic injury: helical CT is diagnostic and antihyperthensive therapy reduces rupture. Ann Surg 227: 666-677
24. Mirvis SE, Kithirkamuganathan S, Buell J, Rodriguez A (1998) Use of spiral computed tomography for the assessment of blunt trauma patients with potential aortic injury. J Trauma 45: 922-930
25. Vignon P, Boncoeur MP, Francois B, et al (2001) Comparison of multiplanal transesophageal echocardiography and contrast-enhanced helical CT in the diagnosis of blunt traumatic cardiovascular injuries. Anesthesiology 94: 615-622
26. Pate JW, Gavant ML, Weiman DS, et al (1999) Traumatic rupture of the aortic isthmus: program of selective management. Worl J Surg 23: 59-63
27. Parodi JC, Palmaz JC, Barone HD (1991) Transfemoral intraluminar graft implantation for abdominal aortic aneurysm. Ann Vasc Surg 5: 491-499
28. Dake MD, Miller DC, Semba CP, et al (1994) Transluminal placement of endovascular stent--grafts for the treatment of descending thoracic aortic aneurysms. N Engl J Med 331: 1729-1734
29. Fujikawa T, Yukioka T, Ishimaru S, et al (2001) Endovascular stent grafting for the treatment of blunt thoracic aortic injury. J Trauma 50: 223-229

Abdominal Trauma

G. Sganga, G. Brisinda, G. Maria

Trauma is the main public health problem in every country regardless of the level of socioeconomic development [1]. The abdomen is frequently injured after both blunt and penetrating trauma, and approximately 25% of all trauma victims require abdominal exploration [2]. *Abdominal trauma* (AT) remains a leading cause of morbidity and mortality among all age groups, accounting for a greater percentage of productive years of life lost than heart disease and cancer combined [1-6].

AT frequency is unknown as is also the incidence of out-of-hospital deaths [6]. Data from the World Health Organization indicate that falls from heights of less than 5 m are the leading cause of injury, and automobile crashes are the next most-frequent cause. One review from the National Pediatric Trauma Registry reported that 8% of 25,310 patients had AT: of those injuries, 83% were from blunt trauma [7]. In adult patients, blunt trauma is the leading cause of AT and motor-vehicle collisions are the leading mode of injury [8]. Furthermore, abdominal injuries have been reported to occur in approximately 25% of major trauma victims, and often involve multiple organ injuries (Table 1). Multiple system injuries involving head and/or thoracic injuries are common, and may complicate the management of AT (Table 2). Enteric trauma is more frequent in the presence of an associated, severe, solid organ injury, particularly to the pancreas [9-12].

Table 1. Incidence of intra-abdominal injuries requiring laparotomy for blunt and penetrating abdominal trauma (AT)

	Blunt AT (%)	Penetrating AT (%)
Spleen	47	7
Liver/biliary	51	28
Pancreas/duodenum	10	11
Large bowel	5	23
Stomach/small bowel	9	42

Table 2. Incidence of regional injuries associated with blunt AT

Regional associated injuries	%
Head	23
Thoracic	15
Axial spine/spinal cord	10
Pelvic fractures	23
Long bone fractures	33

Penetrating AT affects approximately 35% of those patients admitted to urban trauma centers and 1-12% of those admitted to rural centers [2, 6]. The mechanism that underlies the penetrating AT [e.g., gunshot wounds (GSW), stab wounds (SW), impalement] relates to the mode of injury (e.g., accidental or intentional injury, homicide, or suicide). Homicide or intentional injury clearly is the predominant mode of injury in this patient population. Accidental penetrating AT is most common in pediatric patients. Incidence of penetrating injury varies and it is related to the industrialization of developing nations and, significantly, to the presence of military conflicts [6, 11].

Pathophysiology of blunt and penetrating AT

Identification of severe intra-abdominal pathology due to AT is often challenging. Many injuries may not manifest during the initial assessment, and often mechanisms of injury result in other associated injuries that may divert the physician's attention from potentially life-threatening intra-abdominal pathology [1, 6].

In patients with blunt AT, injury to abdominal viscera can be classified into two primary mechanisms of injury: compression forces and deceleration forces. Compression or concussive forces may result from direct blows or external compression against a fixed object, such as the spinal column. Most commonly, these crushing forces cause tears and subcapsular hematomas to the solid viscera. These forces also may deform hollow organs and transiently increase intraluminal pressure, resulting in rupture. Deceleration forces cause stretching and linear shearing between relatively fixed and free segments. Classic deceleration injuries include hepatic tear along the ligamentum teres and intimal injuries to the renal arteries [2, 6, 13]. As bowel loops travel from their mesenteric attachments, thrombosis and mesenteric tears, with resultant splanchnic vessel injuries, can result. The liver and spleen seem the most frequently injured organs, although reports vary. Small and large intestines are the next most injured organs, respectively. Recent studies show an increased number of hepatic injuries, perhaps reflecting increased use of computed tomography (CT) scanning and concomitant identification of more injuries [14].

Penetrating injuries or SWs to the abdomen are caused by a wide variety of instruments, including knives, projectiles, ice picks, and industrial implements. The most commonly injured organs associated with penetrating injuries are the small intestine (29%), liver (28%), and colon (23%). SWs cause injury in the direct path of the offending implement, although only 33% of SWs to the abdomen penetrate the peritoneal envelope. Anatomical site, number of wounds, type and size of weapon, and the wound angle are important considerations. Determination of the likely implement path and whether the peritoneum was violated is crucial [1-6].

GSWs have a much broader injury pattern due to several mechanisms. First, any structure directly in the path of the missile suffers a loss of integrity. Approximately 85% of abdominal wall GSWs penetrate the abdominal cavity, and 95% require a surgical procedure for correction. Injury also is caused by fragmentation of the bullet on impact.

Mortality and morbidity

The principal causes of morbidity and mortality in AT are associated with delays in diagnosis or treatment. They have been identified as (1) hemorrhage, as might occur with hepatic, splenic or mesenteric injuries, and (2) secondary inflammatory injury, sepsis, and multiple organ failure syndromes as may occur with bowel, biliary tract, or pancreas injuries [1-6].

The National Pediatric Trauma Registry reported that 9% of pediatric patients with blunt AT died. Of these, only 22% were reported as having intra-abdominal injuries as the likely cause of death. A review of intestinal injuries in blunt AT reported that 85% of injuries occurred from vehicular accidents, and mortality rate was 6%. In a large review of operating room deaths in which blunt trauma accounted for 61% of all injuries, AT was the primary identified cause of death in 54% of cases [1-6].

Death rate from penetrating AT spans the entire spectrum (0-100%), depending on the extent of injury. Patients with penetrating AT without peritoneal injury have a 0% mortality and morbidity rate, while those with multiorgan injury complexes (hypotension, base deficit less than 15 mEq/l HCO_3, lactate more than 20 mmol/l) and near exsanguination have a nearly 100% mortality rate. An average mortality rate for all patients with penetrating AT is approximately 5%. Several studies reveal that the most-common morbidities following penetrating AT are wound infection (2-8%) and intra-abdominal abscess with or without sepsis (10-80%, depending on presence or absence of bowel injury in combination with major vascular injury).

Delayed diagnosis or treatment of AT represents one of the most-common causes of preventable mortality, and therefore constitutes a critical area of trauma management [1-6]. Death generally occurs within the first 72 h from hypoperfusion and its sequelae. It also may occur 2 or more weeks later from complications related to sepsis, the systemic inflammatory response syndrome (SIRS), or multiple organ dysfunction syndrome (MODS).

Sepsis connotes a spectrum of physiological abnormalities that occur in response to a vast array of cytokine-driven cascades in a susceptible host [15, 16]. This spectrum includes SIRS, compensatory anti-inflammatory response syndrome, mixed antagonist response syndrome, and MODS.

SIRS is manifested by elevated cardiac performance, maldistributed flow, acute lung injury, and intense catabolism. The adaptive response is to reduce the inflammatory cascades to a manageable level once the injury has been controlled [15]. This adaptive response is known as compensatory anti-inflammatory response syndrome; it acts to restore homeostasis. If the anti-inflammatory cascades outweigh inflammation, mixed antagonist response syndrome develops. At this stage, incipient organ failures become evident, and the patient is increasingly susceptible to infection [16]. The result of these processes is known as immunological dissonance. These processes manifests as MODS, which ultimately leads to death of the host [17, 18]. The risk for mortality increases as the number of organ failures increases (3 failures = 85% mortality; 4 failures = 95% mortality; 5 failures = 99% mortality).

Initial management

The initial management of AT begins with the rapid restoration of cardiopulmonary function and the prioritized management of airway, breathing, and circulation. Rapid identification and control of hemorrhage and the identification and treatment of traumatic brain injury are typically the two most-important diagnostic and therapeutic goals [1-6].

With the high risk for AT to result in major blood loss and the frequent absence of specific clinical signs or symptoms, morbidity and mortality from delayed diagnosis and treatment of intra-abdominal hemorrhage are a critical pitfall in the initial management of these patients [1-6]. Several studies have suggested that untreated or inadequately treated hemorrhage remains one of the causes of early death in injured patients.

Regardless of the mode of injury, absolute indications for celiotomy are virtually identical: hemodynamic instability, major vascular injury (including devascularized solid organs), evisceration, peritoneal signs, pneumoperitoneum, evidence of diaphragmatic injury, neurological injury with cord compromise, significant intraperitoneal blood [e.g., positive findings at diagnostic peritoneal lavage (DPL)], and evidence of gastrointestinal perforation [1-6].

Diagnostic evaluation

History and physical examination are usually accurate in determining AT in the responsive patient, although the limitations of the physical examination are significant [1]. It has been considered that an objective abdominal evaluation is necessary and should be obtained by using any of the available diagnostic modalities in addition to the physical examination [1-6,13,14]. Indications for objective evaluation in blunt AT are reported in Table 3. The test of choice depends on the hemodynamic stability of the patient and the severity of associated injuries. The comparison of diagnostic methods for evaluating blunt and penetrating AT is reported in Table 4.

Table 3. Indications for objective evaluation in blunt AT

Clinical factor	Incidence of associated abdominal injury (%)
Spinous process fractures	21
Gross hematuria	24
Altered sensorium	45
Abdominal seatbelt sign	64
Hypotension	27
Pelvic fractures	20

Laboratory studies

In recent years, laboratory evaluation of trauma victims has been a matter of significant discussion [1-6]. Commonly recommended studies include serum glucose, complete blood count, serum chemistries, serum amylase, urinalysis, coagulation studies, blood type and match, arterial blood gas (ABG), blood ethanol, urine drug screens, and a urine pregnancy test (for females of childbearing age).

Normal hemoglobin and hematocrit results do not rule out significant hemorrhage. Patients bleed whole blood [6]. Recently, the usefulness of routine serum chemistries of trauma patients has been questioned. Most trauma victims are younger than 40 years and rarely are taking medications that may alter electrolytes (e.g., diuretics, potassium replacements).

Liver functions tests may be useful in the patient with blunt AT; however,

Table 4. Comparison of diagnostic methods for evaluation of blunt and penetrating AT. DPL = diagnostic peritoneal lavage, CT = computed tomography, SW = stab wound, GSW = gun shot wound

Diagnostic method	Time required (min)	Sensitivity/specificity (%)	Comment
DPL	5-15	85-100/43-99	Fast. Very sensitive. Minimal equipment required. Results are quantitative, objective, and operator-independent. Invasive. Not recommended if prior laparotomy. Not injury specific. May miss retro-peritoneal and diaphragm injuries. Sensitivity and specificity highly dependent on cell count criteria used.
Abdominal CT	30-50	85-99/95-100	Very specific with good sensitivity. Good for evaluation of posterior injuries. Staging of blunt organ injury for nonoperative management. Not useful for most anterior penetrating AT. Require time and patient transport. May miss blunt intestinal injuries and, initially, some pancreatic injuries.
FAST	5-10	82-97/95-100	Fast. Sensitive for haemoperitoneum in experienced hands. Noninvasive and no contrast required. Not useful for penetrating AT. Nonquantitative and operator dependent
Diagnostic laparoscopy	30-90	18-100	Excellent for diagnosis of diaphragmatic injuries. Good for diagnosis of hemo-peritoneum and for determining peritoneal penetration for SW/GSW. Invasive. Poor sensitivity for gastrointestinal and retroperitoneal injuries. Require experience and equipment. General anesthesia may be needed in some cases.

test findings may be elevated for several reasons (e.g., alcohol abuse). It has shown that an aspartate aminotransferase or alanine aminotransferase level more than 130 U corresponds with significant hepatic injury [13]. Lactate dehydrogenase and bilirubin are not specific indicators of hepatic trauma. Controversy surrounds the role of amylase determination in the presence of blunt AT. However, an abnormally elevated amylase level 3-6 h after trauma has a much greater accuracy [6].

Indications for diagnostic urinalysis include gross hematuria, microscopic hematuria in the setting of hypotension, and a significant deceleration mechanism.

Arterial blood gas may provide important information in major trauma victims. In addition to information about oxygenation (e.g., pO_2, SaO_2) and ventilation (pCO_2), this test provides valuable information regarding oxygen delivery.

Imaging studies

Ultrasonography

Ultrasonography (US) is widely used in the initial diagnostic assessment of blunt AT [14,19-23]. Initial studies suggested a relatively high incidence of missed injuries but included both penetrating and blunt AT. US suffers from the same lack of sensitivity in detecting penetrating AT as CT scanning: inability to detect small amounts of fluid or gas associated with gastroenteric injuries.

Use of US in blunt trauma, principally for the detection of hemoperitoneum, has been associated however with good sensitivity as experience has accumulated [1,6].

In the emergency setting, the examination in four standard planes (FAST – *focused abdominal sonogram for trauma*) aims to detect or to exclude free intraperitoneal fluid, indicating organ lacerations [20]. FAST's diagnostic accuracy generally is equal to that of DPL. Studies over the last few years have demonstrated the value of bedside US as a noninvasive approach for rapid evaluation of hemoperitoneum. The studies demonstrate a degree of operator dependence; however, some studies have shown that with a structured learning session, even novice operators can identify free intra-abdominal fluid [6].

In the patient with isolated blunt AT and multisystem injuries, a bedside US performed by an experienced sonographer rapidly can identify free intraperitoneal fluid. The sensitivity for solid organ encapsulated injury is moderate in most studies. Gastrointestinal injury rarely is identified; however, free fluid may be visualized in these cases. For those patients with persistent pain or tenderness or for those developing peritoneal signs, consider FAST as a complementary measure to CT scan, DPL, or exploration [1, 2].

FAST evaluation of the abdomen consists of visualization of the pericardium, the splenorenal and the hepatorenal spaces, such as the Morison pouch, the paracolic gutters, and, in the pelvis, the pouch of Douglas. The Morison pouch view has been shown to be the most sensitive, regardless of the etiology of the fluid [20].

Free fluid, generally assumed to be blood in the setting of AT, appears as a black stripe. Free fluid in a hemodynamically unstable patient indicates exigent laparotomy; however, CT scan may further evaluate the stable patient with free fluid.

The spleen and liver are most frequently affected by blunt AT, with incidences of injury varying between 20 and 60% [24-26]. Modern US equipment enables the detection of fluid collections as small as 10-15 ml close to lacerated viscera. A major concern remains, however, about the reliability of peritoneal effusion as a surrogate marker of organ injury. According to recent reports, frequency of visceral lesions not accompanied by free fluid, ranges from 10 to 30%.

A recent systematic review and meta-analysis has shown that, despite its high specificity, US has an unexpectedly low sensitivity for the detection of both free fluid and organ lesions. In clinically suspected AT, another assessment, such as helical CT scan, must be performed regardless of the initial US findings [14].

Computed tomography

Although expensive and potentially time-consuming, CT scan often provides the most detailed images of traumatic pathology and may assist in determination of operative intervention. CT scanning may miss injuries to the diaphragm and perforations of the gastrointestinal tract [1-6]. Pancreatic injuries may not be identified on initial CT scans but generally are found on follow-up examinations performed on high-risk patients. For selected patients, endoscopic retrograde cholangiopancreatography may complement CT scanning to rule out a ductal injury.

The primary advantage of CT scanning for blunt AT is its high sensitivity and specificity in staging solid organ injuries, thereby permitting expectant nonoperative management of injuries selected, in part, based on the CT scan [13]. Furthermore, injuries to the retroperitoneal structures are usually well defined by the CT scan compared with DPL. A principal pitfall of CT scanning for blunt AT is its ability to miss small amounts of free intraperitoneal fluid associated with blunt intestinal injury and a relatively poor sensibility for these injuries [1, 2, 6]. Drawbacks of CT scanning relate to the need to transport the patient from the trauma resuscitation area and the additional time required to perform CT scanning compared with FAST or DPL [1]. This makes the use of CT relatively contraindicated for patients in decompensated shock [1].

The best CT imagery requires both oral and IV contrast. Recently, some controversy has arisen over the utility of oral contrast and whether the additional information it provides negates the drawbacks of increased time and risk of aspiration. The value of oral contrast in diagnosing bowel injury has been debated, but no definitive answer exists at this time [6].

Diagnostic peritoneal lavage

DPL is used as a method of rapidly determining the presence of intraperitoneal blood. DPL is particularly useful if the history and abdominal examination of a patient who is unstable and has multisystem injuries is either unreliable or equivocal [1-6]. DPL is also useful for those patients in whom serial abdominal examinations cannot be performed (patients in an angiographic suite or operating room during emergent orthopedic or neurosurgical procedures).

The preferred method involves an open or semiopen technique that is performed in an infraumbilical location. In pregnant patients or in those patients with particular risk for potential pelvic hematoma, DPL may be performed superior to the umbilicus.

Following insertion of the catheter into the peritoneum, attempt to aspirate free intraperitoneal blood (at least 15-20 ml). Abdominal exploration is always indicated if approximately 10 ml of blood is aspirated upon insertion of the peritoneal catheter (grossly positive) in the unstable patient. If findings are negative, infuse 1,000 ml saline solution into the peritoneum. Then, allow this fluid to drain by gravity, and perform laboratory analysis. Presence of more than 100,000 RBC/mm^3 or more than 500 WBC/mm^3 is considered a positive finding [1-6, 27]. This has resulted in high sensitivity, and a low incidence of false-negative examinations, with an acceptable incidence of nontherapeutic laparotomy. DPL thresholds for penetrating AT are somewhat more controversial, varying in reported series from 1,000 to as high as 50,000 RBC/mm^3. High thresholds result in higher incidence of delayed diagnoses and potential missed injuries, but a very low incidence of nontherapeutic laparotomy, whereas low cell count threshold miss very few injuries but result in a relatively higher incidence of nontherapeutic laparotomies [2, 27]. Other results from DPL fluid that indicate the need for exploration include the presence of bile or abnormally high amylase (greater than 175 IU/dl), food fibers, or bacteria noted on microscopic examination [1-6 ,27].

In some contexts, DPL may be complemented with a CT scan if the patient has positive lavage results but stabilizes. The only absolute contraindication for a DPL is the patient who will undergo laparotomy regardless of the findings.

Complications of DPL include bleeding from the incision and catheter insertion, infection (wound, peritoneal), and injury to intra-abdominal structures (urinary bladder, small bowel, uterus). These complications may increase the possibility of false-positive examinations. Additionally, injury to other intra-abdominal organs can occur.

Laparoscopy

As recent technical improvements have expanded the use of *laparoscopy*, efforts have been made to apply this minimally invasive technique to the diagnosis and the treatment of AT. Several studies have evaluated the use of diagnostic laparoscopy for AT, with mixed results. Although the specificity is good, the diagnostic sensitivity for hollow viscous or retroperitoneal trauma has been unacceptably low [28].

Sensitivity and specificity depend on DPL cell count criteria, and experience of the laparoscopic operator. Despite the fact that diagnostic laparoscopy may be performed in the emergency department, advantages of the routine application of this more-complex and costly diagnostic technique over DPL in terms of sensitivity, cost, and time have yet to be demonstrated [6].

The use of diagnostic laparoscopy in blunt AT has not been associated with higher sensitivity and specificity than that obtained with CT scan, but does offer the potential for therapeutic intervention for solid organ injuries, and possibly selected diaphragm injuries [6, 28].

Other diagnostic modalities

Almost all other tests relate to (1) a skeletal survey for associated fractures, (2) a CT scan of the brain for coincident head injuries, or (3) a retrograde urethrogram or *cystogram* in a stable patient who has a displaced prostate, symphysis pubis diastasis, or blood at the urethral meatus.

Unstable patents with these findings usually undergo exploration if they have injuries other than an isolated pelvic fracture and receive an on-table cystourethrogram or a suprapubic bladder catheter and subsequent antegrade or retrograde studies.

Nuclear medicine studies have no role in the acutely injured AT patient. Patients who have a concomitant deceleration mechanism with an abnormal mediastinal silhouette in addition to penetrating AT require angiogram or transesophageal echocardiography to exclude an aortic transection.

Proctosigmoidoscopy is indicated for evaluation of suspected rectal or sigmoid injury. Frequent swabbing and suctioning to clear stool is usually necessary, since this is an unprepared examination. Typically, sedation is not required for this procedure. Identification of rectal or low sigmoid colon full-thickness rents, intramural hematoma, or luminal arterial blood loss requires prompt surgical exploration.

Interventional radiology can be extremely useful: (1) to identify active hemorrhage, (2) to evaluate renal artery thrombosis, (3) to manage pelvic hemorrhage in patients with pelvic fractures, and bleeding from non-severe hepatic and splenic injuries, (4) in the diagnosis and treatment of hemobilia, (5) in the treatment of retained collections or *intra-abdominal abscesses* [1-6].

Complications of AT

Complications are fairly frequent in this high-risk patient population [1-6]. They are associated with presence of hypotension, combined solid and hollow viscus injury, major vascular injury, cardiac arrest, re-operation, multiple comorbid diseases, pre-hospital near exsanguination, massive blood component transfusion, and steroid use [6, 29]. Clearly, all of these factors relate to impaired tissue perfusion, wound healing capacity, and immune surveillance. Technical complications directly related to operative procedures and missed injuries set the stage for further injury.

Wound failure

These complications include such diverse elements as wound infection, fascial dehiscence, evisceration, and necrotizing fasciitis [30]. Patients with superficial SWs rapidly treated infrequently develop wound infections following irrigation, debridement, and wound edge approximation. In contrast, victims of abdominal GSWs generally should not undergo wound closure due to contamination and the greater tissue destruction that accompanies the bullet tract [1-6, 29, 30].

Accordingly, after abdominal exploration for penetrating AT in which hollow viscus injury is identified and the peritoneal space may be heavily contaminated or frankly infected, the fascia usually is closed, while the skin remains open to undergo delayed primary closure or healing by secondary intention. If the fascia fails to heal properly due to infection, strangulation, or poor surgical technique, the fascial edges separate as the sutures pull through the fascia. The result is a fascial dehiscence, which occurs in approximately 5% of patients operated on for penetrating AT [30]. The patient with fascial dehiscence and open skin margins is at risk for evisceration until the fascial defect is repaired. These patients should remain at bedrest and should have their abdominal contents protected with moist gauze secured with a sterile dressing.

Necrotizing fasciitis is a potentially devastating complication of wound closure. The condition is an infection of the fascia and is associated with microvascular thrombosis, tissue hypoxemia, and impaired neutrophil function. The patient's wound exudes a thin malodorous fluid rather than thick pus. The fascia easily separates from the underlying muscle. Radical excisional debridement combined with aggressive fluid resuscitation and broad-spectrum antimicrobial therapy is the treatment of choice. This complication carries a mortality rate of at least 50% [29, 30].

Malnutrition

Most patients develop a paralytic ileus. When the patient is likely to require a prolonged intensive care unit (ICU) course, it is prudent to place enteral access. Such access provides luminal nutrients to maintain host gut mucosal barrier integrity [17, 31] and provides metabolic substrate to fuel the cellular reparative processes essential for recovery.

The goal of nutritional therapy must also correct pre-existing protein or protein-calorie malnutrition. Albumin, prealbumin, retinol-binding protein, and/or transferrin levels are good markers of pre-existing malnutrition.

Deep vein thrombosis

Patients who are critically ill or relatively immobilized following therapy for penetrating or blunt AT are at risk for deep vein thrombosis (DVT) [1-6]. Intra-abdominal infectious or inflammatory complications following surgery, particularly when localized to the pelvis, greatly increase this risk [30]. The risk is tremendous with direct injury to one of the major pelvic veins.

Overall risk for clinically significant DVT after penetrating AT requiring hospitalization approaches 20%, but may be as high as 82% after common femoral vein cannulation [6]. Prophylactic therapy includes early mobilization, superficial venous compression stockings, sequential compression devices, and subcutaneous normal or low molecular weight heparin. Diagnosis is established by clinical suspicion (pain, increased circumference, positive Homans' sign) and duplex scanning of the lower extremity deep venous system.

The threat associated with DVT formation is venous thromboembolism with venous obstruction in the pulmonary circuit. Pulmonary embolism (PE) occurs in 35% of all patients with DVT. Diagnosis is established by clinical suspicion and radionuclide ventilation/perfusion scan. Spiral CT scan techniques may be able to reliably detect PE. PE carries a mortality rate of more than 60%, but this rate approaches 95% when the presentation is associated with hemodynamic instability [6].

Stress ulceration

Patients who sustain major stress are at risk for abnormal gastric mucosal blood flow with resultant loss of protective mucous [32]. Absent or reduced mucus production allows proton-induced mucosal damage to occur. This mucosal injury may progress to submucosal involvement of the plexus of vessels and lead to stress ulceration and an upper gastrointestinal hemorrhage. The ulcers may be solitary or diffuse. The best protection against stress ulceration is aggressive correction of the underlying problem and vigorous restoration of end-organ oxygen delivery. Stress ulceration occurs in approximately 20% of ICU patients [6, 32].

Pressure ulceration

Patients at bed rest for a variety of reasons may create untoward pressure across skin that overlies bony protuberances [33]. When the external pressure exceeds the capillary pressure, tissue ischemia, cellular hypoxia, and, ultimately, skin necrosis may result. This necrosis appears as a pressure ulcer, which may progress through the classic four stages (skin erythema, dermal destruction, subcutaneous adipose destruction, muscle necrosis with bony exposure).

These ulcers are a source of pain, disability, and potential infection. According to estimates, pressure ulcers occur in less than 1% of penetrating AT [33], with the vast majority occurring in critically ill ICU patients.

Intestinal injury

Intestinal injury may require a substantial resection to remove nonviable bowel [1, 2, 10]. One consequence may be the development of short gut syndrome. This syndrome develops in patients whose total small intestinal length is 4 feet or less. Malabsorption and multiple nutritional, fluid, electrolyte, vitamin, and mineral deficiencies are the rule. Long-term total parenteral nutrition may provide the only secure route of nutritional supplementation in these patients. Enteral stomas frequently are required following intestinal injury.

Intestinal obstruction secondary to postoperative adhesions requires operative therapy in approximately 2% of early cases without intestinal injury, in 4% of early cases with small bowel injury, and in 14% of late cases [1-6]. Adhesiolysis is the most commonly performed procedure in this circumstance.

Intestinal anastomotic leaks may occur postoperatively. An anastomotic leak occurs in 5% of small bowel anastomoses, 10% of colonic anastomoses, and 18% of rectal anastomoses. Intestinal leaks may lead to intra-abdominal abscess formation or widespread peritonitis [1-6].

Intra-abdominal infection

Any emergency abdominal procedure carries a risk of infection that is related to the nature of the procedure and the bacterial load at the time of operation. Risk factors for development of intra-abdominal abscess include, but are not limited to the following: gastrointestinal perforation, retained or recurrent hemoperitoneum, re-operation, missed injury, anastomotic leak, tissue ischemia, and retained and/or contaminated foreign bodies [1-6].

With preoperative antibiotic therapy, the incidence of postoperative infection is 8.3% for gastrointestinal perforations and 5% without enteric injury [10]. CT scan, US, or magnetic resonance imaging commonly establishes diagnosis. Localized collections may be drained percutaneously and may be definitively managed in this fashion.

Inability to percutaneously drain the entire collection or failure of clinical improvement leads to re-exploration and formal drainage. If the patient manifests signs of sepsis earlier than 5 days postoperatively, a CT scan may not localize a collection, and prompt re-exploration generally is warranted [6].

Severe peritonitis remains a potentially fatal disease in AT patients. Furthermore, these infections resulting from injuries still represent a challenge for surgeons. Although greater understanding of the pathophysiology of intra-abdominal infections, the improvement in critical care and introduction of timed radiological and/or surgical intervention have reduced the mortality associated with severe peritonitis, the rate remains unacceptably high, ranging from 20 to 80% [18].

New operative techniques, such as planned relaparotomies, laparostomies or open packing, have been introduced in effort to improve the results of treatment of severe intra-abdominal infections.

Intra-abdominal infection is defined as an inflammatory response of the peritoneum to microorganisms and their toxins, which results in purulent exudate in the abdominal cavity. They have two major manifestations: generalized peritonitis and intra-abdominal abscess, a late and localized stage [18]. Moreover, peritonitis and intra-abdominal infection are not synonymous.

Many attempts have been made to classify peritonitis in general, and secondary peritonitis in particular, which include a large variety of different pathological conditions ranging in severity from a local problem to a devastating disease. A simplified version is presented in Table 5. It differentiates between the relatively rare forms of primary peritonitis, which usually respond to medical treatment, and tertiary peritonitis, which does not respond to any treatment, from the commonly occurring secondary *peritonitis* that mandates surgical intervention [18].

When timely surgical therapy combined with appropriate antimicrobial treatment is undertaken, most patients are able to resolve the infection. However, when patients are unable to contain the peritoneal infection, whether because of an overwhelming infection and impaired defense mechanism, a diffuse and persistent form of peritonitis – so called tertiary peritonitis – that is often fatal, develops. If patients are able to localize the infection, an intra-abdominal abscess develops [1-6, 16, 18].

Table 5. Classification of intra-abdominal infections

Primary peritonitis
Diffuse bacterial peritonitis in the absence of disruption of gastrointestinal tract
1. Spontaneous peritonitis in children
2. Spontaneous peritonitis in adults
3. Peritonitis in patients with continued ambulatory peritoneal dialysis
4. Tuberculous and other granulomatous peritonitis

Secondary peritonitis
Localised or diffuse peritonitis originating from a defect in abdominal viscus
1. Post-traumatic peritonitis
    A. After blunt AT
    B. After penetrating AT
2. Acute perforation peritonitis
    A. Gastrointestinal perforation
    B. Intestinal ischemia
    C. Pelviperitonitis and other forms
3. Postoperative peritonitis
    A. Anastomotic leak
    B. Accidental perforation and devascularization

Tertiary peritonitis
Late peritonitis-like syndrome due to disturbance in the immune response of the patient
1. Peritonitis without evidence for pathogens
2. Peritonitis with fungi
3. Peritonitis with low-grade pathogenic bacteria

The multifaceted nature of severe abdominal infections makes it difficult to precisely define the disease and to assess its severity, and to evaluate and compare therapeutic progress. Both the anatomical source of infection, and to a greater degree, the physiological compromise it inflicts, affects the outcome of the intra-abdominal infection. A classification system including both the anatomical source of the peritoneal infection and its physiological compromise measured using the acute physiological score, a part of the Acute Physiology And Chronic Health Evaluation II (APACHE-II) scoring system, has been proposed [1-6].

The mortality of intra-abdominal infection is related mainly to the severity of the patient's systemic response and his premorbid physiological reserves [34-36]. APACHE-II score, measuring the severity of disease, age and chronic health status of the patient, has been validated prospectively in a large number of patients and has been considered as the best available method of risk stratification. However, examining this stratification system it has been noted that acute physiological score, malnutrition, and age were noteworthy for predicting outcome, whereas etiology of infection contributed only slightly. Furthermore, APACHE-II score was independently associated with the mortality rate: patients treated for abdominal infection with a score up to 20 had a risk of death of about 50% [18].

In secondary peritonitis, the infection is most commonly polymicrobial with an average of four isolates per patient, with the most frequently encountered combination being *Escherichia coli* and *Bacteroides fragilis*. The number and types of bacteria increase progressively down the gastrointestinal tract. Proximally, it contains a sparse aerobe (coliforms) and oral anaerobe flora, with the stomach and duodenum normally sterile. However, diseases of the stomach – such as carcinoma, gastric outlet obstruction – or acid-reducing drugs may result in its colonization [37]. Distally, the colon contains the largest concentration of bacteria: after a colonic perforation, more than 400 different species of bacteria invade the peritoneal cavity, although only a few are involved in the ensuing infection [38].

Postoperative state, administration of systemic and luminal antibiotics, and the invasive environment of the ICU may drastically modify patients' ecology, resulting in colonization of the proximal gastrointestinal tract with peculiar micro-organisms (fungi, coagulase-negative staphylococci and gram-negative bacteria of low pathogenicity). These are the organisms that may be found in tertiary peritonitis, in ICU infections, and in multiple-organ failure [39-42].

The outcome of peritonitis depends on the results of a struggle between the systemic and peritoneal defenses of the patient, on one hand, and the nature, volume and duration of bacterial contamination on the other. The exact events that follow the invasion of the peritoneal cavity with bacteria and adjuvants of infection, such as blood, bile, barium sulfate, and, subsequently, its translymphatic spread, are clearly defined in recent studies [18, 42-44]. The microorganisms and their products stimulate the host's cellular defenses to activate a myriad of inflammatory mediators that are responsible for the sepsis [39, 44].

The understanding of the cytokine-mediated inflammatory response in peritonitis has been increased by recent studies of molecular biology. During peritonitis, cytokines (tumour necrosis factor, interleukin-1, interleukin-6, elastase, and others) are measurable in the systemic circulation and in the peritoneal exudates [15, 45, 46], and the magnitude of the phenomena is negatively correlated with outcome [46]. Bacterial peritonitis appears to induce an intense compartmentalized inflammatory process. The largest part of peritoneal cytokines probably derives from macrophages exposed to endotoxin liberated from infecting bacteria. Other potential sources are direct translocation of cytokines through the intestinal barrier or production by traumatized tissues [17]. The compartmentalization of the cytokine cascades in peritonitis corroborates the concept that circulating concentrations of cytokines may be misleading and not reflect their tissue concentration or biological activity. Local estimation of cytokines in the peritoneal exudate may thus better reflect the severity of an initially local process. Timely therapeutic intervention is crucial to abort the ensuing, self-perpetuating systemic inflammatory response syndrome, before the overproduced mediator nitric oxide completely blocks the Krebs cycle, inflicting advanced injury at the cellular and microvascular level, leading to sequential multiple organ failure and death [47].

Considerable research effort has been directed, in recent years, at elucidating the role of the gastrointestinal tract and its barrier function in the pathogenesis of severe infections [17]. There is accumulating evidence that sepsis and multiple organ failure in critically ill surgical and injured patients are not always the results of an established infected focus, and that a failure of gut barrier function may fuel the systemic component of the SIRS, sepsis and organ failure. In these conditions the bacterial translocation, due to gut failure, has been advocated as the starter of a self-maintaining process for systemic infection and organs failure.

Goals of management of secondary peritonitis are summarized in Table 6. The three fundamental principles of the surgical management of severe secondary peritonitis are the elimination of the source of the infections, the reduction of bacterial contamination of the peritoneal cavity, and the prevention of persistent or recurrent infections. Nevertheless, intensive measures to support tissue oxygenation and maintain organ function are necessary [18].

The operative approach and the surgical strategy depend on the source of the infection, the degree of peritoneal contamination, the clinical condition of the patient, and the concomitant disease. This approach reduced mortality from 90% to approximately 40% [39, 41]. Ideally, a severe intra-abdominal infection should be cured with a single surgical procedure; unfortunately, infection often persists on recurs in cases of severe peritonitis. The second goal of surgical management of severe peritonitis is the reduction of bacterial contamination. All intraperitoneal fluids should be aspirated, and particulate matter should be removed [17].

Despite gradual improvement in intensive care and antimicrobial therapy, it became clear that if the initial standard operation fails, persisting or recurrent

Table 6. Principles for the management of peritonitis due to AT

Supportive measures
A. To combat hypovolemia and shock and maintain adequate tissue oxygenation
B. To treat bacteria, not eliminated by surgery, with antibiotics
C. To support failing organ systems
D. To provide adequate nutrition
Operative treatment
Repair and/or control the source of infection
Evacuate bacterial inoculum, pus, and adjuvants
Treat abdominal compartment syndrome
Prevent or treat persistent and recurrent infection or verify both repair and purge

intra-abdominal infection sometimes is overlooked or the diagnosis is delayed [1-6]. Waiting for the appearance of signs of persisting infection or organ failure as the indication for abdominal re-exploration *on demand* often proved futile. To improve results, two therapeutic concepts have been introduced: open management, so called laparostomy, and planned relaparotomies, in which multiple operative interventions are planned before or during the first procedure for peritonitis, to return to the abdominal cavity to re-explore, evacuate, debride, or resect. Reoperations are performed at fixed intervals, irrespective of clinical condition of the patient, to prevent development of further septic fluid collections, so precluding their systemic effects. Adverse effects of planned relaparotomies are frequent and include damage to abdominal wall structures and intra-peritoneal viscera, causing bleeding or even enteric fistulas.

Open management facilitates frequent re-exploration and, by treating the entire peritoneal cavity as one large infected collection, continuous exposure for maximal drainage. Furthermore, it serves to decompress the high intra-abdominal pressure caused by peritoneal edema associated with inflammation and fluid resuscitation, thus obviating the deleterious systemic consequences of the abdominal compartment syndrome [48]. Early results of these methods were promising, particularly in the management of infected pancreatic necrosis, but were less favorable in cases of postoperative peritonitis. Simple open management was plagued by intestinal fistulas and abdominal wall defects, problems that were almost eliminated by introduction of temporary abdominal closure devices such as the artificial mesh-zipper techniques. Staged abdominal repair as a conceptual operative approach combines the advantages of planned relaparotomy and of open management with a minimal rate of complications. Prospective nonrandomized attempt to compare closed and open techniques did not demonstrate an advantage of the latter. Furthermore, recent series failed to demonstrate the benefits of planned relaparotomies. However, another prospective study showed the staged abdominal repair approach to be superior to conventional operative therapy when patients at equal mortality risk were compared. It has been shown in trauma cases that repeated operations performed in patients in whom the inflammatory response is already active might precipitate multiorgan dysfunction. Besides, these techniques may be beneficial if initiated early, in well-selected patients, for specific indications (Table 7), performed by a team of dedicated surgeons.

Abscess represents a relatively successful outcome of peritonitis. It may be visceral and nonvisceral, extra- or intra-peritoneal. Nonvisceral abscesses arise after resolution of diffuse peritonitis in which a loculated area of suppuration persists, or after a perforation of a viscus that is effectively localized by peritoneal defenses. Percutaneous, US, or CT-guided drainage is the method of

Table 7. Indications for staged abdominal repair

•	Critical patient's condition, such as hemodynamic instability, precluding definitive repair
•	Excessive peritoneal edema, abdominal compartment syndrome, pulmonary, cardiac, renal, or hepatic dysfunction, and decreased visceral perfusion, preventing abdominal closure without under tension
•	Intra-abdominal pressure 15 mmHg
•	Massive abdominal wall loss
•	Impossibility to eliminate or to control the source of infection
•	Incomplete debridement of necrotic tissue
•	Uncertainty of viability of remaining bowel
•	Uncontrolled bleeding (the need for "packing")

choice for single abscesses. Although retrospective studies attribute no lesser mortality or morbidity rates to percutaneous drainage versus surgical drainage [49], the former represents a minimally invasive procedure that can spare the patient the unpleasantness of another open abdominal operation. Furthermore, percutaneous catheter drainage should be considered as the initial therapy for patients with culture-positive peripancreatic fluid collection [50]. Abscesses mutiloculated, associated with tissue necrosis, enteric communication, or tumor require laparotomy. Failure of percutaneous drainage should prompt an urgent operation.

Intra-abdominal compartment syndrome

Massive visceral and/or vascular injury may result in intense intestinal edema and third spacing of fluid. These injuries also may require the placement of intra-abdominal packs for control of hemorrhage to allow for further resuscitation, warming, and correction of coagulopathy prior to definitive therapy. When these events occur, it may not be possible to close the abdominal wall without vastly increasing the intra-abdominal pressure [1, 2, 6].

Intra-abdominal compartment syndrome (IACS) shifts the diaphragm superiorly, increases peak airway pressures, decreases tidal volumes, and compresses the inferior vena cava and renal veins. These effects cause decreased venous return and decreased renal perfusion and create tremendous tension along the abdominal wall repair [1]. Therefore, a number of methods of creating a temporary abdominal wall closure have been developed, including suturing or towel clipping only the skin closed, placing a prosthetic material between the fascial or skin edges to keep the peritoneal contents from eviscerating, and placing an adhesive drape over the entire abdomen separated from the intestines by laparotomy pads.

In patients with closed abdominal walls (primary or with a temporary closure), IACS may be recognized by the above constellation of findings, but can be monitored with a bladder catheter attached to a pressure transducer to monitor bladder pressure as an indicator of intraperitoneal pressure. In general, a bladder pressure exceeding 30 mmHg, when accompanied by the appropriate clinical signs and symptoms, is indication for re-exploration [1, 2]. Experimentally, intra-abdominal pressures of 25 mmHg or more have been associated with significant decreases in abdominal wall and intra-abdominal organ tissue perfusion [2]. The clinical sequelae of IACS may include renal insufficiency or failure, abdominal wound ischemia, and alterations in gastrointestinal mucosal perfusion potentially leading to SIRS and MODS [1, 2, 6, 17].

References

1. Hoyt DB, Coimbra R, Winchell RJ (2001) Management of acute trauma. In: Townsend CM (ed) Sabiston – textbook of surgery, 16th edn. Saunders, Philadelphia, pp 311-344
2. Mackersie RC (2001) Abdominal trauma. In: Norton JA, Bollinger RR, Chang AE, Lowry SF, Mulvihill SJ, Pass HI, Thompson RW (eds) Surgery. Basic science and clinical evidence. Springer, Berlin Heidelberg New York, pp 825-845
3. Abdominal trauma (2000) www.madsci.com/manu/trau_abd.html
4. American College of Surgeons, ACS Committee of trauma (1997) Advanced trauma life support course. Instructor manual, 6th edn
5. American College of Surgeons, ACS (2000) Abdominal trauma algorithm. Bull Am Coll Surg 80: 6
6. Salomone JA III (2000) Abdominal trauma, blunt. www.emedicine.com/emerg/topic1.html
7. Cooper A, Barlow B, DiScala C (1994) Mortality and truncal injury: the pediatric perspective. J Pediatr Surg; 29: 33-38
8. Meyer AA (1998) Death and disability from injury: a global challenge. J Trauma 44: 1-12.
9. Cayten CG, Nassoura ZE (1996) Abdomen. In: Ivatury RR (ed) The textbook of penetrating trauma, 1st edn. Williams and Wilkins, Baltimore, pp 281-299
10. Talton DS, Craig MH, Hauser CJ (1995) Major gastroenteric injuries from blunt trauma. Am Surg 61: 69-73
11. Murray CJ, Lopez AD (1997) Mortality by cause for eight regions of the world: Global Burden of Disease Study. Lancet 349: 1269-1276
12. Akhrass R, Yaffe MB, Brandt CP (1997) Pancreatic trauma: a ten-year multi-institutional experience. Am Surg 63: 598-604
13. Carrillo EH, Platz A, Miller FB, et al (1998) Non-operative management of blunt hepatic trauma. Br J Surg 85: 461-468
14. Stengel D, Bauwens K, Sehouli J, et al (2001) Systematic review and meta-analysis of emergency ultrasonography for blunt abdominal trauma. Br J Surg 88: 901-912
15. Bone RC (1997) Systemic inflammatory response syndrome: a unifying concept of systemic inflammation. In: Fein A, Abraham EM, Balk RA (eds) Sepsis and multiorgan failure. 1st edn. Lippincott, Williams and Wilkins, Baltimore, pp 3-10
16. Dellinger EP (1997) Surgical infections and choice of antibiotics. In: Sabiston DC, Lyerly UK (eds) Sabiston Textbook of Surgery. 15th edn, Philadelphia, WB Saunders Co: 264-280
17. Sganga G, Saene HK van, Brisinda G, Castagneto M (2001) Bacterial translocation. In: Saene HKF van, Sganga G, Silvestri L (eds) Infections in critically ill: an ongoing challange. Springer, Berlin Heidelberg New York, pp 35-45
18. Sganga G, Brisinda G, Castagneto M (2001) Peritonitis: priorities and management strategies.

In:Saene HKF van , Sganga G, Silvestri L (eds) Infections in critically ill: an ongoing challange. Springe, Berlin Heidelberg New York, pp 23-33
19. Branney SW, Moore EE, Cantrill SV (1997) Ultrasound based key clinical pathway reduces the use of hospital resources for the evaluation of blunt abdominal trauma. J Trauma 42: 1086-1090
20. Chiu WC, Cushing BM, Rodriguez A (1997) Abdominal injuries without hemoperitoneum: a potential limitation of focused abdominal sonography for trauma (FAST). J Trauma 42: 617-623
21. Nichols RL (2001) Preventing surgical site infections: a surgeon's perspective. Em Infect Dis 7:220-224
22. Rozycki GS, Ochsner MG, Schmidt JA (1995) A prospective study of surgeon-performed ultrasound as the primary adjuvant modality for injured patient assessment. J Trauma 39: 492-498
23. Rozycki GS, Shackford SR (1996) Ultrasound, what every trauma surgeon should know. J Trauma 40: 1-4
24. Scalea TM, Rodriguez A, Chiu WC, et al (1999) FAST Consensus Conference Committee. Focused assessment with sonography for trauma (FAST): results from an international consensus conference. J Trauma 46: 466-472
25. Akgur FM, Aktug T, Olguner M, et al (1997) Prospective study investigating routine usage of ultrasonography as the initial diagnostic modality for the evaluation of children sustaining blunt abdominal trauma. J Trauma 42: 626-628
26. Hodgson NF, Stewart TC, Girotti MJ (2000) Autopsies and death certification in deaths due to blunt trauma: what are we missing? Can J Surg 43: 130-136
27. Bellows CF, Salomone JP, Nakamura SK (1998) What's black and white and red (read) all over? The bedside interpretation of diagnostic peritoneal lavage fluid. Am Surg 64: 112-118
28. Brandt CP, Priebe PP, Jacobs DG (1995) Potential of laparoscopy to reduce non-therapeutic trauma laparotomies. Am Surg 60: 416-420
29. Mattox KL, Feliciano DV, Moore EE (1999) Trauma, 4th edn. Mc Graw Hill, New York
30. Ivatury RR, Cayton CG (1996) Textbook of penetrating trauma. Lea and Febiger, Philadelphia
31. Sganga G, Brisinda G, Castagneto M (2000) Nosocomial fungal infections in surgical patients: risk factors and treatment. Minerva Anestesiol 66 [Suppl 1]: 71-77
32. Ivatury RR, Simon RJ, Havriliak D (1995) Gastric mucosal pH and oxygen delivery and oxygen consumption indices in the assessment of adequacy of resuscitation after trauma: a prospective, randomized study. J Trauma 39: 128-134
33. File TM Jr, Tan JS (1995) Treatment of skin and soft-tissue infections. Am J Surg 169: 27S-33S
34. Rotstein OD, Meakins JL (1990) Diagnostic and therapeutic challenges of intra-abdominal infections. World J Surg 14: 159-166
35. Rotstein OD, Simmons RL (1994) Peritonitis and intraabdominal abscess. In: Barie PS, Shires GT (eds) Surgical intensive care. Little Brown, London, pp 1043-1063
36. Knaus WA, Draper EA, Wagner DP, Zimmerman JE (1985) APACHE II: a severity of disease classification system. Crit Care Med 13: 818-829
37. Finegold SM (1982) Microflora of the gastrointestinal tract. In Wilson SE, Finegold SM, Williams RA (eds) Intra-abdominal infection. McGraw-Hill, New York, pp 1-22
38. Krepel CJ, Gohr CM, Edmiston CE, Condon RE (1995) Surgical sepsis: constancy of antibiotic susceptibility of causative organisms. Surgery 117: 505-509
39. Bosscha K, Vroonhoven JMV van, Werken C van der (1999) Surgical management of severe secondary peritonitis. Br J Surg 86: 1371-1377
40. Schein M (1992) Management of severe intra-abdominal infection. Surg Annu 24: 47-68
41. Wittmann DH, Schein M, Condon RE (1996) Management of secondary peritonitis. Ann Surg 224: 10-18
42. Marshall JC, Christou NV, Meakins JL (1993) The gastrointestinal tract: the "undrained abscess" of multiple organ failure. Ann Surg 218: 111-119
43. Maddaus MA, Ahrenholz D, Simmons RL (1988) The biology of peritonitis and implications for treatment. Surg Clin North Am 68: 431-433
44. Parrillo JE (1993) Pathogenic mechanisms of septic shock. N Engl J Med 328: 1471-1477

45. Holzheimer RG, Schein M, Wittmann DH (1995) Inflammatory mediators in plasma and peritoneal exudate of patients undergoing staged abdominal repair (STAR) for severe peritonitis. Arch Surg 130: 1314-1320
46. Gabay C, Kushner I (1999) Acute-phase proteins and other systemic responses to inflammation. N Engl J Med 340: 448-454
47. Palmer RM (1993) The discovery of nitric oxide in the vessel wall. Arch Surg 128: 396-401
48. Schein M, Wittmann DH, Aprahamian C, Condon RE (1995) Abdominal compartment syndrome: the physiological and clinical consequences of elevated intra-abdominal pressure. J Am Coll Surg 180: 745-753
49. Levison MA, Zeigler D (1991) Correlation of APACHE II score, drainage technique and outcome in postoperative intra-abdominal abscess. Surg Gynecol Obstet 172: 89-94
50. Baril NB, Ralls PW, Wren SM, et al (2000) Does an infected peripancreatic fluid collection or abscess mandate operation? Ann Surg 231: 361-367

Visceral Trauma: Diagnostic Imaging and Interventional Radiology

F. POZZI MUCELLI

In clinical practice, physical examination is often unreliable in patients who are sedated, intoxicated, paralyzed, have head injures, or otherwise are unable to communicate symptoms. Moreover, intra-abdominal injury in particular can be present in the absence of signs and symptoms in blunt trauma patients. So for an accurate evaluation of the patient with multiple trauma the utilization of diagnostic modalities is often required. Three diagnostic imaging tools are utilized for the evaluation of thoraco-abdominal visceral trauma: standard X-ray plain film, ultrasonography (US), and computed tomography (CT). Furthermore, we must remember that in the last 10 years interventional radiology has been shown to be able to contribute to the treatment of these conditions due to its low invasiveness.

Ultrasonography

US offers the advantages of short time and easy execution and the possibility of performing the study at the patient's bedside or in the emergency department. Another advantage is the relatively widespread availability of US equipment and the absence of biological risks, and so this technique is used extensively and successfully in many trauma centers in Europe and Asia as the screening test of choice [1]. Limitations are dependent on operator experience, the complexity of some of the findings, and the difficulty in performing the examination in the case of bowel gas or in the presence of skin wounds or bands that can limit a correct approach of the transducer.

A technically correct examination of the abdomen must be done with specific attention to the following areas: Morrison's pouch, right kidney and right paracolic gutter, liver, right dome of the diaphragm and right pleural space, left kidney and left paracolic gutter, spleen, left dome of the diaphragm and left pleural space, bladder and pouch of Douglas/rectovesical pouch and retroperitoneal spaces.

The incidence of non-diagnostic US studies has been a matter of investigation by a group of researchers [2], who wanted to evaluate the frequency, causes, associations, and sequelae of indeterminate (IND) sonograms in blunt trauma. Among adult blunt trauma patients assessed with screening sonography, clinician sonographers recorded the abdominal sonogram as positive, negative, or IND for free fluid. Patients with IND sonograms were further investigated with repeat sonography, CT, or diagnostic peritoneal lavage. Among 417 patients with blunt trauma managed with sonography, there were 28 (6.7%) IND and 389 (93.3%) non-IND sonograms. Sonograms were IND because of patient factors in 71% (20 of 28) and because of operator factors in 29% (8 of 28). None of the 28 patients were managed with repeat sonography alone. All 4 diagnostic peritoneal lavage examinations gave negative results, whereas 8 of 23 CT scans were abnormal (6 of 8 patients underwent laparotomy). The mean time required for diagnostic workup was 117 min in the IND group and 48 min in the non-IND group ($P < 0.001$ in both cases).

This prospective study has demonstrated that IND sonograms are not so common (6.7%), are usually attributable to patient factors, and are associated with greater diagnostic time. Patients with IND sonograms require further investigation because they often have injuries requiring laparotomy.

It must be emphasized that this diagnostic modality is extremely operator dependent. This has been investigated by a group from the Trauma Center and Intensive Care Department of the University of Philadelphia [3]. They decided to establish the ability to detect intraperitoneal fluid in a group of patients under peritoneal dialysis (used as model of injured patients) by different sonographic operators (residents, surgeons, radiologists, and ultrasound technicians), with different levels of experience in such diagnosis (< 30 cases, 30-100 cases, >100 cases). The results of this investigation were that the less-experienced operator had an accuracy between 38 and 45%, while the more-experienced operator was able to detect the presence of intraperitoneal fluid in 90-100% of cases. This result underlines the necessity of specific training to optimize the results on the patient.

Other studies have tried to validate the accuracy of US in the evaluation of blunt abdominal trauma patients by evaluating either its direct contribution in the Emergency Care Unit or by comparing the results of US with more-invasive diagnostic procedures such as peritoneal lavage or CT.

Recently some authors [4] have reported the accuracy of abdominal US in blunt trauma patients requiring in-hospital patient treatment. One thousand and ninety patients with blunt abdominal trauma were assessed with focused abdominal US within 30 min of arrival at the hospital. Focused abdominal US results were positive if intra- or retroperitoneal fluid was detected. Patients with negative US results and no other major injuries were observed in the emergency department for 12 h before discharge. Patients who deteriorated clinically after negative initial US underwent repeat US and/or emergency abdominopelvic CT. Patients with positive or indeterminate US results underwent emergency abdominopelvic CT. Nine hundred and seventy-four (89%) patients had negative focused abdominal US results; 8 of these underwent CT; 66 (6%) had positive US results; 4 (0.4%) had false-negative and 19 (1.7%) had false-positive US results. Twenty-seven (2.5%) had indeterminate US results; of these, 5 (18.5%) had positive CT results. One hundred and twenty-four (11.4%) required emergency CT. After indeterminate cases were excluded, focused abdominal US had 94% sensitivity, 98% specificity, 78% positive predictive value, 100% negative predictive value, and 95% accuracy. The conclusions are that focused abdominal US has a high negative predictive value for major abdominal injury in patients with blunt abdominal trauma.

To determine the utility of emergency abdominal sonography for evaluating patients with blunt abdominal trauma, Lentz et al. [5] designed a prospective study in order to compare US with diagnostic peritoneal lavage. Emergency sonography was performed prior to diagnostic peritoneal lavage on 54 acutely injured patients in the resuscitation area. Their results reveal that US has a sensitivity of 87%, a specificity of 100%, and an overall accuracy of 96% for detecting free intraperitoneal fluid. The conclusions are that US is a reliable method for the emergency evaluation of blunt abdominal trauma and can be used in place of diagnostic peritoneal lavage as the initial indicator of significant intraperitoneal injury requiring surgical intervention.

A recently published study [6] presents a prospective analysis performed to determine the relevance of abdominal CT in multiple trauma patients compared with abdominal US. The authors recorded all multiple trauma patients in the emergency room (N = 248) from August 1996 to July 1997 with an evaluation form and performed abdominal CT subsequent to US whenever the patient was hemodynamically stable and not in need of immediate surgery (n = 105). They documented the results of both methods and their impact on acute therapy. In 27 of 105 patients (25.7%), therapy management was influenced by both US or CT; 76 patients (72.4%) showed normal US findings, followed by a CT that showed additional findings with therapeutic relevance in 5 patients (6.6%). Twenty-nine patients (27.6%) showed abnormal US findings. After US, the subsequent CT led to a change in therapy in 12 patients (41.4%). The conclusions of the authors were that if US is normal, additional CT of the abdomen provides information of therapeutic relevance in only a limited number of cases. If US is abnormal, CT will have an important impact on therapy in a high number of patients.

Another study evaluated the contribution of US in the evaluation of trauma patients in comparison with CT. Rose et al. [7] evaluated whether US would affect clinical decision making as determined by abdominal CT scan use in blunt multiple trauma patients. This study used a prospective randomized format in an urban county Emergency Department (ED) with level II trauma center status. Patients were randomized to receive either abdominal US or no US (control) during initial ED resuscitation. The primary outcome variable was use of abdominal CT scan in patients with and without US. Two hundred and eight patients were enrolled. The mean age was 40 ± 18 years, and 62% were men. Mechanism of injury was motor vehicle crash, 56%; automobile versus pedestrian, 18%; motorcycle crash, 16%; falls, 10%; and other, 10%. One hundred and four US and 104 control patients were analyzed. There were no apparent differences between US and control groups in demographics, injury type, or Injury Severity Score. Of 104,52 (54%) of the control group received abdominal CT scans versus 37 of 104 (36%) abdominal CT scans for the US group; mean difference in proportions was 15.9 ($P< 0.01$, 95% confidence interval 2.6-29.1). This trial shows that the routine use of abdominal US in the evaluation of patients with multiple blunt injuries resulted in significantly fewer abdominal CT scans. A larger trial is needed to more clearly define the clinical and financial impact of US in the management of blunt abdominal trauma.

Another aspect to emphasize is the ability of a diagnostic tool to detect parenchymal lesions to abdominal organs. This aspect has been evaluated in a recent study by Brown et al. [8], which investigated the benefit of screening US for parenchymal abnormalities, as well as free fluid during screening abdominal US in patients with blunt trauma. They examined a total of 2,693 patients with blunt trauma who were triaged to a level 1 at a trauma center and underwent screening abdominal US in the resuscitation suite. Examinations were performed by experienced sonographers and included a screen for free intraperitoneal fluid and evaluation of the abdominal organ parenchyma and heart for traumatic injury. Screening US findings were reviewed and compared with findings from autopsy, laparotomy, diagnostic peritoneal lavage, CT, repeated US, cystography, and clinical outcome. Imaging studies of all patients with confirmed or suspected injuries were reviewed to identify those in whom parenchymal findings aided diagnosis. The results of this study reported that 172 patients were found to have evidence of abdominal injury due to blunt trauma on the basis of clinical data, imaging, laparotomy, or autopsy. Forty-four of these patients had no sonographic evidence of hemoperitoneum at the time of initial US. Screening US findings were positive for injury in 19 of 44 patients on the basis of parenchymal findings or small retroperitoneal collections of fluid thought to be indicative of trauma. In the remaining 25 patients, screening

US showed no abnormalities, and injuries were detected by repeat US, subsequent CT, or diagnostic peritoneal lavage performed for suspected occult injury on the basis of clinical parameters. In addition, 47 of 126 injured patients with sonographically detected free fluid had parenchymal findings that helped localize injury. Sixteen of those patients were taken to the operating room on the basis of clinical and sonographic findings without undergoing CT. In conclusion, the inability to show injuries with no hemoperitoneum or with delayed hemoperitoneum is a limitation of US in patients with blunt trauma. In this series, 26% of all patients with documented injuries had no free fluid visible on screening US. Attention to findings other than free fluid allowed detection in 43% of injured patients without sonographic evidence of hemoperitoneum.

Considering the kidney lesions US is not so convincing, especially for minor lesions. McGahan et al. [9] studied 32 patients with 37 renal injuries retrospectively to identify in how many patients the sonogram detected free fluid or a renal parenchymal abnormality. Free fluid in the abdomen was identified in 19 of 32 patients (59%). However, 12 of these 19 patients had concomitant injury, such as splenic rupture requiring splenectomy, severe liver lacerations, or bowel lacerations requiring repair, which were possible causes of the free fluid. Eliminating these patients, only 7 of 20 patients with isolated renal injuries had free fluid in the abdomen (35%), whereas 13 of 20 patients (65%) had no evidence of free fluid. All 7 patients with free fluid had moderate or severe renal injuries. Renal parenchymal abnormalities were identified by US in 8 of 37 (22%) injured kidneys. The abnormalities were detected more commonly in cases of severe injury (60%). In conclusion, acute injuries of the kidney from blunt abdominal trauma are often associated with significant splenic, hepatic, or bowel trauma. Isolated renal injuries frequently occur without the presence of free fluid in the abdomen. Furthermore, US of the kidney often is normal with acute renal injuries, but it is more likely to be abnormal with severe (grade II or greater) renal injuries. Sonography may be used in the triage of patients with blunt abdominal trauma and possible renal injury. However, negative US does not exclude renal injury, and, depending on clinical and laboratory findings, other imaging procedures such as CT should be performed.

In conclusion how precise and reliable is US as a primary tool for injury assessment in blunt abdominal trauma? Stengel et al. [10] recently tried to answer to this question by making a systematic review and meta-analysis of prospective clinical trials of US for blunt abdominal trauma. Publications were retrieved by structured searching among databases, review articles, and major textbooks. Authors and experts in the field were contacted for original and unpublished data. The results were that 13 of 123 trials enrolling 9,047 patients were eligible for final analysis. With respect to targeting organ lesions, US showed a summary Q* value of 0.91; negative predictive values ranged from 0.72 to 0.99. A similar SROC slope was calculated for screening for free fluid [Q* = 0.89 (95% confidence interval 0.73-1.05)]. US detects the presence of organ lesions, but fails to exclude abdominal injuries [random effects negative LR 0.23 (95% confidence interval 0.18-0.28)]. Given a pre-test probability of 50% for blunt abdominal injury, a post-test probability of nearly 25% remains in the case of a negative sonogram. The conclusions were that despite its high specificity, US has an unexpectedly low sensitivity for the detection of both free fluid and organ lesions. In clinically suspected abdominal trauma, another assessment (e.g., helical CT) must be performed, regardless of the initial US findings.

Computed tomography

The introduction of CT to the diagnostic assesment of the trauma patient is broadly accepted; usually factors that limit its utilisation are frequently connected to organization problems (patient transfer, examination length, staff availability) more than to doubts on its real diagnostic efficacy.

Recently some authors have evaluated the contribution of CT in comparison with US in a series of 25 patients with blunt abdominal trauma in a district general hospital [11]. The hospital records of 25 patients who were admitted with blunt abdominal trauma and who had both US and CT of the abdomen within 48 h of admission were reviewed. US missed 7 lesions in 7 patients (7/25, 28%) compared with CT. Three of these were intestinal lesions that needed laparotomy. US had a usefulness index of 1, 0.76, 0.72, 0.69, and 0, respectively, for detecting lesions of the kidneys, free intraperitoneal fluid, the liver, the spleen, and intestines. Although US can be used as an initial screening method for blunt abdominal trauma, CT is still the imaging modality of choice for detecting intra-abdominal lesions for stable patients in a district general hospital.

Not all authors agree on a routine CT evaluation for all abdominal blunt trauma patients and some suggest limiting its use to relevant clinical cases. A prospective cohort study was carried out that compared a protocol using screening diagnostic peritoneal lavage (DPL) followed by selective use of abdominal CT (DPL/abdominal CT) and the use of abdominal CT alone in the evaluation of hemodynamically stable, adult blunt trauma patients [12]. One hundred and sixty-seven adult blunt trauma patients were initially evaluated by DPL (n = 71) or abdominal CT (n = 96). ED evaluation required less time in the DPL/abdominal CT group than in the abdominal CT alone group (41 min vs. 2.5 h; $P < 0.001$). There were no missed injuries in the DPL/abdominal CT group versus 7 missed injuries in the abdominal CT group (P = 0.02). There were no non-therapeutic celiotomies in either study group. The conclusion of this study is that screening DPL, followed by abdominal CT if positive, is a safe, efficient method of evaluating adult blunt abdominal trauma that reduces the time required to evaluate the abdomen, does not result in increased non-therapeutic celiotomies, results in fewer missed injuries, and reduces the overall use of abdominal CT.

The role of CT in diagnosing hollow viscus injury after blunt abdominal trauma remains controversial, with previous studies reporting both high accuracy and poor results. Recently, Killeen et al. [13] performed a study to determine the diagnostic accuracy of helical CT in detecting bowel and mesenteric injuries after blunt abdominal trauma in a large cohort of patients. This study evaluated 150 patients admitted to a level I trauma center over a 4-year period and evaluated with CT scan or surgical diagnosis of bowel or mesenteric injury. CT scan findings were retrospectively graded as negative, non-surgical, or surgical bowel or mesenteric injury. The CT scan diagnosis was then compared with surgical findings, which were also graded as negative, non-surgical, or surgical. CT had an overall sensitivity of 94% in detecting bowel injury and 96% in detecting mesenteric injury. Surgical bowel cases were correctly differentiated in 64 of 74 cases (86%), and surgical mesenteric cases were correctly differentiated from non-surgical in 57 of 76 cases (75%). The conclusions by Killeen et al. [13] were that helical CT scanning is very accurate in detecting bowel and mesenteric injuries, as well as in determining the need for surgical exploration in bowel injuries. However, it is less accurate in predicting the need for surgical exploration in mesenteric injuries alone.

Diagnostic imaging has an extremely important role in the evaluation of the trauma patient, and correct use has lead to a significant reduction of aggressive therapeutic treatments such as splenectomies and nephrectomies. Recently some authors [14] have demonstrated that mandatory laparotomies could be reduced by a correct evaluation of CT images. This recommendation has been based upon retrospective data and concerns over the potential morbidity from the late diagnosis of blunt intestinal injury. This study examined the rate of intestinal injury in patients with free fluid on abdominal CT after blunt abdominal trauma. Data were collected concurrently at the time of patient enrolment and included demographics, Injury Severity Score, findings on CT scan, and presence or absence of blunt intestinal injury. This database was specifically queried for those patients who had free fluid without solid organ injury. Two thousand two hundred and ninety-nine patients were evaluated. Free fluid was present in 265. Of these, 90 patients had isolated free fluid with only 7 having a blunt intestinal injury. Conversely, 91% of patients with free fluid did not. All patients with free fluid were observed for a mean of 8 days (95% confidence interval 6.1 - 10.4, range 1 - 131). There were no missed injuries. In conclusion, free fluid on abdominal CT scan does not mandate celiotomy. Serial observation with the possible use of other adjunctive tests is recommended.

Recently some authors have stated that a closed follow-up of all trauma patients is not systemically necessary, especially in minor splenic lesions, for which a surveillance approach was established. They have shown that imaging follow-up may be useful only when the clinical picture becomes symptomatic [15].

Interventional radiology

This branch of radiology has developed rapidly over the last ten years and many emergencies can be treated with an interventional radiological approach. In this paper we will only discuss endovascular procedures.

Abdominal trauma can be complicated by vascular lesions such as rupture with bleeding or with the formation of pseudoaneurysm of visceral branches that in their evolution can rupture and cause massive hemorrhage. The endovascular approach to these lesions is to close the damaged vessel making an embolization. This treatment can be done with embolizing agents and covered stents.

Embolizing agents can be solid or liquid agents. Coils are the more frequently used embolic materials in this clinical setting. Coils are short metallic and memory-shaped fragments; sometimes coils also have Dacron filaments to increase thrombogenicity. Coils can be accurately deployed in the targeted artery district by means of an angiographic catheter (in the case of 0.035-0.038 inch coils) or by a microcatheter (0.014-0.018 inch microcoils). When the coil escapes from the catheter, it resumes its tridimensional conformation in the lumen vessel (memory). The diameter of the coil must be defined by the diameter of the vessel to be occluded.

Liquid embolic agents are limited to hemodynamic crises. The more-efficient agent is acrylic glue. This glue must be diluted with a oleous contrast media, the lipiodol and the solution has to be injected with a catheter or a microcatheter into the target vessel. When the solution comes out from the catheter it immediately becomes solid. The catheter must be quickly retracted in order to avoid its adhesion to the vessel wall.

Another option is the covered stent, which can have a role in the treatment of pseudoaneurysmatic lesions. This stent differs from conventional uncovered stent in the presence of a Dacron or PTFE material, which covers the struts of the stent. The limitations of this material are the stiffness of the stent and the difficulty of using it in tortuous vessels.

Embolization treatment in abdominal hemorrhagic visceral injury can be done in three different clinical pictures: acute bleeding, recurrent bleeding, and risk of bleeding. The first situation is the more difficult to treat for the interventional radiologist, because often the severity of the clinical symptoms leaves a very short time for the preparation of the patient and the operator and for the execution of the procedure. The aim is to detect the site of the bleeding and whenever possible to stop the hemorrhage with embolic material. Angiography is able to detect active gastrointestinal bleeding if the blood loss is of about 0.5 ml/min; diagnostic accuracy of angiography in this situation is 71% in the acute form and of 55% in the chronic form.

The therapeutic success of vascular embolization, in a review of different studies [16, 17], is about 90%. More-frequent causes of intestinal haemorrhage are tumors (25%), while the incidence of trauma is about 12% [18].

References

1. Bode PJ, Edwards MJR, Kruit MC, et al (1999) Sonography in a clinical algorithm for early evaluation of 1671 patients with blunt abdominal trauma. AJR 172: 905-911
2. Boulanger BR, Brenneman FD, Kirkpatrick AW, et al (1998) The indeterminate abdominal sonogram in multisystem blunt trauma. J Trauma 45: 52-56
3. Gracias VH, Frankel HL, Gupta R, et al (2001) Defining the learning curve for the focused abdominal sonogram for trauma (FAST) examination: implications for credentialing. Am Surg 67: 364-368
4. Lingawi SS, Buckley AR (2000) Focused abdominal US in patients with trauma. Radiology 217: 426-429
5. Lentz KA, McKenney MG, Nunez DB Jr, Martin L (1996) Evaluating blunt abdominal trauma: role for ultrasonography. J Ultrasound Med 15: 447-451
6. Buhne KH, Zugel N, Mayr E, Haser H (2001) Routine use of abdominal ultrasound and epigastric CT in polytrauma. Analysis of therapeutic relevance in 105 patients. Chirurg 72: 43-48
7. Rose JS, Levitt MA, Porter J, et al (2001) Does the presence of ultrasound really affect computed tomographic scan use? A prospective randomized trial of ultrasound in trauma. J Trauma 51: 545-550
8. Brown MA, Casola G, Sirlin CB, et al (2001) Importance of evaluating organ parenchyma during screening abdominal ultrasonography after blunt trauma. J Ultrasound Med 20: 577-583
9. McGahan JP, Richards JR, Jones CD, et al (1999) Use of ultrasonography in the patient with acute renal trauma. J Ultrasound Med 18: 207-213
10. Stengel D, Bauwens K, Sehouli J, et al (2001) Systematic review and meta-analysis of emergency ultrasonography for blunt abdominal trauma. Br J Surg 88: 901-912
11. Abu-Zidan FM, Sheikh M, Jadallah F, Windsor JA (1999) Blunt abdominal trauma: comparison of ultrasonography and computed tomography in a district general hospital. Australas Radiol 43: 440-443
12. Mele TS, Stewart K, Marokus B, et al (1999) Evaluation of a diagnostic protocol using screening diagnostic peritoneal lavage with selective use of abdominal computed tomography in blunt abdominal trauma. J Trauma 46: 847-852
13. Killeen KL, Shanmuganathan K, Poletti PA, et al (2001) Helical computed tomography of bowel and mesenteric injuries. J Trauma 51: 26-36

14. Livingston DH, Lavery RF, Passannantr MR, et al (2001) Free fluid on abdominal computed tomography without solid organ injury after blunt abdominal injury does not mandate celiotomy. Am J Surg 182: 6-9
15. Uecker J, Pickett C, Dunn E (2001) The role of follow-up radiographic studies in non operative management of spleen trauma. Am Surg 67: 22-25
16. Gordon RL, Ahl KL, Kerlan LK, et al (1997) Selective arterial embolization for the control of lower gastrointestinal bleeding. Am J Surg 174: 24-28
17. Mannella P, Galeotti R (1996) Gli insulti vascolari: l'approccio interventistico. In: Corso monotematico, emergenze addomino-pelviche. XXXVII Congresso Nazionale SIRM, Milano, Grafiche RB, Falconara Marittima, pp 91-97
18. Simonetti G, Rossi P, Passariello R, et al (1986) Valore diagnostico e terapeutico dell'angiografia nel distretto mesenterico. Radiol Med 72: 439-461

Trauma Operative Procedures: Timing of Surgery and Priorities

G. SGANGA, G. BRISINDA, M. CASTAGNETO

Abdominal trauma (AT) remains a leading cause of morbidity and mortality among all age groups. Its true frequency is unknown, as is the incidence of out-of-hospital deaths [1, 2]. Moreover, it has been noted that AT occurs in approximately 25% of major trauma victims, and often involves multiple organ injuries. These involving head and/or thoracic injuries are common, and may complicate AT management [1-8].

The most-common reasons for death in trauma patients are head injury, *exsanguination*, and *multiple organ failure* (MOF) [1-9]. Metabolic derangements during initial operative and resuscitation efforts have been recognized as an equally challenging cause of death in patients with AT. During the past decade, a new surgical approach to patients with devastating AT has emerged. Based on a modified operative sequence using rapid lifesaving techniques – damage control surgery (DCS) is currently the most-common term to describe staged surgery [10-12] – definitive resection and reconstruction are delayed until the patient can be adequately resuscitated and stabilized in the intensive care unit (ICU). This new and innovative surgical strategy requires interdisciplinary collaboration and an understanding of the DCS process, ICU care, and possible complications. This paper reviews the historical perspectives, surgical approach, and complications of DCS.

Historical perspective

Since the 1980s, surgeons have made every attempt to continue aggressive surgical intervention until complex surgical problems were completely resolved. Trauma centers used extreme measures such as extracorporeal support, extensive resections and reconstructions, and aggressive fluid and blood product replacement, and surgeons were able to continue operating until serious metabolic derangements developed, most often characterized as the trauma triad of death: hypothermia, coagulopathy, and acidosis.

Often, the patient survived the initial operation but died in ICU from continued hemorrhage or MOF. During the 1980s, civilian multivisceral trauma increased, and this extensive trauma frequently required lengthy and complex repairs, with bleeding often difficult to control. Traditional operative sequence did not achieve the desired level of success, and other methods to decrease morbidity and mortality were explored [10, 11]. The technique of abdominal packing with planned re-operation was first described in the early 1900s as perihepatic packing [13, 14]. Furthermore, surgeons turned attention to the military model, in which a staged approach to complex injury was thought to be the most-effective way to manage multiple patients during warfare. A similar protocol is used for hemorrhage control and stopping enteric spillage. This concept was further developed during World War II [10]. However, in this era perihepatic packing fell into disfavor because of reports of hemorrhage, sepsis, and hepatic necrosis [15].

In 1981 Feliciano et al.[16] reported the survival in nine of ten patients who underwent temporary laparotomy pad tamponade for hepatic injuries. Moreover, staged laparotomy approach was extended to nonhepatic abdominal injuries, and abdominal packing followed by rapid abdominal closure was used for treatment of severe coagulopathy [17, 18]. One benefit of rapid abdominal closure is the prevention of hypothermia and further heat loss, rather than the tamponade effect caused by early closure [15]. The modern DCS concept with abbreviated laparotomy and planned re-operation allows for interruption of the vicious cycle of the trauma triad of death.

Damage control surgery

DCS is one of the major advances in surgical technique in the past 20 years. Moreover, DCS principles have been slow to be accepted by surgeons. However it is now well recognized that multiple trauma patients are more likely to die from their intraoperative metabolic failure rather than from a failure following complete operative repairs. Patients with major exsanguinating injuries will not survive complex procedures such as hepatectomy or duodenopancreatectomy.

The central tenet of DCS is that patients die from a triad of coagulopathy, hypothermia, and metabolic acidosis. Once this metabolic failure has become established it is extremely difficult to control hemorrhage and correct the derangements. If the patient is to survive the operation must be foreshortened so that they can be transferred to ICU where they can be warmed and the hypothermia and acidosis corrected. Once this is achieved the definitive surgical procedure can be carried out as necessary. Then, principles of DCS procedure are control of hemorrhage, prevention of contamination and protection from further injury. There is no margin for error and no place for careless surgery. DCS can be thought of in three distinct phases: initial laparotomy, resuscitation phase, and definitive operation (Fig. 1).

In these patients, pre-hospital and emergency department times should be minimized. All unnecessary and superfluous investigations that will not immediately affect patient management should be deferred. Cyclic fluid resuscitation prior to surgery is futile and will worsen hypothermia and coagulopathy. Colloid solutions will also interfere with clot quality. These patients should be transferred rapidly to the operating room (OR) without repeated attempts to restore circulating volume [1]. They require operative control of hemorrhage and simultaneous vigorous resuscitation with blood and clotting factors.

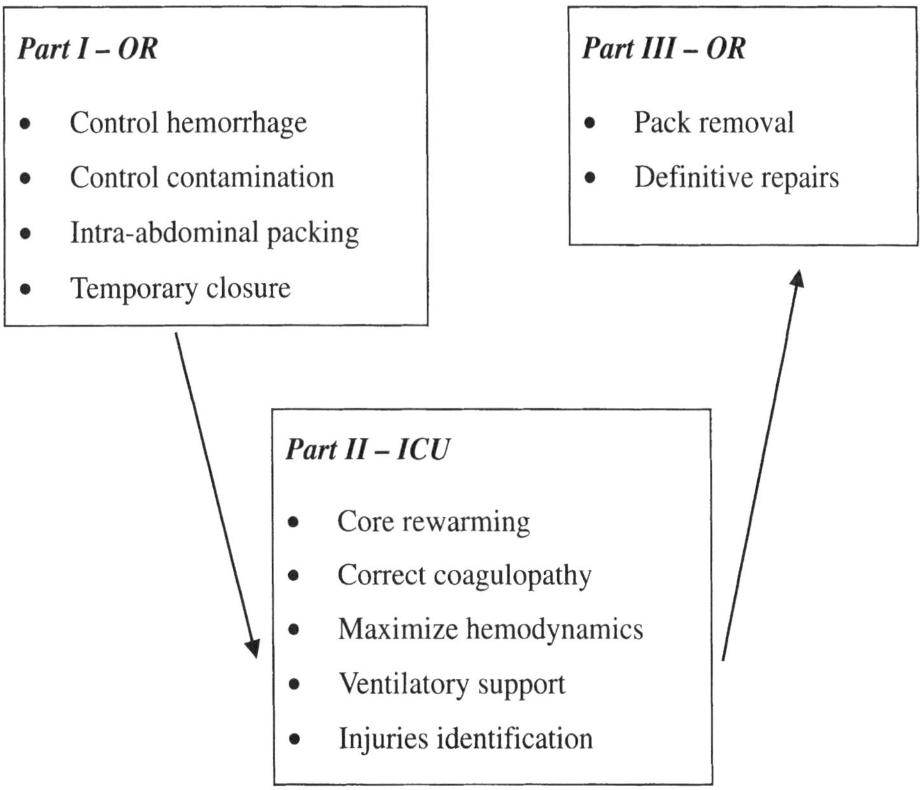

Fig. 1. Three phases of damage control surgery (OR= operating room, ICU= intensive care unit)

Initial laparotomy

The decision to abbreviate the initial surgery for critical injury should ideally be made within the first 15 min of the operation, but this rarely occurs outside the setting of an experienced trauma team that frequently performs DCS [19]. Operative situations that lead the surgeon to choose an abbreviated laparotomy include: the exsanguinating patient with hypothermia and coagulopathy who is hemodynamically unstable, inability to control bleeding by direct hemostasis, and inability to close the abdomen or chest formally without tension because of massive visceral edema [1, 2, 20]. Relative indications for DCS include inconclusive surgical procedures and need to treat other extra-abdominal life-threatening injuries. Preliminary data suggest that this approach to severe and multiple abdominal injuries may improve outcome. Timing for planned re-operations is generally based on the correction of coagulopathy and metabolic derangements and the specific injuries left incompletely treated.

Following preliminary control of severe hemorrhage, several maneuvers may be necessary to completely define all significant injuries (Table 1). The principal technical objective for abdominal exploration for AT is to carefully examines the path of the stab or gunshot wound until:

- (A) the tract is completely defined and all injuries treated,
- or (B) the wound tract is found to pass beyond any vital structures,
- or (C) all structures possibly subject to injury are completely evaluated.

This approach, so-called *trace-the-track*, coupled with a systematic evaluation of all intra-peritoneal and retroperitoneal structures is critical to avoid missed intra-abdominal injuries.

Exclusion criteria for DCS are less well defined. Morris et al. [21] identified three categories of trauma patients who were unsalvageable and therefore ineligible for staged abdominal surgery: aged 70 years or more, fatal closed head injuries, and pre-hospital cardiac arrest after blunt trauma. However, elderly patients are more likely to benefit from staged surgery because of increased sensitivity to physiological instability.

Because no comparative studies have been performed, the choice of temporary closure techniques is left to institutional preference. The towel-clip closure can be performed quickly and is easily reversible in the ICU if necessary. Often, the increased capillary permeability of traumatic shock and concurrent fluid resuscitation produce massive visceral edema. If extensive edema is present, a temporary silo is fashioned from the Bogota bag to cover abdominal wounds [1, 2, 10, 11, 22]. Because there is often considerable fluid loss from the abdominal wound before the definitive closure, closed suction drains under an adhesive drape to allow for fluid collection and protection of the surrounding skin may be used. Advantages of the plastic bag include low cost, availability,

Table 1. Considerations in the operative management of major and severe abdominal trauma (AT)

Incision	Midline for virtually all injuries
Control of severe hypotension	Proximal aortic control may be needed. Options include thoracotomy *vs.* abdominal approach
Initial maneuvers	Pack control for haemorrhage (all 4 quadrants) Immediate solid organ assessment (blunt AT) Immediate assessment of proximal mesentery and retroperitoneum for major vascular injury (penetrating AT)
Exploratory maneuvers	Mobilization of right and left colon and organ block Mobilization of the spleen and pancreatic tail *Kocherisation* of duodenum and pancreatic head Lesser sac exploration Mobilization of the right and left triangular ligaments and falciform ligament Proximal control of renal vessels followed by mobilization of the kidney
Hepatic injuries	Control of hemorrhage and control/containment of biliary drainage Packing. Inflow occlusion. Hepatic mobilization. Sternotomy extension for exposure. Hepatic isolation, including aortic clamp or atrial-caval shunt. Simple hepatorraphy. Packing with planned return to OR. Hepatic artery ligation for selected injuries. Resectional debridement if necessary
Splenic injuries	Control of hemorrhage and preservation of splenic function if possible Complete mobilization of spleen. Proximal hilar control. Splenectomy. Splenorrhaphy: suture, wrapping, partial splenectomy
Pancreatic injuries	Control of associated hemorrhage and exocrine secretions. Complete exposure of area of suspected injury. Assessment of major pancreatic duct injury. Drainage only. Distal resection. Drainage only *vs.* duodenopancreatectomy for severe injuries to pancreatic head
Duodenal injuries	Control of associated hemorrhage. Control of gastrointestinal secretions with reestablishment of duodenal continuity. Suture line durability. Complete mobilization of duodenum (Kocher and ligament of Treitz). Simple repair. Jordan modified diversion. Roux-en-Y jejunoduodenostomy. Resection for combined pancreatic head injury
Colorectal injuries	Reestablishment of gastrointestinal continuity. Prevention of large bowel-related septic complications. Complete mobilization of the involved region of large bowel. Flexible sigmoidoscopy for rectal evaluation. Primary repair for most penetrating large bowel injuries. Diversion and repair/resection reserved for more-severe combined injuries and for rectal injuries

and transparency, which allows the team to assess and monitor for ongoing hemorrhage, necrosis, or uncontrolled leak from the gastrointestinal tract.

Abdominal packing may be used before closure of the abdomen, with laparotomy pads or rolled mesh gauze used to control slow venous bleeding. The hemorrhage is best controlled with placement of packing both above and below the injury, achieving compression from both sides [20]. Difficulties of this technique are that packing may fail to stop the bleeding because of incomplete tamponade or arterial bleeding, and overpacking may cause increased intra-abdominal pressure [20]. Furthermore, balloon catheter tamponade with a Foley catheter or Blakemore tube may be used when sites of bleeding are inaccessible; catheter is then brought through the closure and may be successfully removed in ICU without the need for reoperation [1, 2, 20]. In these patients, when bleeding sites are operatively inaccessible, angiographic embolization may be also helpful.

Resuscitation phase

The challenges facing the interdisciplinary team after the patient's return to the ICU include ongoing resuscitation and frequent reassessment. Primary goals of the resuscitation phase are immediate resuscitation and prevention of the onset of the trauma triad of death: hypothermia, coagulopathy, and acidosis. These derangements become established quickly in the exsanguinating trauma patient and, once established, form a vicious circle that may be impossible to overcome. This in critically ill patients is rapidly fatal if uninterrupted. Thus, rewarming, correction of coagulopathy and acidosis, and optimizing pulmonary functioning are the primary concerns of the resuscitation phase.

Hypothermia

The majority of major trauma patients are hypothermic on arrival in the emergency department due to environmental conditions at the scene. Inadequate protection, intravenous fluid administration, and ongoing blood loss will worsen the hypothermic state. Hemorrhagic shock leads to decreased cellular perfusion and oxygenation and so inadequate heat production. Hypothermia has dramatic systemic effects on the body's functions, but most importantly in this context exacerbates coagulopathy and interferes with blood homeostatic mechanisms.

The major immediate concern after DCS is the correction of hypothermia by extensive rewarming techniques. Heat loss during major trauma laparotomy may be as high as 4.6°C per hour despite aggressive attempts to limit heat loss [19]. Hypothermia, or core temperatures less than 35°C, can affect all systems of the body. Of primary concern in the trauma patient are platelet dysfunction and disruption of the coagulation cascade. Despite aggressive replacement of clotting factors and platelets, normal coagulation may not occur until the core temperature exceeds 34°C [23].

Acidosis

Uncorrected hemorrhagic shock will lead to inadequate cellular perfusion, anaerobic metabolism and the production of lactic acid. This leads to severe *metabolic acidosis,* which also interferes with blood clotting mechanisms, and promotes coagulopathy and blood loss. Persistent metabolic acidosis is generally a sign of hypoperfusion and the need for ongoing volume resuscitation. The goal of resuscitation is adequate oxygen delivery, which is achieved by maximizing cardiac output and ensuring adequate oxygen carrying capacity, with a hematocrit higher than 21%, or slightly higher in patients with coronary artery disease. Packed red blood cells, platelets, and fresh-frozen plasma are administered in addition to crystalloids. Use of inotropic support may be considered, but should be used only after the patient does not respond adequately to volume and hemoglobin loading [24]. Use of sodium bicarbonate to achieve a pH of less than 7.2 is standard at some institutions [15]. Response to therapy is monitored closely by observing vital signs, urine output, arterial pH, serum lactate levels, and correction of coagulopathy [24].

Coagulopathy

Hypothermia, acidosis, and the consequences of massive blood transfusion all lead to the development of a *coagulopathy.* Even if control of mechanical bleeding is achievable, patients may continue to bleed from all cut surfaces. This leads to a worsening of hemorrhagic shock and so a worsening of hypothermia and acidosis, prolonging the vicious cycle.

Some studies have attempted to place threshold levels on these parameters. Some state that conversion to DCS should take place if the pH is below 7.2, core temperature is below 32°C, or the patient has received more than one blood volume transfusion. However, once these levels are reached, it is already too late.

The trauma surgeon must make the decision to convert to a limited procedure within 5 min of starting the operative procedure. This decision is made on the initial physiological state of the patient and the rapid initial assessment of internal injuries. This early decision is imperative to the patient's survival.

In most patients who continue to bleed, the bleeding is obvious in the first hours after the initial laparotomy. Coagulopathy in postoperative patients who have received massive transfusions may be caused by a variety of factors. The most-common cause of coagulopathic bleeding in the trauma patient after massive transfusion is thrombocytopenia. Large volumes of crystalloids and packed red blood cells contribute to coagulopathy by diluting coagulation proteins. A supraceliac cross-clamp time longer than 30 min may cause hepatic dysfunction, and severe brain injury may cause primary fibrinolysis. Ischemic tissue necrosis may cause disseminated intravascular coagulation when major arterial trunks have been ligated [25]. Rewarming the patient is also essential in reversing coagulopathy.

Patients returning to the ICU after DCS are maintained on mechanical ventilation. Goals are to achieve adequate oxygen saturation. Pulmonary artery catheter is used to monitor physiological parameters so that oxygen delivery is maximized. Volume is administered to achieve a pulmonary capillary wedge pressure of more than 15 mmHg.

Definitive operation

Returning a patient to OR after DCS may be planned or more emergent and unplanned and is frequently dictated by clinical circumstances. Ideally, transfer of the patient back to the OR is a well-coordinated, planned event after the patient is hemodynamically stable and normothermic, without coagulopathy.

The indications for planned return to the OR include removal of packing, closure of the chest or abdomen, assessment of viability of and debridement of ischemic or necrotic tissue, and treatment of other injuries previously left untreated. There is no consensus on the timing of re-operation, because physiological endpoints and timing of increased infection from packing are not well defined. Generally, the patient is metabolically prepared to return to the OR by 24 h, with most series reporting re-operation within 18-48 h [21, 25-28]. Early re-operation allows for reduction in local inflammation, which may result in systemic inflammatory response syndrome [15].

Early closure of the wound also allows for early mobilization, which is essential for decreasing pulmonary complications and pressure ulcers and for facilitating rehabilitation efforts. Nutritional needs must be determined, and placement of enteral feeding access may be considered during re-operation. The planned re-operation generally consists of unpacking, new exploration, reconstruction, and definitive abdominal closure. Some patients, because of fascial retraction or abdominal wall loss from infection or trauma, are not candidates for a definitive closure at this time, and a delayed closure may be appropriate. Skin closure with planned fascial reconstruction at a later date may be considered.

When skin closure is still not possible, an absorbable mesh may be sutured to the fascia if sufficient omentum exists to protect the underlying viscera. The mesh is kept moist with normal saline and gauze, and the skin margins are closed gradually over several days using tension devices. In the infected abdomen or an abdomen with a continued gastrointestinal leak, gauze packing with frequent dressing changes is used until the granulation bed matures to allow for skin grafting [15, 22, 25].

Organ-specific techniques

Liver

The liver is the most commonly injured organ after both penetrating and blunt AT [1-8, 29-39]. The variable nature of injuries is the main reason for the several operative alternatives adopted. Currently, *hepatic injuries,* graded according to size, location, and involvement of vascular structures (Table 2), are best described using the classification of the Organ Injury Scaling Committee of the American Association for the Surgery of Trauma (AAST).

Basic DCS technique to control hepatic hemorrhage is perihepatic packing [29-35]. When properly performed, this maneuver will arrest most hemorrhage except for major arterial bleeding. These may be partially controlled by Pringle's maneuver. Further vascular isolation (inferior vena cava above and below the liver) may be hazardous and is generally unnecessary in DCS setting. Full hepatic mobilisation and extension into the chest either through a median sternotomy or left thoracotomy may be required to achieve this [34].

Liver parenchyma can be compressed manually initially, followed by ordered packing. To adequately pack the liver requires compression in the antero -posterior plane. This can only be achieved by mobilization of the right hepatic

Table 2. Liver organ injury scale of American Association for the Surgery of Trauma (AAST)

Grade [a]		**Injury description**
I	Hematoma	Subcapsular, < 10% surface area
	Laceration	Capsular tear, < 1 cm parenchymal depth
II	Hematoma	Subcapsular, 10-50% surface area
		Intraparenchymal, < 10 cm diameter
	Laceration	1-3 cm parenchymal depth, 10 cm length
III	Hematoma	Subcapsular, > 50% surface area or expanding. Ruptured subcapsular or parenchymal hematoma
		Intraparenchymal hematoma > 10 cm or expanding
	Laceration	> 3 cm parenchymal depth
IV	Laceration	Parenchymal disruption involving 25-75% of hepatic lobe or 1-3 Coinaud's segments in a single lobe
V	Laceration	Parenchymal disruption involving > 75% of hepatic lobe or 3 Coinaud's segments within a single lobe
	Vascular	Juxtahepatic venous injuries (retrohepatic vena cava, central major hepatic veins)
VI	Vascular	Hepatic avulsion

[a] Advance one grade for multiple injuries to same organ up to grade III

ligament and systematic placement of packs posterior and anterior to this, as well as one or two in the hepatorenal space. Even retrohepatic venous and inferior vena cava injuries may be controlled in this manner.

Only major arterial bleeds from the parenchyma will require further attention. In this case the injury can be extended using a finger-fracture technique and the bleeding vessels identified and tied or clipped. In some cases, where the injury is not deep and easily accessible, rapid debridement may be possible by placing large clamps along the wound edges, with suture to include the entire raw surface. Furthermore, patients who undergo hepatic packing should be transferred to the angiography suite immediately after the operation to identify any ongoing arterial hemorrhage, which may be controlled with selective embolisation.

Substantial experience with nonoperative management of hepatic injuries has now been accumulated over the past years. The results of this approach are reported in Table 3.

Table 3. Selected clinical experiences with nonoperative management of blunt hepatic trauma.

Author		No. of patients	Results/conclusions
Mirvis et al. [29]	1989	37	83.7% (31 patients) successfully treated nonoperatively. 4 other patients had findings at laparotomy that required no further surgery CT-based grading system was useful in predicting outcome
Hiatt et al. [30]	1990	68	16 patients successfully managed nonoperatively. 2 patients received non-therapeutic laparotomy
Federico et al. [31]	1990	56	16 patients managed nonoperatively. No delayed laparotomies or deaths. 50% required transfusion not exceeding 3 units. Amount of fluid in abdomen did not predict failure of treatment
Hollands and Little [32]	1991	nr	Patients managed nonoperatively were less likely to be in shock, had less severe CT grade of injury, younger in age. Cardiovascular status and abdominal exam, not CT grade of injury, are basis to determine nonoperative management. 30% of the patients in the operative group had non-therapeutic laparotomy
Bynoe et al. [33]	1992	26	All patients managed nonoperatively. 5 patients (19%) developed complications: 2 bowel leaks, 3 subcapsular hematomas
Pachter et al. [34]	1992	404	Mortality was 7%; 0.4% mortality due to hepatic injuries. Complication rate was 5%. 0.7% failure rate (surgery required for haemorrhage), mostly in grades IV and V injuries. Nonoperative management of liver injury is successful in 98.5% without excessive transfusion. Missed hollow viscus injuries in 0.5% of the patients. Hemodynamic instability mandates operative intervention
Meredith et al. [35]	1994	72	70 patients were successfully managed nonoperatively; 2 patients explored had non-therapeutic laparotomy. Grade of injury did not predict need for surgery. No missed bowel or retroperitoneal injuries.
Boone et al. [36]	1995	66	70% successfully managed nonoperatively. 91% of Grade V injuries required surgery
Croce et al. [37]	1995	112	5% failure related to liver injuries. 6% failure from nonhepatic source
Brasel et al. [38]	1997	50	4% failure rate. Transfusion 11.3 vs. 2.7 in operative and nonoperative groups, respectively

nr: Not reported.

Liver trauma may complicate acutely or belatedly as hemobilia [40]. This is one of the more commonly reported causes of obscure gastrointestinal hemorrhage. Origins of hemobilia may be diverse and include the cystic artery, anomalous hepatic artery, and hepatic artery to portal vein fistula [41]. Following ultrasonography, the best diagnostic option is angiography rather than CT scan. Recently, the value of a nonoperative approach to the management of hemobilia by means of interventional radiological therapy has been documented [40]. This approach was invariably beneficial and had an impressive therapeutic success rate (hemobilia successfully controlled by angiographic embolisation in all 23 patients with liver trauma studied) coupled with a negligible morbidity and mortality rate (one death from fulminant hepatic sepsis). Surgery could be reserved for patients who cannot be managed radiologically.

Spleen

These injuries are potentially life-threatening following major AT, and are an important cause of potentially preventable morbidity and mortality [1-6]. *Splenic injuries* are typically described by grade (Table 4).

Splenorrhaphy is generally performed for active splenic hemorrhage and may be accomplished through a variety of technical means, including simple or pledgeted suture, or absorbable mesh wrap, or through the use of topical hemostatic agents [42-50]. The results with this technique have been good, with a low incidence of re-operation and an estimated 70% to 90% intraoperative success rate. Appropriately performed, the re-operative rate for post-splenor-

Table 4. Splenic injury scale of AAST

Grade [a]		Injury description
I	Hematoma	Subcapsular, < 10% surface area
	Laceration	Capsular tear, < 1 cm parenchymal depth
II	Hematoma	Subcapsular, 10-50% surface area Intraparenchymal, < 5 cm diameter
	Laceration	1-3 cm parenchymal depth not involving a parenchymal vessel
III	Hematoma	Subcapsular, > 50% surface area or expanding. Ruptured subcapsular or parenchymal hematoma. Intraparenchymal hematoma > 5 cm Laceration > 3 cm parenchymal depth or involving trabecular vessels
IV	Laceration	Laceration of segmental or hilar vessels producing major devascularization (> 25% of spleen)
V	Laceration	Completely shattered spleen
	Vascular	Hilar vascular injury which devascularized spleen

[a] Advance one grade for multiple injuries to same organ up to grade III

rhaphy hemorrhage should be less than 3%. Although more time consuming, the rationale for splenorrhaphy is related to the observation that splenectomy for trauma compromise immune function and has been associated with a higher incidence of postoperative septic complications [49-55].

In more recent years, the nonoperative management of blunt splenic injuries, practice once confined almost exclusively to children, has been extended to adult patients [5, 42-55]. In several cases, this is the treatment modality of choice in hemodynamically stable patients (Table 5). It is associated with a low overall morbidity and mortality, and does not results in increases in length of stay, need for blood transfusions, and bleeding complications compared with operative management. Patients to be considered candidates for nonoperative management should generally meet the following conditions: (A) no evidence of hypovolemic shock, persistent or recurrent splenic haemorrhage, massive haemoperitoneum or grade V injury; (B) no need for transfusion requirements as the result of splenic trauma; (C) no evidence of active extravasation or splenic vascular injury seen on CT scan; (D) no other indications for laparotomy; (E) age less than 55 years; and (F) no exacerbating factors such as portal hypertension or coagulopathy.

Table 5. Selected clinical experiences with nonoperative management of blunt splenic injuries

Author	No. of patients	Results/conclusions
Malagoni et al. 1984 [42]	77	70% failure rate for observed patients
Bitseff and Adkins 1984 [43]	154	30 managed nonoperatively. 70% failure rate for observed patients. 18 required splenectomy
Mahon and Sutton 1985 [44]	76	11 patients managed nonoperatively. 73% failure rate for observed patients. All required splenectomy
Tom et al. 1985 [45]	53	19 managed nonoperatively. 11% failure rate for observed patients. 2 required splenectomy
Cogbill et al. 1989 [46]	832	112 managed nonoperatively. Nonoperative failure rate: 2% in children, 17% in adults
Elmore et al. 1989 [47]	143	47 managed nonoperatively. 13% failure rate for observed patients. All required splenectomy
Longo et al. 1989 [48]	252	60 patients managed nonoperatively. 8% failure rate for observed patients
Pachter et al. 1990 [49]	193	26 managed nonoperatively. 10% failure rate for observed patients
Koury et al. 1991 [50]	91	23 managed nonoperatively. 9% failure rate for observed patients. All required splenectomy
Schurr et al. 1995 [51]	309	89 nonoperative patients. 67% failure rate for observed patients
Godley et al. 1996 [52]	135	11 patients over 55 years managed nonoperatively. 91% failure rate in this group
Wasvary et al. 1997 [53]	40	26 nonoperative patients. 15% failure rate for observed patients. All required splenectomy
Cocanour et al. 1998 [54]	280	87 nonoperative patients. 6% failure rate for observed patients 3% required splenectomy. 3% treated with embolization.
Davis et al. 1998 [55]	524	344 nonoperative patients. 6% failed nonoperative management with embolization

Pancreas and duodenum

Because of the protected anatomical location, the incidence of significant *injuries to pancreas and duodenum* is relatively low, typically between 3% and 8% [1, 2]. These injuries often occur in conjunction with other abdominal or extra-abdominal injuries [1]. Therapeutic goal with respect to the pancreas is the need to control exocrine secretions in the setting of glandular or ductal disruption and the prevention of secondary hemorrhage or septic complications [56-67].

The specific treatment of pancreatic injuries depends primarily on two factors: (A) presence of injury of the main pancreatic duct; and (B) anatomical location of the injury (Table 6). The results of clinical experience with the operative management of pancreatic and duodenal injuries are reported in Table 7.

Table 6. Pancreas injury scale of AAST

Grade[a]		Injury description
I	Hematoma	Minor contusion without duct injury
	Laceration	Superficial laceration without duct injury
II	Hematoma	Major contusion without duct injury or tissue loss
	Laceration	Major laceration without duct injury or tissue loss
III	Laceration	Distal transection or parenchymal injury with duct injury
IV	Laceration	Proximal transection or parenchymal injury involving ampulla
V	Laceration	Massive disruption of pancreatic head

[a]Advance one grade for multiple injuries to same organ up to grade III
Proximal pancreas is to the right of the superior mesenteric vein

Insufficient data exist allowing the formulation of optimal treatment for injuries at the pancreatic head [60-67]. Patients may suffer from higher complication rates because of normal pancreatic consistency, normal-sized bile duct, or associated injuries. Alternative to pancreatic head resection involves pancreatic endoscopic sphincterotomy or placement of a temporary stent to decompress the otherwise high-pressure pancreatic ductal system. Closed suction drainage of the pancreatic head in association with ductal decompression can be used to control intra-abdominal pancreatic secretions [62].

For combined duodenal and pancreatic injuries, several authors have advocated the use of duodenal exclusion, involving diversion of the gastric stream via a gastrojejunostomy, temporary closure of the pylorus, and primary repair plus drainage of the duodenal and pancreatic injuries. Duodenopancreatectomy is required for severe injuries causing devitalization of pancreatic head or duodenum, and for more focal injuries destroying the ampulla and adjacent pancreas [64-67].

Table 7. Selected clinical experiences with the operative management of duodenal and pancreatic injuries

Author	No. of patients	Site of injury	Results
Stone and Fabian 1979 [56]	321	Duodenum	Dehiscence rate < 1% with indirect duodenal decompression, 8% with no decompression, 23% with decompression via suture line
Stone and Fabian 1981 [57]	283	Pancreas	5 fistulas, 3 deaths
Martin et al. 1983 [58]	313	Duodenum	Duodenal fistula rate 5.5%. Marginal ulcers 3%. Recanalization of pylorus 94%
Oreskovich and Carrico 1984 [59]	10	Duodenum	No deaths. 90% return to functional activity at 3.5-year follow-up
Ivatury et al. 1985 [60]	100	Duodenum	Fistula rates 27% with decompressive enterostomy, 1.6% with repair/resection
Feliciano et al. 1987 [61]	129	Duodenum	24% simple repair, 50% pyloric exclusion, 10% duodenopancreatectomy
Cogbill et al. 1990 [62]	164	Duodenum	117 primary repair, 27 pyloric exclusion, 6 resection/anastomosis, 5 duodenopancreatectomy. Duodenal fistula 6 patients, dehiscence 5 patients
Ivatury et al. 1990 [63]	103	Pancreas	Penetrating injuries. 76 debridement/drainage alone; 19 distal pancreatectomy; 6 duodeno-pancreatectomy. Fistula rate 5%. Pancreatic abscess rate 11%
Cogbill et al. 1991 [64]	74	Pancreas	Distal pancreatectomy. Overall complication rate 45% (fistula 14%, abscess 33%, pancreatitis 8%, pseudocyst 3%)
Madiba et al 1995 [65]	152	Pancreas	Drainage alone. For blunt and penetrating injuries fistula rate was 13% and 23%, respectively
Akhrass et al. 1997 [66]	72	Pancreas	External drainage 13 patients; Laparotomy 22 patients; Distal resection 23 patients; Proximal resection 2 patients. Fistula 11%; Intraabdominal abscess 8%
Young et al. 1998 [67]	62	Pancreas	10 early deaths. 19 main pancreatic duct injury treated with distal resection: 2 fistulas. 33 parenchymal injuries treated with drainage only 3 fistulas.

Stomach, small and large bowel

These injuries occur as the result of penetrating AT. The majority of lacerations are simple lateral or tangential injuries amenable to primary repair. More-severe injuries of the small bowel are generally best managed by resection and primary reanastomosis [1-4].

One of the primary goals in the management of colorectal injuries is the prevention of associated postoperative septic complications [68-73]. The results of clinical experience with the use of primary repair and resection with anastomosis are reported in Table 8.

Table 8. Representative clinical experiences with primary repair and resection with anastomosis in the treatment of penetrating colon injuries

Author	No. of patients	Results
Shannon and Moore 1985 [68]	228	80 primary repairs: 1 leak, 17% septic complications 30 resection/anastomosis: 0 leaks 118 diverted/exteriorised: 48% septic complications
Chappuis et al. 1991 [69]	56	17 primary repairs: 0 leaks, 6 septic complications. 11 resection/anastomosis: 0 leaks 28 proximal colostomy: 5 septic complications
Schultz et al.1993 [70]	100	40 primary repairs: 0 leaks 17 resection/anastomosis: 0 leaks 43 diverted/exteriorised
Ivatury et al. 1993 [71]	252	159 primary repairs: 0 leaks 26 resection/anastomosis: 2 leaks 67 diverted/exteriorised 17% intraabdominal abscess
Sasaki et al. 1995 [72]	71	31 primary repairs: 0 leaks, 8 complications 12 resection/anastomosis: 0 leaks 28 diverted/exteriorised: 10 complications
Gonzalez et al. 1996 [73]	114	56 primary repairs: 1 leak, 11 septic complications 5 resection/anastomosis: 1 leak
53 diverted: 13 septic complications		

Re-operation and complications

The principles of *re-operation* are removal of clots and abdominal packs, complete inspection of the abdomen to detect missed injuries, hemostasis and restoration of intestinal integrity and abdominal wound closure. Timing of re-operation is critical [74, 75]. There is usually a window of opportunity between correction of metabolic failure and the onset of the systemic inflammatory response syndrome and MOF. This window usually occurs at 24-48 h after first DCS. There is a tradeoff between earlier re-operation, when the patient may be less stable and bowel wall edema marked, and delaying the procedure to a point where cardiovascular, respiratory, and renal failures make the procedure hazardous.

Abdominal packs, especially around the liver or spleen, should be removed cautiously as they may be stuck to the parenchyma and removal may lead to further bleeding. Soaking the swabs may aid this process. The bleeding is rarely dramatic, however, and may be controlled with argon-beam diathermy or fibrin glue. Occasionally repacking will be necessary [76].

Any intestinal repairs carried out at the first procedure should be inspected to determine their continued integrity. Bowel ends that were stapled or tied off should be inspected, necrotic tissue debrided, and primary repair with end-to

-end anastomosis undertaken. With a hemodynamically stable, warm patient, colostomy is rarely necessary [75].

Washout should be performed and the abdomen closed with standard mass closure to the sheath and routine skin closure. If the sheath cannot be re-approximated temporary silo closure can be reinstated or an absorbable mesh applied that can be skin grafted at a later stage. The resulting incisional hernia can be closed at a later procedure.

Complications are frequent among patients who survive a staged repair. The most frequent and lethal major complication is MOF [11, 21, 77]. Intra-abdominal abscess has been reported in 12% to 67% of cases, with an increased risk in patients who have undergone multiple procedures, intestinal spillage, and abdominal packing [24, 77]. Abscesses and other septic complications in the chest and abdomen may cause a systemic inflammatory response, which is a marker for poor prognosis [21, 25, 26]. Complications may necessitate early or unplanned return to the OR. Unplanned re-operation is usually preceded by one of the following: abdominal compartment syndrome, continued bleeding, abdominal sepsis and peritonitis, and ischemic tissue causing metabolic derangements [77]. In an urgent re-exploration in the OR, attention is focused on quickly obtaining hemostasis or abdominal decompression followed by rapid return to the ICU.

Abdominal compartment syndrome

Massive visceral and/or vascular injury may result in intense intestinal edema and third spacing of fluid. These injuries also may require the placement of intra-abdominal packs for control of hemorrhage to allow for further resuscitation, warming, and correction of coagulopathy prior to definitive therapy. When these events occur, it may not be possible to close the abdominal wall without vastly increasing the *intra-abdominal pressure* [12,76]. If the abdomen is closed, intra-abdominal pressure may rise to a level (25 cm H_2O) where it leads to significant cardiovascular, respiratory, renal, and cerebral dysfunction [76].

Cardiovascular dysfunction

A rise in the intra-abdominal pressure leads to a fall in cardiac output, due mainly to compression of the inferior vena cava and reduction in venous return to the heart. Cardiac output is reduced despite apparent rises in central venous pressure, pulmonary artery occlusion pressure, and systemic vascular resistance. This makes adequate and appropriate resuscitation difficult.

Respiratory dysfunction

Raised intra-abdominal pressure will effectively splint the diaphragm and lead to a rise in peak airway pressure and intrathoracic pressure, and subsequently a reduced venous return to the heart. The increase in airway pressures may also exacerbate barotrauma and contribute to the development of acute respiratory distress syndrome.

Renal dysfunction

Acute increase in intra-abdominal pressure leads to oliguria and anuria, probably due to compression of the renal vein and renal parenchyma. Renal blood flow and glomerular filtration are decreased, with a corresponding increase in renal vascular resistance.

Cerebral dysfunction

The rise in intra-abdominal pressure and intrathoracic pressure leads to a rise in central venous pressure that prevents adequate venous drainage from the brain, leading to a rise in intracranial pressure and worsening of intracerebral edema.

Diagnosis and management of abdominal compartment syndrome

Abdominal compartment syndrome should be suspected and sought in any multiple trauma patients who have undergone a period of severe shock. Clinically it is characterized by a fall in urine output associated with an elevated central venous pressure. The diagnosis can be confirmed by the measurement of intra-abdominal pressure. This may be done either through a Foley catheter in the bladder or a nasogastric tube in the stomach. Simple water-column manometry is used at 2- to 4-hourly intervals, although it is possible to connect a pressure transducer to a Foley catheter.

Table 9. Grading system for abdominal compartment syndrome

Grade	Bladder pressure measure (cm H_2O)
I	10-15
II	15-25
III	25-35
IV	>35

Normal intra-abdominal pressure is zero or subatmospheric. A pressure of over 25 cm H_2O is suggestive, and over 30 cm H_2O diagnostic, of the abdominal compartment syndrome (Table 9).

It is better to anticipate the development of abdominal compartment syndrome and use an alternate wound closure technique to prevent its occurrence. If the abdomen is at all difficult to close, this procedure should be abandoned and alternative techniques applied. A good rule of thumb is that if, when looking at the abdomen horizontally, the guts can be seen above the level of the wound, the abdomen should be left open and temporary closure utilized. The easiest method to control the open abdomen is to use a silo-bag closure [76].

An alternative technique is the vacuum-pack technique. Here the 3-l bag is opened and placed into the abdomen to protect the gut contents, under the sheath. Two large suction drains are placed over this, and a large adherent steridrape placed over the whole abdomen. The suction catheters are connected to high-displacement suction to provide control of fluid losses and create the vacuum-pack effect.

Sudden release of the *abdominal compartment syndrome* may lead to an *ischemia-reperfusion injury* causing acidosis, vasodilatation, cardiac dysfunction, and arrest. Prior to release the patient should be pre-loaded with crystalloid solution. Mannitol and vasodilators such as dobutamine or the phosphodiesterase inhibitors may have a place here.

References

1. Mackersie RC (2001) Abdominal trauma. In: Norton JA, Bollinger RR, Chang AE, Lowry SF, Mulvihill SJ, Pass HI, Thompson RW (eds) Surgery. Basic science and clinical evidence. Springer, Berlin Heidelberg New York, pp 825-845
2. Hoyt DB, Coimbra R, Winchell RJ (2001) Management of acute trauma. In: Townsend CM (ed) Sabiston – Textbook of surgery. Saunders, Philadelphia, pp 311-344
3. National Center for Injury Prevention and Control (2001) http://www.cdc.gov/ncipc/
4. Fabian TC, Croce MA (1996) Abdominal trauma, including indication for celiotomy. In: Mattox KL, Moore EE, Feliciano DV (eds) Trauma. 3rd edn, Appleton and Lange, Stanford: 441-460
5. Alonso M, Brathwaite C, Garcia V, et al (2000) Practice management guidelines for the nonoperative management of blunt injury to the liver and spleen. Eastern Association for the Surgery of Trauma. http://www.east.org
6. Abdominal trauma (2000) http://www.madsci.com/manu/trau_abd.html
7. American College of Surgeons, ACS (2000) Abdominal trauma algorithm. Bull Am Coll Surg 80: 6
8. Salomone JA (2000) Abdominal trauma. http://www.emedicinecom/ emerg/topic1.html
9. Sauaia A, Moore FA, Moore EE, et al (1995) Epidemiology of trauma deaths. J Trauma 38: 185-193
10. Mattox K (1997) Introduction, background, and future projections of damage control surgery. Surg Clin North Am 77: 753-759
11. Hirshberg A, Mattox KL (1995) Planned reoperation for severe trauma. Ann Surg 222: 3-8

12. Rotondo MF, Schwab CW, McGonial MD, et al (1993) Damage control: an approach for improved survival in exsanguinating penetrating abdominal injury. J Trauma 35: 375-382
13. Halstead WS (1913) The employment of fine silk in preference to catgut and the advantages of transfixing tissues and vessels in controlling hemorrhage. Also an account of the introduction of gloves, gutta-percha tissue and silver foil. JAMA 60: 1119
14. Schroeder WE (1906) The process of liver hemostasis. Reports of cases. Surg Gynecol Obstet 2: 52
15. Moore EE (1996) Staged laparotomy for the hypothermia, acidosis, and coagulopathy syndrome. Am J Surg 172: 405-410
16. Feliciano DV, Mattox KL, Jordan GL, et al (1981) Packing for control of hepatic hemorrhage: a reappraisal. J Trauma 21: 285-290
17. Svoboda JA, Peter ET, Dang CV, et al (1982) Severe liver trauma in the face of coagulopathy: a case for temporary packing early reexploration. Am J Surg 144: 717-721
18. Stone HH, Strom PR, Mullins RJ (1983) Management of the major coagulopathy with onset during laparotomy. Ann Surg 197: 532-535
19. Burch JM, Denton JR, Noble RD (1997) Physiologic rationale for damage control surgery. Surg Clin North Am 77: 779-782
20. Hirshberg A, Walden R (1997) Damage control for abdominal trauma. Surg Clin North Am 77: 813-820
21. Morris JA, Eddy VA, Binman TA, et al (1993) The staged celiotomy for trauma: issues in unpacking and reconstruction. Ann Surg 217: 576-586
22. Moore EE, Burch JM, Franciose RJ, et al (1998) Staged physiologic restoration and damage control surgery. World J Surg 22:1184-1191
23. Reed RL, Bracey AW, Hudson JD, et al (1990) Hypothermia and blood coagulation: Dissociation between enzyme activity and clotting factor levels. Circ Shock 32: 141
24. Gentilello LM, Cobean RA, Offner PJ, et al (1992) Continuous arteriovenous rewarming: rapid reversal of hypothermia in critically ill patients. J Trauma 32: 316-327
25. Martin RR, Byrne M (1997) Postoperative care and complications of damage control surgery. Surg Clin North Am 77: 919-924
26. Burch JM, Ortiz VB, Richardson RJ, et al (1992) Abbreviated laparotomy and planned reoperation for critically injured patients. Ann Surg 215: 476-482
27. Pachter HL, Knudson MM, Esrig B, et al (1996) Status of nonoperative management of blunt hepatic injuries in 1995: a multicenter experience with 404 patients. J Trauma 40: 31-38
28. Burch JM, Moore EE, Moore FA, Franciose R (1996) The abdominal compartment syndrome. Surg Clin North Am 76: 833-842
29. Mirvis SE, Whitley NO, Vainwright JR, Gens DR (1989) Blunt hepatic trauma in adults: CT-base classification and correlation with prognosis and treatment. Radiology 171: 27-32
30. Hiatt JR, Harrier HD, Koenig BV, Ransom KJ (1990) Nonoperative management of major blunt liver injury with hemoperitoneum. Arch Surg 125: 101-103
31. Federico JA, Horner WR, Clark DE, Isler RJ (1990) Blunt hepatic trauma. Nonoperative management in adults Arch Surg 125: 905-909
32. Hollands MJ, Little JM (1991) Non-operative management of blunt liver injuries. Br J Surg 78: 968-972
33. Bynoe RP, Bell RM, Miles WS, et al (1992) Complications of nonoperative management of blunt hepatic injuries. J Trauma 32: 308-315
34. Pachter HL, Spencer FC, Hofstetter SR, et al (1992) Significant trends in the treatment of hepatic trauma. Experience with 411 injuries. Ann Surg 215: 492-502
35. Meredith JW, Young JS, Bowling J, Roboussin D (1994) Nonoperative management of blunt hepatic trauma: The exception or the rule? J Trauma 36: 529-535
36. Boone DC, Federle M, Billiar TR, et al (1995) Evolution of management of major hepatic trauma: identification of patterns of injury. J Trauma 39: 344-355
37. Croce MA, Fabian TC, Menke PG, et al (1995) Nonoperative management of blunt hepatic

trauma is the treatment of choice for hemodynamically stable patients. Results of a prospective trial. Ann Surg 221: 744-753
38. Brasel KJ, DeLisle CM, Olson CJ, Borgstrom DC (1997) Trends in the management of hepatic injury. Am J Surg 174: 674-677
39. Carrillo EH, Platz A, Miller FB, et al (1998) Non-operative management of blunt hepatic trauma. Br J Surg 85: 461-468
40. Moodley J, Singh B, Lalloo S, et al (2001) Non-operative management of haemobilia. Br J Surg 88: 1073-1076
41. Green MHA, Duell RM, Johnson CD, Jamieson NV (2001) Haemobilia. Br J Surg 88: 773-786
42. Malangoni MA, Levine AW, Droege EA, et al (1984) Management of injury to the spleen in adults. Results of early operation and observation. Ann Surg 200: 702-705
43. Bitseff EL, Adkins, Jr RB (1984) Splenic trauma: a trial at selective management. South Med J 77: 1286-1290
44. Mahon PA, Sutton JE (1985) Nonoperative management of adult splenic injury due to blunt trauma: a warning. Am J Surg 149: 716-721
45. Tom WW, Howells GA, Bree RL, et al (1985) A nonoperative approach to the adult ruptured spleen sustained from blunt trauma. Am Surg 51: 367-371
46. Cogbill TH, Moore EE, Jurkovich GJ, et al (1989) Nonoperative management of blunt splenic trauma: a multicenter experience. J Trauma 29: 1312-1317
47. Elmore JR, Clark DE, Isler RJ, Horner WR (1989) Selective nonoperative management of blunt splenic trauma in adults. Arch Surg 124: 581-585
48. Longo WE, Baker CC, McMillen MA, et al (1989) Nonoperative management of adult blunt splenic trauma. Criteria for successful outcome. Ann Surg 210: 626-629
49. Pachter HL, Spencer FC, Hofstetter SR, et al (1990) Experience with selective operative and nonoperative treatment of splenic injuries in 193 patients. Ann Surg 211: 583-589
50. Koury HI, Peschiera JL, Welling RE (1991) Non-operative management of blunt splenic trauma: a 10-year experience. Injury 22: 349-352
51. Schurr MJ, Fabian TC, Gavant M, et al (1995) Management of blunt splenic trauma: computed tomographic contrast blush predicts failure of nonoperative management. J Trauma 39: 507-512
52. Godley CD, Warren RL, Sheridan RL, McCabe CJ (1996) Nonoperative management of blunt splenic injury in adults: age over 55 years as a powerful indicator for failure. J Am Coll Surg 183: 133-139
53. Wasvary H, Howells G, Villalba M, et al (1997) Nonoperative management of adult blunt splenic trauma: a 15-year experience. Am Surg 63: 694-699
54. Cocanour CS, Moore FA, Ware DN, et al (1998) Delayed complications of nonoperative management of blunt adult splenic trauma. Arch Surg 133: 619-624
55. Davis KA, Fabian TC, Croce MA, et al (1998) Improved success in nonoperative management of blunt splenic injuries: embolization of splenic artery pseudoaneurysms J Trauma 44: 1008--1013
56. Stone HH, Fabian TC (1979) Management of duodenal wounds. J Trauma 19: 334-339
57. Stone HH, Fabian TC, Satiani B, Turkleson ML (1981) Experiences in the management of pancreatic trauma. J Trauma 21: 257-262
58. Martin TD, Feliciano DV, Mattox KL, Jordan GL (1983) Severe duodenal injuries. Treatment with pyloric exclusion and gastrojejunostomy. Arch Surg 118: 631-635
59. Oreskovich MR, Carrico CJ (1984) Pancreaticoduodenectomy for trauma: a viable option? Am J Surg 147: 618-623
60. Ivatury RR, Nallathambi M, Gaudino J, et al (1985) Penetrating duodenal injuries. Analysis of 100 consecutive cases. Ann Surg 202: 153-158
61. Feliciano DV, Martin TD, Cruse PA, et al (1987) Management of combined pancreatoduodenal injuries. Ann Surg 205: 673-680
62. Cogbill TH, Moore EE, Feliciano DV, et al (1990) Conservative management of duodenal trauma: a multicenter perspective. J Trauma 30: 1469-1475

63. Ivatury RR, Nallathambi M, Rao P, Stahl WM (1990) Penetrating pancreatic injuries. Analysis of 103 consecutive cases. Am Surg 56: 90-95
64. Cogbill TH, Moore EE, Morris, Jr JA, et al (1991) Distal pancreatectomy for trauma: a multicenter experience. J Trauma 31: 1600-1606
65. Madiba TE, Mokoena TR (1995) Favourable prognosis after surgical drainage of gunshot, stab or blunt trauma of the pancreas Br J Surg 82: 1236-1239
66. Akhrass R, Yaffe MB, Brandt CP, et al (1997) Pancreatic trauma: a ten-year multi-institutional experience. Am Surg 63: 598-604
67. Young PR, Meredith JW, Baker CC, et al (1998) Pancreatic injuries resulting from penetrating trauma: a multi-institution review. Am Surg 64: 838-843
68. Shannon FL, Moore EE (1985) Primary repair of the colon: when is it a safe alternative? Surgery 98: 851-860
69. Chappuis CW, Frey DJ, Dietzen CD, et al (1991) Management of penetrating colon injuries. A prospective randomized trial. Ann Surg 213: 492-497
70. Schultz SC, Magnant CM, Richman MF, et al (1993) Identifying the low-risk patient with penetrating colonic injury for selective use of primary repair. Surg Gynecol Obstet 177: 237-242
71. Ivatury RR, Gaudino J, Nallathambi MN, et al (1993) Definitive treatment of colon injuries: a prospective study. Am Surg 59: 43-49
72. Sasaki LS, Allaben RD, Golwala R, Mittal VK (1995) Primary repair of colon injuries: a prospective randomized study J Trauma 39: 895-901
73. Gonzalez RP, Merlotti GJ, Holevar MR (1996) Colostomy in penetrating colon injury: is it necessary? J Trauma 41: 271-275
74. Cue JI, Cryer HG, Miller FB et al (1990) Packing and planned reexploration for hepatic and retroperitoneal hemorrhage - critical refinements of a useful technique. J Trauma 30: 1007-1013
75. Carvillo C, Fogler RJ, Shafton GW (1993) Delayed gastrointestinal reconstruction following massive abdominal trauma. J Trauma 34: 233-235
76. Schein M, Wittman DH, Aprahamian CC, Condon RE (1995) The abdominal compartment syndrome - the physiological and clinical consequences of raised intra-abdominal pressure. J Am Coll Surg 180:745-753
77. Sganga G, Brisinda G, Castagneto M (2001) Peritonitis: priorities and management strategies. In: Saene HKF van , Sganga G, Silvestri L (eds) Infections in critically ill: an ongoing challenge. Springer, Berlin Heidelberg New York, pp 23-33

Trauma in Children

A.J. SUTCLIFFE

Caring for the injured adult is a challenge because of the huge variety of injury patterns that occur. Caring for the injured child is an even greater challenge because not only do the injuries vary from child to child, but each child's anatomy and physiology changes through childhood to adulthood. Although in some countries, children are treated in Pediatric Trauma Centres because their outcome is said to be better, this is not universally the case. There is some evidence that the staff who normally treat adults manage children more effectively if they have additional qualifications in pediatrics [1]. This implies that an appreciation of the special features of children's trauma improves care. The following text is directed towards doctors who do not specialize in pediatric trauma. In this chapter it is almost inevitable to stress the differences between children and adults. However, we should not forget that there are very many similarities in the management of children and adults and that the principles of management are identical.

The principles of management are the same for children and adults

As for adults, immediately after injury, the diagnosis and treatment of life threatening injuries which compromise airway patency, breathing and circulation are crucial. Time is then needed to take a history of the accident and to obtain a full medical history including illnesses, drugs, allergies and the time of the last meal.Children as well as adults should be undressed and examined from head to toe. Appropriate laboratory studies and radiological examinations should be ordered and when necessary information has been gathered, a treatment plan should be agreed upon between the surgeons, anaesthetists and other staff members.

Although the principles of management are the same, the details differ depending on the child's age. In the following sections, key differences between adults and children will be discussed as well as the appropriate clinical management.

The epidemiology of pediatric trauma

In the United States, one quarter of children, i.e. 25 out of every 100, are injured every year. The annual fatality rate is 38 children per 100 000. Boys are injured more frequently than girls and the injury rate for all children increases with age. Both the injury rate and fatality rate are greater in non-urban areas [2]. This may be because the distances to the hospitals are greater. The injury rate for children in England is also 25 out of 100 [3]. Although the injury rate varies from country to country, the causes of injury seem to be similar in all Western Countries [4]. The different frequencies are accounted for by cultural differences that alter the exposure rate to risks. Falls and road traffic accidents are common causes of injury [5]. Predictors of injury in childhood include maternal education, age and parity [6], recent injury of a sibling [7] and low socio-economic status [8]. Injury to the head and spine is a main determinant of mortality [5] as are gun shot wounds, drowning and non-accidental injury [9]. Certain situations such as the playground [10] or the use of adult seat belts for children younger than 5 years of age [11] are associated with specific injury patterns and may be preventable with suitable parental education, with or without design changes [10, 11]. Multi-faceted prevention programmes have reduced the incidence of injuries for children as pedestrians and bicycle riders [12, 13].

The primary survey

Airway

Young children are particularly prone to airway obstruction. This is partly because due to the child's physiology: small airway, large head, short neck, small mandible, large tongue, narrow nasal passages and adenotonsillar hypertrophy. In addition a higher metabolic rate increases oxygen demand and respiratory rate. Airway obstruction causes grunting or stridor, respiratory distress with the obvious use of accessory muscles of respiration and cyanosis. The chin lift manoeuvre may help but over-extension of the neck may worsen obstruction in infants. The neutral position is better in this age group. If endotracheal intubation is required, an uncuffed tube is used for children up to 10 years of age. In younger children, the cricoid ring is circular (as opposed to the heart shaped in older children and adults) and a correctly sized, uncuffed tube will form an adequate seal. A useful formula is: Internal diameter (mm) = (age / 4) + 4. If the child's age is unknown, the distal phalanx of the little finger frequently approximates to the correct tube size. The length of the tube can be estimated by measurement against the child or by using the formula: Length of tube (mm) = (age / 2) + 12. It is important to remember that the trachea is short. In infants, the carina lies opposite T2 and migrates downwards as the child grows reaching T4 in adults. In infants the bronchi branch off the trachea are at equal angles. Hence, endobronchial intubation occurs with equal frequency on the right and left sides of the chest. Furthermore, if the cheeks are chubby, movement of the endotracheal tube is relatively common unless it is firmly fixed.

Breathing

Difficulty in breathing may be due to fractured ribs but because the bones of children are compliant it is more often related to pulmonary contusion, the pneumothorax, or the haemothorax. Inhalation of stomach contents or blood also cause distress. The child may be cyanosed, using accessory muscles and breathing rapidly (Table 1). In infants, because of the elasticity of the chest wall, intercostal and sternal recession are features of respiratory distress. Respiratory distress associated with hypoxia or hypercarbia is an indication for ventilation. The tidal volume used does not depend on age and is usually 6 $ml.kg^{-1}$. This should mean that chest expansion is visible but does not appear to be excessive. The ventilation rate should be chosen according to the child's age. Sometimes, respiratory distress is caused by gastric dilatation or an over-distended bladder. These causes are rare immediately after injury.

Circulation

Children normally have higher heart rates (Table 1) and smaller stroke volumes than adults. The response to hypovolaemia is usually tachycardia. Hypotension is a late feature and does not occur until 40% of the blood volume has been lost [14] (Table 2). Table 2 also lists other signs of hypovolaemia. In children, the treatment of hypovolaemia is either a crystalloid bolus of 40 $ml.kg^{-1}$ or colloid bolus of 20 $ml.kg^{-1}$. If there is a poor response this may be repeated. If this fails, blood is usually given. Although the absolute volume of blood loss may be small and thus appear to be insignificant, it is important to relate the volume of loss to the child's total blood volume (Table1).

Table 1: Physiological variations throughout childhood

	Infants	Young children	Older children	Adults
Respiratory rate (breaths / min)	40 - 30	30 - 20	20 - 15	15
Tidal volume (ml / kg)	6	6	6	6
Heart rate (beats / min)	160 - 110	140 - 95	120 - 80	90 - 60
Systolic blood pressure (mmHg)	70 - 90	80 - 100	90 - 110	110 - 130
ICP (mmHg)	2 - 6	6 - 13	6 - 13	Up to 15
Blood volume (ml/kg)	80	75	70	70

Table 2: Hypovolaemia in children

Blood loss (% blood volume)	Clinical signs
< 20%	Tachycardia, normal blood pressure, capillary refill 2-3 seconds, urine output < 1 ml/k/h, irritable or fractious
25 -40%	Tachycardia, normal blood pressure, cold peripheries, oliguria, confusion, lethargy
> 40%	Hypotension, tachycardia or bradycardia, pale cold mottled skin, anuria, coma

Disability

The level of consciousness can be rapidly assessed in four categories which are the same as for adults; **a**wake, responds to **v**erbal stimulus, responds to **p**ainful stimulus and **u**nresponsive. If the level of consciousness is such that the airway is poorly protected, endotracheal intubation is indicated.

It is also useful to note the quality of a child's cry. It is normal for a child to cry after an accident. Fear also causes crying, particularly in the hospital environment. Therefore, if a child does not cry, this should be taken seriously because it may indicate a painful thoracic or abdominal injury. Similarly, children who have a head injury often have an abnormal high-pitched cry.

Exposure

As for adults, it is important that the child's clothes are removed so that whole body can be examined. Children have a large surface area in relation to their body weight. They get cold very quickly. Total exposure should be kept as short as possible during a complete physical examination.

Secondary survey and subsequent management

The principles and practice of the secondary survey are the same as for adults. However, frequency of specific injuries is different from adults. For clarity, injuries to each body area are described in the approximate order of their importance.

Head injury

Head injuries are present in 75% of children with trauma and 70% of pediatric traumatic deaths are due to head injury [15]. Significant head injury can result from relatively minor falls in children less than 2 years of age [16] but there is also a high incidence caused by non-accidental injury [17]. Outcome is related to the severity of the primary injury and the severity of subsequent swelling and or hyperaemia [18]. Thus, the Glasgow Coma Scale (GCS) score often predicts outcome but this is no always so [16]. For young children there is a need to modify the method of assessing the GCS score [19] (Table 3). The assessment of verbal response in small children is subjective. Therefore, it is important that when there is a charge of staff members during a shift, the staff makes a verbal assessment together to ensure consistency. Other clinical signs may be dependent on motor development [20]. Bilateral extensor plantar responses and ankle clonus are normal in children less than one year old [20].

A GCS score of eight or less defines a coma and indicates possible airway compromise and the need for intubation and ventilation. Hypoxia should be actively treated. Intubation at the accident scene may improve survival [21]. Unless the child is in cardiopulmonary arrest, drugs should be given prior to intubation to reduce the risk of raising intracranial pressure (ICP). Thiopentone, intravenous lignocaine and succinyl choline are recommended [22]. Hypovolaemia should be treated urgently. There is evidence that hypertonic saline improves cerebral oxygenation without raising ICP [23].

Table 3: Assessment of the Glasgow Coma Scale (GSC)

	< 4 Years	4 – 15 Years	GCS score
Eyes	Open spontaneously	Open spontaneously	4
	React to speech	Verbal command	3
	Pain	Pain	2
	No response	No response	1
Best motor response	Spontaneous or obeys Verbal command	Spontaneous or obeys Verbal command	6
	Localizes pain	Localizes pain	5
	Withdraws to pain	Flexes to pain	4
	Abnormal flexion to pain	Abnormal flexion to pain	3
	Extension to pain	Extension to pain	2
	No response	No response	1
Verbal	Smiles, interacts, follows objects	Orientated and converses	5
	Consolable crying / inappropriate interaction	Disorientated and converses	4
	Inconsistently consolable crying / moaning	Inappropriate words	3
	Inconsolable crying / irritable	Incomprehensible sounds	2
	No response	No response	1

Hypoxia and hypercarbia have similar effects in adults and children but for the latter, the response range is somewhat different. Nonetheless, the principles and practice of head injury management and monitoring are similar in adults and children [20].

Cervical spine injury

In children, the entire spine is flexible. In infants, incomplete ossification of C1 –2 and poor neck muscle tone increase susceptibility to high spinal cord injury [14] and partly explain the high mortality rate in younger children [24]. Of those children who survive a cervical spine injury, 25% suffer permanent neurological deficit [24]. Thus, a high index of suspicion is necessary to prevent spinal cord damage. Fortunately clinical evidence, such as neck pain or limited neck movement, is present in all conscious children with cervical spine fractures [25]. Unfortunately, high spinal cord injuries are often associated with apnoea and hypotension or cardiorespiratory arrest at the scene of the accident. The cause of these signs is often mistaken for head injury [26]. For children who survive, clinical management is similar to adults [14].

Chest injury

Rib fractures are a marker of severe injury in children and the mortality rate is approximately 40% when the fractures occur alone and 70% when they are associated with head injury [27]. Pulmonary contusion is more common, probably because the ribs are springy and injury forces are transmitted to the underlying lung. Pulmonary contusion occurs frequently when associated to motor vehicle and auto-pedestrian accidents [28]. Little has been written about the management of chest injury in children. New approaches to ventilation in children and adults appear to be similar [29].

Abdominal injuries

Abdominal injuries account for less than one percent of childhood injuries and are usually associated with a direct blow such as a seat belt or an infliction when the child is being abused [30]. Diagnosis is difficult. Ultrasonography alone is not a useful screening test [31]. CT helps to diagnose the type of injury but rarely influences the decision for operative intervention [32, 33]. Nonoperative management is becoming popular for some spleen and liver injuries. The presence of a head injury does not change this approach [34].

Anaesthetic and intensive care unit management of the injured child

A variety of anaesthetic techniques are described for children [14, 20, 35]. Injured children are frightened and often cry or struggle. Preoxygenation may not be possible but a rapid sequence technique with cricoid pressure should be used if the stomach is full. The use of topical local anaesthetic cream may reduce the pain associated with the placement of intra-venous cannulae or intra-osseus needles. A wide range of anaesthetic agents can be used for children. Ketamine is popular, particularly in the absence of a head injury for sedation or when profound hypotension may occur at induction. The child should be kept warm. If warming blankets obstruct the surgical field, wrapping the head in bubble wrap, warming intravenous fluids and increasing the environmental temperature may help. Blood loss should be carefully monitored.

Postoperative pain relief is as essential for children as it is for adults. Morphine in appropriate dosage should be given for severe pain. Otherwise paracetamol, non-steroidal anti-inflammatory drugs or regional block may be sufficient. The adequacy of pain relief should be formally and regularly assessed. A pictorial pain assessment tool may be helpful in younger children [19]. Intensive care unit (ICU) management is summarized elsewhere [36].

Conclusion

Not all injured children are able to benefit from care in a specialist centre. With some additional knowledge and skills, the trauma anaesthetist can successfully resuscitate and provide anaesthesia for children. Posters (describing tube sizes, pediatric physiological data and pediatric drug doses) displayed in appropriate places can be a helpful memory aid. Most children make an excellent recovery after injury and this can be a delight to see.

References

1. Potoka DA, Schall LC, Gardner MJ et al (2000) Impact of pediatric trauma centers on mortality in a statewide system. J Trauma 49: 237-245
2. Danseco ER, Miller TR, Spicer RS (2000) Incidence and costs of 1987-1994 childhood injuries: demographic breakdowns. Pediatrics 105: E27
3. Kendrick D, Marsh P (1997) Injury prevention programmes in primary care: a high-risk group or a whole population approach? Inj Prev 3:170-175
4. Roberts I, Carlin J, Bennett C et al (1997) An international study of the exposure of children to traffic. Inj Prev 3: 89-93
5. Snyder CL, Jain VN, Saltzman DA et al (1990) Blunt trauma in adults and children: a comparative analysis. J Trauma 30: 1239-1245
6. Scholer SJ, Mitchel EF, Ray WA (1997) Predictors of injury mortality in early childhood. Pediatrics 100: 342-347
7. Johnston BD, Grossman DC, Connell FA et al (2000) High-risk periods for childhood injury among siblings. Pediatrics 105: 562-568
8. Roberts I, Power C (1996) Does the decline in child injury mortality vary by social class? A comparison of class specific mortality in 1981 and 1991. Br Med J 313: 784-786
9. Peciet MH, Newman KD, Eichelberger MR et al (1990) Patterns of injury in children. J Pediatr Surg 25: 85-91

10. Lillis KA, Jaffe DM (1997) Playground injuries in children. Pediatr Emerg Care 13: 149 – 153
11. Winston FK, Durbin DR, Kallan MJ et al (2000) The danger of premature graduation to seat belts for young children. Pediatrics 105: 1179-1183
12. Durkin MS, Laraque D, Lubman I et al (1999) Epidemiology and prevention of traffic injuries to urban children and adolescents. Pediatrics 103: E74
13. Ytterstad B (1995) The Harstad injury prevention study: hospital-based injury recording used for outcome evaluation of community-based prevention of bicyclist and pedestrian injury. Scand J Prim Health Care 13: 141-149
14. Meyer P, Cuttaree H (1996) Severe trauma in children. Clin Anaesthesiol 10(4): 753-770
15. Lam WH, MacKersie A (1999) Paediatric head injury: incidence, aetiology and management. Paediatr Anaesth 9: 377- 385
16. Gruskin KD, Schutzman SA (1999) Head trauma in children younger than 2 years: are there predictorS for complications? Arch Pediatr Adolesc Med 153: 15-20
17. Goldstein B, Kelly MM, Bruton D et al (1993) Inflicted versus accidental head injury in critically injured children. Crit Care Med 21: 1328-1332
18. Feickert HJ, Drommer S, Heyer R (1999) Severe head injury in children: impact of risk factors on outcome. J Trauma 47: 33-38
19. Lissauer T, Clayden G (1997) Illustrated textbook of paediatrics. Mosby, London
20. Hammer GB, Krane EJ (1996) Perioperative care of the neurosurgical pediatric patient. Int Anesthesiol Clin 34(4): 55-71
21. Suominen P, Baillie C, Kivioja A et al (2000) Intubation and survival in severe paediatric blunt head injury. Eur J Emerg Med 7: 3-7
22. Nakayama DK, Waggoner T, Venkataraman ST et al (1992) The use of drugs in emergency airway management in paediatric trauma. Ann Surg 216: 205-211
23. Peterson B, Khanna S, Fisher B et al (2000) Prolonged hypernatremia controls elevated intracranial pressure in head-injured pediatric patients. Crit Care Med 28: 1136-1143
24. Orenstein JB, Klein BL, Gotcschall CS et al (1994) Age and outcome in pediatric cervical spine injury: 11 year experience. Pediat Emerg Care 10: 132-137
25. Scwartz GR, Wright SW, Fein JA et al (1997) Pediatric cervical spine injury sustained in falls from low heights. Ann Emerg Med 30: 249-252
26. Bohn D, Armstrong D, Becker L et al (1990) Cervical spine injuries in children. J Trauma 30: 463-469
27. Garcia VF, Gotschall CS, Eichelberger MR et al (1990) Rib fractures in children: a marker of severe trauma. J Trauma 30: 695-700
28. Allen GS, Cox CS, Moore FA et al (1997) Pulmonary contusion: are children different? J Am Coll Surg 185: 229-233
29. Martin LD (1995) New approaches to ventilation in infants and children. Curr Opin Pediatr 7: 250-261
30. Canty TG, Brown C (1999) Injuries to the gastrointestinal tract from blunt trauma in children: a 12-year experience at a designated pediatric trauma center. J Trauma 46: 234-240
31. Mutabagani KH, Coley BD, Zumberge N et al (1999) Preliminary experience with focused abdominal sonography for trauma in children: is it useful? J Pediatr Surg 34: 48-52
32. Stein JP, Kaji DM, Eastham J et al (1994) Blunt renal trauma in the pediatric population: indications for radiographic evaluation. Urology 44: 406- 410.
33. Ruess L, Sivit CJ, Eichelberger MR et al (1997) Blunt abdominal trauma in children: impact of CT on operative and non-operative management. Am J Roentgenol 169: 1011-1014
34. Keller MS, Sartorelli KH, Vane DW (1996) Associated head injury should not prevent nonoperative management of spleen or liver injury in children. J Trauma 41: 471-475
35. Berry FA (1990) Perioperative management of the pediatric trauma patient. Crit Care Clin 6(1): 147-163
36. Sutcliffe AJ (1988) Critical Care. In: Alpar EK, Owen R (eds) Paediatric Trauma, Castle House Publications, Tunbridge Wells, 47-62

Trauma in Pregnancy

S. E. LAPINSKY

The pregnant woman is at risk of trauma throughout pregnancy, the most common causes being motor vehicle accidents, falls and physical abuse. Trauma complicates about 6 to 7% of pregnancies, and 0.3 to 0.4% of pregnant women sustain traumatic injuries sufficient to require hospitalisation [1]. The most common cause of traumatic maternal death is head injury and foetal demise usually occurs secondary to maternal hypotension or placental abruption. A review of pregnant women admitted to three Level 1 trauma centres revealed a maternal mortality of 3%, and a foetus death of 15% [1]. Care of the severely injured pregnant patient requires a multidisciplinary approach involving the emergency physician, trauma surgeon, obstetrician, intensivist and neonatologist.

Maternal physiology in pregnancy

Pregnancy is associated with a number of physiological changes which affect the assessment and management of the mother following traumatic injury (Table 1).

Pulmonary physiology

Airway mucosa becomes hyperemic and edematous, with hypersecretion and increased friability. The clinical relevance is that extra care should by taken when inserting nasogastric tubes or nasotracheal tubes due to the increased risk of epistaxis. Intubation may be technically more difficult due to the mucosal edema, requiring the use of a smaller endotracheal tube [2].

The expanding uterus displaces the diaphragm upwards, but diaphragmatic function remains normal. This causes a decrease in functional residual capacity (FRC) by 10% to 25% by term [3]. There is compensatory widening of the anteroposterior and transverse diameters of the thoracic cage so that vital capacity remains unchanged and total lung capacity decreases only minimally.

Table 1. Physiological changes in pregnancy and effects on trauma management

Physiology	Clinical implication
Respiratory	
Reduced FRC	Rapid development of hypoxemia
Increased O_2 consumption	
Elevated diaphragm	Higher positioning of chest tubes
Increased ventilation	Interpretation of ABG's
Cardiovascular	
Increased blood volume	Protection in event of haemorrhage
Increased cardiac output	Interpretation of haemodynamic data
Aortocaval compression	Supine hypotension
Urogenital	
Ureteric dilation	Abnormal intravenous pyelogram
Bladder displacement	Increased risk of injury
Gastrointestinal	
Decreased gastric emptying	Increased risk of aspiration
Peritoneal stretching	Reduced guarding and rebound
Enlarged uterus	Abdominal viscera protected Abnormal positioning of organs

FRC = functional residual capacity; ABG = arterial blood gas

Values of FEV_1 measured through pregnancy are not different from the non-pregnant state. Lung compliance is unchanged but the chest wall and total respiratory compliance are reduced in late pregnancy. These anatomical changes may influence the presentation of traumatic injury. While abdominal viscera may be protected to some degree by the gravid uterus, penetrating injury to the upper abdomen can result in significant bowel injury due to the proximity of organs in this area. The bladder is displaced into an intrabdominal position in the second trimester, increasing the risk of direct injury. Stretching of the peritoneum can blunt the normal response to peritoneal irritation, making physical examination less reliable. Tube thoracostomy should be placed one or two interspaces higher than usual due to the elevated diaphragm.

A significant increase in minute ventilation occurs, beginning in the first trimester and reaching 20 to 40% above baseline at term. This is due to the increase in CO_2 production and stimulation of respiratory drive by the elevated serum progesterone level [4]. The augmented ventilation is produced by an increase in tidal volume of about 30% to 35% while respiratory rate increases only slightly. The arterial carbon dioxide pressure falls to 28 to 32 mmHg [5], with plasma bicarbonate decreasing to 18 to 21 mEq/l to maintain pH in the range of 7.40 to 7.47. Alveolar-to-arterial oxygen tension difference and physiological shunt remain similar to non-pregnant values and mean arterial PO_2 is generally greater than 100 mmHg throughout pregnancy [5]. Mild hypoxemia may develop in the supine position due to airway closure as FRC diminishes. Oxygen consumption increases by 20 to 33% by the third trimester, due to the demands of the foetus and the increased maternal metabolic processes [6]. The combination of a reduced FRC and increased oxygen consumption results in a lowered oxygen reserve, making the pregnant patient susceptible to the development of hypoxia which can occur rapidly in response to hypoventilation or apnea [7].

Cardiovascular physiology

Cardiovascular physiology changes significantly during pregnancy, beginning in the first trimester and continuing into the post-partum period. Maternal blood volume increases progressively, peaking at a value about 40% above baseline by the third trimester [8]. Plasma volume increases more than red cell mass accounting for the relative anaemia of pregnancy. The increase in blood volume provides some protection against blood loss. The average blood loss of 0.6 L following an uncomplicated vaginal delivery and 1.0 L following a cesarean section is usually well tolerated, with no change in the haematocrit [9].

The increased blood volume is associated with an elevation in cardiac output, beginning by 5 weeks gestation and peaking at 30% to 50% above baseline levels by 25 to 32 weeks, due to an increased heart rate and stroke volume, and decreased afterload [10]. Systemic blood pressure decreases slightly during pregnancy. Diastolic pressure falls about 10 to 20% reaching a nadir at 28 weeks. Haemodynamic profiles obtained by pulmonary artery catheter in the near-term patient reveal an increased cardiac output, about 40% higher than baseline levels. Systemic vascular resistance and pulmonary vascular resistance are decreased by 20 to 30%. The central venous pressure and pulmonary capillary wedge pressure remain unchanged compared to nonpregnant values.

Near term, uterine blood flow is estimated at 500ml/min or approximately 10% of cardiac output. The enlarged uterus may compress surrounding vascular structures resulting in aorto-caval compression. Compression of the vena cava in the supine patient results in decreased venous return with a drop in cardiac output, sometimes associated with reflex vasovagal effects - the supine hypotensive syndrome [11]. Compression of the aorta may cause impaired uterine blood flow and foetal distress.

Renal physiology

Significant alterations in renal physiology form part of the maternal adaptation to pregnancy. Renal blood flow increases throughout the first and second trimesters to a level 60 to 80% above baseline. Glomerular filtration rate increases early in the first trimester, reaching a value 50% above pre-pregnancy levels at 16 weeks, and remains elevated throughout pregnancy. As a result, the normal serum creatinine level is in the range of 0.5 to 0.7 mg/dL (45 to 60 umol/L). The bladder, when distended, extends above the pelvis from the second trimester, increasing its risk of injury. As pregnancy progresses, the ureters dilate, as a result of uterine compression and smooth muscle relaxation [12]. A dilated collecting system does not therefore always indicate pathological obstruction.

Gastrointestinal physiology

Pregnancy is associated with a decreased lower oesophageal sphincter pressure, beginning in the first trimester and reaching a nadir at 36 weeks perhaps due to a progressive increase in plasma progesterone. As pregnancy progresses, the position of the stomach is displaced causing a further decrease in the effectiveness of the gastroesophageal sphincter. Basal gastric pH and acid output are unchanged. The pregnant woman should always be considered to be at risk for aspiration of stomach contents, regardless of the time elapsed since her last meal.

Effects of trauma

Maternal Injury

The pregnant woman is susceptible to similar injuries to the non-pregnant patient, but the anatomical and physiological changes of pregnancy may alter the severity or manifestation of trauma. The uterus is protected by the pelvis until 12 weeks gestation after which time it becomes an intrabdominal organ. Blunt abdominal trauma will often primarily affect the uterus, but injury to other viscera should be considered. Uterine injury can produce severe haemorrhage due to the prominent uterine circulation. Penetrating injury to the abdomen predominantly affects the uterus in later pregnancy. However, because intraabdominal viscera are compressed in the upper abdomen, relatively minor injury may produce significant damage [14]. Fractures of the pelvis may result in severe retroperitoneal haemorrhage due to dilation of pelvic veins [1].

Injury to the uterus may precipitate contractions, which are usually self-limited. Ongoing contractions should be an alert for associated placental abruption [14]. Tocolysis is sometimes used, with intensive foetal monitoring. Uterine rupture is rare, manifesting with maternal shock, abdominal pain and palpable foetal parts.

Assessment of the mother includes a history of the mechanism of injury, last menstrual period, uterine contractions and foetal movements. In addition to the usual physical examination, assessment includes palpation of the uterus for contractions and tenderness, sterile speculum examination and ausculation for foetal heart sounds.

Foetal injury

Maternal trauma is associated with a significant increase in foetal loss, secondary to maternal shock or hypoxia, placental injury or direct foetal injury [15]. The foetus is protected to some degree from direct injury by the cushioning effect of amniotic fluid. Poor foetal outcome correlates with the severity of maternal injury as assessed by the Injury Severity Score [1]. Maternal haemodynamic status alone is a poor predictor of foetal outcome, likely due to the physiological changes of pregnancy. Maternal acidemia is an accurate indicator of hypoperfusion and correlates with foetal mortality.

Direct foetal injury due to blunt trauma usually involves head injury secondary to maternal pelvic fracture [16]. Other foetal injuries may occur following blunt trauma, such as a motor vehicle accident, with minimal maternal injury. Penetrating trauma can produce a wide range of foetal injury. Electrical injury to the mother, involving current passing from upper body to the feet, may affect the foetus. A high foetal mortality occurs with maternal burns to greater than 30% of the body surface area, and delivery of the foetus should be considered if the foetus is viable [17].

Placental abruption is an important cause of foetal demise and complicates about 3% of non-catastrophic injuries and up to 38% of major injuries [14, 18]. Abruption may occur as a result of direct blunt trauma, but also follows deceleration forces in a motor vehicle accident and may not be associated with significant maternal injury [19, 20]. Indicators of placental abruption include vaginal bleeding, abdominal cramps, uterine tenderness, amniotic fluid leakage and unexplained foetal distress or maternal hypovolemia. Confirmation is performed by an abdominal ultrasound, which is only about 50% sensitive, foetal monitoring, or MRI [21, 22]. When foetus and mother are stable following partial abruption, expectant management can be considered. However, further placental separation can occur at any time and close observation is essential. Placental abruption is often complicated by coagulopathy due to release of thromboplastin into the maternal circulation.

Foetomaternal haemorrhage

The transplacental haemorrhage of foetal blood into the maternal circulation may complicate abdominal trauma, and can result in foetal exsanguination and maternal Rh sensitisation. This occurs in 28% of traumatic injuries with a mean volume of haemorrhage of 16ml [23]. Foetomaternal haemorrhage (FMH) is detected by the Kleihauer-Betke test, which identifies foetal cells in the maternal blood smear. It has been suggested that all pregnant women after 11 weeks gestation should be screened [14], but the major value is in identifying large haemorrhages in Rh-negative women [24]. The volume of foetal haemorrhage can be calculated by the percentage of red cells of foetal origin, and the test is sensitive to about 5 ml foetal blood (1 foetal red cell in 1000 cells). Rh sensitisation occurs with lesser FMH, and Rh-negative mothers with abdominal trauma should receive Rh immune globulin even in the presence of a negative Kleihauer-Betke test. The dose of Rh immune globulin is related to the volume of FMH - 50ug is sufficient for 5ml and suffices for gestation less than 12 weeks. The usual dose is 300ug, but a dose of 300ug per 25 ml haemorrhage is required for larger volumes [25].

Management

Initial management

Initial resuscitation follows usual management principles with efforts directed primarily at stabilizing the mother [26]. However, it is important to remember that the pregnant woman is at increased risk of aspiration, the upper airway may be edematous and she will desaturate rapidly due to decreased oxygen reserves. Adequate intravenous access and volume resuscitation are essential. It has been recommended that fluid replacement be given more rapidly than in non-pregnant women due to the physiological increase in plasma volume [27]. The foetus is very vulnerable to hypotension and hypoxemia - uterine blood flow will be markedly reduced when maternal circulation is compromised [28]. Due to the expanded circulation, maternal blood pressure and heart rate may not be reliable predictors of the degree of haemorrhage. However, signs of foetal distress may indicate impending maternal shock. Management of shock in a woman beyond 20 weeks gestation should include left lateral positioning to prevent supine hypotensive syndrome.

The secondary survey should include a detailed abdominal examination, remembering that physical signs may be affected by changing organ position and reduced peritoneal sensitivity [27]. In the absence of direct uterine injury, the distance from the symphysis pubis to the fundus of the uterus in centimetres equals gestation age in weeks. Foetal evaluation includes heart rate assessment by auscultation (possible from 20 weeks) or Doppler probe. Continuous foetal cardiotocography is important for evaluating and monitoring the foetus greater than 24 weeks gestation. A minimum of 4 hours monitoring has been suggested to detect intrauterine pathology [14], extended to 24 hours in the presence of contractions, abnormal foetal heart rate, rupture of membranes or vaginal bleeding. Obstetric consultation should be obtained. Foetal monitoring also acts as a sensitive indicator of changes in maternal haemodynamics and oxygenation [27].

Initial investigations include a complete blood count, blood type with Rh and coagulation studies. Ultrasound is a useful investigation for evaluation of the foetus for injury and biophysical profile, and to assess intraabdominal organ damage. Ultrasound guided paracentesis or diagnostic peritoneal lavage (by open technique, above the uterus) may aid in detecting bowel perforation or intraperitoneal haemorrhage [29]. CT scan or MRI may be required in indeterminate cases. Surgical exploration is carried out according to usual surgical principles. In the unstable mother, management of maternal injuries should take precedence over foetal distress, as correction of maternal haemodynamics is beneficial to the foetus. If the mother is stable, caesarean section may be indicated if the foetus is considered viable. Surgical repair of foetal wounds has been performed. The limits of viability are dependent on the level of neonatal care available, but aggressive resuscitation of foetuses over 25 weeks has been suggested.

Radiologic procedures and foetal risk

Despite the potential risk of exposing the foetus to ionising radiation, radiological investigations are often required for the management of the pregnant trauma patient. Foetal well-being depends on maternal recovery and the mistake should not be made of avoiding necessary radiological procedures.

Estimated foetal radiation exposure varies from less than 0.01 rad (0.0001 Gy) for a chest radiograph to 0.05 rad (0.0005 Gy) for a head CT and about 2 to 5 rad (0.02 - 0.05 Gy) for pelvic computed tomography (Table 2)[30, 31]. Techniques such as shielding the abdomen with lead and using a well-collimated x-ray beam can effectively reduce exposure.

The potential adverse effects of uterine exposure to radiation include oncogenicity and teratogenicity. An increased risk of childhood leukemia may occur with relatively low dose radiation (less than 5 rads), increasing the risk of childhood leukemia two-fold [30]. Teratogenicity is thought not to occur at these low radiation doses. Microcephaly and hydrocephaly have been described

Table 2. Estimated foetal radiation exposure during radiographic studies with appropriate shielding [from refs 30,31]

Radiographic study	Estimated foetal dose (rad)
Chest X-ray	< 0.002
Cervical spine series	< 0.002
Lumbosacral spine	0.4
Pelvis	0.1
CT head	0.05
CT chest	0.1 - 1.0
CT abdomen/pelvis	2 - 5

after radiation exposure of 10 to 150 rads [30]. Although radiation exposure in pregnancy carries definite risks, the likelihood of any adverse effect is about 0.1% per rad. Exposure to the foetus of less than 5 rads is therefore associated with a risk far below the spontaneous rate of congenital malformations. Nonetheless, every effort should be made to minimize foetal exposure, particularly in the first trimester.

ICU Management

Drug therapy

Pharmacotherapy during pregnancy requires consideration of the pharmacological and teratogenic effects of drugs on the embryo or foetus. The major risk period for teratogenesis is the first 10 weeks of gestation. A brief review of some drugs used in the critically ill pregnant patient follows.

Catecholamines: In the critically ill patient, an important consideration is the effect of vasoactive drugs on uteroplacental circulation. Commonly used catecholamines, including dobutamine, norepinephrine and epinephrine, adversely affect uterine blood flow. From animal data, only ephedrine has been shown to increase maternal blood pressure as well as increasing uterine blood flow [32]. Limited human data give similar results - dopamine (by infusion), and ephedrine or phenylephrine (given in small boluses) are effective in restoring maternal blood pressure, but decrease umbilical vein oxygenation. Early aggressive administration of ephedrine can reverse the foetal acidosis occurring secondary to maternal hypotension [33]. The rapidity of restoration of blood pressure may be more important than the specific inotropic agent used. Given these potential adverse effects, the importance of non-pharmacological manoeuvres such as adequate volume replacement and left lateral positioning must be stressed.

Sedation, analgesia, paralysis: Few data exist on the preferred drugs for prolonged sedation, analgesia and neuromuscular blockade. Sedation with benzodiazepines has been associated with a small risk of congenital malformations, mainly cleft lip and palate, when used in early gestation. Midazolam crosses the placenta to a lesser degree than diazepam, which can accumulate in the foetus at levels greater than the mother [34]. No significant risk of congenital malformations has been demonstrated for narcotic analgesics such as morphine, meperidine and fentanyl. The majority of non-depolarising neuromuscular blocking agents have been shown to cross the placenta, including pancuronium, vecuronium and atracurium, but transfer occurs at a low level and is unlikely to have clinical effects on the foetus, in the short term. Nevertheless, the use of any of the above agents by the intensivist must be communicated to the neonatologist who should anticipate the need for ventilatory support for the foetus.

Antibiotics: Similar antibiotic regimens to those used in the non-pregnant patient are appropriate in pregnancy, with a few cautions. Clearance and volume of distribution of antibiotics may be increased in pregnancy. Quinolones should probably be avoided due to the potential risk of arthropathy. Tetracyclines produce adverse effects on foetal teeth and bone. Aminoglycosides and sulfonamides should be used with caution. The potential for foetal risk should be considered for any drug administered in the pregnant woman.

Mechanical ventilation

Management of the pregnant patient with respiratory failure is similar to the non-pregnant patient, with some exceptions. The indications for intubation and mechanical ventilation in pregnancy are similar to the non-pregnant patient, but the normal $PaCO_2$ in pregnancy of about 30 mmHg should be considered in the interpretation of arterial blood gases. Endotracheal intubation should be performed via the oral rather than the nasal route, usually using a smaller tube. The pregnant woman's predisposition to rapid arterial desaturation following apnoea must be considered during intubation [7]. Adequate preoxygenation with 100% oxygen is required, avoiding respiratory alkalosis.

Few data exist concerning prolonged mechanical ventilation in pregnancy. In the absence of any acid-base problems or other contraindications, it is reasonable to aim for a $PaCO_2$ of about 30 mmHg, the normal level in pregnancy. Respiratory alkalosis should probably be avoided, since this may reduce uterine blood flow. Foetal pH appears to increase with modest hyperventilation but decreases with marked hyperventilation ($PaCO_2$ 17 mmHg), due to diminished uteroplacental perfusion [35]. While the current recommendations in non-pregnant patients aim at avoiding high ventilatory pressures, the effects of permissive hypercapnia have not been assessed in pregnancy. The decreased chest wall compliance in late pregnancy results in a 25% decrease in total respiratory compliance, and therefore transpulmonary pressures may not be elevated at a plateau pressure of 35 cmH_2O. Higher ventilatory pressures may be acceptable in these patients. Maternal hypercapnia up to 60 mmHg, with adequate supplemental inspired oxygen, does not appear to be detrimental to the foetus [36].

Haemodynamic monitoring

Although invasive monitoring is common critical care practice, controversy exists as to whether this modality improves clinical outcome. Guidelines have been suggested for the use of pulmonary artery catheters in obstetrics [37]. In general, the indications are similar to those in non-obstetric patients and pregnancy is not a contraindication to invasive monitoring. An awareness of the normal cardiovascular physiological changes in pregnancy (discussed above) is necessary in order to correctly interpret the haemodynamic data obtained.

Cardiopulmonary resuscitation

The management of cardiac arrest in the pregnant patient should be according to standard protocols, with some modifications. Cardiac compressions may be technically difficult due to the enlarged uterus and engorged breasts. Electrical cardioversion and defibrillation may be performed in pregnancy, after removal of the foetal monitor to prevent arcing. Appropriate pharmacological therapy should not be withheld when clinically indicated. However, conventional CPR in the supine position may cause significant aorto-caval compression, resulting in impaired venous return and inadequate cardiac output [38]. The use of a table that provides a lateral tilt, a wedge under the right hip, or manual displacement of the uterus to the left, is recommended.

Perimortem caesarean section may be indicated when initial attempts at resuscitation have failed in a woman at 24 to 26 weeks or more of gestation. The duration from the onset of cardiac arrest to the delivery of the infant is the single most important foetal prognostic factor [39]. Data suggest that infant survival without neurological sequelae is highest if the postmortem caesarean section is initiated within four minutes of cardiac arrest. However, operative delivery after four minutes is justified if signs of foetal life are present. Maternal resuscitative efforts must be continued during the caesarean section to maximize utero-placental perfusion. Caesarean section should be performed by the most experienced physician, via a classic midline vertical incision. Performance of a perimortem caesarean section may reverse aorto-caval compression and allow successful resuscitation of both the mother and infant.

Miscellaneous

Several other aspects of the management of the critically ill pregnant patient differ from routine care and deserve mention.

Positioning: As described above, the "supine hypotensive syndrome" should be considered in haemodynamically unstable patients. In the supine position, the gravid uterus produces significant mechanical effects on the vena cava and aorta, reducing central venous return, resulting in decreased cardiac output and blood pressure. It is important to avoid the supine position in the pregnant patient who is haemodynamically unstable or when there is foetal distress. The patient should be positioned on her left side, or at least with the right hip slightly elevated.

Nutrition: Adequate nutrition during pregnancy is an important aspect of management. During starvation, maternal nutrition and body stores are protected at the expense of the foetus and malnutrition may result in intrauterine growth retardation and foetal loss [40]. Growth restriction before 26 weeks gestation may lead to neurological impairment. Caloric requirements in pregnancy increase by only about 300 kcal per day but good control of maternal glucose levels should be maintained. Protein intake should be augmented by 20 - 50% to support increased maternal and foetal protein synthesis. Only a small number of nutrients have a markedly increased requirement in pregnancy, particularly iron, folate and calcium. In the patient in whom enteral nutrition is not possible, total parenteral nutrition (TPN) has been used successfully to provide nutritional support during pregnancy. TPN regimens employed are similar to those used in non-pregnant patients, with attention to increasing the intake of the nutrients described above.

Thrombosis prophylaxis: Pregnancy increases the risks of venous thrombosis due to hypercoagulability and venous stasis (particularly affecting the left leg). The risk is increased throughout pregnancy, but thromboembolism is most likely to occur in the postpartum period. Antithrombotic precautions, including physical interventions and heparin prophylaxis, are important.

References

1. Kissinger DP, Rozycki GS, Morris JA et al (1991) Trauma in pregnancy. Predicting pregnancy outcome. Arch Surg 126:1079-1086
2. Elkus R, Popovich J (1992) Respiratory physiology in pregnancy. Clin Chest Med 13:555-565
3. Baldwin GR, Moorthi DS, Whelton JA, MacDonnell KF (1977) New lung function and pregnancy. Am J Obstet Gynecol 127:235-239
4. Skatrud JB, Bempsey JA, Kaiser DG et al (1978) Ventilatory response to medroxyprogesterone acetate in normal subjects: time course and mechanism. J Appl Physiol 44:939
5. Templeton A, Kelman GR (1976) Maternal blood-gases, (PAO2-PaO2), physiological shunt and VD/VT in normal pregnancy. Br J Anaesth 48:1001-1003
6. Pernall ML, Metcalfe J, Schlenker TL, et al (1975) Oxygen consumption at rest and during exercise in pregnancy. Respir Physiol 25:285-293
7. Archer GW, Marx GF (1974) Arterial oxygen tension during apnoea in parturient women. Br J Anaesth 46:358-360
8. Ueland K (1976) Maternal cardiovascular dynamics. VII. Intrapartum blood volume changes. Am J Obstet Gynecol 126:671-677
9. Pritchard JA, Baldwin RM, Dickey JC, Wiggins KM (1962) Blood volume changes in pregnancy and the puerperium. Am J Obstet Gynecol 84:1271-1281
10. Mabie WC, DiSessa TG, Crocker LG, et al (1994) A longitudinal study of cardiac output in normal human pregnancy. Am J Obstet Gynecol 170:849-856
11. Kinsella SM, Lohmann G (1994) Supine hypotensive syndrome. Obstet Gynecol 83:774-788
12. Marchant DJ (1978) Alterations in anatomy and function of the urinary tract during pregnancy. Clin Obstet Gynecol 21:855-862
13. Dudley DJ, Cruikshank DP (1990) Trauma and acute surgical emergencies in pregnancy. Semin Perinatol 14:42-51
14. Pearlman MD, Tintinalli JE, Lorenz RP (1990) A prospective controlled study of outcome after trauma during pregnancy. Am J Obstet Gynecol 162:665 -671.
15. Drost TF, Rosemurgy AS, Sherman HF, et al (1990) Major trauma in pregnant women: maternal/fetal outcome. J Trauma. 30:574-8.
16. Murdoch Eaton DG, Ahmed Y, Dubowitz LM (1991) Maternal trauma and cerebral lesions in preterm infants. Br J Obstet Gynaecol 98:1292-1294.
17. Gang RK, Bajec J, Tahboub M (1992) Management of thermal injury in pregnancy - an analysis of 16 patients. Burns 18:317-320
18. Dahmus MA, Sibai BM (1993) Blunt abdominal trauma: are there predictive factors for abruptio placentae or maternal-fetal distress? Am J Obstet Gynecol 169:1054-1059
19. Agran PF, Dunkle DE, Winn DG, Kent D (1987) Fetal death in motor vehicle accidents. Ann Emerg Med 16:1355-1358
20. Lane PL (1989) Traumatic fetal deaths. J Emerg Med 7:433-435
21. Kay HH, Spritzer CE (1991) Preliminary experience with magnetic resonance imaging in patients with third-trimester bleeding. Obstet Gynecol 78:424-429
22. Pearlman MD, Tintinalli JE (1991) Evaluation and treatment of the gravida and fetus following trauma during pregnancy. Obstet Gynecol Clin North Am 18:371-381
23. Rose PG, Strohm PL, Zuspan FP (1985) Fetomaternal hemorrhage following trauma. Am J Obstet Gynecol 153:844-847
24. Goodwin TM, Breem MT (1990) Pregnancy outcome and fetomaternal hemorrhage after noncatastrophic trauma. Am J Obstet Gynecol 162:665-671
25. Bowman JM (1985) Controversies in Rh prophylaxis. Who needs Rh immune globulin and when should it be given? Am J Obstet Gynecol 151:289-294
26. Mighty H (1994) Trauma in pregnancy. Crit Care Clin 10:623-634
27. Pearlman MD, Tintinalli JE, Lorenz RP (1990) Blunt trauma during pregnancy. N Engl J Med 323:1609-1613

28. Assali NS (1989) Dynamics of the uteroplacental circulation in health and disease. Am J Perinatol 6:105-109
29. Esposito TJ, Gens DR, Smith LG, Scorpio R (1989) Evaluation of blunt abdominal trauma occurring during pregnancy. J Trauma 29:1628-1632
30. Toppenberg KS, Hill DA, Miller DP (1999) Safety of radiographic imaging during pregnancy. Am Fam Physician 59:1813-1818.
31. Ginsberg JS, Hirsh J, Rainbow AJ, Coates G (1989) Risks to the fetus of radiologic procedures used in the diagnosis of maternal venous thromboembolic disease. Thromb Haemost 6:189-196
32. Lapinsky SE, Kruczynski K, Slutsky AS (1995) State of the Art: Critical care in the pregnant patient. Am J Resp Crit Care Med 152:427-455
33. Datta S, Alper MH, Ostheimer GW, Weiss JB (1982) Method of ephedrine administration and nausea and hypotension during spinal anesthesia for cesarean section. Anesthesiology 56:68-70
34. General anesthesia. In: Drug Evaluations Annual 1994, AMA Division of Drugs and Toxicology. American Medical Association, Chicago, 173-195
35. Moya F, Morishima HO, James LS (1965) Influence of maternal hyperventilation on the newborn infant. Am J Obstet Gynecol 91:76-84.
36. Ivankovic AD, Elam JO, Huffman J (1970) Effect of maternal hypercarbia on the newborn infant. Am J Obstet Gynecol 107:939-946.
37. American College of Obstetricians and Gynecologists (1993) Invasive hemodynamic monitoring in obstetrics and gynecology. Int J Gynecol Obstet 42:199-205. ACOG Technical bulletin number 175.
38. Lee RV, Rodgers BD, White LM, Harvey RC (1986) Cardiopulmonary resuscitation of pregnant women. Am J Med 81:311-318.
39. Strong TH, Lowe RA (1989) Perimortem cesarean section. Am J Emerg Med 7:489-494.
40. Rosso P (1981) Nutrition and maternal-fetal exchange. Am J Clin Nutr 34(suppl 4):744-755.

Trauma in the Elderly

G. Berlot, A. Tomasini

Due to the increased ageing of the population observed in all developed countries, more and more elderly people (that is subjects ≥ 65 years old) are exposed to trauma [1]. Several factors account for this observation, including the prolongation of the active life, the reduction of the visual and acoustic capabilities, the slowing of reflexes, the loss of neuromotor co-ordination, and the effects of age-related diseases such as heart failure, osteoarthrosis, dementia etc. Altogether, these changes cause:

- a peculiar vulnerability of trauma-exposed tissues (i.e., fractures in ostheoporotic bones following minor trauma) [2,3];
- a more or less marked loss of the functional reserve, in terms both of single organ [1] and/or systemic stress response [4];
- altered responses to stressful events due to the effects of drugs that can influence the compensatory mechanisms to trauma (i.e., diuretic-related hypovolaemia, β-blocking agents and/or Ca^{2+} receptor antagonist- induced bradycardia, etc) [5].

Thus, although the mainstay of the treatment of trauma does not change among different age groups, the overall approach to the elderly severely injured patient must take in account these characteristics warranting modulation of the treatment, which should be adapted according to the age-related changes in both the single organ function and systemic response.

Epidemiology and prognosis

Features of trauma in the elderly

Falls

Although elderly people are exposed to the same trauma affecting younger victims, they are particularly prone to some injuries, whose effects are often disproportionate, such as falls from level or from the bed. A number of age-related factors contribute to their occurrence, including the instability of gait and the presence of other risk factors, such as neuropsychic alterations [6], postural hypotension [7] and vertebrobasilar insufficiency [8]. The consequent injuries are constituted mainly by: (a) fractures of the upper limb, of the pelvis and of the femur, which are more common in women, and (b) intracranial hematomas, which appear more common in men. [1].

Road accidents

In absolute terms, elderly people are less exposed to road accidents compared with younger subjects. However, this gap is reduced if the total number of traumatic events is corrected either for the age and the distance, with subjects aged ≥ 85 years having the highest rate of accidents per kilometer [1]. Furthermore, elderly people are often involved in collisions with cars due either to the very same causes responsible for low-level falls or to cognitive dysfunction [1,6].

Burns

In the elderly, as in other age groups, most burns are caused by home fires, whose main risk factors are smoking, the effects of alcohol and other sedatives, and the social conditions [1]. Not dissimilar from other traumatic injuries, burns of identical extension are associated with an increased morbidity and mortality compared with younger patients [9].

Prognosis

On the basis of the previous statements and aiming at a better allocation of the ever-decreasing resources, it appears particularly relevant to decide whether intensive care treatment is justified in elderly people; this particularly applies to those subjects of more-advanced age or with severe chronic underlying conditions. Several investigations have addressed these questions, studying the relationships among the causes of admission to the intensive care unit (ICU), the pre-existing diseases, and the final outcome; this latter point encompasses different categories, including ICU mortality, hospital mortality, and severity of the possible functional impairments after hospital discharge. Kass et al. [10] studied a group of critically ill patients aged ≥ 85 years and demonstrated that the overall mortality was related to the severity of the acute event and not to the pre-existing conditions; moreover, the survivors did not present relevant functional impairments as much as 1 year after ICU admission. Other investigators compared the outcome of two groups of ICU patients aged < and > 65 years, respectively, and, again, were able to demonstrate that the prognosis was more influenced by the cause of ICU admission than by the age per se [11]. Similar studies have been performed in elderly trauma patients, and also in this setting it appears that the outcome is more affected by the kind and severity of the trauma, and that the pre-existing conditions played a marginal role only [12]. However, due to the above reasons, in elderly people (a) traumas of comparable severity are associated with more-severe injuries than in younger subjects; and (b) for identical lesions, either the immediate or late mortality rate is higher [13-15]. Head injuries are associated with a particularly severe prognosis: advanced age is an independent risk factor for death and severe neurological disability even in the absence of extracranial injuries [16, 17].

Systemic stress response in the elderly and the clinical approach

The neuroendocrine response to stress in the elderly

The neurohormonal response to stress and trauma involves a number of complex biochemical and cardiovascular reactions whose ultimate goal is the systemic adaptation to the enhanced metabolic requests aimed at wound repair [4,18,19]. In the elderly, this response is somewhat blunted due either to the normal ageing process or to coexisting cardiovascular disease. This impairment can be clinically appreciated as the failed increase of cardiac output in response to the trauma, ultimately leading to the occurrence of tissue hypoxia [20,21], and/or the impaired elimination of the excess fluids administered during the initial phase of resuscitation [22]. These alterations can account for the increased rate of cardiovascular complications commonly observed in elderly trauma patients compared with younger subjects [23]. At the endocrine level, the secretion of growth hormone, cortisol, and other counter-regulatory hormones is decreased compared with younger patients, causing a reduced supply of substrates for the injured tissues and the immunocompetent cells [24, 25]. Altogether, these findings indicate that the neurohormonal response to stress is blunted in the aged, and this could constitute a prerequisite for the development of immediate and late post-traumatic complications [19, 26].

Respiratory considerations

The process of ageing is associated with a number of respiratory changes that eventually facilitate the occurrence of post-traumatic complications [26]. Even in the absence of pathological changes, the ageing per se is associated with a reduction of all the main respiratory variables (Table 1) [21,27]. At the same time, airway protective reflexes are attenuated, thus facilitating the occurrence of macro- and micro-inhalations [28]. These alterations are further aggravated by surgical procedures involving the chest and the upper abdomen [26]. Prolonged mechanical ventilation, which is often needed in critically ill trauma patients, is associated with severe degenerative changes of the tracheo-bronchial epithelium, including inflammation, atrophy, de-exfoliation, and exposition of the submucosa; these changes impair the clearance of the bronchial secretions, thus predisposing to respiratory tract infections [29]. The main indications and techniques for mechanical ventilation for elderly patients do not differ from those used in other age groups. However, it should be remembered that, due to the degenerative modifications, the risk of baro- and volotrauma is substantially increased [30]. Finally, in the elderly the optimal timing for a tracheostomy has not been defined yet [31].

Renal considerations

Ageing is associated with a reduction of the renal parenchyma, whose weight decreases as much as 30-40 % in subjects aged > 80 years compared with controls aged ≤ 40 years [22]. The cortex appears relatively more involved than the medulla. Whereas the overall glomerular population decreases, glomeruli saved from these degenerative changes undergo a compensatory increase of their volume and workload [32]. Actually, the renal ageing process is associated with marked differences between the cortical and medullary glomeruli. In the cortex, the decrease is associated with the atrophy of both the afferent and efferent arterioles, ultimately leading to the sclerosis of the affected regions. In the medulla, the ongoing reduction of the glomeruli facilitates the opening of shunts between the afferent and efferent arterioles; these neovessels significantly contribute to the maintenance of the medullary blood flow [22]. The total number of sclerotic glomeruli increases with age, ranging from < 5% in the 4th decade up to 30% in subjects aged > 80 years free of kidney disease. At the

Table 1. Age-related changes of the respiratory system. From [21], modified

↑ chest stiffness
↑ work of breathing
↓ muscle straight and endurance
↓ alveolar surface (15 % at 70 years)
↓ response to hypoxemia and hypercapnia
↓ vital capacity (20-40 ml/year)
↑ residual volume (30 % of total pulmonary capacity at 70 years)
↑ closing volume

same time, the renal blood flow (RBF) substantially decreases, particularly in males [22]. Different factors are associated with the reduction of the RBF, including the decrease of the cardiac output (CO) and the increase of the vascular resistances both at systemic and intraparenchymal level [22]. Taken together, these changes can account for the decrease of the glomerular filtration rate (GFR) commonly observed in the elderly. However, this decrease is not always predictable on the basis of age only, and is strongly influenced by individual factors: according to Lindeman et al. [33], the average decrease of the GFR can be approximated to 1 ml / 1.73 m^2 of body surface area for every year > 50; however, in 35% of the elderly people studied by these investigators, the creatinine clearance, which is considered an acceptable marker of the GFR, remained stable during as many as 20 years of observation. Beside the reduction of the RBF, other marked changes of glomerular function have been observed. As the renal plasma flow decreases more than the GFR, the filtration fraction (FF) increases; this increase could be ascribed also to the redistribution of the RBF toward the juxta-medullary glomeruli, whose FF is higher even under normal conditions.

The age-related involutive process is not limited to the glomeruli. The proximal tubules undergo a degenerative process similar to that involving the glomeruli. As a consequence, the ratio between glomerular surface and tubular length remains substantially constant [34].

These alterations are exacerbated by the concomitant presence of diabetes, hypertension, or other pathological processes involving the renal microvascular network, and account for the vulnerability of the critically ill elderly patient to the occurrence of acute renal failure [35].

In elderly trauma patients with a pre-existing non-oliguric chronic renal failure, the occurrence of hypovolemia can exacerbate this condition, leading to the occurrence of an irreversible anuria requiring the use of renal replacement therapies [36].

Cardiovascular considerations

The normal ageing process of the cardiovascular system is associated with a number of biomechanical and physiological changes that are associated with several relevant hemodynamic changes, either at rest and during stress or exercise (Table 2). Even in the absence of coexisting cardiovascular disease, these alterations can determine a failed rise in the CO and oxygen supply (DO_2) in circumstances associated with enhanced oxygen requirements, such as the postoperative or posttraumatic phase [21]. As a consequence, tissue hypoxia can ensue, thus facilitating the occurrence of complications and multi-system

Table 2. Age-related changes in some cardiovascular variables from 20 to 80 years. From [21], modified

Function	At rest	During exercise
Left ventricular end-diastolic volume	↑ men ↔ women	↑ men ↔ women
Left ventricular end-systolic volume	↑ men ↔ women	↓ both sexes
Ejection fraction	↓ both sexes	↔ both sexes
Systolic volume	↑ men ↔ women	↓ both sexes
Heart rate	↓ both sexes	↔ both sexes
Cardiac output	↔ men ↓ women	↓ both sexes
Left ventricular systolic work	↑ both sexes	↑ men ↔ women
Inotropism	↔ both sexes	↓ both sexes
Myocardial oxygen consumption	↔ both sexes	↓ both sexes
Systolic arterial pressure	↑ both sexes	↔ men ↑ women
Diastolic arterial pressure	↔ men ↑ women	↑ both sexes

dysfunctions [20,37]. The use of cardiovascular drugs and the presence of chronic hypertension can complicate the management of elderly trauma patients in different ways. First, anemia and hypovolemia can go undetected, as these patients may not become tachycardic due to the action of β-blocking agents or Ca^2 receptor antagonists; second, in hypertensive subjects the kidney and the brain may become underperfused when the arterial pressure is still in the "normal" range, due to the upward resetting of the intraparenchymal vasoregulatory mechanisms; finally, the use of diuretics facilitate and/or aggravate the occurrence of hypovolemia and predispose to arrhythmias. These considerations induced some authors to advocate the early use of a pulmonary artery catheter in the treatment of elderly trauma patients [38]. The practical management can be facilitated by the use of an algorithm (Fig. 1), which includes the administration of fluids and/or inotropes on the basis of the hemodynamic variables. It should also be remembered that in patients with an ischemic cardiopathy the transfusional threshold must be maintained higher than in normal patients, and that the hemoglobin levels should not be fall below 8-10 g/dl [39].

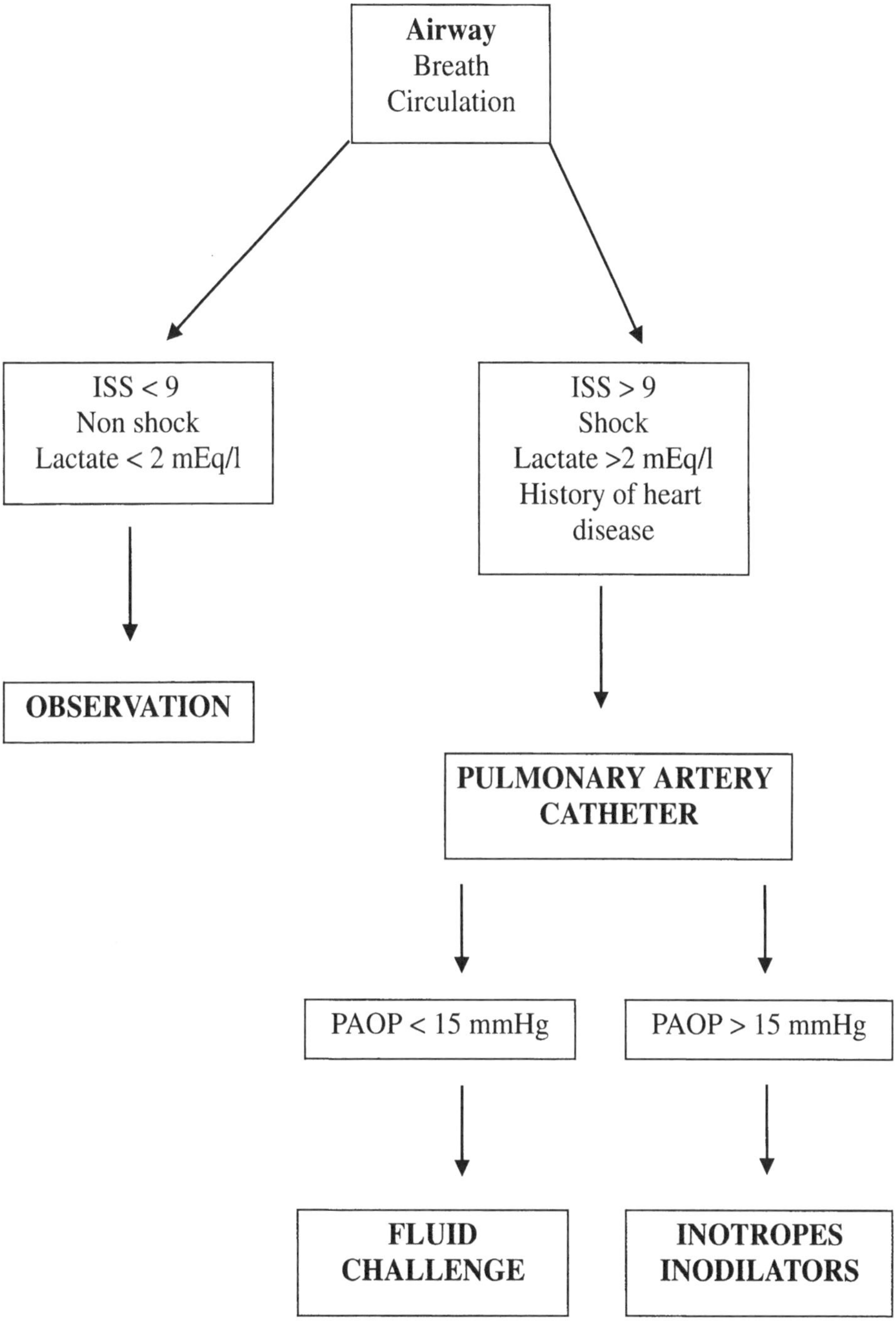

Fig. 1. Practical hemodynamic approach to the critically ill, elderly trauma patient
ISS = Injury Severity Score, PAOP = pulmonary artery occlusion pressure

Pharmacological considerations

In the elderly, the administration of drugs must take into account the relevant age-related changes in pharmacodynamics and pharmacokinetics that are determined by the regressive alteration both in the target and in the depurative organs (Table 3) [40]. In elderly trauma patients this process can be further complicated by the administration of large amounts of fluids during the initial phase of resuscitation and by the possible concomitant disturbances of the acid-base and electrolyte balance. In these circumstances, the monitoring of the blood concentrations of drugs is warranted in order to avoid the occurrence of either under- or overdosage.

Conclusions

The unrelenting improvement of the treatment of several age-related chronic diseases has led to more individuals surviving to an advanced age; as a consequence, more elderly people are exposed to trauma and its complications and sequelae. Although the mainstays of diagnosis and treatment of critically ill trauma patients do not substantially change in the different age groups, it should be remembered that (a) elderly patients suffer from a number of physiological age-related regressive changes that involve all organs and systems, and that these alterations can be further aggravated by the presence of coexisting diseases; (b) the outcome is more influenced by the acute event than by the effects of these changes. As a consequence, an aggressive approach appears justified in elderly trauma patients independent of age.

Table 3. Age-related functional changes affecting the pharmacokinetic and pharmacodynamic properties of drugs in the elderly. From [40], modified

Cause(s)	Effects	Clinical consequences
↓ total body water ↓ lean body mass ↑ fat ↓ albumin ↓ α_1 acid glycoprotein	Altered volume of distribution of drugs	Difficulties of drug titration ↑ drug active fraction ↑ drug T/2
↓ functioning hepatic tissue ↓ hepatic blood flow ↓ microsomal activity	Altered drug hepatic metabolism	↑ drug T/2 ↑ risk of drug toxicity
↓ glomerular filtration ↓ urinary concentration capability ↓ renal blood flow	Reduced drug renal elimination	↑ drug T/2 ↑ risk of drug toxicity

References

1. Santora TA, Schinco MA, Trooskin SZ (1994) Management of trauma in the elderly patient. Surg Clin North Am 74: 163-186
2. Lewy DB, Hanlon DP (1993) Geriatric trauma. Clin Geriatr Med 9: 601-620
3. Lonner JH, Koval KJ (1995) Polytrauma in the elderly. Clin Orthop Rel Res 318: 136-143
4. Weissman C (1990) The metabolic response to stress: an overview and update. Anesthesiology 73: 308-327
5. Watters JM, Bessey PQ (1994) Critical care for the elderly patient. Surg Clin North Am 74: 187-197
6. Lypowski ZJ (1989) Delirium in the elderly patient. N Engl J Med 320: 578-582
7. Lipsitz LA (1989) Current concepts: geriatrics: orthostatic hypotension in the elderly. N Engl J Med 321: 952-957
8. Tinetti ME, Williams CS (1997) Falls, injuries due to falls, and the risk of admission to a nursing home. N Engl J Med 337: 1279-1284
9. Ryan CM, Schoenfeld DA, Thorpe WP, Sheridan RL, Cassem EH, Tompkins RG (1998) Objective estimates of the probability of death from burn injuries. N Engl J Med 338: 362-366
10. Kass JE, Castriotta RJ, Malakoff F (1992) Intensive care outome in the very elderly. Crit Care Med 20: 1666-1671
11. Rockwood K, Noseworthy TW, Gibney RTN, et al (1993) One year outcome of elderly and young patients admitted to intensive care unit. Crit Care Med 21: 678-691
12. Ferrera PC, Bartfield JM, D'Andrea CC (2000) Outcomes of admitted geriatric trauma victims. Am J Emerg Med 18: 575-508
13. Sterling DA, O'Connor JA, Bonadies J (2001) Geriatric falls: injury severity is high and dispoportionate to mechanism. J Trauma 50: 116-119
14. McGwin G, Melton SM, May AK, Rue RW (2000) Long term survival in the elderly after trauma. J Trauma 49: 470-476
15. Sluis CK van der, Klasen MJ, Eisma Wh, Duis HJ ten (1996) Major trauma in young and old: what is the difference? J Trauma 40: 78-82
16. Luerssen TG, Klauber MR, Marshall LF (1988) Outcome from head injury related to patient's age. J Neurosurg 68: 409-416
17. Vollmer DG, Torner JC, Eisemberg HM, et al (1991) Age and outcome following traumatic coma: why do older patients fare worse? J Neurosurg 75: S37-S49
18. Woolf PD (1992) Hormonal response to trauma. Crit Care Med 20: 216-226
19. Weinmann M (2001) Stress induced hormonal alterations. Crit Care Clin 17: 1-10
20. Moore FA, Haenel JB, Moore EE, Whitehill TA (1992) Incommensurate oxygen consumption in response to maximal oxygen availability predicts postinjury multiple organ failure. J Trauma 33: 58-67
21. Priebe HJ (2000) The aged cardiovascular risk patient. Br J Anaesth 85: 763-768
22. Epstein M (1996) Aging and the kidney. J Am Soc Nephrol 7: 1106-1122
23. Horst HM, Obeid FN, Sorensen VJ, Bivins BA (1986) Factors influencing survival of elderly trauma patients. Crit Care Med 14: 681-684
24. Desai D, March R, Watters JM (1989) Hyperglycemia after trauma increases with age. J Am Geriatr Soc 29: 719-725
25. Rudman D, Kutner MH, Rogers CM, et al (1981) Impaired growth hormone secretion. J Clin Invest 67: 1361-1365
26. Watters JM, McClaran JC (1990) The elderly surgical patient. In: Wilmore DW, Brennan MF, Herken AH (eds) Care of the surgical patient. Scientific American/American College of Surgeons, New York
27. Enright PL, Kronmal RA, Higgins M, Schenker M, Haponik EF (1993) Spirometry reference values for women and men 65 to 85 years of age. Am Rev Respir Dis 147: 125-133
28. Marik PE (2001) Aspiration pneumonitis and aspiration pneumonia. N Engl J Med 344: 665-671

29. Stauffer JL, Olson DE, Petty TL (1981) Complications and consequenses of endotracheal intubation and tracheotomy: a prospective study of 150 critically ill adult patients. Am J Med 70: 65-76
30. Schnapp LM, Chin DP, Szaflarsky N, Matthay MA (1995) Frequency and importance of barotrauma in 100 patients with acute lung injury. Crit Care Med 23: 272-278
31. Pryor JP, Relly PR, Shapiro MB (2000) Surgical airway management in the intensive care unit. Crit Care Clin 16: 473-488
32. Goyal VK (1982) Changes with age in the human kidney. Exp Gerontol 17: 312-331
33. Lindeman RD, Tobin JD, Shock NW (1985) Longitudinal studies on the rate of decline of renal function with age. J Am Geriatr Soc 33: 278-285
34. Epstein M, Hollemberg NK (1976) Age as a determinant of renal sodium conservation in normal man. J Lab Clin Med 87: 411-417
35. Macìas-Nunez J, Lòpez-Novoa J, Martinez-Maldonado M (1996) Acute renal failure in the aged. Semin Nephrol 16: 330-338
36. Cacheco R, Millham FH, Wedel SK (1994) Management of the trauma patients with preexisting renal disease. Crit Care Clin 10: 523-536
37. Fiddian-Green RG (1989) Studies in splanchnic ischemia and multiple organ failure. In: Marston A, Bulkley GB, Fiddian-Green RG, et al (eds) Splanchnic ischemia and multi-organ failure. Arnold, London pp 349-363
38. Scalea TM, Simon HM, Duncan AO, et al (1990) Geriatric blunt multiple trauma: improved survival with early invasive monitoring. J Trauma 30: 129-134
39. McFarland J (1999) Perioperative blood transfusions: indications and options. Chest 115: 113S-121S
40. Montamat SC, Cusack BJ, Vestal RE (1989) Management of drug therapy in the elderly. N Engl J Med 321: 303-309

Trauma Anaesthesia and Pain Management

W. LINGNAU

Anaesthesiologists are increasingly involved in the treatment of trauma patients. The trauma anaesthesiologist performs this mission in the field, the emergency room, or the critical care unit, as well as in the operating room. In some parts of the world, anaesthesiologists are actively involved in prehospital (emergency medical service) care and transportation of the trauma patients [1]. Prehospital resuscitation and transportation to an emergency room for further diagnostic assessment as well as aggressive stabilisation of vital organ functions are cornerstones of the initial management of injured patients. The anaesthesiology team aims on circulatory stability and sufficient respiratory function. Surgical intervention to stop haemorrhage and to fix long bone fractures are listed on top of the priority list for subsequent treatment in the operation room. Trauma patients are then referred to a Postanaesthesia Care Unit (PACU) or an Intensive Care Unit (ICU) depending on the severity of injury and the expected duration of impaired organ function. Trauma management, however, includes treatment of pain at the site of an accident, in the emergency room, during surgical procedures, and in the postoperative period. By means of their specialization, anaesthesiologists are perfectly able to cover this task.

Tasks of the anaesthesiologist

Trauma centre organizations recognize trauma as a specific surgical disease, which requires highly trained anaesthesia care for optimal outcomes [2]. It has been demonstrated that there is a wide variation in the duties of anaesthesiologists in trauma care world-wide. In general, the surgeon concentrates on surgical diagnosis and treatment and the anaesthesiologist provides a secure airway, adequate ventilation, appropriate intravenous fluid management, and required sedation, analgesia or anaesthesia for both stress reduction and facilitation of surgical procedures. Potential roles of anaesthesiologists include the trauma team leader, a trauma team member in the emergency room, a disaster planning consultant, a prehospital care physician, an anaesthesiologist in the operating theatre, a pain relief physician or a critical care specialist.

Anaesthesia and pain management on the scene

Prehospital resuscitation, aggressive stabilization of vital organ functions and transportation to an emergency room are cornerstones of the initial management of injured patients. Airway management, fluid resuscitation and pain treatment are pivotal in the treatment of trauma victims. However, the level of measures depends on the type and degree of injury and functional impairment.

Human physiologic response to injury is uniform enough to justify the term traumatic disease despite the myriad causes of trauma [3-5]. However, the mechanism of injury is important, as it determines the pattern of injury, and this knowledge focuses the treatment priorities for that patient. For example, acute oxygen deprivation from drowning requires immediate attention to restoring oxygen delivery to the cardiopulmonary systems to prevent massive cellular necrosis. Penetrating thoracic trauma requires immediate placement of a chest tube to drain extrapulmonary pleural air and blood. Such a patient may often require no further surgery. Blunt chest trauma requires immediate attention to gas exchange because widespread pulmonary contusion complicates instability of the chest wall. Myocardial contusion and traumatic aneurysm of the thoracic aorta must be immediately ruled out. Besides this, a wide scale of pain treatment is warranted including the administration of analgesics or induction of anaesthesia, regional anaesthesia or peripheral nerve blocks. Neurological screening and the level of consciousness should be scored prior to the administration of anaesthetic agents.

Scoring systems

The Injury Severity Score (ISS) [6], an anatomic scale composed of the sum of squares of the Abbreviated Injury Scale (AIS) from the three most severely injured body regions, is used retrospectively to compare outcomes in trauma centres. Prospective physiologic scoring systems such as the Trauma Score (TS) and the Paediatric Trauma Score (PTS) are used to predict outcome and direct patients to appropriate facilities [7,8]. Easy to use Revised Trauma Score (RTS) detects cerebral, cardiovascular and respiratory dysfunction by testing consciousness (GCS), systolic arterial blood pressure and respiratory frequency. The NACA-scale (National Advisory Committee of Aeronautics) used in helicopter rescue systems adequately describes life threat in trauma victims and correlates well with morbidity and mortality. Thus, it is a valuable tool for demographic purposes in emergency medical systems. The Glasgow Coma Scale (GCS) is a useful prognostic tool for patients with acute head injuries [9]. Initial evaluation of the patient's GCS, pupil reactivity, and four-extremity motor function provides a baseline of neurological function prior to extensive therapeutic manoeuvres. Intracranial swelling leading to brain death following trauma is a major cause of traumatic death [10]. Endotracheal intubation and hyperventilation should be initiated on all comatose trauma patients. The indication for immediate endotracheal intubation and hyperventilation varies from trauma centre to trauma centre, ranging from a GCS of 7 or lower to a GCS of 9 or lower. Intubation in the field prior to transport would be most beneficial to comatose patients, as they would receive early airway protection from aspiration as well as hyperventilation with oxygen. Care must be taken to stabilize the cervical spine during intubation because of the increased association of cervical spine injury with head and facial injuries in blunt trauma [11]. However, despite the fear about the unstable cervical spine raised by radiographic post-mortem studies of a few victims who died from devastating total body crush injuries [12], a well conducted oral endotracheal intubation can be performed without spinal cord damage. Cervical spine stabilisation during intubation can be adequately performed with manual immobilization of the head and neck on a long spine board.

Airway control is vital to improve pulmonary gas exchange during resuscitation from haemorrhagic shock as well as to protect the patient from aspiration. The trauma patient who cannot maintain a patent, protected airway should have a cuffed tube placed in the trachea. Oral or nasal airways have no role in the initial management of the unstable trauma patient except to maintain a patent airway temporarily during preparation for endotracheal intubation.

Resuscitation from haemorrhagic shock requires rapid administration of intravenous fluids to ensure the circulation of well-oxygenated blood from the lungs to the brain and other vital organs. If disruption of either the superior or inferior vena cava is suspected, intravenous catheters should be placed to provide infusion into the heart through the other vena cava. Therefore, intravenous catheters should be placed above and below the diaphragm in patients with severe trauma to the chest or abdomen. Warming of intravenous fluids is extremely important if the trauma patient requires several exchanges of blood volume. Hypothermia decreases the effectiveness of haemorrhagic shock resuscitation.

The choice of the initial administered fluid is based on the priority of first restoring intravascular volume, next haemoglobin concentration, and finally coagulation [13-15]. Proponents of crystalloid use claim that such solutions replace extracellular water more effectively than colloidal solutions. Colloidal solutions preserve intravascular volume and microcirculatory blood flow more efficiently than crystalloids and they increase cardiac output and oxygen delivery, as well as blood pressure, at much lower infused volume than do crystalloid solutions. Crystalloid solutions may merely restore blood pressure without increasing cardiac output. In penetrating trauma, it is important to note that surgical procedures to stop blood loss should precede blood and volume replacement [16]. The anaesthesiologist must be aware of the potential for venous air embolism until injured cervical veins are ligated or repaired. The patient should be kept in a flat or slightly head-down position; positive pressure ventilation is used to increase venous pressure in the neck.

Analgesia, sedation, anaesthesia

In most posttraumatic pain situations peripheral nociceptors are activated and normal afferences are conducted via an intact nociceptive system. In contrast, lesions of the nervous system itself cause neuropathic pain. Mechanisms of central sensibilization and involvement of the sympathetic nervous system may lead to chronification of such pain conditions. In posttraumatic pain, a certain number of adjuvant blockades or infiltrations of trigger points may be helpful.

The prehospital approach to the trauma victim includes analgesics in addition to non-pharmacological measures for pain reduction such as immobilisation of fractured bones in splints. In fractures of limb or back, morphine (10 mg i.v.) or piritramide (15 mg i.v.) are effective (Table 1).

Table 1. Properties of commonly used agents

Use for	Drug	Dose (mg/kg i.v.)
Non-opioid analgesia	Diclofenac	1.0
	Naproxen	5-7 (oral)
	Paracetamol	15 (oral)
Opioid analgesia	Morphine	0.05-0.15
	Piritramide	0.07-0.20
	Tramadol	0.5-1.5
	Ketamine (analgetic dose)	0.25-0.5
	S-(+)-Ketamin	0.1-0.2
	Fentanyl for use in ventilated patients during anaesthesia	0.002-0.01
Sedation	Diazepam	0.05-0.15
	Midazolam	0.03-0.05
Anaesthesia	Thiopentone	3.5-5.0
	Propofol	1-2
	Etomidate	0.2-0.4
	Ketamine (anaesthetic dose)	1-2
	S-(+)-Ketamin	0.5-1
Muscle relaxation	Succinylcholine	1.0-1.5
	Vecuronium	0.2-0.3
	Rocuronium	0.6-0.9

Sometimes higher doses are required to relief pain. In multiply injured patients, adequate treatment may not be possible until anaesthesia has been induced. This is especially true in blunt chest trauma and brain injury. Pain induces sympathetic activity and metabolic responses leading to increased oxygen consumption, vasoconstriction and elevated intracranial pressure. This is part of the initial response to haemorrhagic shock. Sedation and sufficient analgesic therapy are essential even in the unconscious patient, and the use of muscle relaxants alone is obsolete. Analgesics, especially opioids blunt the sympathetic stress reaction. Substantial decrease of systemic blood pressure may follow the administration of these drugs. Ketamine or S-(+)- Ketamine may be the drug of choice in haemodynamic instability, in jammed patients, or in triage situations, where the number of patients outweighs medical resources initially available on the scene. Ketamine acts like an analgesic in low doses, but induces anaesthesia in higher doses. Respiratory depression occurs rarely, but systemic blood pressure rises. Psychomimetic side effects are covered by the use of benzodiazepam for sedation. In contrast to earlier recommendations, ketamine is not contraindicated in brain injury, if the patient is ventilated sufficiently.

Acute pain management for wound pain and patients suffering from bone fractures starts with opioids. Despite the fact that this type of pain is treated more efficiently by non-opioids like cyclooxygenase inhibitors (diclofenac, naproxen etc., Table 1) or paracetamol, WHO group three opioids (piritramide, morphine hydrochloride) facilitate fast onset, and, hence, are best at the site of an emergency. For induction of anaesthesia, thiopentone or propofol are the drugs of choice. While the former substance has to be prepared before administration, propofol is ready to use. This is an important advantage at the site of an emergency. Both, however, may produce a decrease of systemic blood pressure in hypovolemic trauma patients. Etomidate is ready for injection, too, but it does not influence blood pressure and myocardial function. Thus, etomidate may be used in the haemodynamically unstable patient. Fentanyl is a 100-times more potent than morphine and should be used for analgesia in ventilated patients. Orotracheal intubation facilitated by the use of muscle relaxants is the technique of choice for intubating the trachea of trauma patients. Succinylcholine (1-1.5 mg/kg) may produce elevation of intracranial and intraocular pressure. Despite the fact that this might be harmful in penetrating eye injury, one should never delay intubation because of this theoretical concern. Succinylcholine may also produce hyperkalemia as a result of asynchronous depolarisation of the muscle cells. Although the elevation in serum potassium is typically below 0.5 mEq/dl, in some pathologic states the hyperkalemic response may exceed 5 mEq/gl. These conditions include severe burns and major muscle trauma. It is important to note, however, that these large elevations will occur only in patients who had significant tissue damage at least 24 hours to a couple of days before succinylcholine administration. Succinylcholine is therefore not contraindicated in the acute phase of trauma management. We do not recommend mivacurium (0.12-0.2 mg/kg) for emergency use since it's metabolism is dependent on pseudocholinesterase, and this substance is a strong histamine liberator. Rocuronium (0.6-0.9 mg/kg) is a relatively fast acting nondepolarising muscle relaxant. This substance is to be used, if endotracheal intubation can be planned and aspiration is not a primary concern. An emergency room comparison of muscle relaxant-facilitated oral intubation and blind nasal intubation demonstrated a high rate of complications, including aspiration, in the blind nasal group [17].

Correctly applied cricoid pressure protects the airway from aspiration of stomach contents. Cricoid pressure prevents insufflating the stomach with air during mask ventilation prior to intubation in addition to preventing regurgitation of gastric contents into the mouth [18]. Administering oxygen via mask-and-bag ventilation, using cricoid pressure to protect the airway, improves oxygenation prior to endotracheal intubation. Ultimately, the best protection from aspiration for the trauma patient is pain treatment and sedation, and a smooth, well-conducted endotracheal intubation.

Anaesthesia during transportation

If the airway is secured, and the patient presents haemodynamically stable, the prehospital trauma team is ready for transportation. Analgesics and sedatives will be effective on transportation as well. For helicopter transportation one should choose a prophylactic agent against nausea and vomiting (metoclopramide, haloperidol, ondasentron, granisetron). For controlled ventilated patients, choices of anaesthesia maintenance are

- Opioide-benzodiazepine-combination, i.e., fentanyl 1-4 µg/kg every 10-30 min plus midazolam 0,05-0,1 mg/kg every 10-30 min administered intravenously (i.v.)
- Ketamine-benzodiazepine-combination (especially in haemorrhagic shock): ketamine 1 mg/kg every 10-15 min or 2-6 mg/h/h; alternatively use S-(+)-ketamine 0,5-3 mg/kg/h, both in combination with midazolam 0,05-0,1 mg/kg every 10-15 min i.v.

One challenge of trauma care is the continuous need to transport critically ill patients throughout the hospital. Patients suffering from multiple blunt trauma frequently have associated head injuries and require multiple brain CT scans for diagnosis and follow-up of treatment regimens. CT, MRI, and radionuclide imaging techniques are used to outline the extent of injury in other body regions beside the head. Because these imaging techniques require fixed specialised equipment, the patients must be moved to the imaging area.

The anaesthesiologist is responsible for anaesthetic technique and adequate level of monitoring throughout transportation and anaesthesia at remote locations. Patients with head injury who have intracranial pressure that is critically sensitive to $PaCO_2$ should be transported with constant ventilation. Portable, battery-powered carbon dioxide monitors facilitate monitoring ventilation during patient transport. Transportation by helicopter or ambulance accentuates all the problems of transportation of critically ill patients and is a frontier of trauma care in which anaesthesiologists can have a vital impact.

Anaesthesia in the emergency room

Diagnostic and therapeutic procedures should be sequentially performed to meet the needs determined by vital functions, type of injury and its severity. The anaesthetist aims on circulatory stability, sufficient respiratory function and pain management. Surgical intervention to stop haemorrhage and to fix long bone fractures are listed on top of the priority list for subsequent treatment in the operation room. Unstable mandibular or maxillofacial fractures may make mask ventilation impossible, and awake intubation frequently relieves life-threatening airway obstruction. Direct laryngoscopy is frequently superior to fiberoptic bronchoscopic intubation in these patients because upper airway bleeding may preclude adequate visualization.

Tracheotomy is reserved for those patients who cannot be intubated translaryngeally. Massive disruption of the floor of the mouth by penetrating injury and disruption of the larynx or cervical trachea are two indications for emergency tracheotomy. However, it is frequently worth one attempt to intubate patients carefully with a small endotracheal tube prior to tracheotomy unless open laryngeal cartilage is seen during direct laryngoscopy. The cricothyrotomy route is the preferred route for an emergency primary tracheotomy [19]. Although the prolonged care of many patients with maxillofacial injuries and brain trauma is improved by an intraoperative tracheotomy, the presence of highly skilled anaesthesiologists in a trauma centre will minimise the number of emergency cricothyrotomies needed for airway control. Anaesthesiologists should be comfortable with the technique of cricothyrotomy with both a needle and a tracheotomy tube.

High-energy fractures of the femur cause the release of large amounts of bone marrow fat into the circulation. Post fracture hypoxic respiratory failure occurs as the circulating fat released from the fracture collects in the pulmonary vascular system. More recently investigational interest has focused on the interaction among platelets, the coagulation system, and fat in the release of vasoactive substances and the triggering of intravascular coagulopathy. Lung surfactant activity is decreased, functional residual capacity is reduced, and diffusion abnormality develops. Early operative stabilization of the fracture under general anaesthesia with positive-pressure ventilation will prevent mild post fracture hypoxia from developing into severe adult respiratory distress syndrome (ARDS).

Many trauma patients, on analysis with pulse oximetry or admission blood gas measurements, exhibit significant degrees of oxygen desaturation because of deranged chest wall mechanics or intrapulmonary ventilation/perfusion abnormalities. Endotracheal intubation is avoidable even in patients with multiple rib fractures. Thoracic epidural catheters are able to provide both pain relief and improved oxygen saturation. Hence, such a patient may only need continuous positive airway pressure (CPAP) therapy by face or nose mask, and the risk of infectious complications due to controlled ventilation is reduced.

Trauma operations: general anaesthesia, regional anaesthesia

Preanaesthetic history

Preanaesthetic history includes information from the scene of the accident, either from the prehospital physician, witnesses or from the patient's own description. Information about how the injury occurred will help the anaesthesiologist to prepare for surgical correction of occult injuries.

Preoperative information concerning allergies, pre-existing diseases, previous operations, and drug therapy is as important in the trauma patient as in any other surgical patient. Although trauma patients must be treated as patients with full stomachs, careful inquiry into time and type of last oral intake will reveal a variable potential for quantity and quality of stomach contents [20]. Self-medication with psychoactive drugs and alcohol is a particular problem with trauma patients. Careful questioning will frequently reveal a pattern of substance abuse followed by injury, which is especially prevalent in chronic alcoholics [21]. Besides ethanol, trauma patients frequently are intoxicated with marijuana, cocaine, phencyclidine (PCP), and opioids. A history of chronic substance abuse or acute intoxication alerts the anaesthesiologist to prepare for unusual responses to anaesthetic drugs [22].

The orderly progression of history, physical examination, diagnosis, and treatment must often be abandoned with trauma patients, as resuscitation has priority over diagnosis to ensure a successful outcome. The anaesthesiologist will be primarily concerned with preserving CNS function, maintaining adequate respiratory gas exchange, and achieving circulatory homeostasis. Patients with minimal impairment on neurological examination may be hiding significant brain pathology that would cause them to decompensate during anaesthesia. Therefore, these patients require a baseline neurological examination, a computed tomography (CT) scan of the brain, and the placement of an intracranial pressure recording device if there is any question about structural brain injury. Ensuring an adequate flow of well-oxygenated arterial blood to the brain and preventing secondary spinal cord damage due to movement of an unstable spinal fracture protect CNS function.

Physical examination

Trauma patients require a physical examination and laboratory testing, as do other surgical patients, but with concentration on the respiratory, circulatory, and nervous systems. The status of the CNS is evaluated with a brief neurological examination, including level of consciousness (GCS), pupil size, pupil reactivity, and motor function of each extremity. If the trachea is not intubated, the examination includes evaluation of the upper airway for potential intubation problems. Immobilization of the cervical spine will increase the difficulty of intubation. The anaesthesiologist should examine the chest for signs of pneumothorax, myocardial contusion, and pericardial tamponade. The circulatory system is evaluated for signs of haemorrhagic shock and blood loss. Arterial blood gases, chest radiographs, cervical spine roentgenograms, haemoglobin and haematocrit measurements, serum glucose, urea nitrogen, creatinine, and electrolytes as well as an electrocardiogram (ECG) round out the laboratory analysis.

Monitoring

Trauma patients require at least basic non-invasive monitoring in accordance with the minimal standards concerning ventilation, oxygenation, circulation and body temperature regardless of the anaesthetizing location - emergency room, diagnostic area, radiology suite, operating room, or critical care unit.

More invasive monitoring is indicated to evaluate the patient's response to therapy. Urinary output via an indwelling urethral catheter (Foley catheter) is an important indicator of fluid balance and renal perfusion modelling organ perfusion in general. The urinary catheter is also a diagnostic tool for trauma to the urinary tract that causes haematuria. Oxygen consumption can be calculated from the pulmonary artery catheter measurements by using the product of cardiac output times the difference between PaO_2 and pulmonary artery oxygen content. Mortality from trauma varies inversely with post-traumatic oxygen consumption [23].

Anaesthesia plan and intraoperative management

General anaesthesia is the technique of choice for patients with multiple injuries. Regional anaesthesia may seem attractive because it causes little interference with the patient's cardiopulmonary function and avoids airway manipulation. However, patients with serious trauma benefit from endotracheal intubation and mechanical ventilation and are unlikely to co-operate with lying still during prolonged surgery. Combined regional and general anaesthesia may be a solution. Sympathetic blockade from spinal or epidural anaesthesia offers the advantage to uncover hidden hypovolemia. Therefore, regional anaesthesia is most useful for isolated limb trauma, for example, brachial plexus block for a forearm fracture.

General anaesthesia can be administered safely in the patient with multiple injuries by choosing drugs that minimize cardiovascular depression and intracranial hypertension. Small doses of highly lipophilic drugs such as thiopental, etomidate, and sufentanil can be titrated to desired anaesthetic effect without producing profound hypotension. Although pharmacokinetic data during haemorrhagic shock are limited, clinically these patients appear to reach desired drug effects from extremely small intravenous doses. The reduction in blood volume probably concentrates the delivered dose at the active site in the brain, and reduced hepatic blood flow may prolong clearance of the drug. However, normal doses of muscle relaxants need to be used to achieve the rapid paralysis necessary for endotracheal intubation. The drugs outlined in table 1 for induction of anaesthesia and endotracheal intubation are useful in both the operating room as well as the emergency room.

Succinylcholine is contraindicated because of exaggerated hyperkalemia more than 24 hours after upper motor neuron (spinal cord) injury and more than 24 hours following major burns. The inadvertent use of succinylcholine in these patients can be treated with intravenous calcium, glucose, and insulin as well as cardiopulmonary resuscitation to support the circulation until the serum potassium falls to levels consistent with normal cardiac function. Short acting, non-depolarizing neuromuscular blocking drugs such as mivacurium have a much longer onset time than succinylcholine but do terminate action rapidly. Large doses (several multiples of the ED_{95}) of vecuronium have been used to decrease onset time for neuromuscular blockade. Drugs such as rocuronium combine rapidity of onset with a short duration of neuromuscular blockade similar to that of succinylcholine.

Nitrous oxide is contraindicated for patients with potentially closed air spaces in which this anaesthetic will accumulate such as patients with pneumothorax, pneumocephaly, and gas-filled bowel loops. Its use for head-injured patients is controversial, but at low concentrations its contribution to cerebral blood flow/metabolism imbalance is probably minimal. Nitrous oxide has also been demonstrated to decrease cardiac output when combined with opioids. Thus, the use of nitrous oxide should be specifically indicated for trauma patients, not used routinely. Anaesthesia machines should be equipped to deliver air, oxygen, and nitrous oxide for use with these patients so that air-oxygen mixtures may be used to decrease the inspired oxygen fraction (FIO_2).

Common intraoperative problems

Despite the complexities of the injuries in a multiple trauma patient, certain intraoperative problems occur frequently. Some problems - prolonged anaesthesia, hypothermia, and massive transfusion - are consequence of long and difficult surgery in a patient with uncontrolled haemorrhage. Other complications, namely, facial trauma, burns, hypoxia, fever, and malignant hyperthermia (MH), are a result of specific injuries or patient characteristics. The pregnant patient, the very young patient, and the very old patient present special problems for trauma anaesthesia. Finally, cardiac arrest (usually electromechanical dissociation) is the terminal event for acute trauma victims who die in the operating room.

Prolonged surgery

Prolonged operations require prolonged anaesthesia. Optimal outcome for an unstable multiply injured patient is achieved if all injuries can be corrected at the time of initial surgery. The blunt trauma victim with multiple fractures will especially benefit from early fracture fixation that reduces ongoing haemorrhage, intravascular release of marrow, and postoperative complications of immobilization. The anaesthesiologist must treat the operating room as an intensive care unit for these patients.

Hypothermia

Maintenance of temperature homeostasis challenges anaesthesiologists caring for multiply injured patients. Many patients enter the trauma centre with low body temperature, and an inverse relationship between temperature and Trauma score has been noted. Prolonged exposure to a cold operating room, evaporative heat loss from the respiratory tract, infusions of cold fluids, and loss of heat production secondary to shock cause decreased core temperature in most patients. Hypothermia can contribute to wound infections both by directly impairing immune function [24] and by triggering thermoregulatory vasoconstriction that in turn decreases wound oxygen delivery [25]. Profound hypothermia (<33°C), finally, can produce unconsciousness. All skin surfaces not in the surgical field should be covered to reduce convective and radiant heat loss. This is especially true for vasodilated skin areas during regional anaesthesia. Convective air heaters help to restore and maintain body temperature. Humidification of inspired gases reduces evaporative heat loss from the lung, and saturation of inspired gases with water heated higher than body temperature produces active warming of the patient. All intravenous fluids should be warmed; modern equipment is available, with heat exchangers capable of warming fluids to 37°C at very rapid infusion rates. Other techniques of temperature maintenance include warming the operating room above 22°C and irrigating open body cavities with warm saline.

Massive blood transfusion

Prolonged surgical attempts to achieve haemostasis require the anaesthesiologist to replace massive amounts of fluids. After their blood volume has been replaced several times, patients frequently develop dilutional thrombocytopenia, prolonged clotting times, and transient reductions in calcium ion concentration. The consumptive coagulopathy is a spectrum of disorders characterised by inappropriate and widespread small vessel thrombosis, associated with generalized bleeding as a result of the consumption of coagulation factors and excessive fibrinolysis. Transfused red cells serve to dilute out patient's native coagulation reserves [26]. These effects are exacerbated by the infusion of dextrans or starch. Coagulopathy is treated with appropriate factor replacement. The anaesthesiologist should monitor the coagulation status to prescribe replacement therapy accurately. Calcium replacement is initiated when ionized calcium levels decrease secondary to citrate chelation or when hypotension occurs despite adequate volume replacement [27]. The bivalent cat ion Ca^{++} is the active form of calcium, and replacement based on calcium concentrations should be based on measured ionized calcium, not total calcium.

Local and regional anaesthesia

Proper wound preparation requires adequate anaesthesia. Local anaesthetic agents may be classified as amides or esters (Table 2). Allergic reactions to these agents are rare and are usually due to preservatives (such as methylparaben). Most often these reactions are seen in response to ester-type local anaesthetics, but amide-type drugs may cause allergic reactions as well [28]. Patients with known allergies to a specific local anaesthetic from one of the groups (for example, procaine) can be treated with an agent from the other group (for example, lidocaine). The use of pure agents without preservatives (for example, cardiac lidocaine) further reduces the risk of an allergic reaction. Diphenhydramine may be used for the rare patient who is allergic to an unknown local anaesthetic agent [29].

Table 2. Properties of commonly used local anaesthetic agents

Agent	Trade name	Class	Recommended concentration Percent	Maximal safe dose mg/kg	Duration of action
Procaine	Novocain	Ester	0.5 –1.0	7	15 –45 min
with epinephrine				9	30 –90 min
Lidocaine	Xylocaine	Amide	0.5 –2.0	4.5	1 – 2 hr
with epinephrine				7	2 – 4 hr
Bupivacaine	Marcaine	Amide	0.125 – 0.25	2	4 – 8 hr
with epinephrine	Carbostesin			3	8 – 16 hr
Ropivacaine	Naropin	Amide	0.2-0.4	8	4 – 6 hr
Levobupivacaine	Chirocain	Amide	0.125 – 0.25	5	4 – 6 hr

There are several ways to reduce the pain associated with local infiltration: adding sodium bicarbonate to the local anaesthetic; using warm solutions of anaesthetic, small needles, and slow rates of infiltration; injecting the agent through the edges of the wound when the wound is not contaminated; and pretreating the wound with topical anaesthetics [30-33]. The change in the local pH of the wound due to buffering does not increase the likelihood of infection [34]. Alternative methods of anaesthesia include topical application and regional nerve blocks.

Regional anaesthesia should be used for large wounds that would otherwise require large, potentially toxic doses of local anaesthetics. In the trauma patient, regional anaesthesia is especially recommended in osteosynthetic stabilization of isolated limb fractures. The practice of any regional anaesthesia technique presumes the intact state of the patient's coagulation mechanism. Creation of compressive haematoma or neural ischaemia is the potential result of an attempted block in a patient with a coagulopathy.

Interscalene, infraclavicular, axillary plexus brachialis block

Interscalene block is effective for surgery and postoperative pain management in the shoulder or upper arm. Reduction of dislocated shoulders is an ideal candidate since this block can be performed with the arm almost in any position. Landmarks of anatomy include the larynx, sternocleidomastoid muscle, and external jugular vein. To insert a catheter for postoperative use, the needle should be inserted in a plain joining the cricoid cartilage to the C6 transverse process, and is then directed in a caudal and posterior direction. The volume of local anaesthetics is 30-40 ml. Potential problems include sparing of the ulnar nerve and its more peripheral distribution to the hand, pneumothorax, and epidural or phrenic block.

Infraclavicular brachial plexus block is often used for trauma patients requiring prolonged analgesia after procedures on the elbow, forearm or hand. The advantage over the axillary approach is the sufficient analgesia for cuffed blood barriers placed on the upper arm during surgery. For performance of both infraclavicular and axillary plexus block, patients must be able to abduct the arm at the shoulder.

Femoral and three-in-one block

This block is ideal for hip fractures. t is a technique for blocking femoral, lateral femoral cutaneous and obturator nerves, hence, providing analgesia in the anterior thigh, both superficial and deep. Since the patient is in supine position when this block is carried out, virtually any patient undergoing a surgical procedure of the lower extremity is a candidate. After identification of the femoral pulse, the needle is advanced slowly cephalic at about 60°. It is easy to insert a catheter, and 20 ml of a local anaesthetic are administered. For superficial and lateral procedures, i.e., skin graft harvesting, the lateral femoral cutaneous nerve may be blocked additionally at a site 2 cm medial and 2 cm caudal to the anterior superior iliac spine.

Intercostal nerve blocks

Intercostal nerve blocks provide excellent analgesia to the body wall. They are appropriate to use for analgesia after unilateral rib fractures or minor surgical procedures. Needle insertion is just lateral to the paraspinous muscles at the angle of the ribs. In each level, the needle is directed onto the rib passing by caudally for an addition centimetre. Volume of local anaesthetic is no more than 1-2 ml.

Neuroaxial blockade

Lumbar spinal is especially useful for any trauma surgery of the lower limb. For hip fractures in the elderly this block is the method of choice. However, patient selection often places too much emphasis on spinal headache than on the applicability of the technique. The incidence of spinal headache correlates inversely with age, and is higher in female gender. It is more important to perform this block on the first pass than to use a small 26-gauge needle. Correct patient position may be difficult due to pain from the injured bone. For trauma patients both the sitting or lateral decubital positions are suitable. The latter allows unilateral block using hyperbaric local anaesthetics. A small dose of ketamine may be given intravenously.

Lumbar epidural and combined spinal epidural (CSE) anaesthesia offer the advantage for postoperative pain management. CSE blocks have the advantages of both techniques when used as the single-space technique. When epidural anaesthesia is used without intrathecal administration, required doses of local anaesthetics make systemic toxicity a concern. We use much lower concentrations for postoperative pain relief.

Thoracic epidural catheters are ideal for isolated chest trauma and multiple rib fractures. While ventilation deteriorates with pain relief due to systemic opioids, epidurals abolish pain and improve respiratory performance.

Postoperative pain management

Non-opioids are sufficient for trauma patients with bone fractures treated in the recovery room or on the ward. Opioids administered by pumps on demand (patient-controlled analgesia, PCA) may be used. We allow boluses of 1.5 mg piritramide every 10 minutes, and we permit a maximum of 30 mg within four hours.

Postoperative pain management by continuous epidural analgesia is an excellent choice for patients with chest trauma, because analgesia is provided without depression of consciousness, thus permitting continuous neurological evaluation. Serious neurological complications caused by spinal haematoma or abscess following central neuraxial block have been reported more often during the last years. In contrast, severe complications are extremely rare associated with peripheral nerve blocks. We encourage the use of peripheral regional techniques for procedures on the lower extremity and especially for postoperative regional analgesia. Motor block due to lumbar epidural anaesthesia using high concentrations of local anaesthetic makes spinal haematoma or abscess difficult to recognize. Therefore, low concentrations of local anaesthetic should be used for postoperative epidural analgesia. Any increase in motor block following neuraxial blockade should raise the suspicion of a spinal compression (e.g. haematoma or abscess). By using low concentrations of these potent drugs, i.e., bupivacain 0.0625% or ropivacaine 0.08%, no toxic plasma levels are seen with the exception of artificial intravasal injections. Additives such as opioids and β_2-sympathomimetics (clonidine) are also used. While the use of opioids is controversial, β_2-sympathomimetics are able to accelerate the onset and to extend the duration of regional anaesthesia and analgesia.

Conclusion

Trauma care is becoming an increasingly important part of modern medical practice. Analgesia is an important part of trauma care. Conscious trauma patients suffer from strong pain from their injuries and from manipulations during transportation and diagnostic procedures. Even in unconscious injured patients analgetics are mandatory to reduce stress. It is routine on the scene and in the emergency room to treat pain after the first survey in almost every injured patient. Endotracheal intubation may be necessary to provide a secure airway and to ensure sufficient ventilation. Intramuscular administration has no place in trauma. In hospital, regional anaesthesia is an elegant method for pain control.

References

1. Grande CM (ed) (1993) Textbook of Trauma Anesthesia and Critical Care. Mosby-Year Book, St. Louis
2. Committee on Trauma of the American College of Surgeons Resources for Optimal Care of the Injured Patient (1990). American College of Surgeons, Chicago
3. Booij LHDJ (1982) Pitfalls in anaesthesia for multiply injured patients. Injury 14:81
4. Burri C, Kreuzer U, Limmer J (1982) Principles and practice of fracture treatment in the multiply injured patient. Injury 14:44
5. Gann DS, Lilly MP (1983) The neuroendocrine response to multiple trauma. World J Surg 7:101
6. Baker SP, O'Neill B, Haddon W, Long WB (1974) The injury severity score: a method for describing patients with multiple injuries and evaluating emergency care. J Trauma 14:187-196
7. MacKenzie EJ (1984) Injury severity scales: overview and directions for future research. Am J Emerg Med 2:537
8. Morris JA, Auerbach PS, Marshall GA et al. (1986) The trauma score as a triage tool in the prehospital setting. JAMA 256:1319

9. Jennett B, Teasdale G (1977) Aspects of coma after severe head injury. Lancet 1:878
10. Committee on Trauma Research Injury in America (1985) A Continuing Public Health Problem. National Academy Press, Washington
11. Lewis VL, Manson PN, Morgan RF et al. (1985) Facial injuries associated with cervical fractures: recognition, patterns and management. J Trauma 25:90
12. Bivins HG, Ford S, Bezmalinovic Z et al. (1988) The effect of axial traction during orotracheal intubation of the trauma victim with an unstable cervical spine. Ann Emerg Med 17:25
13. Lowery BD, Cloutier CT, Carey LC (1971) Electrolyte solutions in resuscitation in human hemorrhage shock. Surg Gynecol Obstet 133:273
14. Modig J (1986) Effectiveness of dextran 70 versus Ringer's acetate in traumatic shock and adult respiratory distress syndrome. Crit Care Med 14:454
15. Hankeln K, Radel C, Beez M et al. (1989) Comparison of hydroxyethyl starch and lactated Ringer's solution on hemodynamics and oxygen transport of critically ill patients in prospective crossover studies. Crit Care Med 17:133
16. Bickell WH, Wall MJ, Pepe PE et al (1994) Immediate versus delayed fluid resuscitation for hypotensive patients with penetrating torso injuries. N Engl J Med 331:1105-1109
17. Dronen SC, Merigian KS, Hedges JR et al. (1987) A comparison of blind nasotracheal and succinylcholine-assisted intubation in the poisoned patient. Ann Emerg Med 16:650
18. Lawes EG, Campbell I, Mercer D (1987) Inflation pressure, gastric insufflation and rapid sequence induction. Br J Anaesth 59:315
19. American College of Surgeons (1988) Advanced Trauma Life Support Manual. Chicago
20. Hardy JF (1988) Large volume gastroesophageal reflux: a rationale for risk reduction in the perioperative period. Can J Anaesth 35:162
21. Soderstrom CA, Dischinger PC, Smith GS et al. (1992) Psychoactive substance dependence among trauma center patients. JAMA 267:2756
22. Pavlin EG (1993) Ethanol and substance abuse in trauma patients. In: Grande CM (ed) Textbook of Trauma Anesthesia and Critical Care. Mosby-Year Book, St.Louis p 744
23. Shoemaker WC, Appel PL, Kram HB (1988) Tissue oxygen debt as a determinant of lethal and nonlethal postoperative organ failure. Crit Care Med 16:1117
24. Van Oss CJ, Absolom DR, Moore LL et al (1980) Effect of temperature on the chemotaxis, phagocytic engulfment, digestion and O_2 consumption of human polymorphonuclear leukocytes. J Reticuloendothel Soc 27:561-564
25. Sheffield CW, Hopf HW, Sessler DI (1993) Local heat reverses the decrease in subcutaneous oxygen tension produced by thermoregulatory vasoconstriction. Anesth Analg 76:S389
26. British Committee for standards in haematology blood transfusion task force (1988) Transfusion for massive blood loss. Clin Lab Haematol 10:265-267
27. Martlew VJ (2000) Perioperative management of patients with coagulation disorders. Br J Anaesth 84:446-455
28. Egglestone ST, Lush LW (1996) Understanding allergic reactions to local anesthetics. Ann Pharmacother 30:851
29. Dire DJ, Hogan DE (1993) Double-blind comparison of diphenhydramine versus lidocaine as a local anesthetic. Ann Emerg Med 22:1419-22
30. Bartfield JM, Gennis P, Barbera J et al (1990) Buffered versus plain lidocaine as a local anesthetic for simple laceration repair. Ann Emerg Med 19:1387-9.
31. Brogan GX Jr, Giarrusso E, Hollander JE et al (1995) Comparison of plain, warmed, and buffered lidocaine for anesthesia of traumatic wounds. Ann Emerg Med 26:121-5.
32. Bartfield JM, Lee FS, Raccio-Robak N et al (1996) Topical tetracaine attenuates the pain of infiltration of buffered lidocaine. Acad Emerg Med 3:1001-5.
33. Kelly A-M, Cohen M, Richards D (1994) Minimizing the pain of local infiltration anesthesia for wounds by injection into the wound edges. J Emerg Med 12:593-5
34. Brogan GX, Singer AJ, Valentine SM et al (1997) Comparison of wound infection rates using plain versus buffer lidocaine for anesthesia of traumatic wounds. Am J Emerg Med 15:25-8

Metabolic Pathways in Trauma

G. Biolo

Glutamine and alanine are the major carriers of nitrogen among body tissues. These amino acids are largely synthesized in skeletal muscle [1]. The carbon skeleton of alanine is derived from glycolysis, through a pyruvate, whereas the carbon skeleton of glutamine is derived from the citric acid cycle, through alpha-ketoglutarate. The nitrogen used to form these amino acids is mainly derived from transamination of the branched chain amino acid (leucine, valine and isoleucine) [2] and from intracellular free ammonia. Alanine and glutamine are constantly released from skeletal muscle into the bloodstream, both in the fasting state and in the postaprandial phase. In the liver, alanine is the major amino acid precursor for gluconeogenesis. Glutamine is actively taken up by several tissues to serve as a precursor of many compounds, including hepatic glucose, urinary ammonia, intracellular gluthatione (through glutamate) and nucleic acids. Furthermore, glutamine is utilized for rapidly dividing cells of the intestinal mucosa and immune system [3].

Critically ill patients are characterized by a number of alterations involving body protein kinetics and intermediary metabolism. These metabolic changes represent a common response in almost every acute illness. The greatest alterations are observed in severe trauma, sepsis or large burns. In skeletal muscle there is a persistent loss of myofibrillar protein that is caused by an acceleration of protein degradation. The branched chain amino acids released from accelerated muscle proteolysis are largely oxidized in this tissue. The rate of muscle glycolysis is also accelerated resulting in increased availability of pyruvate that may enter the citric acid cycle or may form lactate which is released into the bloodstream. In the liver, gluconeogenesis from lactate and amino acid precursors is accelerated. Furthermore, there is an increase in glutamine uptake in certain tissues (e.g., kidneys, intestinal mucosa, and immune cells) and a dramatic decline in muscle free glutamine [4].

We have recently evaluated how the muscle tissue provides the peripheral tissues with alanine and glutamine during severe stress [5]. In this study, the rates of alanine and glutamine de novo synthesis have been determined in skeletal muscle during the postabsorptive state in normal controls and in patients with severe burns during the "flow" phase after injury. The patients exhibited an accelerated protein and amino acid catabolism and a depletion of the intramuscular and circulating glutamine pools. We found that, in muscle, the decrease in glutamine concentration was parallel to a suppression of the rate of net synthesis of this amino acid. Consequently, systemic glutamine availability from de novo muscle synthesis was decreased by about 50% in the patients with burns. This observation supports the concept that in severe stress situations glutamine becomes a conditionally essential amino acid and provides the rationale for glutamine supplementation in trauma patients [6-11]. In contrast to glutamine, muscle alanine de novo synthesis was increased more than three times in the patients with burns. Therefore, these results demonstrate that alanine is the major carrier of nitrogen from skeletal muscle to body tissues in conditions of prolonged severe stress. After severe trauma the rates of glycolysis [12] and oxidation of the branched chain amino acids [13] are increased. This leads to an increase in availability of pyruvate and of amino-nitrogen for transamination. As a result, pyruvate is transaminated to alanine at a rate greater than normal [12]. This mechanism potentially limits the availability of glutamate as a precursor for glutamine de novo synthesis through increased transamination to form alanine (Fig. 1). Several lines of evidence

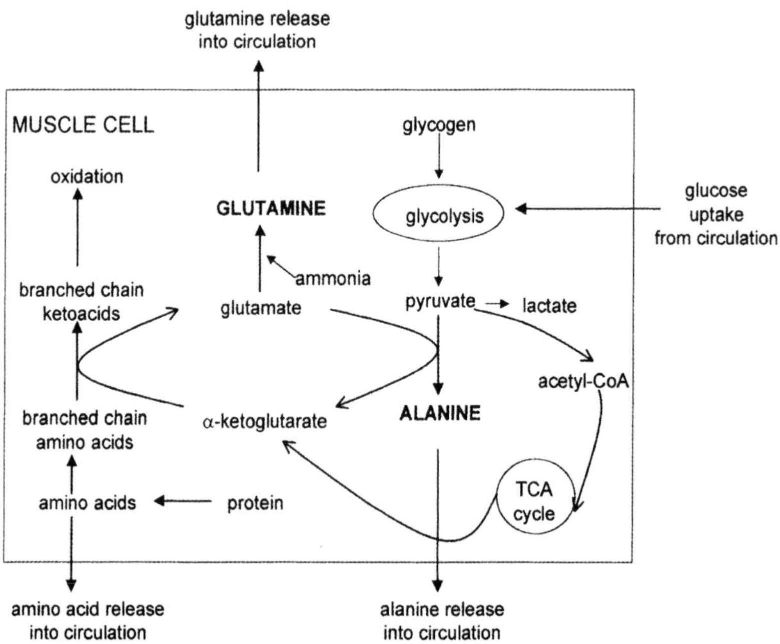

Fig. 1. Schematic presentation of the relation between glutamine and alanine synthesis, branched chain amino acid oxidation, glucose utilization and protein kinetics in skeletal muscle

support this hypothesis: 1) glutamate is decreased in trauma patients [14], and supplementation with alpha-ketoglutarate preserved muscle free glutamine after surgery [15,16]; 2) stimulation of pyruvate oxidation by dichloroacetate administration decreases alanine production [12] and increases muscle glutamine concentration [17] in patients with burns. Finally, muscle free ammonia concentration is elevated in severe stress [18]. Therefore, the reduced glutamine formation in severe burn injury may be the result of a depletion of glutamate, the immediate glutamine precursor, which is preferentially consumed for alanine synthesis. The fact that the activity of the enzyme glutamine synthetase has often been increased in catabolic conditions [19] is consistent with the notion that, whereas the muscle is capable of producing glutamine at an accelerated rate, in the post-absorptive state there are inadequate precursors.

We have further tested in a different study the hypothesis that in trauma the rate of muscle glutamine synthesis is mainly regulated by precursor availability [20]. We have determined the effects of a 24 hour recombinant human growth hormone (rhGH) infusion on muscle protein kinetics and amino acid metabolism in hypercatabolic patients with multiple injuries. We found that rhGH infusion increased muscle protein synthesis. The anticatabolic effect was paralleled by a 50 % suppression of the rate of de novo muscle glutamine production. In contrast, the rate of alanine production did not change during rhGH administration. We also found that the rates of branched chain amino acid oxidation and glutamate utilization were decreased following rhGH infusion. Thus, a decreased glutamine de novo synthesis could be secondary to a decreased glutamate availability from reduced transamination of the branched chain amino acids with Alpha-ketoglutarate. The fact that mRNA levels of glutamine synthetase (i.e., the key enzyme for glutamine synthesis) increased after rhGH infusion, supports the hypothesis that the growth hormone mediated decrease in glutamine synthesis was determined by decreased precursor availability. Gene expression of glutamine synthetase may increase following rhGH infusion to compensate for reduced glutamine precursor availability.

Takala et al. [21] recently reported the results of two large multicenter studies indicating an increased morbidity and mortality in critically ill patients treated with high doses of growth hormone. Multiple organ failure and septic shock or uncontrolled infections were the main causes of death, suggesting that a modulation of the immune system or gut function were involved. However, the reason for such a deleterious effect of growth hormone is still unclear. Our study describes a potential side-effect of rhGH administration in critically ill patients. In these patients, glutamine is an essential substrate for rapidly dividing cells in the immune system and the intestinal mucosa as well as for gluthatione synthesis in the liver. Skeletal muscle is the main tissue involved in glutamine de novo synthesis. In our study [20] whole-body skeletal muscle released about 20 g of glutamine per day into the bloodstream before rhGH administration. Following rhGH administration, glutamine release from skeletal muscle decreased by about 50%, whereas at the whole body level glutamine clearance tended to decrease by about 15%. Therefore, we may speculate that in a clinical setting rhGH therapy could decrease systemic glutamine availability and have negative effects on the immune system and gut function. The obvious solution for this potential side effect of growth hormone treatment in critically ill patients is to simultaneously administer exogenous glutamine to contrast the decreased availability of the endogenous amino acid.

References

1. Biolo G, Fleming RYD, Maggi SP, Wolfe RR (1995) Transmembrane transport and intracellular kinetics of amino acids in human skeletal muscle. Am J Physiol 268:E75-E84
2. Darmaun, D, Dechelotte P (1991) Role of leucine as a precursor of glutamine alpha-amino nitrogen in vivo in humans. Am. J. Physiol. 260: E326-E329
3. Newsholme EA, Crabtree B, Ardawi MSM (1985) The role of high rates of glycolysis and glutamine utilization in rapidly dividing cells. Biosci Rep 5:393-400
4. Askanazi J, Carpentier YA, Michelsen CB, et al (1980) Muscle and plasma amino acids following injury. Ann Surg 192:78-85
5. Biolo G, Fleming RYD, Maggi SP, et al (2000) Inhibition of muscle glutamine formation in hypercatabolic patients. Clinical Science 99: 189-194
6. Stehle P, Mertes N, Puchstein CH, et al (1989) Effect of parenteral glutamine peptide supplements on muscle glutamine loss and nitrogen balance after major surgery. Lancet 1:231-233
7. Ziegler TR, Young LS, Benfell K, et al (1992) Clinical and metabolic efficacy of glutamine-supplemented perenteral nutrition after bone marrow transplantation. Ann Intern Med 116:821-828
8. Van der Hulst RR, van Kreel BK, von Meyenfeld MF, et al (19963) Glutamine and the preservation of gut integrity. Lancet 341:1363-1365
9. Griffiths RD, Jones C, Palmer TEA (1997) Six-months outcome of critically ill patients. Nutrition 13:295-302
10. Houdijk APJ, Rijnsburger ER, Jansen J, et al (1998) Randomized trial of glutamine-enriched enteral nutrition on infectious morbidity in patients with multiple trauma. Lancet 352:772-776
11. Lacey JM, Wilmore DW (1990) Is glutamine a conditionally essential amino acid? Nutr Rev 48:297-309
12. Wolfe RR, Jahoor F, Herndon DN, Miyoshi H (1991) Isotopic evaluation of the metabolism of pyruvate and related substances in normal adult volunteers and severely burned children: effect of dichloroacetate and glucose infusion. Surgery 110:54-67
13. Wolfe RR, Goodenough RD, Burke JF, Wolfe MH (1983) Response of protein and urea kinetics in burn patients to different levels of protein intake. Ann Surg 197:163-171
14. Gamrin L, Essen P, Forsberg AM, et al (1996) A descriptive study of skeletal muscle metabolism in critically ill patients: free amino acids, energy-rich phosphates, protein, nucleic acids, fat, water, and electrolytes. Crit Care Med 24:575-583
15. Hammarqvist F, Wernerman J, von der Decken A, Vinnars E (1991) Alpha-ketoglutarate preserves protein synthesis and free glutamine in skeletal muscle after surgery. Surgery 109:28-36
16. Wernerman J, Hammarqvist F, Vinnars E (1990) Alpha-ketoglutarate and postoperative muscle catabolism. Lancet 335:701-703
17. Ferrando AA, Chinkes DL, Wolf SE, et al (1998) Acute dichloroacetete administration increases

skeletal muscle free glutamine concentrations after burn injury. Ann Surg 228:249-256
18. Ardawi MS, Majzoub MF (1991) Glutamine metabolism in skeletal muscle of septic rats. Metabol 40:155-164
19. Austgen TR, Chakrabarti, Chen MK, Souba WW (1992) Adaptive regulation in skeletal muscle glutamine metabolism in endotoxin-treated rats. J Trauma; 32:600-607
20. Biolo G, Iscra F, Bosutti A, et al (2000) Growth hormone decreases muscle glutamine production and stimulates protein synthesis in hypercatabolic patients. Am J Physiol (Endocrinol Metab) 279:E323-E332
21. Takala J, Ruokonen E, Webster NR, et al (1999) Increased mortality associated with growth hormone treatment in critically ill patients. N Engl J Med 341:785-792

CPR in Trauma and Early Defibrillation

E. CERCHIARI, C. AJMONE CAT

Cardiac arrest is a frequent event ranging from 0.4 to 0.8/1,000 per year [1]. In adults, about 70% of all sudden deaths treated by emergency medical services (EMS) are attributed to presumed cardiovascular diseases [1]; the most-common causes of cardiac arrest of non-cardiac origin are reported to be trauma, non-traumatic bleeding, intoxication, drowning, and pulmonary embolism [2].

In children and young adults (aged 1-45 years) the most-common entities are cardiac diseases (hypertrophic, cardiomyopathy, and myocarditis), airway diseases, epilepsy, hemorrhage, and drug toxicity [3].

According to the Utstein style recommendations [4], the etiology of cardiac arrest is differentiated into (1) of presumed cardiac origin and (2) of origin different from cardiac. However such classification of presumed cardiac origin is not consistently confirmed when compared with the definitive cause as established by clinical evidence or autopsy [5].

In relation to the cause, cardiac arrest may present with a hyperkinetic arrhythmia / ventricular fibrillation (VF) or pulseless ventricular tachycardia (VT) or in a hypokinetic rhythm / asystole or pulseless electrical activity (PEA). The chance of survival is 10 times higher for those patients suffering from VF/VT compared with those with asystole or PEA [6]. In the numerous reports on out-of-hospital cardiac arrest there is wide variation in the reported incidence of VF [7] and in survival, ranging between 2 and 26% - mean 7% [7,8]. In almost all these reports the calculation is based on the first rhythm analysis after the arrival of the ambulance, with various delays in the time from cardiac arrest.

In a recent study [9] aimed at studying the incidence of VF at the time of arrest compared with that on first ECG and the duration of VF, the first ECG showed VF in 43% of all patients, the incidence at the time of arrest was estimated to be 60-70% in all patients and 80-85% in the cases with presumed heart disease. The estimated deterioration rate from VF to asystole was slow, with 40% of patients still in VF 30 min after collapse. Interestingly, in the 10% of patients where arrest was witnessed by the EMS crew, the incidence of VF was very low (42%) in spite of the fact that there was no delay in ECG recording.

Non-VF/VT rhythms are being reported with increasing frequency by acute cardiac life support providers as the first electrocardiographic finding in out-of-hospital cardiopulmonary arrest, although it is still unclear whether the arrest starts in VF/VT evolving into another rhythm or the non VF/VT was the primary arrhythmia responsible for the arrest [10]. Cardiac arrest in non-VF/VT rhythm can also be determined by a variety of causes ranging from respiratory, metabolic, toxic, traumatic, and other [5]. The very low survival rate (0-2%), significantly worse than VF/VT [6-10], is of utmost importance in relation to the reported increased rate of these rhythms.

Treatment algorithms are universally [11] well standardized and besides the common support interventions of CPR, airway securement, and epinephrine, are differentiated based on the presenting ECG rhythm: *FV/pulseless VT* where early defibrillation is the priority and most-effective intervention and *non--VF/VT* (asystole/pulseless electrical activity) where the defibrillation option is not available – probably contributing to the decreased chances of survival – and treatment focuses on correction of reversible causes.

Organization of response to cardiac arrest: the chain of survival

The sequence of interventions required for the treatment of cardiac arrest by any cause are well established and have been summarized since the 1990s in the "chain of survival" [12]: early access, early *CPR*, *early defibrillation*, early advanced life support *(ALS)*.

If all links in the chain come together quickly, there is a good chance of successful resuscitation [1,13]. Early access requires prompt recognition of emergencies that require time-critical interventions. Early access of the EMS system should quickly alert EMS providers and lead callers through the steps of CPR until EMS arrive.

Early CPR is the best treatment for cardiac arrest until the arrival of an AED (automatic external defibrillator) and ALS care. Early CPR generates a cardiac output of 30-50% normal and thereby slows VF deterioration to asystole, may increase the chances of defibrillation, contributes to preservation of heart and brain function, and significantly improves survival [1,9].

Early defibrillation is the single greatest determinant of survival for adult victims of cardiac arrest. Since the development of CPR, public access defibrillation (PAD), made possible by the development of automated external defibrillators (AEDs), holds promise to be the single greatest advance in the treatment of VF arrest doubling the resuscitation rates previously achieved by the most-successful EMS programs [1,9,13].

Early ALS (definitive airway control and pharmacological therapy) is often necessary to sustain a perfusing rhythm once restoration of spontaneous circulation (ROSC) is achieved.

The single variables that proved to be associated with survival from cardiac arrest are type of EMS system (one-tier vs. two-tier), incidence of bystander CPR, and time to defibrillation [14]. Survival is maximum when call-to-shock interval is less than 6 min, inversely related to response time when call-to-shock interval lies in the range between 6 and 11 min, and becomes futile for call-to-shock interval longer than 11 min [13-15].

Since the chain is as strong as its weakest link, each community should identify weaknesses in its chain of survival and strengthen the single links by single initiatives. The evidence on the effectiveness of interventions to improve the single links has been recently reviewed [16].

Early access

Ways to improve early access have focused on reducing the delay in summoning EMS care for persons with chest pain. Several randomized studies of specific interventions designed to heighten community awareness have not shown any improvement in reducing the delay and thus improving early access [17, 18]. The multicenter rapid early action for coronary treatment (REACT) study of community interventions to reduce the time that people with chest pain wait before accessing the EMS system did not show any benefit of the interventions tested [19]. At the time, no interventions have been proved to enhance early access.

Early CPR

Strategies to improve the likelihood of bystander CPR are equally disappointing. Several randomized community intervention trials, including one that involved the distribution of a short CPR training video to households, have failed to show an increased likelihood of either CPR being performed or EMS being summoned [20]. Another study showed that targeting relatives of high-risk individuals did not increase the likelihood of CPR being performed in an emergency [21, 22]. The method used to reach mass audiences and the frequency of the message seem to be potentially crucial determinants of uptake in a targeted audience. So far, no community interventions have been proved to improve the likelihood of CPR being performed in an emergency.

Early defibrillation

This has been clearly shown to be effective in a number of studies, its implementation represents the single most-important possibility of intervention to improve survival and will be discussed in detail.

Early ALS

The single components of ALS have to be analyzed to determine intervention, but indirect data on its effectiveness derive from the superiority of two-tiered systems over single-tier systems [14,15].

It has been proposed [16] to extend the chain of survival by adding three links: (1) early prevention, (2) early recognition, and (3) rehabilitation as a class IIa recommendation.

Prevention strategies are cost-effective and significantly reduce the incidence of heart disease and encompass both primary prevention - before the onset of disease (healthy lifestyle including not smoking, eating an appropriate diet, exercising regularly, and treatment with anticoagulants, antiplatelets, angiotensin-converting enzyme inhibitors, beta-blockers, hydroxymethylglutaryl coenzyme A reductase inhibitors, amiodarone) and secondary prevention - of a second or subsequent event- (implantation of cardioverter defibrillators in patients without comorbid illness and beta-blocker therapy).

Early recognition is implied in the early access link of the chain of survival but is not specifically addressed, whereas the time to treatment is one of the strongest predictors of survival after acute myocardial infarction [23].

Participating in a cardiac rehabilitation program, beginning before discharge and continuing as hospital- or community-based and maintaining life-style changes are two of the most-effective ways to improve quality of life and reduce the risk of additional heart problems after a cardiac event.

However the chain of survival represents the emergency response to an acute event and the proposal of extending it has correctly not been accepted in the ILCOR consensus on science [11].

Early defibrillation

The important considerations relating to the implementation of early defibrillation programs invest the recommendations for response time, type of defibrillator waveform, and identification of potential rescuers who can perform defibrillation.

Guidelines recommendations for defibrillation

The ILCOR 2000 Guidelines [11] identify as a high priority goal:
for in-hospital cardiac arrest:

- early defibrillation, defined as call-to-shock interval less than 3 min in all areas of the hospital and ambulatory care facilities (class I)
- early defibrillation capability defined as trained first responders and appropriate equipment available throughout hospitals and affiliated outpatient facilities (class IIa)
- accurate reporting of response time intervals (class IIa)

for out-of-hospital cardiac arrest:

- early defibrillation, defined as shock delivery within 5 minutes of EMS call receipt
- training, equipment and authorization to perform defibrillation for all healthcare providers with a duty to perform CPR (class IIa)

In *out-of-hospital cardiac arrest* granting defibrillation within 5 min requires, at least in areas where EMS response is expected to be longer, the implementation of PAD programs.

Defibrillation waveforms

The utilization of defibrillators by non-health care personnel has been made possible by the development of automatic/semiautomatic defibrillators that reliably recognize (sensitivity 99%, specificity 96%) shockable rhythms (VF and tachycardia) and indicate the need for shock.

Monophasic waveforms, either damped sinusoidal (MDS) or truncated exponential (MTE), are the conventional waveforms used for transthoracic defibrillation with both manual defibrillators and AEDs. The recommended energy levels with monophasic waveforms are initially 200-J shock with increases in energy levels to either 200 or 300 J and then to 360 J for subsequent shocks.

During the past two decades, biphasic waveform defibrillation has been examined in experimental and clinical settings. Biphasic waveforms deliver both a positive and a negative current that together result in successful defibrillation with significantly less delivered energy than monophasic waveforms when VF is of short duration (< seconds) [24, 25]. The advantages of low-energy biphasic defibrillation in the design of ICDs are widely recognized [26, 27]. By the early 1990s, all implantable defibrillators were designed to use biphasic waveforms.

In the human electrophysiology laboratory or operating room, impedance

-compensating biphasic waveforms with energy levels of 115 or 130 J are as effective as monophasic waveforms with energy levels of 200 to 360 J for induced VF of short duration (15 s) [25, 28, 30].

In a multicenter, randomized clinical study, 150-J biphasic (BTE) waveform and monophasic waveform shock delivery (80% MTE) were compared in victims of out-of-hospital cardiac arrest. Biphasic waveform defibrillation with a fixed energy of 150 J significantly improved the efficacy of defibrillation (98% vs. 67%, P<0.0001). This was associated with a significantly greater rate of ROSC (76% vs. 55%, P<0.02). There were no statistical differences in survival-to-hospital admission and survival-to-hospital discharge between the two groups [31].

PAD programs

Evidence supports establishment of PAD programs in the following cases:

(1) the frequency of cardiac arrest events is such that there is a reasonable probability of 1 AED use in 5 years (estimated event rate of 1 sudden cardiac arrest per 1,000 person-years);

(2) an EMS call-to-shock time interval of less than 5 min cannot be reliably achieved with conventional EMS services.

In many communities, this EMS call-to-shock time interval can be achieved by training and equipping laypersons to function as first responders in the community, recognize cardiac arrest, activate the EMS system at appropriate times, provide CPR; and attach/operate an AED safely.

The 2000 ILCOR guidelines identify three levels of rescuers that can be trained in the use of automatic defibrillators:

level I – BLS responders such as police, fire-fighters, security personnel, etc (class IIa)

level II – targeted responders such as citizens at worksites or in public places (class indeterminate)

level III – family or friends of patients at high risk (class indeterminate)

The existing literature supports as class II evidence only PAD programs utilizing level I rescuers. Although there are no randomized clinical trials on PAD by other levels of responders, several case series with and without historical control subjects conducted among flight attendants, casino workers, and airport personnel have documented the ability of properly trained "layperson" first responders to use AEDs appropriately, safely, and effectively [32-35].

The areas where to locate AED have to be identified on the basis of EMS response times, number of people present, and expected frequency of events. For example, a retrospective analysis of site of occurrence of cardiac arrests in

Seattle King County over 5 years showed that only 16% of cardiac arrests occurred in public locations. The analysis of the public locations sites identified higher incidence sites, including international airports, county jails, shopping malls, with an estimated need of 276 defibrillators to save an estimated number of 8-32 lives in 5 years [36].

In decision models comparing the potential cost-effectiveness of standard EMS systems with that of EMS supplemented by PAD, the implementation of PAD by lay responders would lead to a median incremented survival of 0.7% with a median cost of U.S. $ 44,000 per additional quality adjusted life year, indicating that lay responders' PAD can be cost-effective over a broad range of model assumptions [37, 38].

To satisfy the need to respond to cardiac arrests occurring in private locations, the over-the-counter sale of defibrillators has been proposed. AEDs are small, safe and easy to use, have long-lasting batteries and are cheap, but must be prescribed by a physician. In a consumer scenario, an official deregulation of defibrillators as applications would be needed and could be expected to lead to a significant cost reduction, further improving cost-effectiveness. [39] Against such hypothesis speaks the lack of evidence supporting the effectiveness of widespread home defibrillators and the risk that investment in home defibrillators would induce the risk of resource diversion from EMS systems and prevention [40]. The debate is still ongoing.

Traumatic cardiac arrest

Traumatic cardiac arrest is characterized by a dismal survival, even worse than the corresponding ECG rhythms by non traumatic causes [41].

The presenting ECG rhythm may be VF/VT [5] and the major mechanism by which trauma can determine VF cardiac arrest is believed to be myocardial contusion from thoracic trauma [42].

However, the majority of traumatic cardiac arrests present in non-VF/VT ECG rhythms, secondary to hypoxia, hypovolemia, hypothermia, tension pneumothorax, and cardiac tamponade [11], and thereby, therapeutic interventions, besides support measures (oxygenation, CPR, cardioactive drugs etc), are limited to correction of reversible causes, including control of hemorrhage.

The best-reported results are in *penetrating trauma*, in which rapid transport to a nearby trauma center with pre-arrival notification of the trauma surgical team may be lifesaving [43].

In *blunt trauma*, after aggressive pre-hospital treatment and emergency department thoracotomy, survival was achieved only in patients who either responded to pre-hospital treatment [44] or presented with a heart rate greater than 40 beats /min [45].

The organization of response varies from non-traumatic cardiac arrest and a different chain of survival has been proposed for traumatic cardiac arrest including: (1) access and dispatch, (2) on-field definition of priorities, (3) pre-hospital treatment, (4) triage and hospital selection, (5) in hospital treatment [46].

Therapeutic recommendations for traumatic cardiac arrest interventions are not different from standard cardiac arrest except [11]:

- In the case of multiple patients' events treatment of traumatic cardiac arrest is not indicated
- All interventions require immobilization of head and neck.

Open thoracotomy does not improve outcome from out-of-hospital blunt trauma cardiac arrest, but can be lifesaving for patients with penetrating chest trauma, particularly penetrating wounds of the heart [47].

Recently, a minimally invasive device inserted via a limited thoracic incision, allowing provision of hemodynamic performance comparable to open--chest CPR and epicardial defibrillation, has been developed. Preliminary human studies proved the device to be effective, to allow defibrillation with lower energies, and to be feasible to use in the pre-hospital setting. Further studies are ongoing and the results are needed before final recommendations can be made [48].

The dismal survival of traumatic cardiac arrest and the high human and economic costs of aggressive treatment have stimulated discussion on the desirability of starting resuscitation at all in traumatic cardiac arrest - the cost of futility [41]. The debate is still ongoing and has reasons in favor and against.

Starting aggressive pre-hospital treatment may offer the opportunity of treating reversible causes of cardiac arrest and, thereby, avoid the situation where a less than aggressive treatment may lead to the self-fulfilling prophecy of dismal survival. In a recent workshop, the need to enhance aggressive treatment of trauma cardiac arrest and research to maintain viability has been strongly underlined and promoted [49].

Some authors have proposed aggressive resuscitation of traumatic cardiac arrest in order to offer the best chance of survival and take into consideration that resuscitation of trauma arrest may allow maintenance of the patient for organ donation. However, success was low for ROSC (32/111), for intact survival (2) and for donation (3) [50]. This therapeutic strategy, however, conflicts with the ethical consideration of applying invasive maneuvers being aware of their uselessness for the patient and the risk of inducing false hope in the family. Furthermore, even overlooking the very high costs, the negative effect of repeated resuscitation failures on the resuscitating team should be taken into account.

References

1. Eisenberg MS, Mengert TJ (2001) Primary care: cardiac resuscitation N Engl J Med 344: 1304-1313
2. Kuisma M, Alaspaa A (1997) Out-of-hospital cardiac arrests of non-cardiac origin: epidemiology and outcome. Eur Heart J 18: 1122-1128
3. Richman PB, Nashed AH (1999) The etiology of cardiac arrest in children and young adults: special considerations for ED management Am J Emerg Med 17: 264-270
4. Cummins RO, Chamberlain DA (1991) Recommended guidelines for uniform reporting of data from out-of-hospital cardiac arrest: the Utstein style: a statement for health professionals from a task force of the American Heart Association, the European Resuscitation Council, the Heart and Stroke Foundation of Canada, and the Australian Resuscitation Council. Circulation 84:960--975
5. Kurkciyan I, Meron G, Beheringer W, et al (1998) Accuracy and impact of present causes in patients with cardiac arrest. Circulation 98: 766-771
6. Pepe PE (1993) Cardiac arrest presenting with rhythms other than VF: contribution of resuscitative efforts towards total suvivorship. Crit Care med 21:1813-1814
7. Eisenberg MS (1990) Cardiac arrest and resuscitation: a tale of 29 cities. Ann Emerg Med 19: 179-186
8. Kette F, Sbrojavacca R, Rellini G, et al (1998) Epidemiology and survival rate of out-of-hospital cardiac arrest in north-east Italy: The F.A.C.S. study. Resuscitation 36: 153-159
9. Holmberg M, Holmberg S, Herlitz J, et al (2000) Survival after cardiac arrest outside the hospital in Sweden. Resuscitation 44: 7-17
10. Stratton SJ, Niemann JT (1998) Outcome from out-of-hospital cardiac arrest caused from non ventricular arrhythmias: contribution of successful resuscitation to overall survivorship supports the current practice of initiating out-of-hospital ACLS. Ann Emerg Med 32: 448-453
11. International Guidelines 2000 for CPR and ECC – A Consensus on Science (2000) Resuscitation, 46: 1-447
12. Cummins RO, Ornato JP, Thies WH, Pepe (1991) Improving survival from sudden cardiac arrest: the "chain of survival" concept: a statement for health professionals from the Advanced Life Support Subcommittee and the Emergency Cardiac Care Committee, American Heart Association Circulation 83: 1832-1847
13. Stiell IG, Wells GA, Field BJ, et al (1999) Improved out-of-hospital cardiac arrest survival through the inexpensive optimization of an existing defibrillation program: OPALS Study Phase II. JAMA 281: 1175-1181
14. Nichol G, Stiell IG, Laupacis A (1999) A cumulative meta-analysis of the effectiveness of defibrillator-capable emergency medical services for victims of out-of-hospital cardiac arrest. Ann Emerg Med 34: 517-525
15. Nichol G, Detsky AS, Stiell IG, et al (1996) Effectiveness of emergency medical services for victims of out-of-hospital cardiac arrest: a metaanalysis Ann Emerg Med, 27:700-710
16. Jacobs I, Callanan V, Nichol G, et al (2001) The chain of survival. Ann Emerg Med. 37:S5-S16
17. Bilger MC, Giesen BC, Wollan PC, et al (1997) Improved retention of the EMS activation component (EMSAC) in adult CPR. Resuscitation 35:219-224.
18. Meischke H, Dulberg EM, Schaeffer SS, et al (1997) 'Call fast, Call 911': a direct mail campaign to reduce patient delay in acute myocardial infarction. Am J Public Health 87:1705-1709
19. Simons-Morton DG, Goff DC, Osganian S, et al (1998). Rapid early action for coronary

treatment: rationale, design, and baseline characteristics: REACT Research Group. Acad Emerg Med 5:726-738
20. Eisenberg M, Damon S, Mandel L, et al (1995) CPR instruction by videotape: results of a community project. Ann Emerg Med 25:198-202
21. Dracup K, Moser DK, Taylor SE, et al (1997) The psychological consequences of cardiopulmonary resuscitation training for family members of patients at risk for sudden death. Am JPublic Health 87:1434-1439
22. Dracup K, Moser DK, Doering LV, et al (1998) Comparison of cardiopulmonary resuscitation training methods for parents of infants at high risk for cardiopulmonary arrest. Ann Emerg Med 32:170-177
23. Fibrinolytic Therapy Trialists' (FTT) Collaborative Group (1994) Indications for fibrinolytic therapy in suspected acute myocardial infarction: collaborative overview of early mortality and major morbidity results from all randomised trials of more than 1000 patients. Lancet 343:311--322
24. Jones JL, Swartz JF, Jones RE, et al. (1990) Increasing fibrillation duration enhances reltive asymmetrical biphasic versus monophasic defibrillator waveform efficacy. Circ Res 67:376-384
25. Bardy GH, Marchlinski FE, Sharma AD, et al (1996) Multicenter comparison of truncated biphasic shocks and standard damped sine wave monophasic shocks for transthoracic ventricular defibrillation. Circulation 94:2507-2514
26. Chapman PD, Vetter JW, Souza JJ, et al (1989) Comparison of monophasic with single and dual capacitor biphasic waveforms for nonthoracotomy canine internal defibrillation. J Am Coll Cardiol 14:242-245
27. Bardy GH, Ivey TD, Allen MD, et al (1989) A prospective randomized evaluation of biphasic versus monophasic waveform pulses on defibrillation efficacy in humans. J Am Coll Cardiol 14:728-733
28. Bardy GH, Gliner BE, Kudenchuk PJ, et al (1995) Truncated biphasic pulses for transthoracic defibrillation. Circulation 91:1768-1774
29. Greene HL, DiMarco JP, Kudenchuk PJ, et al (1995) Comparison of monophasic and biphasic defibrillating pulse waveforms for transthoracic cardioversion. Biphasic Waveform Defibrillation Investigators. Am J Cardiol 75:1135-1139
30. Reddy RK, Gleva MJ, Gliner BE, et al (1997) Biphasic transthoracic defibrillation causes fewer ECG ST-segment changes after shock. Ann Emerg Med 30:127-134
31. Schneider T, Martens PR, Paschen H, et al (2000) Multicenter, randomized, controlled trial of 150-J biphasic shocks compared with 200- to 360-J monophasic shocks in the resuscitation of out-of-hospital cardiac arrest victims. Circulation 102:1780-1787
32. O'Rourke MF, Donaldson E, Gedden JS (1997) An airline cardiac arrest program. Circulation 96: 2849-2853
33. Valenzuela TD, Roe DJ, Nichol G, et al (2000) Outcomes of rapid defibrillation by security officers after cardiac arrest in casinos. N Engl J Med 343:1206-1209
34. Page RL, Joglar JA, Kowal RC, et al (2000) Use of automated external defibrillators by a U.S. airline N Engl J Med 343:1210-1216
35. Wassertheil J, Keane G, Fisher N, et al (2000) Cardiac arrest outcomes at the Melbourne Cricket Ground and shrine of remembrance using a tiered response strategy – a forerunner to public access defibrillation. Resuscitation 44: 97-104
36. Becker L, Eisenberg M, Faharenbruch C, et al (1998) Public locations of cardiac arrest: implications for public access defibrillation. Circulation 97: 2106-2109
37. Nichol G, Hallstrom AP, Ornato JP, et al (1998) Potential cost-effectiveness of public access defibrillation in the United States. Circulation 97:1315-1320
38. Valenzuela TD, Roe DJ, Cretin S, et al (1997) Estimating effectiveness of cardiac arrest interventions: a logistic regression survival model. Circulation 96:3308-3313
39. Eisenberg MS (2000) Is it time for over-the-counter defibrillators? JAMA 284:1435-1438
40. Brown J, et al (2000) The shocking truth about automated external defibrillators. JAMA 284: 1438-1441

41. Rosemurgy AS, Norris PA, Olson SM, et al (1993) Prehospital traumatic cardiac arrest: the cost of futility. J Trauma 35: 473-474
42. Mc Lean RF, Devitt JH, Dubbin J, et al (1991) Incidence of abnormal RNA studies and dysrhythmias in patients with blunt chest trauma. J Trauma 31: 968-970
43. Bickell WH, Wall MJ, Pepe PE, et al (1994) Immediate versus delayed resuscitation for hypotensive patients with penetrating torso injuries. N Engl J Med 331: 1105-1109
44. Kellerman AL, Hackman BB, Somes G (1993) Predicting the outcome of unsuccessful prehospital advanced cardiac life support. JAMA 270: 1433-1436
45. Battistella F, Nugent W, Owings JT, et al (1999) Field triage of the pulseless trauma patient. Arch Surg 134: 742-746
46. Albanese P, Cattarossi A, Diani A, et al (1998) Prehospital trauma care manual. Italian Resuscitation Council, Bologna
47. Durham LA, Richardson RJ, Wall MJ, et al (1992) Emergency center thoracotomy: impact of prehospital resuscitation. J Trauma 32: 775-779
48. Enyon CA (2000) Minimally invasive direct cardiac massage and defibrillation. Resuscitation 47:325-328
49. Weil MH, Becker L, Budinger T, et al (2001) Workshop executive summary report: postresuscitative and initial utility in life-saving efforts (PULSE). Crit Care Med 29: 878-882
50. Kette F, Nardi G, Sanson G (1997) L'arresto cardiaco nel politraumatizzato. In: Cattaneo F (ed) Tuttoquantofaemergenza. Riva del Garda, Parma, pp 43-45

Printed by Printforce, the Netherlands